IMMUNOTHERAPY IN ASTHMA

LUNG BIOLOGY IN HEALTH AND DISEASE

Executive Editor

Claude Lenfant
Director, National Heart, Lung and Blood Institute
National Institutes of Health
Bethesda, Maryland

1. Immunologic and Infectious Reactions in the Lung, *edited by C. H. Kirkpatrick and H. Y. Reynolds*
2. The Biochemical Basis of Pulmonary Function, *edited by R. G. Crystal*
3. Bioengineering Aspects of the Lung, *edited by J. B. West*
4. Metabolic Functions of the Lung, *edited by Y. S. Bakhle and J. R. Vane*
5. Respiratory Defense Mechanisms (in two parts), *edited by J. D. Brain, D. F. Proctor, and L. M. Reid*
6. Development of the Lung, *edited by W. A. Hodson*
7. Lung Water and Solute Exchange, *edited by N. C. Staub*
8. Extrapulmonary Manifestations of Respiratory Disease, *edited by E. D. Robin*
9. Chronic Obstructive Pulmonary Disease, *edited by T. L. Petty*
10. Pathogenesis and Therapy of Lung Cancer, *edited by C. C. Harris*
11. Genetic Determinants of Pulmonary Disease, *edited by S. D. Litwin*
12. The Lung in the Transition Between Health and Disease, *edited by P. T. Macklem and S. Permutt*
13. Evolution of Respiratory Processes: A Comparative Approach, *edited by S. C. Wood and C. Lenfant*
14. Pulmonary Vascular Diseases, *edited by K. M. Moser*
15. Physiology and Pharmacology of the Airways, *edited by J. A. Nadel*
16. Diagnostic Techniques in Pulmonary Disease (in two parts), *edited by M. A. Sackner*
17. Regulation of Breathing (in two parts), *edited by T. F. Hornbein*
18. Occupational Lung Diseases: Research Approaches and Methods, *edited by H. Weill and M. Turner-Warwick*
19. Immunopharmacology of the Lung, *edited by H. H. Newball*
20. Sarcoidosis and Other Granulomatous Diseases of the Lung, *edited by B. L. Fanburg*
21. Sleep and Breathing, *edited by N. A. Saunders and C. E. Sullivan*
22. *Pneumocystis carinii* Pneumonia: Pathogenesis, Diagnosis, and Treatment, *edited by L. S. Young*
23. Pulmonary Nuclear Medicine: Techniques in Diagnosis of Lung Disease, *edited by H. L. Atkins*
24. Acute Respiratory Failure, *edited by W. M. Zapol and K. J. Falke*
25. Gas Mixing and Distribution in the Lung, *edited by L. A. Engel and M. Paiva*

26. High-Frequency Ventilation in Intensive Care and During Surgery, *edited by G. Carlon and W. S. Howland*
27. Pulmonary Development: Transition from Intrauterine to Extrauterine Life, *edited by G. H. Nelson*
28. Chronic Obstructive Pulmonary Disease: Second Edition, *edited by T. L. Petty*
29. The Thorax (in two parts), *edited by C. Roussos and P. T. Macklem*
30. The Pleura in Health and Disease, *edited by J. Chrétien, J. Bignon, and A. Hirsch*
31. Drug Therapy for Asthma: Research and Clinical Practice, *edited by J. W. Jenne and S. Murphy*
32. Pulmonary Endothelium in Health and Disease, *edited by U. S. Ryan*
33. The Airways: Neural Control in Health and Disease, *edited by M. A. Kaliner and P. J. Barnes*
34. Pathophysiology and Treatment of Inhalation Injuries, *edited by J. Loke*
35. Respiratory Function of the Upper Airway, *edited by O. P. Mathew and G. Sant'Ambrogio*
36. Chronic Obstructive Pulmonary Disease: A Behavioral Perspective, *edited by A. J. McSweeny and I. Grant*
37. Biology of Lung Cancer: Diagnosis and Treatment, *edited by S. T. Rosen, J. L. Mulshine, F. Cuttitta, and P. G. Abrams*
38. Pulmonary Vascular Physiology and Pathophysiology, *edited by E. K. Weir and J. T. Reeves*
39. Comparative Pulmonary Physiology: Current Concepts, *edited by S. C. Wood*
40. Respiratory Physiology: An Analytical Approach, *edited by H. K. Chang and M. Paiva*
41. Lung Cell Biology, *edited by D. Massaro*
42. Heart–Lung Interactions in Health and Disease, *edited by S. M. Scharf and S. S. Cassidy*
43. Clinical Epidemiology of Chronic Obstructive Pulmonary Disease, *edited by M. J. Hensley and N. A. Saunders*
44. Surgical Pathology of Lung Neoplasms, *edited by A. M. Marchevsky*
45. The Lung in Rheumatic Diseases, *edited by G. W. Cannon and G. A. Zimmerman*
46. Diagnostic Imaging of the Lung, *edited by C. E. Putman*
47. Models of Lung Disease: Microscopy and Structural Methods, *edited by J. Gil*
48. Electron Microscopy of the Lung, *edited by D. E. Schraufnagel*
49. Asthma: Its Pathology and Treatment, *edited by M. A. Kaliner, P. J. Barnes, and C. G. A. Persson*
50. Acute Respiratory Failure: Second Edition, *edited by W. M. Zapol and F. Lemaire*
51. Lung Disease in the Tropics, *edited by O. P. Sharma*
52. Exercise: Pulmonary Physiology and Pathophysiology, *edited by B. J. Whipp and K. Wasserman*
53. Developmental Neurobiology of Breathing, *edited by G. G. Haddad and J. P. Farber*
54. Mediators of Pulmonary Inflammation, *edited by M. A. Bray and W. H. Anderson*

55. The Airway Epithelium, *edited by S. G. Farmer and D. Hay*
56. Physiological Adaptations in Vertebrates: Respiration, Circulation, and Metabolism, *edited by S. C. Wood, R. E. Weber, A. R. Hargens, and R. W. Millard*
57. The Bronchial Circulation, *edited by J. Butler*
58. Lung Cancer Differentiation: Implications for Diagnosis and Treatment, *edited by S. D. Bernal and P. J. Hesketh*
59. Pulmonary Complications of Systemic Disease, *edited by J. F. Murray*
60. Lung Vascular Injury: Molecular and Cellular Response, *edited by A. Johnson and T. J. Ferro*
61. Cytokines of the Lung, *edited by J. Kelley*
62. The Mast Cell in Health and Disease, *edited by M. A. Kaliner and D. D. Metcalfe*
63. Pulmonary Disease in the Elderly Patient, *edited by D. A. Mahler*
64. Cystic Fibrosis, *edited by P. B. Davis*
65. Signal Transduction in Lung Cells, *edited by J. S. Brody, D. M. Center, and V. A. Tkachuk*
66. Tuberculosis: A Comprehensive International Approach, *edited by L. B. Reichman and E. S. Hershfield*
67. Pharmacology of the Respiratory Tract: Experimental and Clinical Research, *edited by K. F. Chung and P. J. Barnes*
68. Prevention of Respiratory Diseases, *edited by A. Hirsch, M. Goldberg, J.-P. Martin, and R. Masse*
69. *Pneumocystis carinii* Pneumonia: Second Edition, *edited by P. D. Walzer*
70. Fluid and Solute Transport in the Airspaces of the Lungs, *edited by R. M. Effros and H. K. Chang*
71. Sleep and Breathing: Second Edition, *edited by N. A. Saunders and C. E. Sullivan*
72. Airway Secretion: Physiological Bases for the Control of Mucous Hypersecretion, *edited by T. Takishima and S. Shimura*
73. Sarcoidosis and Other Granulomatous Disorders, *edited by D. G. James*
74. Epidemiology of Lung Cancer, *edited by J. M. Samet*
75. Pulmonary Embolism, *edited by M. Morpurgo*
76. Sports and Exercise Medicine, *edited by S. C. Wood and R. C. Roach*
77. Endotoxin and the Lungs, *edited by K. L. Brigham*
78. The Mesothelial Cell and Mesothelioma, *edited by M.-C. Jaurand and J. Bignon*
79. Regulation of Breathing: Second Edition, *edited by J. A. Dempsey and A. I. Pack*
80. Pulmonary Fibrosis, *edited by S. Hin. Phan and R. S. Thrall*
81. Long-Term Oxygen Therapy: Scientific Basis and Clinical Application, *edited by W. J. O'Donohue, Jr.*
82. Ventral Brainstem Mechanisms and Control of Respiration and Blood Pressure, *edited by C. O. Trouth, R. M. Millis, H. F. Kiwull-Schöne, and M. E. Schläfke*
83. A History of Breathing Physiology, *edited by D. F. Proctor*
84. Surfactant Therapy for Lung Disease, *edited by B. Robertson and H. W. Taeusch*

85. The Thorax: Second Edition, Revised and Expanded (in three parts), *edited by C. Roussos*
86. Severe Asthma: Pathogenesis and Clinical Management, *edited by S. J. Szefler and D. Y. M. Leung*
87. *Mycobacterium avium*–Complex Infection: Progress in Research and Treatment, *edited by J. A. Korvick and C. A. Benson*
88. Alpha 1–Antitrypsin Deficiency: Biology • Pathogenesis • Clinical Manifestations • Therapy, *edited by R. G. Crystal*
89. Adhesion Molecules and the Lung, *edited by P. A. Ward and J. C. Fantone*
90. Respiratory Sensation, *edited by L. Adams and A. Guz*
91. Pulmonary Rehabilitation, *edited by A. P. Fishman*
92. Acute Respiratory Failure in Chronic Obstructive Pulmonary Disease, *edited by J.-P. Derenne, W. A. Whitelaw, and T. Similowski*
93. Environmental Impact on the Airways: From Injury to Repair, *edited by J. Chrétien and D. Dusser*
94. Inhalation Aerosols: Physical and Biological Basis for Therapy, *edited by A. J. Hickey*
95. Tissue Oxygen Deprivation: From Molecular to Integrated Function, *edited by G. G. Haddad and G. Lister*
96. The Genetics of Asthma, *edited by S. B. Liggett and D. A. Meyers*
97. Inhaled Glucocorticoids in Asthma: Mechanisms and Clinical Actions, *edited by R. P. Schleimer, W. W. Busse, and P. M. O'Byrne*
98. Nitric Oxide and the Lung, *edited by W. M. Zapol and K. D. Bloch*
99. Primary Pulmonary Hypertension, *edited by L. J. Rubin and S. Rich*
100. Lung Growth and Development, *edited by J. A. McDonald*
101. Parasitic Lung Diseases, *edited by A. A. F. Mahmoud*
102. Lung Macrophages and Dendritic Cells in Health and Disease, *edited by M. F. Lipscomb and S. W. Russell*
103. Pulmonary and Cardiac Imaging, *edited by C. Chiles and C. E. Putman*
104. Gene Therapy for Diseases of the Lung, *edited by K. L. Brigham*
105. Oxygen, Gene Expression, and Cellular Function, *edited by L. Biadasz Clerch and D. J. Massaro*
106. $Beta_2$-Agonists in Asthma Treatment, *edited by R. Pauwels and P. M. O'Byrne*
107. Inhalation Delivery of Therapeutic Peptides and Proteins, *edited by A. L. Adjei and P. K. Gupta*
108. Asthma in the Elderly, *edited by R. A. Barbee and J. W. Bloom*
109. Treatment of the Hospitalized Cystic Fibrosis Patient, *edited by D. M. Orenstein and R. C. Stern*
110. Asthma and Immunological Diseases in Pregnancy and Early Infancy, *edited by M. Schatz, R. S. Zeiger, and H. N. Claman*
111. Dyspnea, *edited by D. A. Mahler*
112. Proinflammatory and Antiinflammatory Peptides, *edited by S. I. Said*
113. Self-Management of Asthma, *edited by H. Kotses and A. Harver*
114. Eicosanoids, Aspirin, and Asthma, *edited by A. Szczeklik, R. J. Gryglewski, and J. R. Vane*
115. Fatal Asthma, *edited by A. L. Sheffer*
116. Pulmonary Edema, *edited by M. A. Matthay and D. H. Ingbar*

117. Inflammatory Mechanisms in Asthma, *edited by S. T. Holgate and W. W. Busse*
118. Physiological Basis of Ventilatory Support, *edited by J. J. Marini and A. S. Slutsky*
119. Human Immunodeficiency Virus and the Lung, *edited by M. J. Rosen and J. M. Beck*
120. Five-Lipoxygenase Products in Asthma, *edited by J. M. Drazen, S.-E. Dahlén, and T. H. Lee*
121. Complexity in Structure and Function of the Lung, *edited by M. P. Hlastala and H. T. Robertson*
122. Biology of Lung Cancer, *edited by M. A. Kane and P. A. Bunn, Jr.*
123. Rhinitis: Mechanisms and Management, *edited by R. M. Naclerio, S. R. Durham, and N. Mygind*
124. Lung Tumors: Fundamental Biology and Clinical Management, *edited by C. Brambilla and E. Brambilla*
125. Interleukin-5: From Molecule to Drug Target for Asthma, *edited by C. J. Sanderson*
126. Pediatric Asthma, *edited by S. Murphy and H. W. Kelly*
127. Viral Infections of the Respiratory Tract, *edited by R. Dolin and P. F. Wright*
128. Air Pollutants and the Respiratory Tract, *edited by D. L. Swift and W. M. Foster*
129. Gastroesophageal Reflux Disease and Airway Disease, *edited by M. R. Stein*
130. Exercise-Induced Asthma, *edited by E. R. McFadden, Jr.*
131. LAM and Other Diseases Characterized by Smooth Muscle Proliferation, *edited by J. Moss*
132. The Lung at Depth, *edited by C. E. G. Lundgren and J. N. Miller*
133. Regulation of Sleep and Circadian Rhythms, *edited by F. W. Turek and P. C. Zee*
134. Anticholinergic Agents in the Upper and Lower Airways, *edited by S. L. Spector*
135. Control of Breathing in Health and Disease, *edited by M. D. Altose and Y. Kawakami*
136. Immunotherapy in Asthma, *edited by J. Bousquet and H. Yssel*

ADDITIONAL VOLUMES IN PREPARATION

Chronic Lung Disease of Early Infancy, *edited by R. D. Bland and J. J. Coalson*

Diagnostic Pulmonary Pathology, *edited by P. T. Cagle*

Multimodality Treatment of Lung Cancer, *edited by A. T. Skarin*

Cytokines in Pulmonary Infectious Disease, *edited by S. Nelson and T. Martin*

Asthma's Impact on Society: The Social and Economic Burden, *edited by K. B. Weiss, A. S. Buist, and S. D. Sullivan*

Asthma and Respiratory Infections, *edited by D. P. Skoner*

New and Exploratory Therapeutic Agents for Asthma, *edited by M. Yeadon and Z. Diamant*

Particle–Lung Interactions, *edited by P. Gehr and J. Heyder*

Pulmonary and Peripheral Gas Exchange in Health and Disease, *edited by J. Roca, R. Rodriguez-Roisen, and P. Wagner*

Environmental Asthma, *edited by R. K. Bush*

Tuberculosis: A Comprehensive International Approach, Second Edition, *edited by L. B. Reichman and E. S. Hershfield*

Sleep and Breathing in Children: A Developmental Approach, *edited by G. M. Loughlin, J. L. Carroll, and C. L. Marcus*

The opinions expressed in these volumes do not necessarily represent the views of the National Institutes of Health.

IMMUNOTHERAPY IN ASTHMA

Edited by

Jean Bousquet
*Montpellier University and Montpellier University Hospital
Montpellier, France*

Hans Yssel
*Hôpital Arnaud de Villeneuve
Montpellier, France*

MARCEL DEKKER, INC. NEW YORK • BASEL

ISBN: 0-8247-0176-3

This book is printed on acid-free paper.

Headquarters
Marcel Dekker, Inc.
270 Madison Avenue, New York, NY 10016
tel: 212-696-9000; fax: 212-685-4540

Eastern Hemisphere Distribution
Marcel Dekker AG
Hutgasse 4, Postfach 812, CH-4001 Basel, Switzerland
tel: 41-61-261-8482; fax: 41-61-261-8896

World Wide Web
http://www.dekker.com

The publisher offers discounts on this book when ordered in bulk quantities. For more information, write to Special Sales/Professional Marketing at the headquarters address above.

Current printing (last digit):
10 9 8 7 6 5 4 3 2 1

PRINTED IN THE UNITED STATES OF AMERICA

INTRODUCTION

The great merit of a new theory is not to be true, because there is no such thing as a true theory, but to be fruitful.

Emile Duclaux

Emile Duclaux, an associate of Louis Pasteur, made this statement on the occasion of one of his lectures at the Sorbonne in 1880. By then, immunology was already developing as a specialized discipline that was broadly defined as the "act of self defense." It is reported that Paul Ehrlich was the first to use the term *immunotherapy* in 1906. At that time, there was great hope that diseases could be effectively treated, if not cured, by such therapy. Although some had developed doubts that immunotherapy would be as fruitful as expected, significant successes were reported.

Over the centuries, many great names have been associated with the development of what eventually became immunotherapy, but Leonard Noon and then his colleague John Freeman stand out as having accepted its concept and its application to allergy and to asthma. In the *Lancet* article "Prophylactic Inoculation Against Hay Fever" (1911), Noon and Cantor described the course of immunizations in patients receiving injections of pollen extracts and concluded that the "susceptibility of hay fever patients may be decreased . . . but it remains to be seen whether the immunity thus attained is sufficient to carry the patients through a season without suffering from their annual attack of hay fever." Because by then Noon had developed tuberculosis, he ended this paper by announcing that Freeman would carry on the observations during his enforced absence, and he did so successfully!

Eventually, the work of Noon, Freeman, and others led to, and culminated with, the important observations of many contemporary investigators. Some of these "pioneers" are contributors to this volume.

Today, the therapy of asthma is quite different from what it was in the earlier years of this century: it includes new classes of medications such as bronchodilators, anti-inflammatory compounds, and, just introduced, inhibitors of inflammatory mediators. Does this mean that immunotherapy has lost the place that it deserves in the treatment of asthma! Certainly not! In fact one can safely predict that recent understanding of the immune reaction will create an important new role for this therapy.

In this volume, *Immunotherapy in Asthma*, the editors, Jean Bousquet and Hans Yssel, rebuild the case for immunotherapy with the participation of a cadre of contributors whose expertise is unchallenged. The last section of the volume poses the question: “Prevention of Allergic Asthma: Is It Possible?” The authors and contributors have made their case and the answer is “yes.” Immunotherapy is no longer a theory, it is a validated therapy and, unquestionably, as the readership will find, it will be fruitful for many!

As the Executive Editor of the Lung Biology in Health and Disease series, I want to express my deepest appreciation to the editors and authors for their contributions.

Claude Lenfant, M.D.
Bethesda, Maryland

PREFACE

Allergen immunotherapy is the practice of administering gradually increasing quantities of an allergen extract to an allergic subject to ameliorate the symptoms associated with subsequent exposure to the causative allergen. Allergen immunotherapy was introduced to treat "pollinosis" or allergic rhinitis by Noon and Freeman in 1911 (1). For more than 80 years, immunotherapy has been used to treat allergic diseases caused by inhalant allergens, and there is good evidence that immunotherapy, using inhalant allergens to treat seasonal or perennial allergic rhinitis and asthma, is clinically effective when optimally used.

Over the past years, guidelines and indications for immunotherapy with inhalant allergens have been published by WHO (2–4), the European Academy of Allergy and Clinical Immunology (EAACI) (5), the International Consensus Report on Asthma (6), the Global Strategy for Asthma Management and Prevention (7), the British Society for Allergy and Clinical Immunology (8), and the American Academy of Allergy, Asthma and Immunology (AAAAI) (9). These reports provide guidelines for a better understanding of the use of allergen immunotherapy. Immunotherapy is the only treatment that may affect the natural course of allergic diseases, and it may prevent the onset of asthma.

The indications of immunotherapy in asthma and rhinitis have been separated and this has led to unresolved discussions (10,11), possibly because the IgE-mediated reaction has not been considered as multiorgan involvement. Therefore, it is important to consider immunotherapy, depending on the allergen sensitization, rather than on the disease itself.

Considerable progress has been made in better understanding the mechanisms of allergy, such as the involvement of Th1 and Th2 cells or the role of cytokines in regulation of the immune response, and specific inhibition of immune responses is being scrutinzed in both animals and humans. In the future, these advances should result in new, safer, and substantially more effective methods of manipulating the human immune response. Several approaches may be used, such as the development of nonanaphylactic allergens, as allergen fragments or peptides for active immunotherapy (12,13); IgE-binding haptens of major allergens for passive saturation of effector cells and induction of blocking antibodies (14); allergen-specific antibodies and antibody fragments for passive therapy in the allergic effector organs (15,16); plasmid DNA immunization (17); and anti-IgE-humanized monoclonal antibodies (18).

In the present book, various aspects of current allergen immunotherapy are discussed that attempt to link an old, but still largely used, therapy with a promising future.

Jean Bousquet
Hans Yssel

References

1. Noon L. Prophylactic inoculation against hay fever. Lancet 1911; i:1572–1573.
2. The current status of allergen immunotherapy (hyposensitisation). Report of a WHO/IUIS working group. Allergy 1989; 44:369–379.
3. Current status of allergen immunotherapy. Shortened version of a World Health Organisation/International Union of Immunological Societies Working Group Report. Lancet 1989; 1:259–261.
4. Bousquet J, Lockey D, Malling H. WHO Position Paper. Allergen immunotherapy: therapeutic vaccines for allergic diseases. Allergy 1998; 53(suppl 54).
5. Malling H, Weeke B. Immunotherapy. Position Paper of the European Academy of Allergy and Clinical Immunology. Allergy 1993; 48(suppl 14):9–35.
6. International Consensus Report on Diagnosis and Management of Asthma. International Asthma Management Project. Allergy 1992; 47:1–61.
7. Global strategy for asthma management and prevention. WHO/NHLBI workshop report. In: National Institutes of Health, National Heart, Lung and Blood Institute, Publication No. 95-3659, 1995.
8. Frew AJ. Injection immunotherapy. British Society for Allergy and Clinical Immunology Working Party. Br Med J 1993; 307:919–923.
9. Nicklas R, Bernstein I, Blessing-Moore J, et al. Practice parameters for allergen immunotherapy. J Allergy Clin Immunol 1996; 6:1001–1011.
10. Norman P. Is there a role for immunotherapy in the treatment of asthma? Yes. Am J Respir Crit Care MEd 1996; 154:1225–1228.
11. Barnes P. Is there a role for immunotherapy in the treatment of asthma? No. Am J Respir Crit Care Med 1996; 154:1227–1228.
12. Ferreira F, Hirthenlehner K, Briza P, et al. Isoforms of atopic allergens with reduced allergenicity but conserved T cell antigenicity: possible use for specific immunotherapy. Int Arch Allergy Immunol 1997; 113:125–127.
13. Yssel H, Fasler S, Lamb J, de-Vries JE. Induction of non-responsiveness in human allergen-specific type 2 T helper cells. Curr Opin Immunol 1994; 6:847–852.
14. Ball T, Vrtala S, Sperr WR, et al. Isolation of an immunodominant IgE hapten from an epitope expression cDNA library. Dissection of the allergic effector reaction. J Biol Chem 1994; 269:28323–28328.
15. Visco V, Dolecek C, Denepoux S, et al. Human IgG monoclonal antibodies that modulate the binding of specific IgE to birch pollen Bet v1. J Immunol 1996; 157:956–962.
16. Lebecque S, Dolecek C, Laffler S, et al. Immunologic characteristizations of monoclonal antibodies which modulate human immunoglobulin E binding to the major birch pollen allergen Bet v1. J Allergy Clin Immunol 1997; 99:374–384.

17. Raz E, Tighe H, Sato Y, et al. Preferential induction of a Th1 immune response and inhibition of specific IgE antibody formation by plasmid DNA immunization. Proc Natl Acad Sci USA 1996; 93:5141–5145.
18. Fahy J, Fleming H, Wong H, et al. The effect of an anti-IgE monoclonal antibody on the early and late phase responses to allergen inhalation in asthmatic subjects. Am J Respir Crit Care Med 1997; 155(6):1828–1834.

CONTRIBUTORS

Michael J. Abramson, M.B., Ph.D., F.R.A.C.P., F.A.F.P.H.M. Associate Professor, Department of Epidemiology and Preventive Medicine, Monash Medical School, Alfred Hospital, Prahran, Victoria, Australia

Pamela J. Amelung, M.D. Assistant Professor, Center for the Genetics of Asthma and Complex Diseases, University of Maryland School of Medicine, Baltimore, Maryland

Tanja Ball, M.Sc. Department of General and Experimental Pathology, University of Vienna, Vienna General Hospital, Vienna, Austria

Jean-Claude Bessot, M.D. Staff Physician, Service de Pneumonologie et d'Allergologie, Pavillon Laennec, Hôpitaux Universitaires de Strasbourg, Strasbourg, France

Eugene R. Bleecker, M.D. Professor, Center for the Genetics of Asthma and Complex Diseases, University of Maryland School of Medicine, Baltimore, Maryland

Jean Bousquet, M.D., Ph.D. Professor, Montpellier University, and Service des Maladies Respiratoires–INSERM U454, Montpellier University Hospital, Montpellier, France

Yvan Boutin, Ph.D. Research Associate, Section of Immunobiology, Yale University School of Medicine, New Haven, Connecticut

Giorgio Walter Canonica, M.D. Professor, Division of Allergy and Respiratory Diseases, Department of Internal Medicine, University of Genoa, Genoa, Italy

Pascal Chanez, M.D., Ph.D. Service des Maladies Respiratoires–U454 Montpellier University Hospital, Montpellier, France

Martin D. Chapman, Ph.D. Professor, Asthma and Allergic Diseases Center, University of Virginia School of Medicine, Charlottesville, Virginia

Richard W. Chapman, Ph.D. Senior Research Fellow, Department of Allergy, Schering–Plough Research Institute, Kenilworth, New Jersey

Francis M. Cuss, M.D. Vice President, Biological Research–Allergy and Immunology, Department of Discovery Research, Schering–Plough Research Institute, Kenilworth, New Jersey

Frédéric de Blay, M.D. Associate Professor, Department of Pulmonology, Service de Pneumonologie and Allergology, Pavillon Laennec, Hôpitaux Universitaires de Strasbourg, Strasbourg, France

Pascal Demoly, M.D., Ph.D. Assistant Professor, Montpellier University, and Service des Maladies Respiratoires–INSERM U454, Montpellier University Hospital, Montpellier, France

Robert W. Egan, Ph.D. Presidential Fellow, Department of Allergy, Schering–Plough Research Institute, Kenilworth, New Jersey

Petra Eibensteiner, M.Sc. Department of General and Experimental Pathology, University of Vienna, Vienna General Hospital, Vienna, Austria

Sabine Fischer, M.Sc. Department of General and Experimental Pathology, University of Vienna, Vienna General Hospital, Vienna, Austria

Sabine Flicker, M.Sc. Department of General and Experimental Pathology, University of Vienna, Vienna General Hospital, Vienna, Austria

Anthony J. Frew, M.A., M.D., F.R.C.P. Department of University Medicine, Southampton General Hospital, Southampton, England

Erwin W. Gelfand, M.D. Chairman, Department of Pediatrics, National Jewish Medical and Research Center, and the University of Colorado Health Sciences Center, Denver, Colorado

Jorrit Gerritsen, M.D., Ph.D. Associate Professor, Department of Pediatric Pulmonary Medicine, Beatrix Children's Hospital, University Hospital Groningen, Groningen, The Netherlands

Philippe Godard, M.D., Ph.D. Professor, Montpellier University, and Service des Maladies Respiratoires–INSERM U454, Montpellier University Hospital, Montpellier, France

Hannah J. Gould, Ph.D. Professor of Biophysics, The Randall Institute, King's College London, London, England

Marion H. Grol, M.D. Department of Pediatric Pulmonary Medicine, Beatrix Children's Hospital, University Hospital Groningen, Groningen, The Netherlands

Jacques Hébert, M.D. Department of Allergy–Immunology, Laval University, and Department of Medicine, Centre Hospitalier de l'Université Laval, Centre Hospitalier Universitaire de Québec, Sainte Foy, Quebec, Canada

Patrick G. Holt, D.Sc., F.R.C.Path., F.R.C.P.I. Professor, Division of Cell Biology, TVW Telethon Institute for Child Health Research, Perth, Western Australia, Australia

Dany Jaffuel, M.D. Montpellier University, and Service des Maladies Respiratoires–INSERM U454, Montpellier University Hospital, Montpellier, France

Marie-Hélène Jouvin, M.D. Instructor, Department of Pathology, Harvard Medical School and Beth Israel Deaconess Medical Center, Boston, Massachusetts

A. Barry Kay, D.Sc., Ph.D., F.R.C.P., F.R.S.E. Professor, Department of Allergy and Clinical Immunology, Imperial College School of Medicine, National Heart and Lung Institute, London, England

Jean-Pierre Kinet, M.D. Professor, Department of Pathology, Harvard Medical School and Beth Israel Deaconess Medical Center, Boston, Massachusetts

Dietrich Kraft, M.D. Professor, Department of General and Experimental Pathology, University of Vienna, Vienna General Hospital, Vienna, Austria

Franz Kricek, Ph.D. Laboratory Head, Novartis Research Center, Vienna, Austria

Nanna S. Kristensen Institute for Medical Microbiology and Immunology, University of Copenhagen, Copenhagen, Denmark

Gideon Lack, M.B., B.Ch. Consultant, Division of Pediatric Allergy and Immunology, Department of Pediatrics, Imperial College, St. Mary's Medical School, London, England

Sylvia Laffer, Ph.D. Department of General and Experimental Pathology, University of Vienna, Vienna General Hospital, Vienna, Austria

Jonathan R. Lamb, Ph.D. Respiratory Medicine Unit, University of Edinburgh Medical School, Edinburgh, Scotland

Donald Y. M. Leung, M.D., Ph.D. Professor and Head, Department of Pediatric Allergy–Immunology, National Jewish Medical and Research Center, and the University of Colorado Health Sciences Center, Denver, Colorado

Richard F. Lockey, M.D. Professor, Joy McCann Culverhouse Professor, and Director, Division of Allergy and Immunology, Department of Internal Medicine, University of South Florida College of Medicine, Tampa, Florida

Hans-Jørgen Malling, M.D. Associate Professor, Allergy Unit, Medical Department TA, National University Hospital, Copenhagen, Denmark

Marc Mathieu, Ph.D. Senior Researcher, Service des Maladies Respiratoires–INSERM U454, Montpellier University Hospital, Montpellier, France

François-Bernard Michel, M.D. Professor, Montpellier University, and Service des Maladies Respiratoires–INSERM U454, Montpellier University Hospital, Montpellier, France

Sylvia Margaret Miescher, Ph.D. Institute of Immunology and Allergology, University of Bern, Inselspital, Bern, Switzerland

Michael Minnicozzi, Ph.D. Senior Scientist, Department of Allergy, Schering–Plough Research Institute, Kenilworth, New Jersey

Irene Mittermann, Ph.D. Department of General and Experimental Pathology, University of Vienna, Vienna General Hospital, Vienna, Austria

Shyam S. Mohapatra, Ph.D. Associate Professor, Division of Allergy and Immunology, Department of Internal Medicine, University of South Florida College of Medicine, and VA Hospital, Tampa, Florida

Christopher F. Nicodemus, M.D. Vice President, Medical Affairs, Diatide, Inc., Londonderry, New Hampshire

Philip S. Norman, M.D. Professor, Division of Clinical Immunology, Department of Medicine, Johns Hopkins University School of Medicine, Baltimore, Maryland

Martine Ott, B.Sc. Consultant in Indoor Environment, Service de Pneumonologie et d'Allergologie, Pavillon Laennec, Hôpitaux Universitaires de Strasbourg, Strasbourg, France

Giovanni Passalacqua, M.D. Clinical Researcher, Division of Allergy and Respiratory Diseases, Department of Internal Medicine, University of Genoa, Genoa, Italy

Gabrielle Pauli, M.D. Professor, Department of Pulmonology, Service de Pneumonologie et d'Allergologie, Pavillon Laennec, Hôpitaux Universitaires de Strasbourg, Strasbourg, France

Jérôme Pène, Ph.D. Director of Research, INSERM U454–Physiology of Asthma, Hôpital Arnaud de Villeneuve, Montpellier, France

George Philip, M.D. Associate Director, Medical Services, Merck and Company, Inc., West Point, Pennsylvania

Thomas A. E. Platts-Mills, M.D., Ph.D. Professor, Department of Internal Medicine, and Head, Asthma and Allergic Diseases Center, University of Virginia, Charlottesville, Virginia

Dirkje S. Postma, M.D., Ph.D. Professor, Department of Pulmonary Diseases, University Hospital Groningen, Groningen, The Netherlands

Robert M. Puy, M.B., F.R.A.C.P., F.R.C.P.A. Department of Allergy and Clinical Immunology, Alfred Hospital, Prahran, Victoria, Australia

Douglas S. Robinson, M.A., M.D., M.R.C.P. Senior Lecturer, Department of Allergy and Immunology, Imperial College School of Medicine, National Heart and Lung Institute, London, England

Michael P. Rudolf, Ph.D. Research Associate, Oncology Institute, Loyola University Medical Center, Maywood, Illinois

Jean-Marie R. Saint-Remy, M.D., Ph.D. Professor, Center for Molecular and Vascular Biology, University of Leuven, Campus Gashuisberg, Leuven, Belgium

Jan P. Schouten, M.Sc. Assistant Professor, Department of Epidemiology and Statistics, Faculty of Medicine, University of Groningen, and University Hospital Groningen, Groningen, The Netherlands

Gian Enrico Senna, M.D. Head, Allergy Unit, Verona General Hospital, Verona, Italy

Alisa M. Smith, Ph.D. Assistant Professor, Asthma and Allergic Diseases Center, University of Virginia School of Medicine, Charlottesville, Virginia

François Spirlet, M.D. Staff Physician, Pavillon Laennec, Hôpitaux Universitaires de Strasbourg, Strasbourg, France

Susanne Spitzauer, M.D. Institute of Medical and Chemical Laboratory Diagnostics, University of Vienna, Vienna General Hospital, Vienna, Austria

Beda M. Stadler, Ph.D. Professor, Institute of Immunology and Allergology, University of Bern, Inselspital, Bern, Switzerland

Peter Steinberger, Ph.D. Department of General and Experimental Pathology, University of Vienna, Vienna General Hospital, Vienna, Austria

Brian J. Sutton, D.Phil. Reader in Molecular Biophysics, The Randall Institute, King's College London, London, England

Shelby P. Umland, Ph.D. Section Leader, Department of Allergy, Schering–Plough Research Institute, Kenilworth, New Jersey

Rudolf Valenta, M.D. Professor, Department of General and Experimental Pathology, University of Vienna, Vienna General Hospital, Vienna, Austria

Erkka Valovirta, M.D., Ph.D. Senior Medical Officer, Pediatric Allergist, Turku Allergy Center, Turku, Finland

Ronald van Ree, Ph.D. Department of Allergy, Central Laboratory of the Netherlands Red Cross Blood Transfusion Service, Amsterdam, The Netherlands

Antonio M. Vignola, M.D., Ph.D. Institute of Respiratory Physiopathology, Consiglio Nazionale delle Richerche, Palermo, Italy

Erika von Mutius, M.D. Department of Allergology and Pulmonology, University Children's Hospital, Munich, Germany

Monique Vogel, Ph.D. Institute of Immunology and Allergology, University of Bern, Inselspital, Bern, Switzerland

Susanne Vrtala, Ph.D. Department of General and Experimental Pathology, University of Vienna, Vienna General Hospital, Vienna, Austria

John M. Weiner, M.B., F.R.A.C.P., F.R.C.P.A. Department of Medicine, Monash Medical School, Alfred Hospital, Prahran, Victoria, Australia

Lisa M. Wheatley, M.D. Assistant Professor, Department of Internal Medicine, University of Virginia, Charlottesville, Virginia

Hans Yssel, Ph.D. Director of Research, INSERM U454–Hôpital Arnaud de Villeneuve, Montpellier, France

Adrian Walter Zuercher, M.Sc. Institute of Immunology and Allergology, University of Bern, Inselspital, Bern, Switzerland

CONTENTS

Part Two ALLERGEN-SPECIFIC IMMUNOTHERAPY

Current Knowledge

Part One

MECHANISMS OF ALLERGIC ASTHMA

1

Human T Helper Type 1 and Type 2 Subsets

HANS YSSEL

INSERM U454
Hôpital Arnaud de Villeneuve
Montpellier, France

I. Introduction

About a decade ago, Mosmann and co-workers reported that CD4$^+$ mouse T helper cell clones could be divided into two mutually exclusive subpopulations, called T helper type (Th1) and Th2 cells, based on the cytokines that they secrete, as well as on their functional properties (1). Mouse Th1 clones produce interleukin (IL)-2, interferon (IFN)-γ, tissue necrosis factor (TNF)-β, but no IL-4 or IL-5, whereas Th2 clones produce IL-4, IL-5, IL-6, but no IL-2 or IFN-γ (reviewed in Ref. 2). Initial studies on cytokine production of human CD4$^+$ T-cell clones yielded mostly cells with a Th0 cytokine production profile, producing IL-4, as well as IFN-γ following activation (3,4). However, subsequent analysis of T-cell clones obtained from patients with chronic infections or various immunological diseases have confirmed the notion that subsets with different cytokine production profiles can also be demonstrated in human CD4$^+$ T cells. T-cell clones obtained from atopic patients generally display a Th2-like phenotype (5), whereas those specific for intracellular pathogens, such as *Mycobacterium leprae* or *Borrelia burgdorferi*, or for purified protein derivative (PPD) derived from *M. tuberculosis*, have a Th1-like cytokine production profile (6–8). However, several differences in the cytokine production profile between mouse and human CD4$^+$ T-cell clones have been observed. For example, the production of IL-10, which in the mouse is produced by Th2 clones, is not associated with a Th2 cytokine production profile in humans (9,10). Similarly, IL-13, a cytokine typically produced by mouse Th2 clones, is secreted by human Th1, Th0, and Th2 cell clones (11). In addition, likely because of culture conditions, human T-cell clones, especially of the Th2 type, seem to be less polarized than their murine counterparts. For example, stimulation of most human allergen-specific Th2 clones with phorbol ester and calcium ionophore, by a pathway that does not involve the triggering of the T-cell receptor (TCR)–CD3 complex, induces not only high levels of Th2 cytokines, but also the production of IFN-γ (12). Moreover, in many instances IL-12 can induce, albeit transiently, the production of IFN-γ by cultured human Th2 cell clones (13,14). These observations indicate that different modes of activation, as well as relative, rather than absolute, cytokine secretion levels are important in determining the cytokine production profiles of T cells.

The heterogeneity of cytokine production profiles observed among cloned human and mouse T-cell lines has prompted some researchers to question the categorization of discrete Th1 and Th2 subsets by arguing that the expression of cytokine genes is independently regulated in individual cells (15,16) and that Th1 and Th2 cytokine production profiles represent only two extremes of phenotypes among a continuous spectrum of possible combinations of cytokine production (17). However, transcripts representing Th1 and Th2 cytokine production profiles have been detected in whole tissue (18,19) under experimental conditions that exclude the possible bias introduced by culture and cloning procedures, giving additional support for the notion that the degree of polarization of cytokine production may reflect the nature of the antigenic stimuli to which the cells have been exposed.

The original concept of the Th1–Th2 differentiation is based on early clinical observations in mice that showed striking pathological features following infection with parasite antigens, such as those of *Leishmania major*. Mice strains, such as Balb/c, susceptible to *L. major* infection, generally had elevated antibody titers, especially of the IgG1 and IgE isotype, and a strong Th2 response, with high IL-4 production. In contrast, the development of IFN-γ cytokine production in strains of mice, such as D10 or Bl/6, was associated with cell-mediated immune responses and conferred protection on reinfection with the parasites (reviewed in Ref. 20). These results have led to the hypothesis that Th1 cells induce cell-mediated responses, such as delayed type of hypersensitivity (DTH) reactions, whereas Th2 cells are more involved in humoral immunity, giving optimal help for antibody production by B cells, although this classification seems to be rather oversimplified.

For example, whereas both the Th2 cytokines IL-4 and IL-13 are switch factors for IgG_1 and IgE production in the mouse (IgG_4 and IgE in human), IFN-γ, which is the hallmark Th1 cytokine, induces the switching of murine B lymphocytes to several IgG isotypes and thus must be involved in at least some humoral immune responses. Therefore, in a somewhat different concept, it has been proposed that Th1 cells, by means of their production of IFN-γ, are involved mainly in the protective immunity toward intercellular microorganisms, stimulating the production of complement-fixing and opsonizing antibodies, and activating macrophages to enhance their microbicidal effector functions. As a consequence, Th1-mediated responses are generally characterized by inflammatory reactions that often lead to tissue damage and destruction.

In contrast, Th2 cells give help to B cells for the production of non–complement fixing IgG_1 (in the mouse), IgG_4 (in human) antibodies, as well as IgE antibodies; induce recruitment and infiltration of eosinophils; and are, therefore, likely to play a role in the elimination of extracellular parasites, such as helminths, and furthermore, they are involved in allergic reactions. In addition, IL-4, IL-13, and IL-10 produced by Th2 cells have strong anti-inflammatory properties, thereby counteracting the tissue-damaging effects induced by the protective immune reactions mediated by Th1 cells. Given the functional activities of the Th1 and Th2 cytokines, Th1-mediated responses are likely to dominate in early immune responses, whereas the Th2 type of reactions accumulate later during the immune response. This notion is supported by clinical observations in human diseases, such as leprosy, in which the healing (tuberculoid) form, dominated by a strong DTH response, gradually makes way for the uncontrolled lepromatous form, characterized by weak DTH responses and high antibody levels.

Rather than being derived from separate committed lineage, Th subsets are thought to differentiate from the same precursor cell, which is a mature T cell capable of producing mainly IL-2 on antigenic stimulation. Many factors are involved in this differentiation process, such as the route of antigen entry, the dose of antigen, the strength of the signal received through the interaction of the major histocompatibility complex (MHC)–MHC class II peptide and the TCR–CD3 complex (21), and the presence of different costimulatory molecules, implicating an important role for antigen-presenting cells. However, cytokines themselves have been recognized to be the most potent differentiation-inducing factors.

II. Role of Cytokines in the Differentiation of Th1 and Th2 Helper Subsets

It has been conclusively demonstrated, in in vitro and in vivo experimental mouse models, that the presence of IL-4 is critical for the generation of IL-4 producing Th2 cells (22,23; reviewed in Ref. 24). The strongest evidence of the pivotal role of IL-4 in the induction of Th2 differentiation comes from experiments with IL-4 mutant mice ($IL\text{-}4^{-/-}$) in which the gene for IL-4 has been disrupted by homologous recombination. Infection of these mice with the nematode *Nippostrongylus brasiliensis* results in strongly reduced levels of IL-4, IL-5, and IL-9, as well as reduced eosinophilia, the presence of which is characteristic for Th2 responses (25,26). Similarly, mutant mice deficient for STAT-6 (for signal transducers and activators of transcription), a tyrosine kinase that is specifically phosphorylated following the interaction of IL-4 with its receptor, show deficient Th2 responses, including impaired Th2 helper T-cell differentiation, and immunoglobulin class-switching to IgG1 and IgE, following nematode infection. (27–29). However, although Th2 responses in IL-4($^{-/-}$) mice are strongly reduced, compared with wild-type mice, they are not completely absent, indicating that other, as yet unidentified, factors may be involved in Th2 differentiation.

In humans, IL-4 specifically and directly induces the differentiation of immunologically naive cord blood (10,30) or fetal thymocytes (Yamamaguchi E, de Vries J E, Yssel H, unpublished results) into IL-4-producing Th cells, following CD3-mediated stimulation. In view of the failure to detect IL-4 production by naive T cells (31), an as yet unresolved problem is the origin of IL-4, which is required to be present at the priming of these cells for successful Th2 differentiation. It has been proposed that other types of cells, notably mast cells and basophils, which produce IL-4 following triggering of their high-affinity FcεR by IgE and antigen, might be involved in the priming of naive cells for IL-4 production. However, studies with mice that carried a functional IL-4 gene in either Th cells or non-Th cells have questioned the role of these cells in Th2 differentiation. Mice in which only $CD4^+$ Th cells were able to express IL-4 produce antigen-specific IgE in a T-cell–dependent manner. In contrast, mice that carried a functional IL-4 gene, expressed only in non-Th cells, were unable to mount an IgE response, suggesting that Th cells are the primary, if not the only source of IL-4 for initial induction of IgE synthesis (32). Therefore, it seems likely that some T cells themselves can produce IL-4, following their initial activation, and this will increase following subsequent stimulation with antigen. In addition, in mice, a population of cells, that recognize the CD1 molecule and that are characterized by the expression of the $NK1.1^+$ molecule, have been identified as a source of IL-4, produced early during immune responses (33,34). However, a human homologue has not yet been identified, whereas the importance of $NK1.1^+$ cells in in vivo Th2 responses remains to be established.

In contrast with the involvement of only one cytokine in Th2 differentiation, several cytokines play a role in differentiation of naive cells via the Th1 pathway. Interleukin-12, produced by macrophages and dendritic cells, is the dominant cytokine, inducing the differentiation of IFN-γ–producing Th1 cells from naive precursor T cells (35,36). The production of IL-12 is induced by adjuvants that activate macrophages; by microbial components, such as bacterial endotoxin; by intracellular bacteria, such as *Listeria* or mycobateria; and by protozoa, such as *Toxoplasma,* resulting in the induction of Th1 immune responses that are dominated by the production of IFN-γ (reviewed in Ref. 37). IL-12 can act directly on T cells, as shown by the observation that IL-12–mediated Th1 differentiation of naive human T cells (10), as well as of naive T cells from transgenic mice (38), could not be inhibited by the addition of neutralizing anti–IFNγ monoclonal antibodies (MAbs), indicating a direct effect of IL-12 on T cells. Interaction of IL-12 with its receptor results in the activation and phosphorylation of three putative transcription factors: STAT-2, STAT-3, and STAT-4, from which only STAT-4 seems to be specific for IL-12–mediated signal transduction (39). The important role of IL-12 in

Th1 differentiation is underscored by the observations that mice, deficient in the gene coding for STAT-4 (27,40), or IL-12 (41), show impaired Th1 responses.

Until recently, there has been some controversy over the role of IFN-γ in the process of Th1 differentiation. In many in vitro culture systems IFN-γ is unable to drive Th1 differentiation by itself when added to primary cultures (42). In addition, IFN-γ($^{-/-}$) mice produce efficient antiviral cytolytic responses (43), whereas IFN-γR($^{-/-}$) mice are still able to generate Th1 cells, despite an increased susceptibility to infection with *L. major* (44). Whereas in one study, using experimental transgenic mice model, IL-12–mediated Th1 differentiation was dependent on the presence of IFN-γ (42), in a similar model, the Th1–inducing effects of IL-12 could not be blocked by the addition of a neutralizing anti–IFN-γ MAB (38). Moreover, different results, relative to the involvement of IFN-γ in Th1 differentiation, have been reported between mouse and human. Successful Th1 differentiation requires the expression of a functional IL-12R, consisting of two chains, designated IL-2R-β_1 and IL-12R-β_2 (45). The expression of a functional IL-12R seems to be restricted to recently activated, uncommitted, T cells and to Th1 cells, but is no longer expressed on fully differentiated Th2 cells (46,47); consequently, polarized Th2 cells are no longer able to respond to IL-12 (48). Interferon-γ, but not IFN-α, was able to render naive mouse T cells more responsive to the Th1 differentiation–inducing effects of IL-12 (42,48) by maintaining the expression of IL-12R-β_2 chain on differentiating Th1 cells (47). In contrast, however, only IFN-α and not IFN-γ induced IL-12R-β_2 chain mRNA transcription in human cord blood cells (46), giving support to earlier studies showing that IFN-γ has little or no effect on the differentiation of human CD4$^+$ cord blood T cells into populations of Th1 cells (10,30). The mechanisms underlying this difference between human and mouse cells remain to be elucidated. Finally, an additional, albeit indirect, role for IFN-γ has been demonstrated through its capacity to enhance the production of IL-12 by macrophages in response to infection with intracellular pathogens, thus creating a positive feedback loop (37) and acting in concert with IL-12 in the induction of Th1 responses required for the elimination of these pathogens.

Recently, another cytokine has been identified, originally in the mouse (49) and later in human (50), called IFN–γ–inducing factor (IGIF) or IL-18, which is likely to play an important role in Th1 cell differentiation. IL-18, which is produced by Kupffer cells, activated macrophages, and most likely by dendritic cells, seems to have stronger IFN-γ–inducing capacities than IL-12, apparently through a separate pathway. In addition, IL-18 strongly synergizes with IL-12 in the induction of IFN-γ by T and NK cells, and IL-18, together with IL-12, can even induce the production of high levels of IFN-γ by B cells, thereby inhibiting their production of IgE (51). Interestingly, IL-18 has a strong homology with IL-1, and the name IL-1γ has been proposed for this cytokine (52).Whether signal transduction pathways through the IL-18 receptor are shared with other cytokine receptors has not yet been reported.

III. Effect of Antigen Concentration of Th Differentiation

Several studies have demonstrated that the concentration or dose of antigen used to induce an immune response may have a strong effect on the cytokine production profile of the responding T cells. In general, low concentrations of antigens, or low-dose infections in experimental animals, seem to induce Th1 responses, whereas high concentrations of antigen tend to result in the generation of Th2 cells (21,53). For example, naive transgenic T cells, expressing a human TCR Vβ gene product, that were induced to specifically differentiate in an antigen-specific manner, produced increasing amounts of IL-4 and reduced levels of IFN-γ when very high or very low doses of antigen peptide were used (53).

Similar findings were reported in humans, showing that $CD4^+$ T cells from allergic donors produced high levels of IL-4 when stimulated with low concentrations of allergen, particularly when B-cell–enriched populations presented the antigen. In contrast, the same responding $CD4^+$ T-cell population produced little IL-4 when stimulated with high concentrations of allergen in the presence of monocytes as antigen-presenting effects (APC) (54). The mechanism underlying the effect of antigen dose on the differentiation of T cells is not yet clear. It is possible that, on uptake of low doses of antigen, macrophages or dendritic cells will produce IFN-γ–inducing cytokines, such as IL-12 or IL-18, whereas at high doses of antigen, lower levels of such cytokines are secreted. Alternatively, at high concentrations, antigens may be processed and presented by APC, such as B cells, that do not produce IL-12 or IL-18. Moreover, other factors produced by APC may complicate this picture, such as prostaglandin E_2 (PGE_2), produced by activated macrophages, but not by B cells, which may favor the development of Th2 responses by means of their specific inhibition of IFN-γ production by T cells.

One other published study on the effect of antigen dose on the cytokine production profile of human T cells has yielded somewhat different results. Carballido et al. reported that human T-cell clones, specific for the venom phospholipase A_2 (PLA), derived from allergic and hyposensitized individuals, required higher critical amounts of antigen for IFN-γ-induction and produced increasing IL-4/IFN-γ ratios following stimulation with increasing concentrations of PLA (55). Additional studies, however, are required to substantiate this observation and to point out possible differences among the different experimental models.

IV. Effect of Different Costimulatory Molecules

In view of the important role of APC in the generation of an immune response following antigenic challenge, it is likely that in addition to cytokines produced by these cells, the expression of certain costimulatory molecules may promote the differentiation of Th subpopulations. Among the most studied costimulatory molecules to date are two structurally related members of the immunoglobulin superfamily CD80 (B7.1, BB-1) and CD86 (B7.2). Both molecules are involved in T-cell activation by binding to their specific receptor CD28, which is constitutively expressed on many, but not all, T cells (reviewed in Ref. 56). Both CD80 and CD86 are expressed on activated B cells, dendritic cells, macrophages, as well as on activated T cells and NK cells. However, unlike CD80, CD86 is constitutively expressed on resting human monocytes. Optimal activation and differentiation of T cells requires interaction of CD28 with its ligands (57), and CD28–deficient mice have impaired proliferative responses to antigens (58). It has been demonstrated in various mouse experimental systems that the Th1 and Th2 pathways may be differentially activated through costimulation by CD80 or CD86, respectively, and that interaction of CD28 with either one of its ligands may result in a different clinical outcome in response to antigenic challenge (59,60). For example, in a model of experimental allergic encephalitis (EAE), a disease that is regulated by antigen-specific T cells, blockade of CD28–CD86 interactions increased disease severity. In contrast, administration of neutralizing anti-CD80 MAbs during immunization resulted primarily in generation of Th2 clones in vitro, the transfer of which into mice both prevented induction of EAE and abrogated established disease (60). However, evidence for the notion that costimulation by either CD80 or CD86 may directly affect initial cytokine secretion has not been confirmed in humans. Lanier et al. (61) have reported that stimulation of human peripheral blood T cells with CD86-expressing L-cell transfectants induced similar levels of Th1- and Th2-type cytokines. Furthermore, no differences in cytokine production profiles could be detected between human $CD45RA^+$ or $CD45RA^-$ T cells that were stimulated with transfectants, expressing comparable levels of CD80 or CD86 (62). The latter results underscore the notion that there is as yet no evidence that stimulation by either CD80 or CD86 will result in different biochemical signals to T cells. Nevertheless, it cannot be excluded that subsets of human T cells also have different requirements for costimulation by CD28 during various stages of differentiation or activation.

Another important molecule in T-cell activation is CD40L, which is expressed on T cells following activation. Interaction of CD40L with its ligand CD40, which is constitutively expressed on B cells and other APC, is required for T-cell development (63). However, CD40–CD40L interactions have not been reported to play a role in the differentiation of Th subsets.

V. Stability of Differentiated T Subpopulations

An important question, with important therapeutic implications, is whether the cytokine production profile of differentiated T cells is stable or whether it can revert under opposing polarizing conditions. Studies using transgenic mice have indicated that early in their differentiation mouse Th1 and Th2 populations may revert to the opposite phenotype, but that during further differentiation the cells become irreversibly committed to a particular cytokine production profile (64–66). In particular, differentiated mouse Th2 cell clones seem to be resistant to the IFN-γ–inducing effects of IL-12. A molecular basis for this loss of IL-12 responsiveness is that fully differentiated Th2 cells have lost the expression of a functional IL-12R, lacking the IL-12R β_2-chain and, therefore, they are no longer able to signal by STAT-4 (47,65). Evidence for this notion has been presented in the human system as well (46). However, several other studies have indicated that the phenotype of human Th2 populations is less stable. $CD4^+$ cord blood T cells that had been differentiated into a population of IL-4–producing Th2 cells, following repetitive stimulation in the presence of IL-4 and neutralizing anti-IFN-γ MAbs, reverted to a Th0/Th1 phenotype after a single stimulation and subsequent culture for 4 days in the presence of IL-12 (10). Similarly, when strongly polarized allergen-specific Th2 cells, obtained from skin biopsies of patients with atopic dermatitis following the induction of late-phase cutaneous reactions, were stimulated and cultured with antigen in the presence of IL-4 and IL-12, about 50% of the cells produced IFN-γ, as shown by an intracellular-staining method (67). In contrast to supernatants of activated skin-derived T cells, generated in the presence of IL-4 only, those generated in the presence of IL-4 and IL-12 were no longer able to induce the synthesis of IgE by purified B cells in vitro, indicating that IL-12 is still able to functionally revert a population of human highly differentiated Th2 cells into a population containing Th1 and Th0 cells, in addition to Th2 cells.

It has been argued that the presence of IFN-γ during the initial priming may maintain the expression of the IL-12R β_2-chain on mouse T cells, thereby creating a condition in which even differentiating Th2 cells can revert into IFN-γ producers by the action of IL-12 (47). However, the presence of IFN-γ during priming of human naive T cells had little effect on the transcription of the IL-12R β_2-chain; therefore, some fundamental differences, which remain to be elucidated, seem to exist between human and mouse populations. On the other hand, the aforementioned studies have all been carried out with populations and not with single cells; consequently, it cannot be excluded that the observed changes in phenotype are the result of outgrowth of uncommitted Th cells, rather than a true reversal of differentiated cells. Indeed, a recent report has shown that IL-12, when given together with a standard drug to reduce the parasitic load could reverse established Th2 responses to chronic injection with *L. major* to healing Th1 responses, favoring the hypothesis of reversal by outgrowth and, furthermore, indicating that polarized mouse Th2 responses still can be modulated under certain conditions (68). Although the mechanisms underlying the differentiation of Th cells are not yet completely understood, the ability to manipulate established population of Th cells with a polarized cytokine production profile, will be of therapeutic importance for the treatment of infectious, autoimmune, and allergic diseases.

VI. Phenotypic Differences Between Th1 and Th2 Populations

In spite of their functional differences, as well as the ability to distinguish Th1 and Th1 populations based on their cytokine production profile, until recently, no phenotypic distinction between both subsets had been reported. Obviously, the availability of cell-surface markers that could distinguish Th1 and Th2 cells would be of use for the development and monitoring of clinical therapies as well as for the isolation of polarized Th subsets for research purposes. An elegant method has been described, permitting the identification of individual cytokine-producing Th cells, by flow cytometry. However, this procedure is rather insensitive, requires prior activation of the cells, and does not permit isolation of viable cells. Other methods to isolate different Th cells, based on membrane-linked expression of cytokines are applicable only when cytokines are expressed at high levels; therefore, they are likely to be of little value using antigen-stimulated peripheral blood T cells.

In spite of extensive efforts to identify cell surface molecules that would distinguish polarized Th populations in both mouse and man, few such markers have bene characterized. Whereas in the mouse $CD4^+$ naive precursors cells are $CD44^{high}$, $CD45RA^{high}$, $CD45RB^{high}$, $CD45RO^{low}$, and LECAM-1^{high}, they differentiate into effector cells with a $CD44^{low}$, $CD45RA^{low}$, $CD45RB^{low}$, $CD45R^{high}$, and LECAM-1^{low} cell surface phenotype, irrespective of their cytokine production profile (69). In humans, it has been reported that expression levels of the Reed–Sternberg-specific molecule CD30 enable distinction between Th1, Th0, and Th2 cells (70), although this observation is controversial (71–73). In view of the finding that Th1 clones, in contrast to Th2 clones, have cytotoxic activity (74), levels of expression of cell surface molecules involved in the lytic process might be useful to distinguish both populations of cells. However, it is unclear whether a possible differential expression of cell surface molecules, such as CD95 or its ligand (FasL) will permit the identification and isolation of human Th2 cells or T-cell clones.

In view of the [absence of] regulatory effects of cytokines on differentiated Th cells, much attention has been given lately to the differential expression of cytokine receptors on these cells. Recently, it was reported by Pernis et al. that murine Th1 clones, in contrast with Th2 clones, do not express transcripts for the β-chain of the IFN-γR (75), which is primarily involved in signaling and not in binding of IFN-γ (76–77). These results have not only provided a molecular basis for the longstanding observation that IFN-γ inhibits the proliferation of murine Th2, but not that of Th1 cells (78,79), but, for the first time they also offered the possibility to specifically tag Th subsets. However, it was reported by a different group that IFN-γ, produced during the differentiation of mouse Th1 cells, was able to downregulate the expression of the IFN-γR β-chain on these, as well as Th2 cells (80), which implied that inactivation of IFN-γ signaling in T cells is a dynamic process, depending on the cytokine environment and that the presence or absence of the IFN-γRβ-chain does not discriminate between murine Th1 and Th2 cells per se. The latter results, however, differ from findings in humans indicating that mRNAs for IFN-γR α- and β-chains are indeed expressed in polarized Th2, but not in Th1 clones (81). The expression of a nonfunctional IFN-γR on Th1 cells was confirmed by the inability of IFN-γ to induce the *IFR-1* gene in Th1 clones. Moreover, human Th0 clones, producing IL-4, as well as IFN-γ, express a functional IFN-γR, demonstrating that, in human T cells, IFN-γ does not seem to have a long-lasting down-regulatory effect on IFN-γ-R β-chain expression. Human naive $CD4^+$, $CD45RA^+$ cells express the IFN-γR β-chain as well, which was lost after stimulation and culture of the cells in the presence of rIL-12, but not rIL-4. Together, these results demonstrated that, in humans, the loss of IFN-γ-R β-chain expression is not only intrinsic to the Th1 differentiation process, but it can also be used as a marker of phenotype, distinguishing between differentiated Th1 and Th0/Th2 cells, respectively, confirming the original observation of Pernis et al. (75).

Polarized human Th2 cells, in contrast with Th1 cells, no longer express a functional IL-12 R, owing to the loss of the IL-12R β_2-chain, and similar to the results obtained with the signaling chain of the IFN-βR, this observation could potentially be useful to distinguish both subsets. All these studies have been carried out by analyzing the expression of both receptor components at the transcriptional level, and no information is yet available about the usefulness of MAbs to identify and isolate polarized Th subsets. It must be remembered, however, that similar to the IFN-γR β-chain (81), the IL-12R β_2-chain might also be expressed on populations of Th0 cells. Because it has been argued that populations of Th cells form a continuous spectrum in which the Th1 and Th2 phenotypes are only two of the extremes (17), cytokine receptors are very likely to be expressed on "intermediate" subsets as well, making the identification of polarized Th1 or Th2 cells very difficult, if not impossible.

Alternative receptors that may be differentially expressed on Th subsets are chemokine and "homing" receptors. For example, the observation that Th2 and Th0 cells seem to be more sensitive to infection with human immunodeficiency virus (HIV) than Th1 cells (82), together with the property of CXCR4 to function as coreceptors for HIV entry into T cells (83), might be the result of differential expression of such, and other, chemokine receptors.

Recently, it has been reported that homing of mouse Th1, but not of Th2, cells into sites of inflammation is mediated by the adhesion molecules E-selectin and P-selectin (84), which might be due to differential expression of their ligand, such as CLA on these T-cell subsets. However, no evidence for this notion has yet been reported in humans.

VII. The Subsets in Disease

Given the results obtained from numerous animal models and human studies, there seems to be a direct association between the involvement of Th subsets and susceptibility to infectious, autoimmune, and allergic disorders. Th1 responses are thought to play an important role in the protection against intracellular microbes, inducing cell-mediated inflammatory reactions, as well the production of antibodies that bind to Fcγ receptors on APC and that fix complement. In contrast, Th2 cells include the production of IgE and the recruitment of eosinophils into locations infiltrated by extracellular parasites. Importantly, Th2 cells, owing to the nature of the cytokines that they produce, also limit the damage caused by Th1 cell-mediated

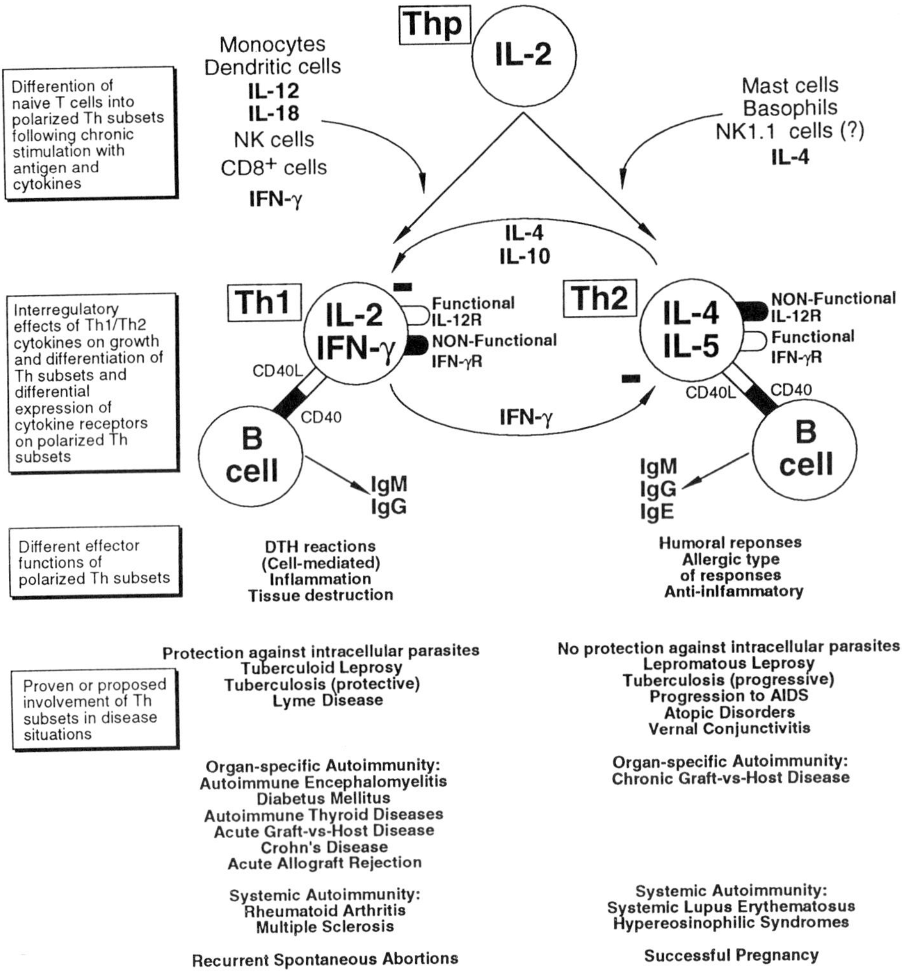

Figure 1 Polarized human Th1 and Th2 subsets.

inflamation. In addition to giving protection to various invading microorganism, Th1 and Th2 cells also play a critical role in the induction and maintenance of other pathological conditions (Fig. 1).

Evidence from animal models has strongly suggested that both Th1 and Th2 responses are implicated in the induction or organ-specific autoimmune diseases, such as insulin-dependent diabetes mellitus, autoimmune thyroid diseases, and systemic autoimmune diseases, such as rheumatoid arthritis, experimental allergic encephalitis (EAE; all Th-1 dominated), and systemic lupus erythematosus (SLE; Th-2 associated). Evidence from related diseases in humans has shown an accumulation of a predominant Th1 response in the target organs of patients with autoimmune thyroid diseases and multiple sclerosis and in those suffering from granulomatous inflammation, such as arthritis and Crohn's disease. In the latter, the host tissue damage seems to originate from the defective Th1-suppressing effect of cytokines, such as IL-10 and TGF-β, as illustrated by the increased susceptibility of IL-10 knockout mice to inflammatory bowel diseases (85).

A complicated issue is the involvement of Th subsets in allograft rejection. Whereas the Th1-dependent effector cells' mechanisms, such as DTH reactions and cytotoxic activity, seem to play a central role in acute graft-versus-host disease (GVHD), Th2 responses have been proposed to be associated with chronic GVHD (reviewed in Ref. 86). Interestingly, maternal–fetal interactions, which because of the presence of paternal alloantigens, should give rise to rejection of the fetus, seem to be governed by a predominant Th2 response, resulting in the fetal survival (87). This notion is underscored by the observation that $CD4^+$ and $CD8^+$ T-cell clones obtained from the decidua of women with recurrent spontaneous abortions showed defective IL-4 and IL-10 production, in contrast with those obtained from women with successful pregnancies (88).

An important role for the Th2 cells has been demonstrated in the induction and maintenance of atopic disorders, which is not surprising in view of the functional capacities of the signature Th2 cytokines IL-4, IL-13, and IL-5, involved in the induction of IgE synthesis and the recruitment, differentiation, and proliferation of eosinophils, respectively. Allergen-specific Th2 cells can readily be isolated from the peripheral blood or from skin and bronchial biopsies from patients with atopic diseases, suggesting an accumulation of such cells in their target organs, whereas allergen-specific T cells, isolated from the peripheral blood of nonatopic individuals, generally show a Th0/Th1 cytokine production profile. Moreover, as described in Chapter 7 of this book, successful immunotherapy of allergic diseases seems to be associated with a conversion from a prevalent Th2 to a Th0/Th1 cytokine production profile of allergen-specific T cells.

The mechanism(s) underlying the genetic predisposition for atopic disease have not yet been identified, but are likely to be the result of molecular changes in genes, coding for the production of Th1 and Th2 cytokines, as well as their receptors. Asthma and other atopic disorders are multifactorial diseases; therefore, multiple gene products are likely to be implicated in the pathology of these diseases. Much attention has focused human chromosome 5 (with its murine homologue chromosome 11) in view of the cluster of Th2 cytokine genes, including IL-4, IL-5, and IL-13, as well as of the genes encoding for the IL-12 p40 chain and IFN-γ response factor 1 (IRF-1) on this chromosome, and although many genetic loci seem to predispose to asthma (89), the genetic control of this disease, including the Th1/Th2 balance and the production of IgE, still remains unclear. In addition to the genetic background of atopic individuals, another outstanding question is the contribution of antigenic environment to the balance of Th1 and Th2 responses. In a recent epidemiological study, an inverse correlation between DTH responses against tuberculin and the presence of asthma and serum IgE concentrations (90), suggests that infections, such as those with *M. tuberculosis*, might have a protective effect on Th2-cell mediated allergic disorders. Moreover, the results of this study suggest that vaccination to induce Th2 responses may be effective against atopic disorders.

VIII. Conclusions

Since the recognition of the dual nature of the immune response and the classification of Th1 and Th2 cytokines, much progress has been made in our understanding of the importance of cytokines in the control of normal and pathological immune responses. Although many questions still have to be resolved, in many experimental models, modulation of the Th1/Th2 balanced has altered the outcome of disease, providing the basis for future therapeutic interventions in human pathophysiological conditions.

References

1. Mosmann TR, Cherwinsky H, Bond MW, Giedlin MA, Coffman RL. J Immunol 1986; 136:2348–2357.
2. Mosmann TR, Coffman RL. Th1 and Th2 cells: different patterns of lymphokine secretion lead to different functional properties. Annu Rev Immunol 1989; 7:145–173.
3. Paliard X, de Waal Malefijt R, Yssel H, Blanchard D, Chretien I, Abrams J, de Vries J, Spits H. Simultaneous production of IL-2, IL-4, and IFN-γ by activated human $CD4^+$ and $CD8^+$ T cell clones. J Immunol 1988; 141:849–855.
4. Maggi E, Del Prete G, Macchia D, Parronchi P, Tiri A, Chrétien I, Ricci M, Romagnani S. Profiles of lymphokine activities and helper function for IgE in human T cell clones. Eur J Immunol 1988; 18:1045–1050.
5. Wierenga EA, Snoek M, de Groot C, Chrétien I, Bos JD, Jansen HM, Kapsenberg M. Evidence for compartmentalization of functional subsets of $CD4^+$ T lymphocytes in atopic patients. J Immunol 1990; 144:4651–4656.
6. Haanen JBAG, de Waal Malefijt R, de Vries RRP, Spits H. Selection of a human Th-1 like T cell subset by *Mycobacterium leprae* antigens. J Exp Med 1991; 174:583–592.
7. Yssel H, Shanafelt M-C, Soderberg C, Schneider PV, Anzola J, Peltz G. *B. burgdorfi* activates T cells to produce a selective pattern of lymphokines in Lyme arthritis. J Exp Med 1991; 174:593–601.
8. Del Prete GF, De Carli M, Mastromauro C, Biagotti R, Macchia D, Falangiani P, Ricci M, Romagnani S. Purified protein derivative of *Mycobacterium tuberculosis* and excretory–secretory antigen(s) of *Toxcara canis* expand in vitro human T cells with stable and opposite (type 1 helper or type 2 helper) profile of cytokine production. J Clin Invest 1991; 88:346–350.
9. Yssel H, De Waal Malefyt R, Roncarolo M-G, Abrams JS, Lahesmaa R, Spits H, de Vries JE. IL-10 is produced by subsets of human $CD4^+$ T cell clones and peripheral blood T cells. J Immunol 1992; 149:2378–2384.
10. Sornasse T, Larenas P, Davis KA, de Vries JE, Yssel H. Differentiation and stability of Th1 and Th2 cells derived from naive human neonatal $CD4^+$ T cells, analyzed at the single-cell level. J Exp Med 1996; 184:473–483.
11. de Waal Malefyt R, Abrams JS, Zurawski SM, Lecron J-C, Mohan-Peterson S, Sanjanwala B, Bennett BF, Silver J, de Vries JE, Yssel H. Differential regulation of IL-4 and IL-13 expression by human T cell clones and EBV-transformed B cells. Int Immunol 1995; 7:1405–1416.

12. Yssel H, Johnson KE, Schneider PV, Wideman J, Terr A, Kastelein R, de Vries JE. T cell activation inducing epitopes of the house dust mite allergen Der p I. Induction of a restricted cytokine production profile of Der p I-specific T cell clones upon antigen-specific activation. J Immunol 1992; 148:738–745.
13. Manetti R, Gerosa F, Giudizi MG, Biagiotti R, Parronchi P, Piccinni M-P, Sampognaro S, Maggi E, Romagnani S, Trinchieri G. Interleukin 12 induces stable priming for interferon γ (IFN-γ) production during differentiation of human T helper (Th) cells and transient IFN-γ production in established Th2 cell clones. J Exp Med 1994; 179:1273–1283.
14. Yssel H, Fasler S, de Vries JE, de Waal Malefyt R. Interleukin 12 (IL-12) transiently induces IFN-γ transcription and protein synthesis in human $CD4^+$ allergen-specific helper type 2 (Th2) T cell clones. Int Immunol 1994; 6:1091–1096.
15. Schmitz J, Assenmacher M, Radbruch A. Regulation of T helper cell cytokine expression: functional dichotomy of antigen-presenting cells. Eur J Immunol 1993; 23:191–199.
16. Bucy RP, Panoskaltsis-Mortari A, Huang GQ, Li J, Karr L, Ross M, Russell JH, Murphy KM, Weaver CT. Heterogeneity of single cell cytokine gene expression in clonal T cell populations. J Exp Med 1994; 180:1251–1262.
17. Kelso A, Groves P, Troutt AB, Francis K. Evidence for the stochastic acquisition of cytokine profile by $CD4^+$ T cells activated in a T helper type 2-like response in vivo. Eur J Immunol 1995; 25:1168–1175.
18. Yamamura M, Uyemura K, Deans RJ, Weinberg K, Re TH, Bloom BR, Modlin RL. Defining protective responses to pathogens: cytokine profiles in leprosy lesions. Science 1991; 254:277–279.
19. Robinson DS, Hamid Q, Ying S, Tsicopoulos A, Barkans J, Bentley AM, Corrigan C, Durham SR, Kay AB. Predominant TH2-like bronchoalveolar T-lymphocyte population in atopic asthma. N Engl J Med 1992; 326:298–304.
20. Reiner SL, Locksley RM. The regulation of immunity to *Leishmania major*. Annu Rev Immunol 1995; 13:151–177.
21. Bretscher PA, Wei G, Menon JN, Bielefeldt-Ohmann H. Establishment of stable, cell-mediated immunity that makes “susceptible” mice resistant to *Leishmania major*. Science 1992; 257:539–542.
22. Swain SL, Weinberg AD, English M, Huston G. IL-4 directs the development of Th2-like helper effectors.. J Immunol 1990; 145:3796–3806.
23. Le Gros G, Ben-Sasson SZ, Seder R, Finkelman F, Paul WE. Generation of interleukin 4 (IL-4)-producing cells in vivo and in vitro: IL-2 and IL-4 are required for in vitro generation of IL-4 producing cells. J Exp Med 1990; 172:921–929.
24. Seder RA, Paul WE. Acquisition of lymphokine-producing phenotype by $CD4^+$ T Cells. Annu Rev Immunol 1994; 12:635–673.
25. Kühn R, Rajewsky K, Muller W. Generation and analysis of interleukin-4 deficient mice. Science 1991; 254:707–710
26. Kopf M, Le Gros G, Bachman M, Larners M, Blüthmann, Kohler G. Disruption of the murine IL-4 gene blocks Th2 cytokine responses. Nature 1993; 362:245–248.
27. Kaplan MH, Schindle RU, Smile YST, Grusby MJ. Stat 6 is required for mediating responses to IL-4 and for development of Th2 cells. Immunity 1996; 4:313–319.
28. Shimoda K, van Deursen J, Sangste RMY, Sarawar SR, Carson RT, Tripp RA, Chu C, Quelle F, Nosaka T, Vignali DA, Doherty P, Grosveld G, Paul WE, Ihle JN. Lack of IL-4-induced Th2 response and IgE class switching in mice with disrupted Stat 6 gene. Nature 1996; 380:630–633.
29. Takeda K, Tanaka T, Shi W, Matsumoto M, Minami M, Kashiwamura S, Nakanishi K, Yoshida N, Kishimoto T, Akira S. Essential role of Stat 6 in IL-4 signaling. Nature 1996; 380:627–630.
30. Demeure CE, Wu CY, Shu U, Schneider PV, Heusser C, Yssel H, Delespesse. In vitro maturation of human neonatal CD4 T lymphocytes. II. Cytokines present at priming modulate the development of lymphokine production. J Immunol 1994; 152:4775–4782.
31. Ehlers S, Smith KA. Differentiation of T cell lymphokine gene expression: the in vitro acquisition of T cell memory. J Exp Med 1991; 173:25–36.

32. Schmitz J, Thiel A, Kuhn R, Rajewsky K, Müller W, Assenmacher M, Radbruch A. Induction of interleukin 4 (IL-4) expression in T helper (Th) cells is not dependent on IL-4 from non-Th cells. J Exp Med 1994; 179:1349–1353.
33. Bendelac A, Lantz O, Quimby ME, Yewdell JW, Bennink JR, Brutkiewicz RR. CD1 recognition by mouse NK 1^+ T lymphocytes. Science 1995; 268:863–865.
34. Yoshimoto T, Paul WE. $CD4^+$, $NK1.1^+$ T cells promptly produce interleukin 4 in response to in vivo challenge with anti-CD3. J Exp Med 1994; 179:1285–1295.
35. Manetti R, Parronchi P, Giudizi MG, Piccinni M-P, Maggi E, Trinchieri G, Romagnani S. Natural killer cell stimulatory factor (interleukin 12 [IL-12]) induces T helper type 1 (T1)-specific immune response and inhibits the development of IL-4 producing cells. J Exp Med 1993; 177:199–204.
36. Hsieh C-S, Mactaonia SE, Tripp CS, Wolf SF, O'Garra A, Murphy KM. Development of TH1 $CD4^+$ T cells through IL-12 produced by *Listeria*-induced macrophages. Science 1993; 260:547–549.
37. Trinchieri G. Interleukin-12: a proinflammatory cytokine with immunoregulatory functions that bridge innate resistance and antigen-specific adaptive immunity. Annu Rev Immunol 1995; 13:251–276.
38. Seder RA, Gazzinelli R, Sher A, Paul WE. Interleukin 12 acts directly on $CD4^+$ T cells to enhance priming of interferon gamma production and diminishes interleukin 4 inhibition of such priming. Proc Natl Acad Sci USA 1993; 90:10188–10192.
39. Jacobson NG, Szabo SJ, Weber-Nordt RM, Zhong Z, Schreiber RD, Darnell JEJ, Murphy KM. Interleukin 12 signaling in T helper type 1 (Th1) cells involves tyrosine phosphorylation of signal transducer and activator of transcription (Stat) 3 and Stat 4. J Exp Med 1995; 181:1755–1762.
40. Thierfelder WE, van Deursen JM, Yamamoto K, Tripp RA, Sarawar SR, Carson RT, Sangster MY, Vignali DA, Doherty PC, Grosvel GC, Ihle JN. Requirement for Stat 4 in interleukin-12-mediated responses of natural killer and T cells. Nature 1996; 382:171–174.
41. Magram J, Connaughton SE, Warrier RR, Carvajal DM, Wu CY, Ferrante J, Stewart C, Sarmiento U, Faherty DA, Gately MK. IL-12-deficient mice are defective in IFN-γ production and type 1 cytokine responses. Immunity 1996; 4:471–481.
42. Wenner CA, Macatonia SA, O'Garra A, Murphy KM. Common roles for IFN-α and IFN-γ in promoting Th1 differentiation induced by IL-12. J Immunol 1996; 156:1442–1447.
43. Graham MB. Response to influenza infection in mice with a targeted disruption of the IFN-γ gene. J Exp Med 1993; 178:1725.
44. Swihart K, Fruth U, Messmer N, Hug K, Behin R, Huang S, Del Guidice G, Aguet M, Louis JA. Mice from a genetically resistant background lacking the interferon gamma receptor are susceptible to infection with *Leishmania major* but mount a polarized T helper cell 1-type $CD4^+$ T cell response. J Exp Med 1995; 181:961–971.
45. Presky DH, Yang H, Minetti LJ, Chua AO, Nabavi N, Wu CY, Gately MK, Gubler U. A functional interleukin 12 receptor complex is composed of two β-type cytokine receptor subunits. Proc Natl Acad Sci USA 1996; 93:14002–14007.
46. Rogge L, Barberis-Maino L, Biffi M, Passini N, Presky DH, Gubler U, Sinagaglia F. Selective expression of an interleukin-12 receptor component by human T helper 1 cells. J Exp Med 1997; 185:825–831.
47. Szabo SJ, Dighe AS, Guebler U, Murphy KM. Regulation of the interleukin (IL)-12R β_2 subunit expression in developing T helper 1 (Th1) and Th2 cells. J Exp Med 1997; 185:817–824.
48. Güler ML, Gorham JD, Hsieh CS, Macke AJ, Steen RG, Dietrich WF, Murphy KM. Genetic susceptibility to *Leishmania*: IL-12 responsiveness in TH1 cell development. Science 1996; 271:984–987.
49. Okamura H, Tsutsi H, Komatsu T, Yutsudo M, Hakura A, Tanimoto T, Torigoe K, Okura T, Nukada Y, Hattori K, Akita K, Namba M, Tanabe F, Fukuda S, Kurimoto M. Cloning of a new cytokine that induces IFN-γ production by T cells. Nature 1995; 378:88–91.
50. Ushio S, Namba M, Okura T, Hattori K, Nukada Y, Akita K, Tanabe F, Konishi K, Micalle M, Fujii M, Torigoe K, Tanimoto T, Fukuda S, Ikeda M, Okumura H, M. K. Cloning of

the cDNA for human IFN-γ-inducing factor, expression in *Escherichia coli*, and studies on the biologic activities of the protein. J Immunol 1996; 156:4274–4279.
51. Yoshimoto T, Okamura H, Tagawa Y-I, Iwakura Y, Nakanishi I. Interleukin 18 together with interleukin 12 inhibits IgE production by induction of IFN-γ production from activated B cells. Proc Natl Acad Sci USA 1997; 94:3948–3953.
52. Bazan JF, Timans JC, Kastelein RA. A newly defined interleukin-1? Nature 1996; 379:591.
53. Hosken NA, Shibuy K, Heath AW, Murphy KM, O'Garra A. The effect of antigen dose on $CD4^+$ T helper cell phenotype development in a T cell receptor–αβ-transgenic model. J Exp Med 1995; 182:1579–1584.
54. Secrist H, DeKruyff RH, Umetsu DT. Interleukin 4 production by $CD4^+$ T cells from allergic individuals is modulated by antigen concentration and antigen-presenting cell type. J Exp Med 199; 181:1081–1089.
55. Carballido JM, Carballido-Perrig N, Terres G, Heusser CH, Blaser K. Bee venom phospholipase A_2-specific T cell clones from human allergic and non-allergic individuals: cytokine patterns change in response to the antigen concentration. Eur J Immunol 1992; 22:1357–1363.
56. Lenschow DJ, Walunas TL, Bluestone JA. CD28/B7 system of T cell costimulation. Annu Rev Immunol 1996; 14:259–274.
57. Schwartz RH. A cell culture model for T lymphocyte clonal anergy. Science 1990; 248:1349–1356.
58. Green JM, Noel PJ, Sperling AI, Walunas TL, Gray GS, Bluestone JA, Thompson CB. Absence of B7-dependent responses in CD28-deficient mice. Immunity 1994; 1:501–508.
59. Freeman GJ, Boussiotis VA, Anumanthan A, Bernstein GM, Ke XY, Rennert PD, Gray GS, Gribben JG, Nadler LM. B7-1 and B7-2 do not deliver identical costimulatory signals, since B7-2 but not B7-1 preferentially costimulates the initial production of IL-4. Immunity 1995; 2:523–532.
60. Kuchroo VK, Das MP, Brown JA, Ranger AM, Zamvil SS, Sobel RA, Weiner HL, Nabavi N, Glimcher H. B7-1 and B7-2 costimulatory molecules activate differentially the Th1/Th2 developmental pathways: application to autoimmune disease therapy. Cell 1995; 80:707–718.
61. Lanier LL, O'Fallon S, Somoza C, Phillips JH, Linsley PS, Okumura K, Ito D, Azuma M. Cd80 (B7) and CD86 (B70) provide similar costimulatory signals for T cell proliferation, cytokine production, and generation of CTL. J Immunol 1995; 154:97–105.
62. Levin BL, Ueda Y, Craighead N, Huang ML, June CH. CD28 ligands CD80 (B7.1) and CD86 (B7.2) induce long-term autocrine growth of $CD4^+$ T cells and induce similar patterns of cytokine secretion in vitro. Int Immunol 1995; 7:891–904.
63. Grewall IS, Xu J, Flavell RA. CD40L. Nature 1995; 378:617–620.
64. Perez VL, Lederer JA, Lichtman AH, Abbas AK. Stability of T_h1 and T_h2 populations. Int Immunol 1995; 7:869–875.
65. Szabo SL, Jacobson NG, Dighe AS, Gubler U, Murphy KM. Developmental commitment to the Th2 lineage by extinction of IL-12 signaling. Immunity 1995; 2:665–675.
66. Murphy E, Shibuya K, Hosken N, Openshaw P, Maino VC, Davis K, Murphy K, O'Garra A. Conversion of T helper 1 and T helper 2 cytokine profiles in antigen-specific CD^+ T cell populations. J Exp Med 1996; 183:901–911.
67. Carballido JM, Aversa G, Kaltoft K, Cocks BG, Punnonen J, Yssel H, Thestrup-Pedersen K, de Vries JE. Reversal of human allergen-specific Th2 responses by engagement of signaling lymphocytic activation molecule. J Immunol 1997; 159:4316–4321.
68. Nabors GS, Afonso LC, Farrell JP, Scott P. Switch from a type 2 to a type 1 T helper cell response and cure of established *Leishmania major* infection in mice is induced by combined therapy with interleukin 12 and Pentostam. Proc Natl Acad Sci USA 1995; 92:3142–3146.
69. Swain SL, Weinberg AD, English M. $CD4^+$ T cell subsets. Lymphokine secretion of memory cells and of effector cells that develop from precursors in vitro. J Immunol 1990; 144:1788–1799.
70. Del Prete G, De Carli M, Almerigogna F, Daniel CK, D'Elios MM, Zancuogh IG, Vinante

F, Pizzolo G, Romagnani S. Preferential expression of CD30 by human CD4+ T cells producing Th2-type cytokines. FASEB J 1995; 9:81–86.
71. Alzona M, Jack HM, Fisher RI, Ellis TM. CD30 defines a subset of T cells that produce IFN-γ and IL-5 and exhibit enhanced B cell helper activity. Immunol 1994; 153:2861–2867.
72. Alzona M, Jack HM, Fisher RI, Ellis TM. IL-12 activates IFN-γ production through the preferential activation of CD30+ T cells. J Immunol 1995; 154:9–16.
73. Hamann D, Hilkens CM, Grogan JL, Lens SM, Kapsenberg ML, Yazdanbakhsh M, van Lier RA. CD30 expression does not discriminate between human Th1- and Th2-type T cells. J Immunol 1996; 156:1387–1391.
74. Del Prete G, De Carli M, Ricci M, Romagnani S. Helper activity for immunoglobulin synthesis of TH and TH human T cell clones: the help of TH1 clones is limited by their cytotoxic activity. J Exp Med 1991; 174:809–813.
75. Pernis A, Gupta S, Gollob KJ, Garfein E, Coffman RL, Schindler C, Rothman P. Lack of interferon γ receptor β chain and the prevention of interferon γ signaling in TH1 cells. Science 1995; 269:245–247.
76. Hemmi S, Merlin G, Aguet M. Functional characterization of a hybrid human–mouse interferon γ receptor: evidence for species-specific interaction of the extracellular receptor domain with a putative signal transducer. Proc Natl Acad Sci USA 1992; 89:2737–2741.
77. Soh J, Donnelly RJ, Kotenko S, Mariano TM, Cook JR, Wang N, Emanuel S, Schwartz B, Miki T, Pestka S. Identification and sequence of an accessory factor required for activation of the human interferon γ receptor. Cell 1994; 76:793–802.
78. Gajewski TF, Fitch FW. Anti-proliferative effect of IFN-γ in immune regulation. I. IFN-γ inhibits the proliferation of Th2 but not Th1 murine helper T lymphocyte clones. J Immunol 1988; 140:4245–4252.
79. Gajewski TF, Joyce J, Fitch FW. Antiproliferative effect of IFN-γ in immune regulation. III. Differential selection of TH1 and TH2 murine helper T lymphocyte clones using recombinant IL-2 and recombinant IFN-γ. J Immunol 1989; 143:15–22.
80. Bach EA, Szabo SJ, Dighe AS, Ashkenazi A, Aguet M, Murphy KM, Schreiber RD. Ligand-induced autoregulation of IFN-γ receptor β chain expression in T helper cell subsets. Science 1995; 270:1215–1218.
81. Groux H, Somasse T, Cottrez F, de Vries JE, Coffman RL, Roncarolo M-G, Yssel H. Induction of human Th1 cell differentiation results in loss of IFN-γ receptor β-chain expression. J Immunol 1997; 158:5627–5631.
82. Maggi E, Mazzetti M, Ravina A, Annunziato F, de Carli M, Piccinni M, Manetti R, Carbonari M, Pesce AM, del Prete G, Romagnani S. Ability of HIV to promote a TH1 to TH0 shift and to replicate preferentially in TH2 and TH0 cells. Science 1994; 265:244–248.
83. Feng Y, Broder CC, Kennedy PE, Berger EA. HIV-1 entry cofactor: functional cDNA cloning of a seven-transmembrane, G protein-coupled receptor. Science 1996; 272:872–877.
84. Austrup F, Vestweber D, Borges E, Lohning E, Brauer R, Renz H, Hallmann A. P- and E-selectin mediate recruitment of T-helper-1 but not T-helper-2 cells into inflamed tissues. Nature 1997; 385:81–83.
85. Kuhn R, Lohler J, Rennick D, Rajewsky K, Muller W. Interleukin-10-deficient mice develop chronic enterocolitis. Cell 1993; 75:263–274.
86. Ferrara JLM. Cytokine dysregulation as a mechanism of graft versus hot disease. Curr Opin Immunol 1993; 5:794–799.
87. Wengmann TG, Lin H, Guilbert L, Mosmann TR. Bidirectional cytokine interactions in the maternal–fetal relationship: is successful pregnancy a Th2 phenomenon? Immunol Today 1993; 14:353–356.
88. Romagnani S. The Th1/Th2 paradigm. Immunol Today 1997; 18:263–266.
89. Daniels SE, Bhattacharrya S, Jame A, Leaves NI, Young A, Hill MR, Faux JA, Ryan GF, le Souef PN, Lathrop GM, Musk AW, Cookson WO. A genome-wide search for quantitative trait loci underlying asthma. Nature 1996; 383:247–250.
90. Shirakawa T, Enomoto T, Shimazu S-I, Hopkin JM. The inverse association between tuberculin responses and atopic disorder. Science 1997; 275:77–79.

2

Mechanisms of Allergic Asthma

A Th2 Disease

DOUGLAS S. ROBINSON and A. BARRY KAY

Imperial College School of Medicine
National Heart and Lung Institute
London, England

I. Introduction

Up to the mid-1980s asthma, particularly atopic asthma, was believed to result essentially from intermittent type I (immediate-type hypersensitivity) reactions involving the IgE-dependent release of pharmacological mediators from mast cells. Mast cell degranulation consequent on physical or other stimuli accounted for nonatopic ("intrinsic") asthma (1). Set against the "leaky mast cell" hypothesis was the observation that corticosteroids, a mainstay in asthma treatment since the 1950s, had no effect on IgE-dependent histamine release from dispersed mast cells obtained from human lung tissue (2). Furthermore, agents such as antihistamines that antagonize the effects of mast cell mediators have little effect in asthma. In addition, it was recognized that, even between acute attacks, the asthmatic airways were hyperresponsive to nonspecific stimuli, such as histamine, even when the patient was asymptomatic. Thus, the concept of asthma as a chronic inflammatory disease emerged. The application of fiberoptic bronchoscopy (3) soon established that eosinophils and activated T cells were a feature of asthmatic airways even in the absence of symptoms. By 1987, asthma definitions included eosinophilic airway hyperresponsiveness, airway inflammation, and desquamative bronchial eosinophilia as characteristics of the disease (4).

There were several reasons for turning to the T cells for clues to what "drives" the asthma process—not the least being the exquisite sensitivity of T cells to the antiproliferative action of corticosteroids. There had also been improved understanding of the allergic response in terms of the essential role of T cells in both antibody-mediated and cell-mediated hypersensitivity reactions. The concept of antigen processing and presentation of antigen-derived peptides complexed with major histocompatibility complex (MHC) on antigen-presenting cells (APCs), such as macrophages and dendritic cells, to specific T-cell receptors (TCRs) had also been confirmed by the elucidation of the crystal structure of MHC class II molecules (5).

$CD4^+$ T cells bind class II MHC molecules on antigen-presenting cells and are principally concerned with handling exogenous antigens (6). After engagement with the T-cell receptor and in the presence of a second signal delivered by costimulatory molecules, CD4 T cells are activated either by direct cell–cell contact, as in "help" for B-cell antibody synthesis, or by production of soluble messenger molecules, termed cytokines. With the identification of IgE as the "reaginic factor" involved in anaphylaxis and immediate hypersensitivity (7), it became clear that control of IgE synthesis was T-cell–dependent, and that T-cell–derived cytokines were involved in the maturation, activation and recruitment of granulocytes, monocytes, and other inflammatory cells. In experimental animals, eosinophil production is T-cell–dependent (8). Because different cytokines were shown to direct immunoglobulin responses of differing isotypes and different patterns of inflammatory cells, it was suggested that different patterns of T-cell cytokine response might determine the nature of immune responses, and that T-cell cytokine profiles might be an important determinant between either antibody-predominant responses or the cellular immune response, as seen in delayed-type hypersensitivity (DTH; 9). This idea was given substantial impetus by the demonstration by Mosmann et al. (10) and Fong and Mosmann (11) that $CD4^+$ murine T-cell clones, could be divided into Th1 (producing interleukin-2 [IL-2] and interferon γ [IFN-γ]), which mediate DTH, and Th2 clones that produced IL-4 and IL-5, but not IL-2 or IFN-γ. With the demonstration that IL-4 was an essential cofactor for IgE synthesis (which is inhibited by IFN-γ), and that IL-5 is a specific eosinophil-acting cytokine, the potential relevance of this dichotomy to allergic asthma, which IgE and eosinophil mechanisms predominate, was clear. Further work established that Th1 and Th2-like CD4 T cells can be identified in humans (12,13), and has extended the concept of a "type 1" and type 2" cytokine profile to CD8 T cells (also called T-cytotoxic [Tc] type 1 and type 2; 14). Thus, it seemed reasonable to speculate that eosinophil, mast cell (and basophil) growth, differentiation and activation, as well as IgE synthesis, all may be a consequence of T-cell activation.

II. T-Cell Activation in Asthma

The T-cell hypothesis of asthma, particularly chronic asthma, is based around the concept that the disease is "driven" and maintained by persistence of a specialized

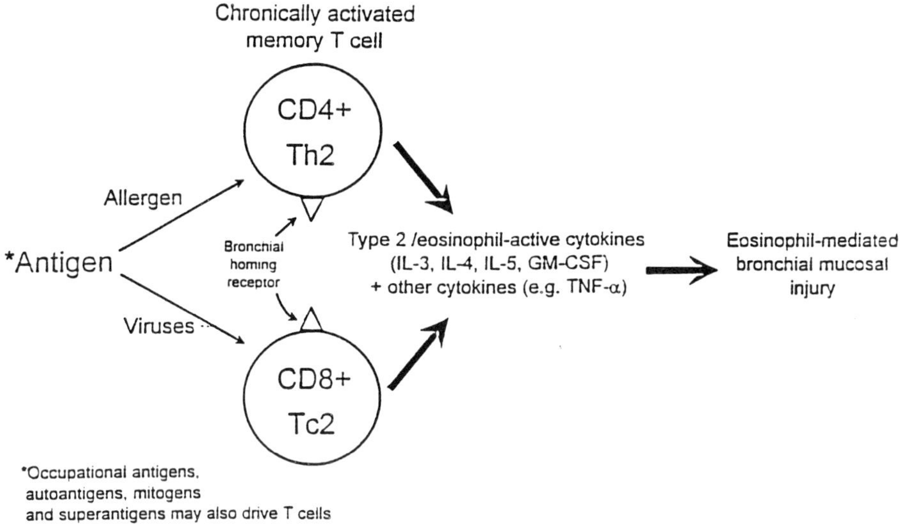

Figure 1 The T-cell hypothesis of chronic asthma.

number of chronically activated T memory cells, sensitized against an array of allergenic, occupational, and viral antigens that "home" to the lung after appropriate antigen exposure or viral infection (Fig. 1). Allergens induce a $CD4^+$ T helper (Th) cell response, whereas $CD8^+$ cytotoxic cells recognize virally infected cells. Superantigens and mitogens may also be involved. In the asthmatic airways, $CD4^+$ and $CD8^+$ cells have a Th2-type cytokine profile producing IL-5, IL-3, and granulocyte–macrophage colony-stimulating factor (GM-CSF) that mobilize and activate eosinophils for subsequent mucosal tissue injury, as well as IL-4 that is an essential cofactor for local or general IgE production. These events lead to eosinophilic desquamative bronchitis, with epithelial shedding, mucous hypersecretion, and bronchial smooth muscle contraction. Thus, although the eosinophil is largely responsible for asthma symptoms, its formation, function, and fate appear to be largely under T-cell control.

In support of the T-cell hypothesis, the numbers of activated T cells in peripheral blood were markedly elevated in patients admitted to hospital with acute severe asthma ("status asthmaticus") when compared with control subjects (15). Cells expressing CD25 (the IL-2 receptor (R) α chain), HLA-DR, and very late antigen-1 (VLA1) were confined almost exclusively to the $CD4^+$ population of cells, and the numbers of $CD4–CD25^+$ cells decreased after successful treatment with corticosteroids. Furthermore, there was a direct correlation between the numbers of activated peripheral blood T cells and airway narrowing, as measured by the peak expiratory flow rate (PEFR). Serum concentrations of the soluble IL-2R were also elevated in patients with acute severe asthma, compared with controls, and the values decreased after clinical improvement with corticosteroid therapy.

Bronchoscopy of asthmatic subjects demonstrated marked epithelial fragility even in mild asthmatics (16). This was confirmed by Jeffery et al. (17), who also observed that epithelial fragility was closely liked to airway hyperreactivity. In the same study (in which cell counts were performed on transmission electron microscopy sections), a striking increase in the number of "irregularly shaped" lymphocytes in the lamina propria and submucosa of symptomatic asthmatics was observed. Immunohistochemical studies demonstrated a significant increase in the numbers of CD25$^+$ cells in bronchial biopsies from asthmatics, compared with nonasthmatic atopic and normal control subjects (18). At the same time an increase in the numbers of eosinophils in asthma compared with controls was confirmed. Bradley et al. (19) extended these observations by demonstrating positive correlations between the total numbers of T cells (CD3$^+$) and activated EG2$^+$ eosinophils, between CD3$^+$ and CD25$^+$ cells, and between CD25$^+$ and EG2$^+$ cells. Furthermore, the ratio of EG2$^+$ to CD45$^+$ cells (total leukocytes) cells correlated with the methacholine PC_{20}. Therefore, this study supported the hypothesis that activated (CD25) T cells released products that regulated recruitment of eosinophils into the airway wall, and thereby disease severity. By double immunofluorescence it was possible to establish that most (>85%) CD25$^+$ cells were indeed CD3$^+$ T cells (20).

The increase in activated airway T cells in atopic asthma, as compared with normal controls, was also confirmed by flow cytometric analysis of bronchoalvelolar lavage (BAL) cells, and a correlation was shown between CD4$^+$–CD25$^+$ lymphocytes and eosinophils in BAL fluid (21).

These studies, in relatively mild asthmatics, had failed to reveal increases in the local numbers of *total* (CD3$^+$) T cells or either CD4$^+$ or CD8$^+$ subsets. Evidence for an overall increase in bronchial mucosal T-cell numbers in severe disease was obtained from the study of Azzawi et al. (22), who measured T and B cells in postmortem cases of fatal asthma and compared their findings with cystic fibrosis (CF) and nonasthmatic cases of sudden death matched for age and sex. Tissue eosinophilia was significantly greater in asthma when compared with CF or with the nonasthmatic controls. The mean numbers of T cells (MT-1$^+$) in the asthma and CF groups were approximately twice those of the controls. B-cell (MB2$^+$) numbers were similar in the asthma and sudden death groups, but were increased in CF. Thus, the immunopathology of death from asthma was characterized by a high T/B-cell ratio and the presence of relatively large numbers of activated (EG2$^+$) eosinophils. This suggested that increases in the total numbers of CD3$^+$ cells, as opposed to activated T lymphocytes, may become apparent only in severe disease.

Several studies have shown that successful treatment of asthma by inhaled corticosteroids or allergen avoidance was associated with decreased expression of bronchial mucosal T cells. In an open study Djukanovic et al. (23) demonstrated a significant decrease in mucosal T-cell, eosinophil, and mast cell numbers after 6 weeks of therapy with inhaled beclomethasone dipropionate (BDP). This was accompanied by clinical improvement. When using a similar experimental design, Wilson et al. (24) demonstrated decreases in CD25$^+$ and HLA-DR$^+$ cells, but not in the total numbers of $CD3^+$, $CD4^+$, or $CD8^+$ cells after treatment with BDP. Similarly, high-altitude climate therapy reduced both the numbers of activated T cells in peripheral blood as well as the degree of airway obstruction in children with house dust mite allergic asthma (25).

III. Immunoglobulin E Regulation

Over the last few years, evidence has accumulated that both IgE synthesis and eosinophil accumulation and activation at sites of allergic inflammation are dependent on activation of Th2 and Tc2-type cells that produce IL-4 and IL-5, but not IL-2 or IFN-γ (26,27). B-cell switching to IgE synthesis is dependent on IL-4 (or IL-13; discussed later), and T-cell help is enhanced by IL-5 and IL-6 and is inhibited by IFN-γ (28–30), whereas IL-5 acts specifically in eosinophil maturation, adhesion, tissue survival, and activation (31–34).

Interleukin-4 is an essential factor in IgE synthesis, switching B-cell immunoglobulin genes to a sterile immature ε-germline mRNA transcript (27,35). A second signal is required for this step to proceed to productive mature IgE mRNA synthesis, and this may be provided by ligation of CD40 on the B-cell surface by CD40 ligand on T lymphocytes (30). In 1993, the human cytokine IL-13 was cloned and was shown to share many of the actions of IL-4, except for those on T cells (36,37). IL-13 is produced by both CD4 and CD8 cells, and by Th0, Th1, and Th2 CD4 T-cell clones (38). The time course of IL-13 production differs from IL-4, in that IL-13 production is sustained after T-cell activation for up to 72 hr, whereas IL-4 mRNA is short-lived and undetectable after 24 hr (39). Similar to IL-4, IL-13 switches human B cells toward production of both IgE and IgG4. IL-13 also induces upregulation of CD23 and MHC class II molecules on the surface of B cells and has effects similar to IL-4 on macrophages. However, although the two cytokines share a receptor chain, IL-13 does not affect T cells and, thus, unlike IL-4, will not favor expansion of a Th2 phenotype (38). IL-13 mRNA has recently been demonstrated in nasal biopsies from patients with perennial allergic rhinitis (40) and in BAL fluid 24 hr after allergen challenge (41), raising the possibility that IL-13 might contribute to IgE synthesis in human allergic disease. Whether IL-13 regulation differs from that of IL-4, and what the relative importance of these two cytokines is in vivo remains to be defined. However, of relevance and importance, are the findings of Ying et al. (42) in which IL-13, but not IL-4, mRNA and protein products correlated with vascular cell adhesion molecule (VCAM)-1 upregulation in eosinophil infiltration in allergen-induced late-phase reaction in the skin of atopic individuals.

The production of IL-4 by non-T cells, particularly basophils, mast cells, and eosinophils, raised the possibility that these cells might interact with B cells to favor IgE synthesis. IL-4 alone is unable to cause IgE production by B cells, and a second signal is required. More recently, Gauchat et al. showed that isolated human lung mast cells and peripheral blood basophils express CD40L and have the capacity for IgE induction from B cells in vitro (43). Basophils stimulated with ionophore and phorbol myristate acetate (PMA) could induce IgE synthesis in this system without exogenous IL-4, presumably through release or synthesis of IL-4 from the basophil, whereas exogenous IL-4 was required to induce IgE switching by mast cell CD40L. The same group showed that eosinophil cell lines and peripheral blood eosinophils also express CD40L and, in the presence of IL-4, were able to support B-cell proliferation, although not IgE synthesis (44). More recently, eosinophils were also shown to express CD40 (45), and because these cells are capable of antigen presentation by MHC class II in vitro (46), it is possible that CD40–CD40L pathway might have a role in T-cell costimulation by eosinophils.

IV. T-Cell Cytokine Production in Asthma

Interleukin-5, of which the T cell is an important source, promotes terminal differentiation of the committed eosinophil precursors and enhances the effector capacity of the mature eosinophil (reviewed in Ref. 47). IL-5 also prolongs the survival of eosinophils in vitro and anti-IL-5 inhibits allergen-induced bronchial hyperresponsiveness and eosinophilia in a primate model of asthma (48). If T cells are activated in the airway mucosa in asthmatics, is there evidence that these cells are producing IL-4 and IL-5? Higher numbers of IL-5 mRNA$^+$ cells were found in endobronchial mucosal biopsies from asthmatics than in controls (49). Within the subjects who demonstrated detectable IL-5 mRNA, there was a correlation between IL-5 mRNA expression and the number of CD25$^+$ and EG2$^+$ cells and total eosinophil counts. When the wider cytokine profile in atopic asthma was studied, Robinson et al. (13) showed that, compared with cells from nonatopic control subjects, there were increased numbers of BAL cells encoding mRNA$^+$ for IL-3, IL-4, IL-5, and GM-CSF, a pattern compatible with predominant activation of the Th2-type T-cell population. Messenger RNA for IL-4 and IL-5 was localized to T cells within the BAL cell population. These findings were confirmed using CD4$^+$- and CD8$^+$-enriched peripheral blood T cells isolated from patients with severe asthma (50). These patients, but not controls, showed spontaneous expression of mRNA for Th2-type cytokines localized to CD4, but not CD8$^+$ cells. This was accompanied by spontaneous elaboration of the eosinophil-active cytokines, IL-3, IL-5, and GM-CSF. These results were also confirmed in part by Kamei et al. (51), who observed allergen-induced release of IL-5 and GM-CSF protein from blood T cells of asthmatics. Similarly, del Prete et al. (52) found that T-cell clones raised in vitro from bronchial mucosal biopsies of asthmatics had predominantly the type 2 T-helper cell cytokine profile.

Further studies showed that atopic asthma, provoked by allergen inhalation, was associated with local increases in activated T cells, eosinophils, and cells expressing mRNA for IL-4, IL-5, and GM-CSF (53,54). Again, these data supported the hypothesis that allergen-induced late asthmatic reactions are accompanied by

T-cell activation and increased expression of cytokines, such as IL-5 and GM-CSF, and local recruitment and activation of eosinophils in the bronchial mucosa.

Conversely, prednisolone treatment in asthmatics was associated with reduction in BAL cells expressing mRNA for IL-4 and IL-5 (55,56). This was accompanied by decrease in BAL eosinophils and clinical improvement, as shown by an increase in the methacholine PC_{20}. Interestingly, there was an increase in the number of cells expressing mRNA for IFN-γ, indicating that prednisolone treatment favors enhancement of a cytokine that downregulates IgE production.

By using the technique of in situ hybridization, it was shown, in a group of atopic asthmatics with a range of disease severity, that there were significant associations between the numbers of cells expressing mRNA for IL-4, IL-5, and GM-CSF and airflow restrictions, bronchial hyperresponsiveness, and an asthma symptom score (57). These results have recently been confirmed (for IL-5) using a more precise semiquantitative reverse transcriptase–polymerase chain reaction (RT–PCR) technique (58). Furthermore, Virchow et al. (59), who used a segmental allergen challenge, found a correlation between IL-5 concentrations, eosinophil numbers, and activated T cells.

V. Non–T-Cell Cytokines in Asthma

Production of IL-3, IL-5, GM-CSF, and tumor necrosis factor-alpha (TNF-α) from mast cells was described in 1989 (60,61), and basophils were a potent source of IL-4 (62), whereas eosinophils can be induced to produce IL-3 and GM-CSF (63,64). A wide variety of cell types have now been shown to be capable of producing a vast array of cytokines following in vitro stimulation. In particular, production of TNF-α, IL-1, and IL-4 by mast cells (65), basophils, and eosinophils (66,67) may be relevant to the upregulation of endothelial adhesion molecules, whereas IL-3, IL-5, and GM-CSF may promote basophil and eosinophil recruitment and activation in a positive-feedback manner. Production of IL-4 from these cells may be particularly relevant both in IgE synthesis and because IL-4 favors development of stimulated primary T cells, toward a Th2 phenotype (68). Thus IL-4 from non–T-cell sources may be relevant to the maintenance, although probably not initiation, of the Th2-type T-cell response to allergens. These in vitro observations probably are of relevance in vivo, because eosinophil and mast cell IL-3, IL-4, IL-5, and GM-CSF have been demonstrated in BAL fluid cells after local allergen challenge and in nasal tissue 24 hr after allergen challenge (69,70).

By double in situ hybridization–immunohistochemistry, Sun Ying et al. showed that T cells are the major source of mRNA encoding IL-4 and IL-5 in asthmatics, compared with controls (71). Eosinophils and mast cells also contribute to the overall cytokine profile, although the numbers of $mRNA^+$ cells were about one-fifth those of the $CD4^+$ T cells. In contrast with mRNA, the expression of the IL-4 and IL-5 protein product in bronchial biopsies from atopic and nonatopic asthmatics appeared to be associated more with eosinophils and mast cells, rather than T cells (72). There are difficulties in demonstrating intracytoplasmic staining of cytokines in nongranular cells, such as T cells, presumably because of the limitations of sensitivity of current immunostaining methods. On the other hand, the eosinophil appears to concentrate several cytokines in its cell granule, with granule-associated cytokines being readily detectable by immunocytochemistry (73,74). Despite these limitations of immunocytochemical detection of cytokines, it seems likely that T cells are an important source of IL-4 and IL-5 in asthma, although the relative contribution of the different cell types to the overall cytokine profile remains uncertain.

VI. Nonatopic ("Intrinsic") Asthma

Several studies have confirmed that other "variants" of the disease, such as occupational asthma and intrinsic asthma, were also associated with elevated numbers of activated T cells in BAL and bronchial biopsies. Bentley et al. (75) were able to establish that activated T cells and eosinophils were features of both nonatopic intrinsic asthma as well as occupational (isocyanate-induced) asthma (76). By flow cytometry, Walker et al. (77) demonstrated activation of both CD4 and CD8 subsets in BAL from subjects with intrinsic asthma, whereas only CD4 T-cell activation was seen in atopic asthma. These observations are compatible with the hypothesis that unidentified antigens, possibly viral in origin, as well as allergens, may be operative in this so-called intrinsic form of the disease. Furthermore, we have been able to establish, using a combination of semiquantitative PCR, in situ hybridization, and immunohistochemistry, that the amount and cellular origin of IL-4 and IL-5 expression was similar in bronchial biopsies taken from atopic and nonatopic asthmatics with, in general, IL-5 being significantly higher in asthmatics than in atopic, nonasthmatic, normal controls, whereas IL-4 was elevated in asthma and atopic nonasthmatics compared with normal nonatopic controls (58). The detection of elevated IL-4 mRNA-bearing cells in atopic nonasthmatic bronchial mucosal biopsies by the sensitive technique of RT-PCR raises the possibility that, in general, IL-5 is related more closely to clinical expression of asthma, whereas IL-4 is related to overproduction of IgE. In both atopic and nonatopic asthmatics, mRNA for IL-4 and IL-5 colocalized, primarily to $CD4^+$, but also to $CD8^+$ T cells (72), findings in agreement with those of Till et al. (78), who found that $CD8^+$ as well as $CD4^+$ T-cell lines from BAL fluid from asthmatics elaborated the IL-5 protein. Our finding of elevated IL-4 expression at both the mRNA and protein levels in intrinsic asthma was in contrast with those of Walker et al. (79), who measured protein product in concentrated BAL fluid. These authors detected increased concentrations of IL-2 and IL-5 (but not IL-4) in BAL fluid from nonatopic asthmatics, compared with control subjects, whereas IL-4 and IL-5 were increased in atopic asthmatics. There still is no satisfactory explanation for these apparent discrepancies, except the possibility that IL-4 is stored, but not secreted, in cytokine-producing cells from nonatopic asthmatics, or that there is some abnormality in IL-4 receptor expression in the intrinsic form of the disease. The role of Th2-type cells in intrinsic asthma, as well as that of local IgE-dependent mechanisms, as suggested by Humbert et al. (79), is unlikely to be resolved until the putative antigen(s) have been identified.

Maestrelli et al. (81) cloned T cells from cells isolated from bronchial biopsy fragments from patients with asthma induced by toluene diisocyanate. They found that most clones were IL-5 and IFN-γ–producing $CD8^+$ cells. Whether these findings are related specifically to this form of occupational asthma, or to the method of cloning, is unclear. Thus, the relative contributions of CD4 and CD8 T cells and the precise cytokine profile of different forms of asthma still remain to be firmly established.

VII. Glucocorticoid Resistance in Asthma

Glucocorticosteroids are remarkably effective in most asthmatics, in controlling symptoms. In vitro, very low doses inhibit T-cell–proliferative responses to mitogens; concentrations of methylprednisolone as low as 10^{-10}M being effective in inhibiting human T-cell expansion (82). A small proportion of asthmatic subjects do not show clinical improvement with glucocorticoid treatment (83). Formal definitions vary, but most would encompass failure to show a 10% or more increase in forced expiratory volume in 1 sec (FEV_1) after 2 weeks of treatment with 40 mg/day of prednisolone or equivalent in subjects with asthma symptoms and demonstrated reversibility of airflow obstruction of at least 15% to inhaled β-agonists. It is unclear whether this is a distinct group or a continuum of clinical responsiveness, but glucocorticoid resistance is also seen in other inflammatory diseases. Peripheral blood mononuclear cells from patients with corticosteroid-resistant asthma proliferated to phytohemagglutinin in the presence of relatively high doses of methylprednisolone (84,85), and a clear relationship was shown between clinical responsiveness to steroids and the in vitro effect of steroids on mitogen-driven colony counts. This adds support to the T-cell hypothesis of asthma, because both T-cell proliferation and cytokine production are exquisitely sensitive to steroid inhibition, and the in vitro responsiveness of T-lymphocyte proliferation and cytokine production was closely correlated with clinical response to glucocorticoids.

The mechanisms of steroid resistance are unclear. Sher et al. (86) found that most patients with steroid-resistant (SR) asthma had a reversible defect in glucocorticoid receptor (GR)-binding affinity that could be sustained in vitro by the addition of the combination of IL-2 and IL-4, but not the individual cytokines. Furthermore, in vitro incubation of normal T cells with the combination of IL-2 and IL-4, in the absence of IFN-γ, reduced their GR-binding affinity to the levels seen in SR asthma (87). On this basis they suggested two types of glucocorticosteroid resistance: a reduced affinity of GR binding confined to T lymphocytes that reverted to normal after 48 hr in culture, and a much less common reduction in GR density (in only 2 of the 17 SR patients) that did not normalize with prolonged incubation

(86). This supports the concept that there may be different types of steroid resistance in asthma. These in vitro data suggested that the pattern of cytokine gene expression may play a role in determining steroid resistance. For this reason, Leung et al. (88) used the technique of in situ hybridization to examine whether airway cells from SR asthmatics versus steroid-sensitive (SS) asthmatics expressed different patterns of mRNA for cytokines, particularly after treatment with oral steroids. They confirmed the findings of Robinson et al. (55) in that SS asthmatics responded well to glucocorticoids, and this response was accompanied by decrease in the numbers of cells expressing mRNA for IL-4 and Il-5 and an increase in IFN-γ transcripts. In contrast, after prednisolone therapy, SR asthmatics had no significant changes in the number of BAL cells expressing mRNA for either IL-4 or IL-5. Furthermore, instead of a decrease, there was an increase in the numbers of IFN-γ mRNA$^+$ cells. These findings suggested that SR asthma is associated with dysregulation of expression of the genes encoding Th2 and Th1 cytokines in airway cells and is compatible with the concept that a combination of IL-2 and IL-4 induced GR-binding affinity and T-cell responsiveness to glucocorticoids.

Studies by Adcock et al. (89) have suggested dysregulation of transcription factors in glucocorticoid-resistant asthma, with increase expression of the proinflammatory AP-1 interfering with steroid actions by cytoplasmic binding to the glucocorticoid receptor. Small alterations in glucocorticoid pharmacokinetics and ligand-binding affinity are also seen in these subjects, but are probably insufficient to account for the clinical features.

VIII. Cyclosporine

It is generally accepted that the primary mode of action of cyclosporine is through inhibition of T-cell activation secondary to blocking early calcium-dependent transcription of a mRNA encoding several cytokines (90). Experience with the use of cyclosporine in chronic steroid-dependent asthma supports the T-cell hypothesis, although it is accepted that this agent also has effects on cytokine synthesis and release from granulocytes, including basophils, mast cells, and eosinophils.

In a group of severe steroid-dependent asthmatics, treatment over a 12-week period with cyclosporine at low dosage (5 mg/kg per day) was associated with improvement in lung function and a reduction in the numbers of disease exacerbations requiring an increase in corticosteroid dosage (91). Cyclosporine also has a corticosteroid-sparing effect in steroid-dependent asthmatics (92). In both studies lung function concurrently improved, despite the reduction in corticosteroid dose, although in one study this improvement was small.

The late-phase asthmatic reaction (LAR), provoked by inhaled allergen, represents a model of asthmatic airway inflammation, because the pathogenesis of the disease is, at least partly, believed to involve the mobilization and local influx of eosinophils subsequent to the release of IL-5, IL-3, and GM-CSF from activated T cells. In contrast, mediators released from IgE-sensitized mast cells have been implicated in the pathogenesis of the allergen-induced early-phase asthmatic response (EAR). Because cyclosporine inhibits both cytokine mRNA transcription by T cells and mast cell degranulation in vitro, it might be expected to inhibit both the EAR and LAR as well as the associated elevation in blood eosinophils. Sihra et al. (93) have recently demonstrated in a double-blind, placebo-controlled, randomized crossover trial that, compared with placebo treatment, cyclosporine reduced the magnitude of the LAR, but not that of the EAR, after allergen challenge. This provides strong indirect evidence that cyclosporine is effective in this model of asthmatic allergen inflammation through its effects on the T cell as opposed to mast cells and basophils.

IX. Animal Models

Although there is controversy over the clinical relevance of animal models of asthma, it is of interest that several groups have established that airway hyperresponsiveness in sensitized animals is dependent on T cells and cytokines. Enander and colleagues (94–96) developed a model of delayed-type hypersensitivity, in the lungs of mice that had been immunized with picryl chloride (PC), characterized by a peribronchial and perivascular mononuclear cell infiltrate and an increase in mucus-producing cells. Garssen and coworkers (97) established that mice with PC-induced pulmonary DTH developed T-cell–dependent, antigen-specific airway hyperreactivity, as determined by measurements of pulmonary resistance in vitro and tracheal reactivity to carbachol in vitro. However, doubts have been cast on the relevance of a DTH-like model that is centered on Th1-type cytokines and events involving predominantly macrophage activation. Clearly, animal models involving IL-4 and IL-5 together with eosinophils, mast cells, and IgE production would have more relevance to the human situation. In a guinea pig model of airway inflammation, Frew et al. (98) established that the allergen-induced late-phase asthmatic reaction was associated with increases in mucosal T cells and eosinophils. More appropriate models may be those of protein sensitization in mice or guinea pigs, using agents such as ovalbumin, and some studies have used allergens such as house dust mite extract to sensitize mice (99,100). Depletion of $CD4^+$ T cells before airway challenge of ovalbumin-sensitized mice prevented antigen-induced airway hyperresponsiveness and pulmonary eosinophilia (101). In this model, and in guinea pigs sensitized to ovalbumin, blocking antibodies to IL-5 also abrogated hyperresponsiveness and eosinophilia to airway challenge (102,103).

The groups of Martin and of Haczku developed models in Brown Norway rats of airway hyperresponsiveness that was associated with elevations of serum-specific IgE and activation of T cells following allergen exposure (104–106). This was associated with activated T cells having a Th2-type cytokine profile. Watanabe et al. (107) and Haczku et al. (108) were successfully able to transfer antigen-induced airway bronchoconstriction and eosinophilia in Brown Norway rats by adoptive transfer of antigen-primed CD4, but not CD8 T cells. Although the degree of airway hyperresponsiveness that can be induced experimentally in rodent models is relatively small, these studies are clearly of interest and are in the mainstream of the T-cell hypothesis of asthma.

More recent experiments on the role of IL-4 and use of IL-5 knockout mice in studies of ovalbumin-induced airway hyperresponsiveness have been conflicting. Foster and colleagues (102) showed that IL-5 knockout mice failed to develop the airway hyperresponsiveness seen in wild-type mice of the same strain after airway challenge, suggesting that this cytokine and eosinophils were central mediators in the pathogenesis of allergic disease. On the other hand, Corry and co-workers (109), using blocking antibodies, found that IL-4, but not IL-5 or eosinophils, was required in a murine model of acute airway hyperreactivity using the Balb/c mouse strain. Differences in the various strains of mice used in these experiments have been used to explain these discrepancies (110).

To delineate further the critical role of T cells on asthma, Kaminuma et al. (111) tested the possibility whether eosinophilic inflammation of the bronchial mucosa is induced by transferred T-cell clones, in the absence of antigen-specific immunoglobulins (IgE, IgA, and IgG). Ovalbumin-specific Th2 clones were established, and cytokine profiles were determined. Eosinophilic inflammation accompanied with airway hyperresponsiveness occurred only when unprimed mice were transferred with IL-5–producing Th2 clones and challenged by the inhalation of relevant antigen. Increase of IL-5 concentration in BAL fluid was detected after the challenge, indicating the local production of cytokines by the transferred T cells, and preceded the appearance of the airway eosinophilia. Eosinophil infiltration was completely suppressed by the administration of anti-IL-5–neutralizing antibody, indicating the essential role of IL-5 in this model. The intensity of the eosinophilic accumulation in vivo correlated well with the capacity of the T-cell clones to produce IL-5 in vitro. Kaminuma and colleagues concluded that the existence of IL-5–producing helper T cells is sufficient for the development of the eosinophilic inflammation as the bronchial mucosa after inhalation challenge of the relevant antigen.

Evidence to support the role of $CD8^+$ T cells in the production of airway eosinophilia comes from the work of Coyle et al. (112), who demonstrated that IL-4 could switch virus-specific $CD8^+$ cells to IL-5 production. The role of IL-5 in asthma was further supported by blocking antigen-induced bronchial hyperreactivity and eosinophilia in monkey treated with humanized antibodies to IL-5. Furthermore, the effect of this treatment was sustained for up to 3 months (48).

X. Determinants of the Th2 Response in Asthma

The factors leading up to a Th2 pattern of T-cell cytokine response in asthma are uncertain. A substantial body of work on human and murine T-cell clones has shown that the cytokine environment during primary expansion, antigen dose, antigen-presenting cell, costimulatory signal, and hormonal environment, all might play a role during the initial activation of a T-cell response (113). The current basic premise is that IL-4 favors expansion of a Th2 phenotype (114), whereas IL-12 expands a Th1 effector population (115). Mast cells, basophils, and eosinophils are potential sources of IL-4 in amplification of allergic responses, but it is difficult to see how these cells would become primed without an initial Th2 T-cell response. Perhaps a better candidate for an initiating cell is the CD4 NK 1.1 cell in the mouse (116), or a small subset of native T cells that seem to produce IL-4 on stimulation (117). Whether a human equivalent of NK 1.1 cells exists is uncertain, and there is no information on how these might be activated by allergen (118).

Recent examination of IL-12 mRNA expression in bronchial biopsies from asthmatic subjects and controls suggests that there may be defective IL-12 response in asthma; this might also favor a Th2 environment (119). This would be in keeping with the observation of increase IL-2 mRNA-encoding cells in cutaneous late responses after immunotherapy, for which it was suggested that induction of an IL-12 response might be protective (120).

In addition to activation by the T-cell receptor, productive T-cell activation requires a second signal. The best-characterized costimulatory pathway is by CD28 on the T-cell surface and the B7 counterreceptors B7-1 (CD80) and B7-2 (CD86) on the surface of antigen-presenting cells (121). Recent evidence suggests that it is possible that selective use of the B7-2 costimulation pathway favors expansion of IL-4 producing T lymphocytes (122). The B7 receptors also interact with a T-cell molecule related to CD28, termed CTLA4. This interaction is of higher affinity than that with CD28 and appears to give a negative signal, inhibiting T-cell proliferation (123). A solubilized form of CTLA4 (CTLA4Ig) was produced by fusion with immunoglobulin. CTLA4Ig has profound immunosuppressive properties in animals, presumably by blocking CD28 activation (124).

The postreceptor-signaling cascade in T-cell signaling that leads to either Th1 or Th2 expansion is not yet fully elucidated, although it is possible that differences in use of IFN-γR may have a role (125). Similarly, differences in IL-12 responsiveness seem to occur in T cells expanded from mouse strains that tend to mount either Th1 (B10.D2) or Th2 (Balb/c) responses to *Leishmania* infection, with an early loss of IL-12 responsiveness in Balb/c cells. This may relate to differences in chromosome 11 (syntenic with human chromosome 5), in the region of the IFN-γ response element IRF 1 (126).

Different parts of the TCR may transduce different signals, as shown by the elegant work of Evavold et al. (127), who showed that amino acid substitution in T-cell–activating peptides could differentially affect proliferation or IL4 production by T-cell clones in vitro. More recent data from work in experimental allergic encephalopathy suggests that such altered peptide ligands may have application in vivo (128).

XI. Chemokines in Asthma

Accumulation of inflammation cells at sites of injury or antigen stimulation presents the integration of various events, including differentiation and release from bone marrow, adhesion and transmigration of vascular endothelium, interaction with extracellular matrix, and survival within the tissue environment. Cells may migrate along a chemoattractant gradient whereby substances released from the inflamed site initiate directed polarization and mobility of the cell toward the initiating stimulus (129). The first chemoattractant agents described were complement fragments, such as C5a; lipid mediators, such as PAF; and nonphysiological peptides, such as fMLP. However, more recently, attention has focused an an ever-increasing family of peptide chemoattractants termed chemokines (129). These 84- to 14-kDa peptides have been divided into two subfamilies, with a structural motif involving two adjacent cysteine residues (C–C), or separated cysteines (C–X–C). Chemokines are of interest because of their selectivity in chemoattractant properties for certain cell types, or groups of cell types. For example, IL-8 is a potent neutrophil chemoattractant. A variety of C–C chemokines have potent chemoattractant activity for eosinophils, basophils, and T cells, including RANTES and methyl-accepting chemotaxis protein (MCP)-3 (130,131). In addition, RANTES, MCP-3, MCP-1, and MIP-1α stimulate leukotrien C_4, (LTC_4) synthesis and histamine release from basophils and stimulate eosinophilic-degranulation (129).

RANTES and MCP mRNA were detected in allergen-induced late cutaneous responses, and subsequently, this was localized to eosinophils within the reaction (132,133). IL-8, MIP-1α, and RANTES were detected in nasal lavage fluid following allergen challenge (134), and MIP-1α and IL-16 (an eosinophil and CD4 T-cell chemoattractant of a novel C chemokine family), but not RANTES, were detected in BAL fluid 6 hr after local allergen challenge of sensitized asthmatic subjects (135). Increased levels of MCP-1, RANTES, and MIP-1α mRNA were detected in BAL cells from atopic asthmatic subjects at baseline when compared with nonasthmatic control subjects, and BAL fluid showed eosinophil chemoattractant activity that was blocked by antibodies to RANTES and MCP-3 (136).

Recently, a novel eosinophil-selective chemokine, termed eotaxin, has been cloned, initially from antigen-challenged lungs of guinea pigs, but more recently in humans (137). Eotaxin mRNA was demonstrated in human nasal polyp tissue, and binding studies suggest that it binds to a novel CCR-3 receptor shared with RANTES and MCP-3 on eosinophils (137). Interestingly, recent animal experiments suggest that eotaxin acts in a cooperative manner with IL-5 in eosinophil accumulation in the skin in guinea pigs: IL-5 acted to release a bone marrow pool of cells that were then attracted to the site of intradermal eotaxin injection (138).

Chemokine production has been described from a wide variety of cell types, and the stimulus to chemokine production in human allergic disease is unclear. However, the profile of chemokines produced may integrate with the Th2 pattern

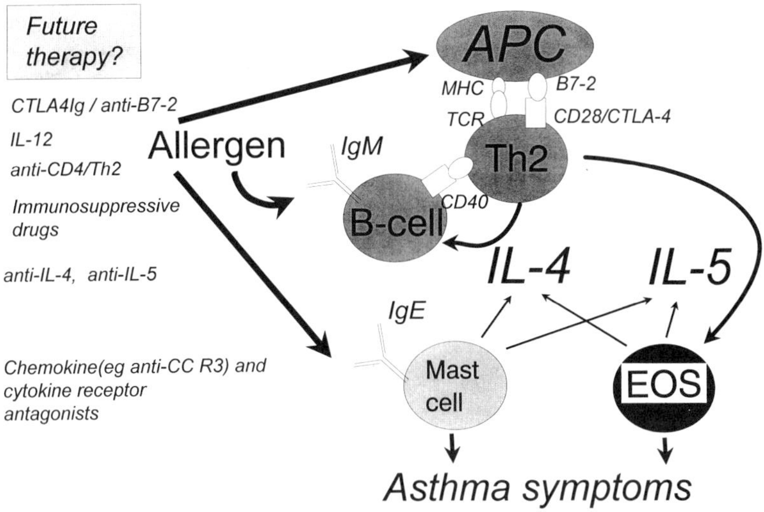

Figure 2 Possible future therapeutic strategies in asthma based on the T-cell hypothesis: Approaches include blocking of costimulation with agents such as CTLA-4 Ig, which may inhibit T-cell activation; or coadministration of IL-12 (possibly together with allergen in immunotherapy), which may enhance switching from a Th2- to a Th1- predominant T-cell response. Direct blocking antibodies to IL-4 and IL-5 may have therapeutic efficacy. Other possible strategies include T-cell–directed antibody therapy with monoclonal antibodies directed against CD4, or immunosuppressants such as tacrolinus (FK506), rapamycin, and mycophenalate mofetil.

of cytokines to result in the characteristic pattern of cellular infiltration and activation seen in allergic disease.

XII. Conclusions

There is now persuasive evidence to support the hypothesis that activation of Th2 cells or Tc2 cells is pivotal to the asthma process. The hypothesis is supported by numerous lines of evidence, particularly studies of bronchoalveolar lavage and bronchial biopsies from asthmatic subjects, in treatment studies and in experimental animal models.

The T-cell hypothesis of chronic asthma has lead to the possibility of a number of novel therapeutic approaches (Fig. 2). These include (1) a range of immunosuppressive drugs that are active in inhibiting mitogen-driven T cells from corticosteroid-resistant asthmatics, in vitro; (2) humanized antibodies against CD4; (3) anticytokine antibodies, particularly against IL-4 and IL-5; (4) cytokine receptor antagonists; (5) agents that modulate the Th2 response (e.g., IL-12); and (6) strategies to inhibit costimulatory pathways (e.g., CTLA4 Ig and anti-B7-2).

References

1. Austen KF. The mast cell. In: Kay AB, Austen KF, Lichtenstein LM, eds. Asthma. Physiology, Immunopharmacology and Treatment. London: Academic Press, 1984:425–445.
2. Schleimer RP, Schulman ES, MacGlashan DR Jr, Peters SP, Adams GK III, Lichtenstein LM, Adkinson NJ Jr. Effects of dexamethasone on mediator release from human lung fragments, and purified human lung mast cells. J Clin Invest 1983; 71:1830–1835.
3. Godard P, Chaintreuil J, Danon M, Coupe M, Flandre O, Crastes de Paulet A, Michel FB. Functional assessment of alveolar macrophages: comparison of cells from asthmatics and normal subjects. J Allerg Clin Immunol 1982; 70:88–93.
4. American Thoracic Society. Standards for the diagnosis and care of patients with chronic obstructive pulmonary disease (COPD) and asthma. Am Rev Respir Dis 1987; 136:225–244.
5. Bjorkmann PJ, Saper MA, Samraoui B, Bennet WS, Stromiger JL, Wiley DC. Structure of the human class I histocompatibility antigen HLA-A2. Nature 1987; 329:506–518.
6. Meuer SC, Hodgson JC, Hussey RC, Protensis JP, Schlossman SF, Reinherz EL. Antigen-like effects of monoclonal antibodies directed at receptors on human T cells. J Exp Med 1983; 158:988–993.
7. Ishizaka K, Isizaka T. Identification of γE-antibodies as a carrier of reaginic activity. J Immunol 1967; 99:1187–1198.
8. Basten A, Beeston PB. Mechanisms of eosinophilia. II. Role of the lymphocyte. J Exp Med 1970; 131:1288–1305
9. Tada T, Toshitada T, Okumura K, Nonaka M, Tokuhisa T. Two distinct types of helper T cells involved in the secondary antibody responser: independent and synergistic effects of Ia^- and Ia^+ helper T cells. J Exp Med 1978; 147:446–458.
10. Mosmann TR, Cherwinski H, Bond MW, Gieldin MA, Coffman RL. Two types of murine helper T cell clones. J Immunol 1986; 136:2348–2357.
11. Fong TAT, Mosmann TR. The role of IFNγ in delayed type hypersensitivity mediated by Th1 clones. J Immunol 1989; 143:2887–2893.
12. Romagnani S. Human Th1 and Th2: doubt no more. Immunol Today 1991; 12:256–257.
13. Robinson DS, Hamid Q, Sun Ying, Tsicopoulos A, Barkans J, Bentley AM, Corrigan CJ, Durham SR, Kay AB. Predominant Th2-like bronchoalveolar T-lymphocyte population in atopic asthma. N Engl J Med 1992; 326:298–304.
14. Mosmann TR, Sad S. The expanding universe of T-cell subsets: Th1, Th2 and more. Immunol Today 1996; 17:139–146.
15. Corrigan CJ, Hartnell A, Kay AB. T lymphocyte activation in acute severe asthma. Lancet 1988; 1:1129–1132.
16. Laitinen LA, Heino M, Laitinen A, Kava T, Haahtela T. Damage of the airway epithelium and bronchial reactivity in patients with asthma. Am Rev Respir Dis 1985; 131:599–606.
17. Jeffery PK, Wardlaw AJ, Nelson FC, Collins JV, Kay AB. Bronchial biopsies in asthma: an ultrastructural, quantitative study and correlation with hyperreactivity. Am Rev Respir Dis 1989; 140:1745–1753.
18. Azzawi M, Bradley B, Jeffery PK, Frew A, Wardlaw AJ, Knowles G, Assoufi B, Collins JV, Durham S, Kay AB. Identification of activated T lymphocytes and eosinophils in bronchial biopsies in stable atopic asthma. Am Rev Respir Dis 1990; 142:1407–1413.
19. Bradley BL, Azzawi M, Jacobson M, Assoufi B, Collins JV, Irani A-MA, Schwartz LB, Durham SR, Jeffery PK, Kay AB. Eosinophils, T-lymphocytes, mast cells, neutrophils and macrophages in bronchial biopsy specimens from atopic subjects with asthma: comparison with biopsy specimens from atopic subjects without asthma and normal control subjects and relationship to bronchial hyperresponsiveness. J Allergy Clin Immunol 1990; 88:661–674.
20. Hamid Q, Barkans J, Robinson DS, Durham SR, Kay A. Co-expression of CD25 and CD3 in atopic allergy and asthma. Immunology 1992; 75:659–663.

21. Robinson DS, Bentley AM, Hartnell A, Kay AB, Durham SR. Activated memory T helper cells in bronchoalveolar lavage from atopic asthmatics. Relationship to asthma symptoms, lung function and bronchial responsiveness. Thorax 1993; 48:26–32.
22. Azzawi M, Johnston PW, Majumdar S, Kay AB, Jeffery PK. T lymphocytes and activated eosinophils in airway mucosa in fetal asthma and cystic fibrosis. Am Rev Respir Dis 1992; 145;1477–1482.
23. Djukanovic R, Wilson JW, Britten KM, Wilson SJ, Walls AF, Roche WR, Howarth PH, Holgate ST. Effect of an inhaled corticosteroid on airway inflammation and symptoms in asthma. Am Rev Respir Dis 1992; 145:669–674.
24. Wilson JW, Djukanovic R, Howarth PH, Holgate ST. Inhaled beclomethasone dipropionate downregulates airway lymphocyte activation in atopic asthma. Am J Respir Crit Care Med 1994; 149:86–90.
25. Simon HU, Grotzer M, Nikolaizik WH, Blaser K, Schoni MH. High altitude climate therapy reduces peripheral blood T lymphocyte activation, eosinophilia, and bronchial obstruction in children with house-dust mite allergic asthma. Pediatr Pulmonol 1994; 17:304–311.
26. Wierenga EA, Snoek M, de Groot C, Chretien I, de Bos J, Jansen HM, Kapsenberg ML. Evidence compartmentalization of functional subsets of $CD4^+$ T lymphocytes in atopic patients. J Immunol 1990; 144:4651–4656.
27. Del Prete GF, Maggi E, Parronchi P, Chretien I, Tiri A, Macchia D, Ricci M, Banchereau J, de Vries J, Romagnani S. IL-4 is an essential factor for the IgE synthesis induced in vitro by human T cell clones and their supernatants. J Immunol 1988; 140:4193–4198.
28. Vercelli D, Jabara HH, Arai K, Yokota T, Geha RS. Endogenous IL-6 plays an obligatory role in IL-4-induced human IgE synthesis. Eur J Immunol 1989; 19:1419–1422.
29. Pene J, Rousset F, Briere F, Chretien I, Wideman J, Bonnefoy JY, de Vries JE. Interleukin 5 enhances interleukin 4-induced IgE production by normal human B cells. The role of soluble CD23 antigen. Eur J Immunol 1988; 18:929–935.
30. Geha RS. Regulation of IgE synthesis in humans. J Allergy Clin Immunol 1992; 90:143–150.
31. Clutterbuck EJ, Hirst EM, Sanderson CJ. Human interleukin 5 (IL-5) regulates the production of eosinophils in human bone marrow cultures: comparison and interaction with IL-1, IL-3, Il-6, and GM-CSF. Blood 1989; 73:1504–1512.
32. Lopez AF, Sanderson CJ, Gamble JR, Campbell HD, Young IG, Vadas MA. Recombinant human interleukin 5 is a selective activator of human eosinophil function. J Exp Med 1988; 167:219–224.
33. Sanderson CJ. Interleukin 5, eosinophils and disease. Blood 1992; 79:3101–3109.
34. Walsh GM, Hartnell A, Wardlaw AJ, Kurihara K, Sanderson CJ, Kay AB. IL-5 enhances the in vitro adhesion of human eosinophils, but not neutrophils, in a leucocyte integrin (CD11/CD18)-dependent manner. Immunology 1990; 71:258–265.
35. Gauchat J-F, Lebman DA, Coffman RL, Gascan H, de Vries JE. Structure and expression of germline ε transcripts in human B cells induced by interleukin 4 to switch to IgE production. J Exp Med 1990; 172:463–468.
36. Mckenzie ANJ, Culpepper JA, de Waal Malefyt R, Briere F, Punnonen J, Aversa G, Sato A, Dang W, Cocks BG, Menon S, de Vries JE, Banchereau J, Zurawski G. Interleukin 13, a T cell derived cytokine that regulates human monocyte and B-cell function. Proc Natl Acad Sci USA 1993; 90:3735–3739.
37. Zurawski G, de Vries JE. Interleukin 13, an interleukin 4-like cytokine that acts on monocytes and B cells but not on T cells. Immunol Today 1994; 15:19–26.
38. de Waal Malefyt R, Abrams JS, Zurawaski G, Lecron S, Mohan-Peterson S, Sanjanwala B, Bennet B, Silver J, de Vries JE, Yssel H. Differential regulation of IL-13 and IL-4 production by human $CD8^+$ and $CD4^+$ Th0, Th1 and Th2 cell clones and EBV transformed B cells. Int Immunol 1995; 7:1405–1416.

39. Jung T, Wijdenes J, Neumann C, de Vries JE, Yssel H. Interleukin 13 is produced by activated human CD45RA and CD45RO T cells: modulation by interleukin 4 and interleukin 12. Eur J Immunol 1996; 26:571–577.
40. Pawankar RU, Okuda M, Hasegawa S, Suzuki K, Yssel H, Okubo K, Okumura K, Ra C. Interleukin 13 expression in the nasal mucosa of perennial allergic rhinitics. Am J Respir Crit Care Med 1995; 152:2059–2067.
41. Huang SK, Xiao HQ, Kleine-Tebbe J, Paciotti G, Marsh DG, Lichtenstein LM, Liu MC. IL-13 expression at the sites of allergen challenge in patients with asthma. J Immunol 1995; 155:2688–2694.
42. Ying S, Meng Q, Barata LT, Robinson DS, Durham SR, Kay AB. IL-13, but not IL-4, correlates with upregulation of VCAM-1 and infiltration of eosinophils, macrophages and T cells in the allergen-induced late-phase cutaneous response in atopic subjects. J Immunol 1997; 158:5050–5057.
43. Gauchat J-F, Henchoz S, Mazzei G, Aubry J-P, Brunner T, Blasey H, Life P, Talabot D, Flores-Romo L, Thompson J, Kishi K, Butterfield J, Dahinden C, Bonnefoy J-Y. Induction of human IgE synthesis in B cells by mast cells and basophils. Nature 1993; 365:340–343.
44. Gauchat J-F, Henchoz S, Fattah D, Mazzei G, Aubry J-P, Jomotte T, Dash L, Page K, Solari R, Aldebert D, Capron M, Dahinden C, Bonnefoy J-Y. CD40 ligand is functionally expressed on human eosinophils. Eur J Immunol 1995; 25:863–865.
45. CD40 expression by human peripheral blood eosinophils. J Clin Invest 1996; 97:1761–1766.
46. Del Pozo V, De Andres B, Martin E, Cardaba B, Fernandez JC, Gallardo S, Tramon P, Leyva-Cobian F, Palomino P, Lahoz C. Eosinophil as antigen presenting cell: activation of T cell clones and T cell hybridoma by eosinophils after antigen processing. Eur J Immunol 1992; 22:1919–1925.
47. Wardlaw AJ, Moqbel R, Kay AB. Eosinophils: biology and role in disease. Adv Immunol 1996; 60:151–266.
48. Mauser PJ, Pitman AM, Fernandez X, et al. Effects of an antibody to interleukin-5 in a monkey model of asthma. Am J Respir Crit Care Med 1995; 152:467–472.
49. Hamid Q, Azzawi M, Sun Ying, Moqbel R, Wardlaw AJ, Corrigan CJ, Bradley B, Durham SR, Collins JV, Jeffery PK, Quint DJ, Kay AB. Expression of mRNA for interleukin-5 in mucosal bronchial biopsies from asthma. J Clin Invest 1991; 87:1541–1546.
50. Corrigan CJ, Hamid Q, North J, Barkans J, Moqbel R, Durham S, Kay AB. Peripheral blood CD4, but not CD8 T lymphocytes in patients with exacerbation of asthma transcribe and translate messenger RNA encoding cytokines which prolong eosinophil survival in the context of a Th2-type pattern: effect of glucocorticoid therapy. Am J Respir Cell Mol Biol 1995; 12:567–578.
51. Kamei T, Ozaki T, Kawaji K, Banno K, Sano T, Azuma M, Ogura T. Production of interleukin-5 and granulocyte/macrophage colony-stimulating factor by T cells of patients with bronchial asthma in response to *Dermatophagoides farinae* and its relation to eosinophil colony-stimulating factor. Am J Respir Cell Mol Biol 1993; 9:378–385.
52. Del Prete GF, De Carli M, D'Elios MM, Maestrelli P, Ricci M, Fabbri L, Romagnani S. Allergen exposure induces the activation of allergen-specific Th2 cells in the airway mucosa of patients with allergic respiratory disorders. Eur J Immunol 1993; 23:1445–1449.
53. Bentley AM, Qui Meng, Robinson DS, Hamid Q, Kay AB, Durham SR. Increases in activated T lymphocytes, eosinophils, and cytokine messenger RNA expression or IL-5 and GM-CSF in bronchial biopsies after allergen inhalation challenge in atopic asthmatics. Am J Respir Cell Mol Biol 1993; 8:35–42.
54. Robinson DS, Hamid Q, Bentley AM, Sun Ying, Kay AB, Durham SR. $CD4^+$ T cell activation, eosinophil recruitment and interleukin-4 (IL-4), IL-5 and GM-CSF in messenger RNA expression in bronchoalveolar lavage afer allergen inhalation challenge of atopic asthmatics. J Allergy Clin Immunol 1993; 92:313–324.
55. Bentley AM, Hamid Q, Robinson DS, Schotman E, Meng Q, Assoufi B, Kay ABA,

Durham SR. Prednisolone treatment in asthma. Reduction in the numbers of eosinophils, T cells, tryptase-only positive mast cells, and modulation of IL-4, IL-5, and interferon-gamma cytokine gene expression within the bronchial mucosa. Am J Respir Crit Care Med 1996; 153:551–556.

56. Robinson DS, Hamid Q, Sun Ying, Bentley AM, Assoufi B, North J, Qui Meng, Durham SR, Kay AB. Prednisolone treatment in asthma is associated with modulation of bronchoalveolar lavage cell interleukin-4, interleukin-5 and interferon-gamma cytokine gene expression. Am Rev Respir Dis 1993; 148:401–406.
57. Robinson DS, Sun Ying, Bentley AM, Qiu Meng, North J, Durham SR, Kay AB, Hamid Q. Relationships among numbers of broncholalveolar lavage cells expressing messenger ribonucleic acid for cytokines, asthma symptoms, and airway methacholine responsiveness in atopic asthma. J Allergy Clin Immunol 1993; 92:397–403.
58. Humbert M, Durham SR, Ying S, Kimmitt P, Barkans J, Assoufi B, Pfister R, Menz G, Robinson DS, Kay AB, Corrigan CJ. IL-4 and IL-5 mRNA and protein in bronchial biopsies from atopic and non-atopic asthmatics: evidence against "intrinsic" asthma being a distinct immunopathological entity. Am J Respir Crit Care Med 1996; 154:1497–1504.
59. Virchow JC Jr, Walker C, Hafner D, Kortsik C, Werner P, Matthys H, Kroegel C. T cells and cytokines in bronchoalveolar lavage fluid after segmental allergen provocation in atopic asthma. Am J Respir Crit Care Med 1995; 151:960–968.
60. Plaut M, Pierce JH, Watson CJ, Haney-Hyde J, Nordan RP, Paul WE. Mast cell lines produce lymphkines in response to cross-linkage of FceRI or calcium ionophore. Nature 1989; 329:64–67.
61. Wodnar-Filipowicz A, Heuser CH, Moroni C. Production of the haemopoeitic growth factors GM-CSF and interleukin 3 by mast cells in response to IgE receptor-mediated activation. Nature 1989; 339:150–152.
62. Brunner T, Heusser CH, Dahinden CA. Human peripheral blood basophils primed by interleukin 3 (IL-3) produce IL-4 in response to immunoglobulin E receptor stimulation. J Exp Med 1993; 177:605–610.
63. Kita H, Ohnishi T, Okubo Y, Weiler D, Abrams JS, Gleich GJ. GM-CSF and interleukin 3 release from human peripheral blood eosinophils and neutrophils. J Exp Med 1991; 174:745–748.
64. Moqbel R, Hamid Q, Ying S, Barkans J, Hartnell A, Tsicopoulos A, Wardlaw AJ, Kay AB. Expression of mRNA for the granulocyte macrophage colony-stimulating factor by activated human eosinophils. J Exp Med 1991; 174:749–751.
65. Gordon JR, Galli SJ. Release of both preformed and newly synthesized tumor necrosis factor α (TNFα/cachectin) by mouse mast cells stimulated via the FcεRI. J Exp Med 1991; 174:103–108.
66. Del Pozo V, Andres B, Martin E, Maruri N, Zubeldia JM, Palomino P, Lahoz C. Murine eosinophils and IL-1: αIl-1 mRNA detection by in situ hybridization. production and release of IL-1 from peritoneal eosinophils. J Immunol 1990; 144:3117–3122.
67. Maggi E, Parronchi P, Manetti R, Simonelli C, Piccini MP, Rugiu FS, Romagnani S. Reciprocal regulatory effects of IFNγ and IL-4 on the vitro development of human Th1 and Th2 clones. J Immunol 1992; 148:2142–2147.
68. Broide DH, Paine MM, Firestein GS. Eosinophils express interleukin 5 and granulocyte macrophage colony stimulating factor mRNA at sites of allergic inflammation in asthmatics. J Clin Invest 1992; 90:1414–1424.
69. Ying S, Durham SR, Jacobson MR, Rak S, Lowhagen O, Kay AB, Hamid Q. T lymphocytes and mast cells express messenger RNA for interleukin 4 in the nasal mucosa in allergen-induced rhinitis. Immunology 1994; 82:200–206.
70. Sedgwick JB, Calhoun WJ, Gleich GJ, Kita H, Abrams JS, Schwartz LB, Volovitz B, Ben-Yaakov M, Busse W. Immediate and late airway response of allergic rhinitis patients to segmental antigen challenge. Am Rev Respir Dis 1991; 144:1274–1281.
71. Ying S, Durham SR, Corrigan CJ, Hamid Q, Kay AB. Phenotype of cells expressing

mRNA for TH2-type (interleukin-4 and interleukin-5) and TH1-type (interleukin-2 and interferon-γ) cytokines in bronchoalveolar lavage and bronchial biopsies from atopic asthmatics and normal control types. Am J Respir Cell Mol Biol 1995; 12:477–487.

72. Ying S, Humbert M, Barkans J, Corrigan CJ, Pfister R, Menz G, Meng Q, Robinson DS, Durham SR, Kay AB. Expression of IL-4 and IL-5 mRNA and protein product by $CD4^+$ and $CD8^+$ T cells, eosinophils and mast cells in bronchial biopsies obtained from atopic and non-atopic (intrinsic) asthmatics. J Immunol 1997; 158:3539–3544.
73. Levi-Schaffer F, Lacey P, Severs NJ, Newman TH, North J, Gomperts B, Kay AB, Moqbel R. Association of granulocyte–macrophage colony-stimulating factor with the crystalloid granules of human eosinophils. Blood 1995; 85:2579–2586.
74. Moqbel R, Ying S, Barkans J, Newman TM, Kimmitt P, Wakelin M, Taborda-Barata L, Meng Q, Corrigan CJ, Durham SR, Kay AB. Identification of mRNA for interleukin-4 in human eosinophils with granule localization and release of the translated product. J Immunol 1995; 155:4939–4947.
75. Bentley AM, Menz G, Storz CHR, Robinson DS, Bradley B, Jeffery PK, Durham SR, Kay AB. Identification of T-lymphocytes, macrophages and activated eosinophils in the bronchial mucosa in intrinsic asthma: relationship to symptoms and bronchial responsiveness. Am Rev Respir Dis 1992; 146:500–506.
76. Bentley AM, Maestrelli P, Saetta M, Fabbri LM, Robinson DS, Bradley BL, Jeffery PK, Durham SR, Kay AB. Activated T-lymphocytes and eosinophils in the bronchial mucosa in isocyanate-induced asthma. J Allergy Clin Immunol 1992; 89:821–829.
77. Walker C, Kaegi MK, Braun P, Blaser K. Activated T cells and eosinophila in bronchoalveolar lavages from subjects with asthma correlated with disease severity. J Allergy Clin Immunol 1991; 88:935–942.
78. Till S, Li B, Durham S, Humbert M, Assoufi B, Huston D, Dickason R, Jeannin P, Kay AB, Corrigan CJ. Secretion of the eosinophil-active cytokines interleukin-5, granulocyte/macrophage colony-stimulating factor and interleukin-3 by bronchoalveolar lavage $CD4^+$ and $CD8^+$ T cell lines in atopic asthmatics, and atopic and non-atopic controls. Eur J Immunol 1995; 25:2727–2731.
79. Walker C, Bode E, Boer L, Hansel TT, Blaser K, Virchow J-C Jr. Allergic and non-allergic asthmatics have distinct patterns of T-cell activation and cytokine production in peripheral blood and bronchoalveolar lavage. Am Rev Respir Dis 1992; 146:109–115.
80. Humbert M, Grant JA, Taborda-Barata L, Durham SR, Pfister R, Menz G, Barkans J, Ying S, Kay AB. High affinity IgE receptor (FcεRI)-bearing cells in bronchial biopsies from atopic and nonatopic asthma. Am J Respir Crit Care Med 1996; 153:1931–1937.
81. Maestrelli P, Del Prete GF, De Carli M, D'Elios MM, Saetta M, Di Stefano A, Mapp CE, Romagnani S, Fabbri LM. CD8 T-cell clones producing interleukin-5 and interferon-gamma in bronchial mucosa of patients with asthma induced by toluene diisocyanate. Scand J Work Environ Health 1994; 20:376–381.
82. Krajewski AS, Wyllie AH. Inhibition of human T lymphocyte colony formation by methylprednisolone. Clin Exp Immunol 1981; 46:206–213.
83. Carmichael J, Paterson IC, Diaz P, Crompton GK, Kay AB, Grant IWB. Corticosteroid resistance in chronic asthma. Br Med J 1981; 282:1419–1422.
84. Poznansky MC, Gordon ACH, Douglas JG, Krajewski AS, Wyllie AH, Grant IWB. Resistance to methylprednisolone in cultures of blood mononuclear cells from glucocorticoid-resistant asthmatic patients. Clin Sci 1984; 67:639–645.
85. Poznansky MC, Gordon ACH, Grant IWB, Wyllie AH. A cellular abnormality in glucocorticoid resistant asthma. Clin Exp Immunol 1985; 61:135–142.
86. Sher E, Leung DYM, Surs W, Kam JC, Zieg G, Kamada AK, Szefler SJ. Steroid-resistant asthma. Cellular mechanisms contributing to inadequate response to glucocorticoid therapy. J Clin Invest 1994; 93:33–39.
87. Kam J, Szefler SJ, Surs W, Sher E, Leung DYM. The combined effects of IL-2 and IL-4 alter the binding affinity of the glucocorticoid receptor. J Immunol 1993; 151:3460–3466.
88. Leung DYM, Martin RJ, Szefler SJ, Sher ER, Ying S, Kay AB, Hamid Q. Dysregulation

of interleukin 4, interleukin 5, and interferon γ gene expression in steroid-resistant asthma. J Exp Med 1995; 181:33–40.
89. Adcock IM, Lane SJ, Brown CR, Lee TH, Barnes PJ. Abnormal glucocorticoid receptor-activator protein 1 interaction in steroid resistant asthma. J Exp Med 1995; 182:1951–1958.
90. Schreiber SL, Crabtree GR. The mechanism of action of cyclosporin A and FK 506. Immunol Today 1992; 13:136–141.
91. Alexander AG, Barnes NC, Kay AB. Trial of cyclosporin A in corticosteroid-dependent chronic severe asthma. Lancet 1992; 339:324–328.
92. Lock SH, Kay AB, Barnes NC. Double-blind, placebo-controlled study of cyclosporin A as a corticosteroid-sparing agent in corticosteroid-dependent asthma. Am J Respir Crit Care Med 1996; 153:509–514.
93. Sihra BS, Durham SR, Walker S, Kon OM, Barnes NC, Kay AB. Effect of cyclosporin A on the allergen-induced late asthmatic reaction. Thorax 1997; 52:447–452.
94. Enander I, Ahlstedt S, Nygren H. Mononuclear cells, mast cells and mucous cells as part of the delayed hypersensitivity response to aerosolized antigen in mice. Immunology 1984; 51:661–668.
95. Enander I, Ahlstedt S, Nygren H, Bjorksten B. Sensitizing ability of derivatives of picryl chloride after exposure of mice on the skin and in the lung. Int Arch Allergy Appl Immunol 1983; 72:59–66.
96. Enander I, Ulfgren A, Nygren H, Larsson P, Holmdahl R, Klareskog L, Ahlstedt S. Regulation by T cells of delayed hypersensitivity reaction in mouse lung as reflected by mononuclear cells, mast cells and mucus-producing cells. Int Arch Allergy Appl Immunol 1988; 85:374–380.
97. Garssen J, Nijamp FP, Van der Vliet H, Van Loveren H. T-cell mediated induction of airway hyperreactivity in mice. Am Rev Respir Dis 1991; 144:931–938.
98. Frew AJ, Moqbel R, Azzawi M, Hartnell A, Barkans J, Jeffery PK, Kay AB, Scheper RJ, Varley J, Church MK, Holgate ST. T lymphocytes and eosinophils in allergen-induced late-phase asthmatic reactions in the guinea pig. Am Rev Respir Dis 1990; 141:407–413.
99. Jose PJ, Griffiths-Johnson DA, Collins PD, Walsh DT, Moqbel RM, Totty NF, Hsuan JJ, Williams TJ. Eotaxin: a potent eosinophil chemoattractant cytokine detected in a guinea pig model of allergic airways disease. J Exp Med 1994; 179:881–887.
100. Hoyne GF, O'Hehir RE, Wraith DC, Thomas WR, Lamb JR. Inhibition of T cell and antibody responses to house dust mite allergen by inhalation of the dominant T cell epitope in naive and sensitized mice. J Exp Med 1993; 178:1783–1788.
101. Gavett SH, Chen X, Finkelman F, Wills-Karp M. Depletion of murine $CD4^+$ T lymphocytes prevents antigen-induced airway hyperreactivity and pulmonary eosinophilia. Am J Respir Cell Mol Biol 1994; 10:587–593.
102 Foster PS, Hogan SP, Ramsay AJ, Matthaei KI, Young IG. IL-5 deficiency abolishes eosinophilia, airways hyperreactivity, and lung damage in a mouse asthma model. J Exp Med 1995; 183:195–201.
103. Chand N, Harrison JE, Rooney S, Pillar J, Jkubicki R, Nolan K, Diamantis W. Sofia D. Anti-IL-5 monoclonal antibody inhibits allergic late phase bronchial eosinophila in guinea pigs: a therapeutic approach. Eur J Pharmacol 1992; 211:121–123.
104. Haczku A, Chung KF, Sun J, Barnes PJ, Kay AB, Moqbel R. Airway hyperresponsiveness, elevation of serum-specific IgE and activation of T cells following allergen exposure in sensitized Brown-Norway rats. Immunology 1995; 85:598–603.
105. Haczku A, Moqbel R, Jacobson M, Kay AB, Barnes, PJ, Chung KF. T-cell subsets and activation in bronchial mucosa of sensitized Brown-Norway rats after single allergen exposure. Immunology 1995; 85:591–597.
106. Eidelman DH, Bellofiore S, Martin JG. Late airway responses to antigen challenge in sensitized inbred rats. Am Rev Respir Dis 1988; 137:1033–1037.
107. Watanabe A, Mishima H, Renzi PM, Hamid Q, Martin JG. Adoptive transfer of allergic airway responses with antigen-primed $CD4^+$ T cells in rats [abstract]. Am J Respir Crit Care Med 1995; 151:A347.

108. Haczku A, Moqbel R, Sun J, North J, Kay AB, Barnes PJ, Chung KF. T cells mediate eosinophilic inflammation and airway hyperresponsiveness in Brown-Norway rats [abstract]. Am J Respir Crit Care Med. 1995; 151:A347.
109. Corry DB, Folkesson HG, Warnock ML, Erle DJ, Matthay MA, Wiener-Kronish JP, Locksley RC. Interleukin-4, but not interleukin-5 or eosinophils, is required in a murine model of acute airway hyperreactivity. J Exp Med 1996; 183:109–117.
110. Drazen JM, Arm JP, Austen KF. Sorting out the cytokines of asthma. J Exp Med 1996; 183:1–5.
111. Kaminuma O, Mori A, Ogawa K, Nakata A, Kikkawa H, Naito K, Suko M, Okudaira H. Successful transfer of late phase eosinophil infiltration in the lung by infusion of helper T cell clones. Am J Resp Cell Mol Biol 1997; 16:448–454.
112. Coyle AJ, Erard F, Bertrand C, Walti S, Pircher H, Le Gros G. Virus-specific $CD8^+$ cells can switch to interleukin 5 production and induce airway eosinophilia. J Exp Med 1995; 181:1229–1233.
113. O'Garra A, Murphy K. Role of cytokines in determining T-lymphocyte function. Curr Opin Immunol 1994; 6:458–466.
114. Maggi E, Parronchi P, Manetti R, Simonelli C, Piccini M-P, Rugiu FS, de Carli M, Ricci M, Romagnani S. Reciprocal regulatory effects of IFNγ and IL-4 on the in vitro development of human Th1 and Th2 clones. J Immunol 1992; 148:2142–2147.
115. Manetti R, Parronchi P, Guidizi MG, Picini M-P, Maggi E, Trinchieri G, Romagnani S. Natural killer cell stimulatory factor (interleukin 12 [IL-12]) induces T helper type 1 (Th1)-specific immune responses and inhibits the development of IL-4 producing cells. J Exp Med 1993; 177:1199–1204.
116. Yoshimoto T, Paul WE. $CD4^+$, $NK1.1^+$ T cells promptly produce interleukin 4 in response to in vivo challenge with anti-CD3. J Exp Med 1994; 179:1285–1295.
117. Bendelac A, Matzinger P, Seder RA, Paul WE, Schwartz RH. Activation events during thymic selection. J Exp Med 1992; 175:731–742.
118. Vicari A, Zlotnik A. Mouse NK1.1 T cells: a new family of T cells. Immunol Today 1996; 17:71–76.
119. Naseer T, Leung DYM, Song Y, Martin R, Hamid Q. Expression of IL-12 mRNA in baseline asthma and in response to steroid therapy [abstract]. Am J Respir Crit Care Med 1995; 151:A701.
120. Hamid QA, Schotman E, Jacobson MR, Walker SM, Durham SR. Increases in interleukin-12 (IL-12) messenger RNA^+ ($mRNA^+$) cells accompany inhibition of allergen induced late skin responses following successful grass pollen immunotherapy. J Allergy Clin Immunol 1997; 99:254–260.
121. Schwartz R. Co-stimulation of T lymphocytes: the role of CD28, CTLA4 and B7/BB1 in interleukin 2 production and immunotherapy. Cell 1992; 71:1065–1068.
122. Thompson CB. Distinct roles for the co-stimulatory ligands B7-1 and B7-2 in T helper cell differentiation? Cell 1995; 81:979–982.
123. Krummel MF, Allison JP. CD28 and CTLA4 have opposing effects on the response of T cells to stimulation. J Exp Med 1995; 182:459–465.
124. Linsley PS, Wallace PM, Johnson J, Gibson MG, Greene JL, Ledbetter JA, Singh C, Tepper MA. Immunosuppression in vivo by a soluble form of the CTLA4 T cell activation molecule. Science 1992; 257:792–795.
125. Pernis A, Gupta S, Gollob KJ, Garfein E, Coffman RL, Schindler C, Rothman P. Lack of interferon γ receptor β chain and the prevention of interferon γ signaling Th1 cells. Science 1995; 269:245–247.
126. Guler ML, Gorham JD, Hsieh CY Mackey AJ, Steen RG, Dietrich WF, Murphy KM. Genetic susceptibility to *Leishmania*: IL-12 responsiveness in Th1 cell development. Science 1996; 271:984–987.
127. Evavold BD, Sloan-Lancaster J, Allen PM. Tickling the TCR: selective T cell functions stimulated by altered peptide ligands. Immunol Today 1993; 14:602.
128. Nicholson LB, Greer JM, Sobel RA, Lees MB, Kuchroo VK. An altered peptide ligand

mediates immune deviation and prevents autoimmune encephalomyelitis. Immunity 1995; 3:397–405.

129. Baggiolini M, Dahniden CA. CC chemokines in allergic inflammation. Immunol Today 1994; 15:127–133.
130. Kameyoshi Y, Dorschner A, Mallet AI, Christophers E, Schroder J-M. Cytokine RANTES released by thrombin stimulated platelets is a potent attraction for human eosinophils. J Exp Med 1992; 176:587–592.
131. Lukacs NW, Strieter RM, Shklee CL, Chensue SW, Kunkel SL. Macrophage inflammatory protein 1α influences eosinophil recruitment in antigen-specific airway inflammation. Eur J Immunol 1995; 25:245–251.
132. Ying S, Taborda Barata L, Meng Q, Humbert M, Kay AB. The kinetics of allergen-induced transcription of messenger RNA for monocyte chemotactic protein 3 and RANTES in the skin of human atopic subjects: relationship to eosinophil, T cell, and macrophage recruitment. J Exp Med 1995; 181:2153–2159.
133. Ying S, Meng Q, Taborda Barata L, Corrigan CJ, Barkans J, Assoufi B, Moqbel R, Durham SR, Kay AB. Human eosinophils express messenger RNA encoding RANTES and store and release biologically active RANTES protein. Eur J Immunol 1996; 26:70–76.
134. Sim TC, Reece LM, Hilsmeier KA, Grant JA, Alam R. Secretion of chemokines and other cytokines in allergen-induced nasal late responses: inhibition by topical steroid treatment. Am J Respir Crit Care Med 1995; 152:927–933.
135. Cruikshank WW, Long A, Tarpy RE, Kornfeld H, Carrol MP, Teran L, Holgate ST, Center DM. Early identification of interleukin 16 (lymphocyte chemoattractant factor) and macrophage inflammatory protein Iα in bronchoalveolar lavage fluid of antigen challenged asthmatics. Am J Respir Mol Cell Biol 1995; 13:738–747.
136. Alam R, York J, Boyars M, Stafford S, Grant JA, Lee J, Forsythe P, Sim T, Ida N. Increased MP-1, RANTES and MIP-1α in bronchoalveolar lavage fluid of allergic asthmatic patients. Am J Respir Crit Care Med 1996; 153:1398–1404.
137. Ponath PD, Qin S, Ringler DJ, Clark-Lewis I, Wang J, Kassam N, Smith H, Shi X, Gonzalo J-A, Newman W, Guiterrez-Ramos J-C, Mackay CR. Cloning of the human eosinophil chemoattractant, eotaxin. J Clin Invest 1996; 97:604–612.
138. Collins PD, Marleau S, Griffiths-Johnson DA, Jose PJ, Williams TJ. Cooperation between interleukin 5 and the chemokine eotaxin to induce eosinophil accumulation in vitro. J Exp Med 1995; 182:1169–1174.

3

Mechanisms of Asthma

Asthma Is an Allergic Disease

LISA M. WHEATLEY and THOMAS A. E. PLATTS-MILLS

University of Virginia
Charlottesville, Virginia

I. Introduction

Most of our knowledge of the pathophysiology of asthma has come from investigating cases where the etiology is known. The best understood cause of asthma is immediate hypersensitivity or allergy to common proteins in the environment. Asthma is a disease defined by three criteria: reversible airflow obstruction, bronchial hyperreactivity, and inflammation. The first is a result of the latter two, and all can be manifestations of allergic airway disease. Allergy is the result of complex genetic traits that result in a specific and characteristic immune response to foreign proteins. The clinical syndromes of hay fever, atopic dermatitis, and asthma are constellations of signs and symptoms associated with the presence of antigen-specific IgE. The tissue response in asthma is a result of diverse elements that are either triggered by IgE (such as release of histamine and leukotrienes from mast cells) or that are produced during the same immunological response (T cells that produce interleukin [IL-4] as well as eosinophil chemotaxis and survival factors). In addition, even when asthma is not obviously the result of a specific IgE reaction to environmental proteins, these same elements may be involved, as are mast cells in exercise-induced bronchospasm, or eosinophils in "intrinsic" asthma. There are presumably multiple factors in the environment that influence the expression of this genetic trait, and the combined effects of exposure and other factors are now producing an epidemic of asthma. Although we are increasingly able to predict who is at risk of developing allergy and, therefore, asthma, by using family history, IgE levels, and possibly, response to vaccinations such as bacillus Calmette-Guerain (BCG), we still do not understand the exact sequence of events nor how to interrupt the process (1,2). The evidence for the importance of allergy in asthma has come from a number of different sources including epidemiology, bronchial challenge models, and allergen avoidance studies.

II. Epidemiology

Although the recognition of seasonal asthma demonstrated the existence of allergic asthma long before the demonstration of IgE, it was not until the mid 1980s that the relevance of allergy in asthma and its importance in large populations became widely appreciated. This involved two related charges. First, the recognition that perennial exposure to indoor allergens (e.g., dust mite) was strongly associated with asthma and, second, the realization that most asthmatics are unaware of the role that allergen exposure plays in producing their symptoms. Dust mites are the prime example of an indoor allergen because they are widely distributed and can produce high concentrations of allergen in dust. Patients are often ignorant of the existence of dust mites; therefore, the patients cannot connect the mites with their asthma. Several case–control studies demonstrated the association between sensitization to mite and asthma. Perhaps the most dramatic studies were those that originated in Papua New Guinea. In the South Fore region of Papua New Guinea, the prevalence of asthma rose from 0.1% in the mid-1970s to 7.5% in the mid-1980s, while remaining low in other parts of the island nation (asthma prevalence in adjacent Asaro remained 0.3%). This increase in asthma in the adult population was traced to the introduction of blankets to this region in the 1950s. The blankets proved to be a fertile breeding ground for dust mites. The relative number of dust mites per gram dust was much higher in the South Fore region (1371 mites versus 283 in Asaro). More significantly, the asthmatics of South Fore had a much higher level of mite-specific IgE (108.6 units/mL) than the asymptomatic in South Fore (3.4 units/mL) or a random sample in Asaro (4.4 units/mL) (3). These reports were particularly important because the increase in asthma was seen predominantly in adults. When the role of allergy in asthma is discussed, it is often perceived to be a risk for children, but not for adults, whereas allergy may be a significant contributor in as many as half of adult asthmatics (4). In addition, these reports are interesting because this increase in asthma was seen in an area relatively untouched by modernization, whereas the "epidemic" of asthma has been seen in the Westernized world.

While dust mites have proved to be a major allergen in many parts of the world, including North and South America, Europe, Taiwan, Japan, and Australia, there are many other important sources of allergens related to asthma. For example, there is an annual increase in hospital visits for asthma in the area around Sacramento during the grass pollen season (5). Similarly, in the Midwest of the United States, there is an increase in admissions during peak periods of airborne *Alternaria*, and, during this "season," sensitivity to *Alternaria* is a risk factor for fatal and near-fatal asthma (6). In cooler, dryer climates, such as Northern Sweden and the mountains of New Mexico, allergens derived from house pets are the dominant sensitizers for asthma (7,8). For the urban poor of large cities of the Northeastern United States, cockroaches are the largest contributor to the allergen load (9). Recently, the National Cooperative Inner City Asthma Study has demonstrated that poor, urban African–American children who are skin test–positive to cockroach allergens are twice as likely to be admitted to the hospital for asthma if they are exposed to cockroach allergen in their bedroom than if they are not exposed (10).

It would have been easier to recognize allergen exposure as a dominant cause of asthma if there were a simple dose–response relation between allergen exposure and symptoms of asthma. However, the distribution of allergens is largely a function of the physical and social environment (temperature, humidity, agriculture, or the lack thereof, and poverty, all tend to be homogenous for a given area). Therefore, exposure is likely to be similar for asthmatics and nonasthmatics within a community. This also explains why the most important allergens differ from community to community, depending on the local environment. Several studies have shown a dose–response relationship between exposure and the development of sensitization, with an increasing percentage of sensitization among children living in houses with higher levels of allergen. In addition, there are different thresholds for different people. A longitudinal study of the acquisition of dust mite–specific IgE showed that children with an allergic diathesis, as predicted by positive skin tests to an allergen other than dust mites at the start of the study, had a threshold for sensitization of 2 μg of group 1 allergen per gram of dust. The threshold of sensitization for children without other positive skin tests was 80 μg or more per gram of dust (11). It is probable that at least a portion of the increase in the prevalence of asthma is due to increased exposure to indoor allergens. Houses are warmer and less drafty, are filled with more upholstered furniture, and are more fully carpeted. Pets are more common, and more commonly kept inside the home. All these changes would be likely to increase allergen levels of mite, pet, and cockroach origin. In addition, persons spend more time indoors, on average more than 23 out of 24 hr. In Australia, an increase in dust mite levels and a parallel increase in sensitization and asthma has been documented over a 10-year period (12). This increase has not been universal. In Great Britain, high levels of dust mites were measured in the mid-1970s, but there is no evidence that levels have risen in step with the rising prevalence of asthma since then (13).

Although exposure is necessary, it is not sufficient for the development of specific IgE. Environmental exposure is "filtered" through the genetic background of the individual. Genetically predisposed individuals develop the typical allergic response with a predominance of T cells producing the cytokines IL-4 and IL-5, rather than interferon (IFN)-γ; B cells producing IgE, rather than IgG; and inflammation typified by eosinophils, rather than the apparent immunological tolerance of the majority of the population. Furthermore, it is the combination of specific IgE and continued exposure to the relevant allergen that is crucial for the development of asthma. Even then an unknown step or steps remain. Although exposure leads to specific IgE, and specific IgE precedes asthma in both adults and children, there are numerous individuals who have positive skin tests and live in houses with a relevant allergen, but they have no symptoms (14,15). When symptoms are present, what makes an atopic individual develop asthma on exposure, rather than rhinitis or dermatitis, for example, is unclear. As the incidence of asthma continues to rise, our inability to understand the link between specific IgE and symptoms is disturbing because at least 20% of the U.S. population is atopic. This means that there is a large pool of people who are asymptomatic or who have only trivial symptoms, yet have the potential to become asthmatic.

III. Characteristics of the Allergic Immune Response and Its Relationship to Asthma

In general, immune responses are influenced by dose, scheduling of doses, age at first exposure, route of administration, and the presence of adjuvants, in addition to genetic background. All of these variables are probably acting in the development of the immune response associated with asthma. For example, the source and timing of allergen exposure may influence the outcome. Allergic asthma in England among 11-year-old children was better correlated with household dust mite allergen levels when the subjects were 2 years of age than with current exposure (13). Whether the early sensitization occurred as a result of increased susceptibility because of an immature and developing immune system, or owing to the extent of exposure (small children spend most of their time indoors, and in close proximity to mattresses, blankets, and carpets), has not been determined. Adults can develop new specific IgE antibody responses; therefore, immunological immaturity is not necessary, although it may facilitate the development of an IgE response. In laboratory experiments, cytokines released from Th2 cells in vitro, skew subsequent responses toward the Th2 phenotype; hence, it is possible that early exposure to one allergen would predispose a child to subsequent allergic responses to other antigens. In support of the idea that a Th2 response to one antigen increases the risk of further allergic responses, a study on mite avoidance in the first 9 months of life showed a decreased risk for any allergy in the cases versus the controls. The cases who were exposed to cats (pet ownership was not controlled) were at increased risk for sensitization to other allergens. At 1 year of age, children in the control arm were at significantly higher risk for all forms of allergy, eczema, and asthma. A follow-up at 2 years of age, revealed that the children in the control arm had more asthma, although the children in the avoidance arm were no longer at an advantage from rhinitis or eczema (16).

IV. Indoor and Perennial Allergens

Except for *Alternaria*, most of the major allergens associated with chronic asthma are found indoors, and exposure is perennial. For instance, in central Virginia, sensitization to seasonal pollens does not correlate with symptomatic bronchial hyperreactivity (17). Similarly, for Australian schoolchildren living in suburban Sydney, bronchial hyperreactivity is associated with dust mite sensitivity, not with *Alternaria* or rye grass (12). Because sensitization to *Alternaria* is a risk factor for asthma in some communities and not in others, study of this relationship may help answer whether the important feature of the allergens associated with asthma is indoor exposure, perennial exposure, or whether the two are inextricably linked. The perennial nature of the exposure to indoor allergens may contribute to the development of asthma and also may pose problems in establishing the etiology. Patients are generally unaware of the relationship and, therefore, do not actively avoid the allergen. The windborne outdoor allergens, such as pollens, are often high dose and impact prominently on the nasal mucosa and the conjunctiva, with easily recognizable symptoms, such as itching and sneezing. Contact with indoor allergens is likely to be insidious, rather than dramatic. The exposure to most indoor allergens is thought to be relatively low dose, but persists on a daily basis for much of the year. Exposure to mite and cockroach allergens is limited by poor aerodynamic properties. Only a small amount of allergen becomes airborne during disturbance, and most of it falls rapidly in the low airflow rates typical of most houses (18,19). The inflammatory response may also be patchy. A mite fecal particle could release a large dose of allergen in the area of impact, but a limited number of fecal particles would be inhaled, so only a small portion of the lung would be involved after any single exposure. In addition, because of the consistent nature of the exposure, symptoms are overlapping; today's response is superimposed on an ongoing response from yesterday's exposure, and so on, such that the inflammation and bronchial hyperreactivity becomes continuous. In the setting of chronic bronchial hyperreactivity, responses to nonspecific stimuli, such as cigarette smoke, household cleaners, methacholine, or histamine become more prominent. These characteristics make it difficult for the patient to recognize the contribution that exposure from a specific source makes to symptoms, and the consequent failure to recognize and avoid further exposure allows the inflammatory cycle to continue. The chronic nature of exposure also makes physician-elicited histories unreliable as a diagnostic tool. At least two other situations exist where asthma develops in the context of persistent exposure, even when symptoms attributable to exposure may be manifest. One is asthma in the workplace, for which there is a financial disincentive to limit exposure, and the other is in a home with a pet for which there is an emotional disincentive to recognize the source of symptoms. In occupational asthma, a longer duration of symptoms before diagnosis correlates with a decreased probability of total resolution of asthma after cessation of exposure (20). This suggests that bronchial hyperreactivity induced by natural exposure to allergens may eventually become irreversible, at least in adults.

Other possible explanations in addition to dose or period of exposure, would be that another agent is required for the expression of asthma in an allergic individual. For instance, it has been proposed that it is the combination of cedar pollen and motor vehicle pollution that associate with cedar allergy in Japan (21). Similarly, in children seen in an emergency room setting, it is the combination of upper respiratory viral infection and allergen sensitivity that increases the risk of wheezing (22). However, the interaction of viral infection with the development of atopy is likely to be complex. In contrast with evidence about the role of viral infection in precipitating acute asthma attacks in school-aged children, the relative lack of upper respiratory infections in early childhood has also been postulated to predispose to atopy (23). The rate of atopy among only children and eldest children is higher than in younger children of larger families (younger siblings would be expected to have more viral infections at an earlier age) (24). Similarly, the rate of asthma is higher in cities in the former West Germany than in East Germany where family sizes are larger (25). In both of these cases, the children with more asthma would be expected to have had fewer upper respiratory viral infections, suggesting that, at least in some cases, viral infections may be protective and decrease the likelihood of developing asthma.

Although the main allergens associated with asthma are inhaled, other sources, such as food allergens and colonizing organisms, may also be important. Allergic bronchopulmonary aspergillosis (ABPA) is a subset of allergic asthma notable for the type of allergen exposure and for the chronicity and severity of the disease. In ABPA, there is a large IgE response to an allergen residing in the lung. This response involves the production of *Aspergillus*–specific IgE, but also nonspecific IgE, with levels being elevated to approximately tenfold higher than normal levels. In addition, there is peripheral eosinophilia and eosinophilic infiltration of the lungs, bronchiectasis, and pulmonary fibrotic changes. The standard treatment for ABPA is suppression of the immune response with prednisone, for treatment with antifungals to remove the allergen has not been proved to be effective.

V. Experimental Studies

Allergen challenge studies have demonstrated the two phases of the asthmatic response to inhaled allergen. The immediate bronchoconstrictive response begins within the first 10 min after allergen inhalation. This is coincident with IgE-triggered release of mediators from mast cells, including histamine, tryptase, and the leukotrienes, all of which are increased in bronchoalveolar lavage (BAL) fluid (26). The immediate response is followed by a return to baseline lung function in about 1 hr. The late-phase response (LPR) is a second obstructive period, beginning between 4 and 8 hr after allergen challenge and is temporally related to a cellular influx, an increased edema, and a hypersecretion of mucus. The late-phase response is often more severe and generally more prolonged than the immediate response. It may take up to 24 hr to resolve clinically, and the presence of eosinophils and $CD4^+$

T cells can persist for at least 96 hr (27). This dual response is dose-dependent and is seen in about half of allergic asthmatics.

Bronchial challenge studies have also demonstrated bronchial hyperreactivity to histamine or methacholine that follows a single exposure to allergen and persists for some period thereafter (28). If exposure is seasonal, rather than a single dose of allergen, bronchial hyperreactivity may persist for several months after the end of a pollen season (29). Segmental allergen challenge has helped document the cellular influx that is part and parcel of the late-phase response, with its domination by eosinophils and by $CD4^+$ T cells, with the characteristic cytokine secretion profile of Th2-type cells (30). However, many questions remain unanswered. For instance, patients with allergic rhinitis who undergo segmental allergen challenge of the lung show a cellular infiltration similar in type and magnitude to asthmatics (31). Studies of bronchoalveolar lavage fluid in patients with "intrinsic" asthma have shown eosinophil and $CD4^+$ T-cell infiltrates and the presence of IL-5, suggesting an allergic response in the absence of identifiable allergen (32). It is possible that although a foreign antigen had established the type of immune response, the response has become self-maintaining. In some patients, it may be that the relevant allergen has not been identified or investigated. For example, *Trichophyton* sensitivity was found in steroid-dependent asthmatics who had previously been evaluated for common inhalant allergen sensitivity, of whom half were negative on skin testing to common inhalant allergens. Treatment aimed at eradicating the source of the relevant antigens, in this instance the patients' onychomycosis, resulted in control of disease, with a concomitant decrease in the reliance on systemic steroids (33).

VI. Treatment

It is now apparent from bronchoscopy that even mild asthma has an inflammatory component. In addition, the improvement in airflow obstruction with anti-inflammatory therapy is better the shorter the period the person has been symptomatic (34). Therefore, the first-line of treatment for anyone with symptoms occurring more than three times a week, is an anti-inflammatory agent. Anti-inflammatories widely in use include the mast cell-stabilizing cromones, the leukotriene antagonists, and inhaled and oral corticosteroids. All of these agents interrupt the allergic inflammatory cascade to some degree.

The recognition of the importance of allergy in asthma has led to the wider acceptance of a truly anti-inflammatory therapy—avoidance. With strict avoidance, symptoms and bronchial hyperreactivity can be reduced. This was demonstrated when children from the Netherlands were taken to Davos, Switzerland, where dust mite levels were approximately 20 mites per gram dust versus levels of 100–1000 in the children's homes (35). After avoidance, the children also had a decrease in nonspecific bronchial hyperreactivity to histamine. In addition, this type of radical avoidance decreases eosinophils and eosinophilic products in the lungs of children (36). Techniques have also been devised to limit exposure to allergens in patient homes with varying success. Reductions in dust mite allergen levels have been the most successful. Use of mite-impermeable encasings on bedding, controlling humidity levels, and the removal of carpets, all are associated with substantial drops in mite levels (37). Moreover, some studies have demonstrated a concomitant and sustained decreased in bronchial hyperreactivity (38). Measures employed for reducing the concentrations of pet-derived allergens are somewhat more complicated as well as less effective. In addition to encasing the bedding and removing the carpet, the animals must be excluded from the bedroom and a high-efficiency particulate air (HEPA) filter employed. These methods have shown reduction in airborne and reservoir allergen load, but have not been sufficient to improve symptoms by themselves (39). However, the combination of environmental control and pharmacotherapy was better than pharmacotherapy alone in the control of rhinitis (40). It is unclear whether frequently washing the animal might also improve the effect. Measures to effectively control cockroach allergens have not yet been published.

Unfortunately, many of the recommendations are expensive or involve a substantial initial cash outlay that is often not reimbursed by insurance (dust mite covers, changing floor coverings, even hot water for the poor), and require considerable and sustained effort. And, in some sense, allergen avoidance is generally too late when it is initiated. As with other anti-inflammatory therapies, such as inhaled corticosteroids, leukotriene antagonists, or cromolyns, it is disease-suppressive, rather than disease-modifying, and the effect lasts only as long as the avoidance continues. It might be that altering housing conditions within an entire community would be helpful, but not in the near-term. The advantage of allergen immunotherapy is that it alters the immune response and, therefore, offers the prospect of long-term control of allergic asthma (41). The difficulty, of course, is that it entails a greater immediate risk than either pharmacological treatment or allergen avoidance. In the studies of immunotherapy deaths, one of the risk factors was the presence of brittle or unstable asthma (42). Thus, achieving maximum control of asthma using a combination of avoidance and anti-inflammatories should be standard practice before initiating immunotherapy.

VII. Conclusions

Allergy is the major identifiable cause of asthma. Exposure to allergens causes not only immediate bronchospasm, but also eosinophilic inflammation of the airways and prolonged bronchial hyperreactivity and, sometimes, irreversible changes to the airways. The major allergens involved are found inside the home, and effective avoidance protocols have been devised for at least some of these allergens. The dominance of the inflammatory response to allergens in the pathophysiology of asthma focuses attention on altering this response with immunotherapy as well as avoiding or suppressing it.

Acknowledgments

Supported by grants RO1-A1-30840, 1U01-A1-34607, K08-A1-01416-10.

References

1. Martinez FD, Wright AL, Taussig LM, Holberg CJ, Halonen M. Asthma and wheezing in the first six years of life. N Engl J Med 1995; 332:133–138.
2. Shirakawa T, Enomoto T, Shimazu S-I, Hopkin JM. The inverse association between tuberculin responses and atopic disorder. Science 1997; 275:77–79.
3. Turner KJ, Stewart GA, Woolcock AJ, Green W, Alpers MP. Relationship between mite densities and the prevalence of asthma: comparative studies in two populations in the Eastern Highlands of Papua New Guinea. Clin Allergy 1988; 18:331–340.
4. Gelbert LE, Seltzer LH, Bouzoukis JK, Pollart SM, Chapman MD, Platts-Mills TAE. Sensitization and exposure to indoor allergens as risk factors for asthma among patients presenting to hospital. Am Rev Respir Dis 1993; 147:573–578.
5. Pollart SM, Reid MJ, Fling JA, Chapman MD, Platts-Mills TAE. Epidemiology of emergency room asthma in northern California: association with IgE antibody to ryegrass pollen. J Allergy Clin Immunol 1988; 82:224–230.
6. O'Hallaren MT, Yunginger J, Offord KP, Somers MJ, O'Connell EJ, Ballard DJ, Sachs MI. Exposure to an aeroallergen as a possible precipitating factor in respiratory arrest in young patients with asthma. N Engl J Med 1991; 324:359–363.
7. Sporik RB, Ingram JM, Price W, Sussman JH, Honsinger RW, Platts-Mills TAE. Association of asthma with serum IgE and skin-test reactivity to allergens among children living at high altitude: tickling the dragon's breath. Am J Respir Crit Care Med 1995; 151:1388–1392.
8. Ehnert B, Lau-Schadendorf S, Weber A. Sensitization to indoor allergens in infants at age 1. J Allergy Clin Immunol 1993; 91:324.
9. Call RS, Smith TF, Morris E, Chapman MD, Platts-Mills TAE. Risk factors for asthma in inner-city children. J Pediatr 1992; 121:862–866.
10. Rosenstreich DL, Eggleston P, Kattan M, Baker D, Slavin RG, Gergen P, Mitchell H, McNiff-Mortimer K, Lynn H, Ownby D, Malveaux F. The role of cockroach allergy and exposure in causing morbidity among inner-city children with asthma. N Engl J Med 1997; 336:1356–1363.
11. Kuehr J, Frischer J, Meiner R. Mite exposure is a risk factor for the incidence of specific sensitization. J Allergy Clin Immunol 1994; 94:44–52.
12. Peat JK, Gray EJ, Mellis CM, Leeder SR, Woolcock AG. Differences in airway responsiveness between children and adults living in the same environment. Eur Respir J 1994; 7:1805–1813.
13. Sporik RB, Holgate ST, Platts-Mills TAE, Cogswell J. Exposure to house dust mite allergen (Der p I) and the development of asthma in childhood: a prospective study. N Engl J Med 1990; 323:502–507.
14. Peat JK, van den Berg RH, Green WF, Mellis CM, Leeder SR, Woolcock AG. Changing prevalence of asthma in Australian children. Br Med J 1994; 308:1591–1596.
15. Ohman JL, Sparrow D, MacDonald M. New onset wheezing in an older male population: evidence of allergen sensitization in a longitudinal study. J Allergy Clin Immunol 1993; 91:252–257.
16. Hide DW, Matthews S, Matthews L, Stevens M, Ridout S, Twiselton R, Gant C, Arshad SH. Effect of allergen avoidance in infancy on allergic manifestations at 2 years. J Allergy Clin Immunol 1994; 93:842–846.
17. Squillace SP, Sporik RB, Rakes G, Couture N, Lawrence A, Merriam S, Zhang J, Platts-Mills TAE. Sensitization to dust mites as a dominant risk factor for asthma among adoles-

cents living in central Virginia: multiple regression of a population-based study. Am J Respir Crit Care Med 1997; 156:1760–1764.
18. Saroong SB, Wood RA, Eggleston PA. Aerodynamic properties of cockroach allergens. J Allergy Clin Immunol 1995; 95:262.
19. De Blay F, Heymann PW, Chapman MD, Platts-Mills TAE. Airborne dust mite allergens: comparison of group II allergens with group I mite allergen and cat allergen Fed d I. J Allergy Clin Immunol 1991; 88:77–82.
20. Chan-Yeung M, MacLean L, Paggiaro PL. Follow-up study of 232 patients and occupational asthma caused by western red cedar (*Thuja plicata*). J Allergy Clin Immunol 1987; 79:792–796.
21. Miyamoto T, Takafuji S, Suzuki S, Tadokoro A, Muranaka A. Allergy and changing environments—industrial/urban pollution. In: Pichler W, Staedler B, Dakindeu C, et al, eds. Progress in Allergy and Clinical Immunology. Toronto: Hay Refe & Huber, 1988: 265–270.
22. Rakes GP, Arruda E, Ingram JM, Hoover GE, Hayden FG, Platts-Mills TAE, Heymann PW. Human rhinovirus in wheezing children: relationship to serum IgE and nasal eosinophil cationic protein. J Allergy Clin Immunol 1995; 95:260.
23. Johnston SL, Pattemore PK, Sanderson G, Smith S, Lampe F, Josephs L, Symington P, O'Toole S, Myint SH, Tyrrel DAJ, Holgate ST. Community study of role of viral infections in exacerbations of asthma in 9–11 year old children. Br Med J 1995; 310:1225–1229.
24. Strachan DP, Harkins LS, Johnston ID, Anderson HR. Childhood antecedents of allergic sensitization in young British adults. J Allergy Clin Immunol 1997; 99:6–12.
25. Von Mutius E, Martinez FD, Fritzsch C, Nicolai T, Reitmeir P, Thurmann HH. Skin test reactivity and number of siblings. Br Med J 1994; 308:692–695.
26. Holgate ST, Hardy CC, Robinson C, Aguis RM, Howarth PH. The mast cell as a primary effector in asthma. J Allergy Clin Immunol 1986; 77:274–282.
27. Metzger WJ, Zavala D, Richerson HB, Mosely P, Iwamota P, Monick M, Sjoerdsma K, Hunninghake GW. Local allergen challenge and bronchoalveolar lavage of allergic lungs: description of the model and local airway inflammation. Am Rev Respir Dis 1987; 135:433–440.
28. Cockcroft DW, Ruffin RB, Dolovich J, Hargreave FE. Allergen-induced increase in nonallergic bronchial reactivity. Clin Allergy 1977; 7:503–513.
29. Altounyan RE. Changes in histamine and atropine responsiveness as a guide to diagnosis and evaluation of therapy in obstructive airways disease. In: Pepys J, Frankland AW, eds. Disodium Chromoglycate in Allergic Airways Disease. London: Butterworth, 1970: 47–53.
30. Robinson DS, Hamid Q, Ying S, Tsicopoulos A, Barkans J, Bentley AM, Corrigan C, Durham S, Kay AB. Predominant TH2-like bronchoalveolar T-lymphocyte population in atopic asthma. N Engl J Med 1992; 326:298–304.
31. Calhoun WJ, Dick EC, Schwartz LB, Busse WW. A common cold virus, rhinovirus 16, potentiates airway inflammation after segmental antigen bronchoprovocation in allergic subjects. J Clin Invest 1994; 94:2200–2208.
32. Till S, Li B, Durham S, Humbert M, Assoufi B, Huston D, Dickason R, Jeannin P, Kay AB, Corrigon C. Secretion of the eosinophil-active cytokines interleukin-5, granulocyte/macrophage colony-stimulating factor and interleukin-3 by bronchoalveolar lavage $CD4^+$ and $CD8^+$ T cell lines in atopic asthmatics, and atopic and non-atopic controls. Eur J Immunol 1995; 25:2727–2731.
33. Ward GW, Hayden ML, Rose G, Call RS, Platts-Mills TAE. *Trichophyton* asthma: response to oral antifungal therapy with fluconazole. J Allergy Clin Immunol 1993; 91:226.
34. Selroos O, Peitinalho A, Lofroos AB, Riska H. Effect of early vs late intervention with inhaled corticosteroids in asthma. Chest 1995; 108:1228–1234.
35. Kerrebijn KF. Endogenous factors in childhood CNSLD: methodological aspects in population studies. In: Orie NGM, van der Lende R, eds. Bronchitis III. The Netherlands: Royal Vangorcum Assen, 1970: 38–48.

36. Simon HU, Grotzer M, Nikolaizik WH, Blaser K, Schouni MH. High altitude climate therapy reduces peripheral blood T lymphocyte activation, eosinophilia, on bronchial obstruction in children with house-dust mite allergic asthma. Pediatr Pulmonol 1994; 17: 304–311.
37. Hill DJ, Thompson PJ, Stewart GA, Corlin JB, Nolan TM, Kemp AS, Hosking CS. The Melbourne House dust mite study: eliminating house dust mites in the domestic environment. J Allergy Clin Immunol 1997; 99:323–329.
38. Ehnert B, Lau-Schadendorf S, Weber A, Buettner P, Schou C, Wahn U. Reducing domestic exposure to dust mite allergen reduces bronchial hyperreactivity in sensitive children with asthma. J Allergy Clin Immunol 1992; 90:135–138.
39. Wood RA, Flanagan E, Van Natta M, Chen PH, Eggleston PA. The effect of a HEPA room air cleaner on cat-induced asthma and rhinitis. J Allergy Clin Immunol 1997; 99:S388.
40. Bjornsdottir US, Jakobinudottir S, Runarsdottir V, Blondal TH, Juliusson S. Environmental control with cat in situ, reduces cat allergen (Fel d I) in house dust samples—but does it alter clinical symptoms? J Allergy Clin Immunol 1997; 99:S389.
41. Norman PS. An overview of immunotherapy: implications for the future [review]. J Allergy Clin Immunol 1980; 65:87–96.
42. Lockey RF, Benedict IM, Turkeltaub PC, Bukantz SC. Fatalities from immunotherapy (IT) and skin testing (ST). J Allergy Clin Immunol 1987; 79:660–677.

4

Inflammation and Airway Remodeling in Asthma

JEAN BOUSQUET and PHILIPPE GODARD

Montpellier University and
Service des Maladies Respiratoires–INSERM U454
Montpellier University Hospital
Montpellier, France

ANTONIO M. VIGNOLA

Institute of Respiratory Physiopathology
Consiglio Nazionale delle Ricerche
Palermo, Italy

PASCAL CHANEZ

Service des Maladies Respiratoires–INSERM U454
Montpellier University Hospital
Montpellier, France

I. Introduction

Inflammation was recognized in asthma several decades ago (1), but it is within the past 15 years that it became the major pathological mechanism of asthma. The understanding of the pathophysiology of asthma has been improved by the pathological examination of bronchi in living asthmatics, made easily available by fiberoptic bronchoscopy, and the information obtained has been considerably enhanced by using electron microscopy and immunohistochemistry techniques, and, more recently, those of molecular biology. Thus, by combining results of bronchoalveolar lavage (BAL) and biopsies, it is possible to better examine the inflammation and the remodeling of the bronchi. However, in 1997, our knowledge is mostly targeted toward the deleterious effects of inflammatory cells, and very little is known about their contributory role in the processes of healing following inflammation.

Inflammation can be demonstrated in allergic (2), nonallergic (3), and occupational asthma (4). Chronic inflammation may be acutely increased by exposure to allergens, pollutants (5,6), or a virus infection (7,8).

II. Origin and Site of Inflammatory Cells in the Airways

A. Cell Recruitment and Survival in the Airways

The inflammatory cells pertinent to airway inflammation are generated in the bone marrow. They then transit through the circulation and migrate rapidly into tissues. The recruitment of peripheral blood cells, including eosinophils, lymphocytes, and monocytes, into inflamed airways results from adhesive interactions between blood and endothelial cells within the microcirculation. Endothelial cells have a major role in inflammatory cell recruitment into the airway submucosa (9–11). This mechanism appears to be of great importance because replication of inflammatory cells in the airways of asthmatics has not yet been confirmed (12,13). The nature and magnitude of leukocyte–endothelial cell adhesion are determined by several factors, among which expression of adhesion molecules on leukocytes play a key role. Rolling along the vessel wall is the first step of the cell recruitment process and is mediated by selectin molecules (14,15). Firm adherence of cells to endothelium is the second step and involves other adhesion molecules such as CD11a, CD11b, CD18, or very late activation antigen (VLA)-4 on blood cells and intracellular adhesion molecule (ICAM)-1 or vascular cell adhesion molecule (VCAM-1) on endothelial cells (9,14,16,17).

Recruitment of cells into the airways is also dependent on cytokines, such as interleukin (IL)-5 (18) and granulocyte–macrophage colony-stimulating factor (GM–CSF) acting on eosinophil recruitment, maturation (19), and increased survival (20). Chemokines such as RANTES also act on eosinophils for enhanced recruitment and activation (21). Once at the site of the airway inflammation, cells are activated, and their survival is increased by a reduced apoptosis, in which GM-CSF is of importance (22), and by the expression of adhesion molecules (23).

B. Site of the Inflammation in Asthma

The bronchial tree is not the only target organ presenting an inflammatory pattern. The whole mucosal immune system appears to be involved in bronchial asthma. Although devoid of gastrointestinal symptoms, asthmatics and asymptomatic asthmatics have duodenal pathological abnormalities mimicking those observed in the bronchial mucosa (24) and an increased intestinal permeability (25). Histological abnormalities have also been observed in a minor salivary gland in patients with bronchial asthma. The main pathological features were T-lymphocyte infiltration, partly degranulated mast cells, basement membrane thickening, and endothelial cell changes (26). The reasons for the preferential involvement of the airways in asthma is not unknown, but it may be related to allergen exposure. Only minute amounts of aeroallergens are inhaled, and they can directly activate mast cells and FcεRI-bearing cells in the airways, leading to a cascade of the inflammatory reaction. On the other hand, aeroallergens may be destroyed by digestive enzymes or such amounts cannot activate cells present in the digestive tract. Thus, only food allergy can trigger asthma (27), whereas some components of inflammation can be detected without inducing symptoms in inhalant allergy.

In the bronchial tree, the site of the airway inflammation is still a matter of controversy. It is accepted that both central and peripheral airways present inflammation, but a recent report focused on the importance of lower airway inflammation (28), whereas two other studies showed that inflammation was no more prominent in the peripheral than in the central airways (29,30). Differences between these studies may relate to the sampling procedure, because Kraft et al. (28) used transbronchial biopsies, whereas the two latter ones (29,30) studied excised lung specimens. The site of the airway inflammation is of importance for the optimal target delivery of anti-inflammatory drugs.

Postmortem studies, as well as transbronchial biopsies studies, showed that the peribronchial tissue as well as the alveoli may be involved in the lung inflammation in asthmatics (28).

III. Epithelium

For many years epithelial cells were considered to have the simple role of a barrier participating in mucous secretion and removal of noxious agents by their cilia. More recently, these cells were found to have a much broader activity.

In patients who died of an asthma attack, bronchial epithelium is mostly shed with separation of the mucosal cells, leaving an intact basal cell layer (31). Changes in the epithelium have been found almost constantly in living asthmatic patients, but more often in patients with moderate to severe asthma than in those with mild disease (32). Epithelial cells recovered by brushing are significantly less viable in asthmatics than in normal subjects. The loss of the bronchial epithelium layer produces a denudation of nerves and mast cells, as shown by electron microscopy. The consequences of epithelial shedding are likely to be important. Epithelial shedding and epithelial damage, characterized by an increase in intracellular space, have been correlated with bronchial hyperreactivity (33).

Bronchial epithelial cells are activated in asthma, as shown by the increased expression of membrane markers, such as ICAM-1 or HLA-DR (23,34), and an increased spontaneous release of proinflammatory mediators (35). Epithelial cells obtained by bronchial brushing were shown to release a greater amount of 15-hydroxyeicosatetraenoic (HETE) acid and prostaglandin (PG)E_2. Endothelin-1 influences the airway caliber, and endothelial expression was found in the epithelium of the airways of asthmatics, but not in normal subjects (36). Moreover, endothelin-1 release was observed by stimulation of the low- and high-affinity receptor for IgE (FcεRI and FcεRII) (37). These findings may partly explain the increased bronchial tone of the asthmatic airways.

Regenerative changes are sometimes observed, as demonstrated by varying stages of ciliogenesis in the nonciliated "metaplastic" surface epithelium. Bronchial mucosal injury initiates a complex series of repair mechanisms, one of which is the reepithelization of a denuded luminal surface, but the regeneration of epithelium in asthma is usually normal, in contradistinction to other bronchial inflammatory diseases, such as chronic bronchitis. In asthma, epithelial cells do not appear to present an increased proliferative rate, but have an increased expression of c-*fos*, a protooncogene regulating the transcription of many genes that play a critical role in cell differentiation (38). It is likely that bronchial epithelial cells initially affected by bronchial injury may be able to initiate repair of an injured area by producing chemotactic factors for epithelial cells and adhesion molecules, such as fibronectin (37).

Epithelial cells can be activated through different mechanisms. It has been recently observed that epithelial cells of asthmatics, but not those of normal subjects, bear the FcεRI and FcεRII receptors (37) and that they can be directly activated by anti-IgE. Therefore, it is possible that cells can be directly triggered by allergens. Pollutants including NO_2 and ozone can activate bronchial epithelial cells (39). Finally, indirect mechanisms have been demonstrated. Also, viruses can directly damage epithelial cells. Histamine (40), platelet-activating factor (PAF), or cytokines can activate bronchial epithelial cells. Other mediators, such as cysteinyl leukotrienes enhance growth of bronchial epithelial cells in vitro.

Epithelial cells bear class II antigens (34), and studies in normal individuals have suggested that they can present antigen to lymphocytes (41). In asthma, studies of cells obtained by brushing or by biopsies have shown that there is an increased expression of class II antigens, but data are lacking to determine whether the presentation of antigen is enhanced.

IV. Submucosal Infiltrate

The bronchial submucosa often shows edema, blood vessel dilation, and a mixed cell infiltrate. These inflammatory cells include eosinophils, mast cells, and mononuclear cells, but in some patients, the infiltrate cannot be found by hematoxylin and eosin (H&E) staining, because the cells may be completely degranulated and can be seen only by immunohistochemistry or electron microscopy.

A. Eosinophils

In acute asthma, eosinophils are activated. During allergen challenge, there is an increase in eosinophil numbers and in levels of their proteins in the BAL fluid. In chronic asthma, eosinophils have been found in increased numbers in bronchial biopsies (42). These cells are usually located beneath the basement membrane and are in an activated stage. Most allergic and nonallergic asthmatics, including those with mild asthma, have eosinophils in their bronchi, and there is a significant correlation between the activation of eosinophils and the severity of the asthma (42). Bronchial eosinophilia, however, is not a characteristic of asthma, for eosinophils can be observed in many diseases, including chronic bronchitis (43).

Eosinophils appear to play a major deleterious role in asthma by the release of highly toxic products (major basic protein [MBP], eosinophil cationic protein [ECP], eosinophil-derived neurotoxin [EDN], oxygen free radicals), inducing the shedding of the epithelium, and thereby confirming the hypotheses of eosinophil-induced damage of the bronchi (44,45). However, other mechanisms are required for epithelial shedding because, in rhinitis, eosinophils can be found degranulated in the epithelium without any shedding. Eosinophils also release cysteinyl leukotrienes possessing vasoactive properties, cytokines (46), and growth factors (47); but their role in the regulation of airway inflammation and of tissue remodeling is still poorly understood.

B. Lymphocytes

T lymphocytes represent another major cell type of the mixed cell infiltrate present in the airways of patients who died of an asthma exacerbation or in asthmatics of variable etiology (48). They often bear CD4 receptors, whereas CD8-positive cells are more rarely identified. There is a correlation between the severity of asthma and the number of CD4-positive cells in biopsies. In acute asthma, an increase in cells bearing IL-2 receptors was observed, indicating that they are in an activated stage. However, T cells are also present in the airway inflammatory infiltrate of chronic bronchitis patients (49). On the other hand, very few B cells are present in the bronchi of asthmatics.

T cells are likely to play an important role in asthma. When using in situ hybridization technique, a T helper cell type 2 (Th2)-phenotype of T cells has been observed in the BAL fluid of asthmatics. In bronchial biopsies or BAL fluid after allergen challenge, many allergen-specific T cells bear the Th2 phenotype (48,50), whereas in chronic asthmatics in whom cells have been removed without allergen challenge, T cells are more of the Th0 or Th1 phenotype (51). Differences between allergic and nonallergic asthma have been observed in the BAL fluid. In the allergic form of the disease IL-4, IFN-γ, and IL-5 are measurable, whereas in the nonallergic form IL-2, IFN-γ, and IL-5 are found (52). Therefore, it seems likely that T cells may be responsible for initiating and possibly maintaining chronic inflammation of allergic and nonallergic origin.

C. Macrophages

Mononuclear phagocytes have a fundamental role in specific immunity by their accessory cell function, and they are metabolic cells that play a major role in chronic inflammation. The presence of activated macrophages in alveolar and bronchial tissues in asthma is a hallmark of chronic inflammation. Activated macrophages have the potential to secrete a wide variety of products, many of which are active in inflammation and play a major role in the pathogenesis of injury and repair. Macrophages can synthetize and secrete elastase and a group of metalloproteases, that have the capacity to degrade various extracellular matrix (EDM) macromolecules, including elastin. Macrophages may also be involved in the regulation of the airway inflammation through the secretion of cytokines, and growth factors. In interstitial lung diseases, alveolar macrophages (AM) are activated and release cytokines, plasminogen activator, and a fibrinolytic inhibitor, as well as macrophage inflammatory protein-1a (MIP-1a).

Bronchoalveolar macrophages (AM) recovered by BAL have been extensively studied and found to be hyperactive in asthma (53). The AM from asthmatics are hypodense by comparison with those of normal subjects and their level of activation is significantly correlated with the severity of asthma (54). Segmental allergen challenge induces a rapid activation of AM (55). Immunohistochemistry with different monoclonal antibodies and electron microscopy (34) showed increased numbers of macrophages, often presenting activation patterns, and the phenotype of the blood monocytes suggested that they were recently recruited.

The activation and regulation of airway macrophages in asthma needs further investigation. Mononuclear phagocytic cells possess low-affinity receptors for IgE (FcεRII or CD23) and AM can be activated by an IgE-mediated mechanism (56). Airway macrophages appear to be in an activated stage and may release enzymes, eicosanoids, platelet-activating factor (PAF), oxygen free radicals, and cytokines that might be deleterious for the bronchi. They can also synthetize and secrete a group of metalloproteases that have the capacity to degrade various ECM macromolecules, including elastin. Macrophages may also be involved in the regulation of the airway inflammation through the secretion of cytokines and growth factors, such as transforming growth factor-beta (TGF-β; 57,58), and in the priming of mast cell or eosinophil secretory processes (59). Finally, macrophages modulate the immune response (60,61). Thus, the macrophage might well be the key cell in bronchial inflammation and repair.

D. Metachromatic Cells

Mast cells have been found in the bronchi of normal subjects and asthmatic patients (62). They are activated both in allergic and nonallergic asthma, as suggested by the presence of increased levels of tryptase, histamine, and PGD_2 in the BAL fluid, as shown by electron microscopy and immunocytochemistry. However, a significant correlation between the severity of asthma and histamine or tryptase levels in the BAL fluid has only rarely been observed. Besides histamine and PGD_2, mast cells can release neutral proteases, including tryptase, and cytokines that may amplify the vasoactive phase of the allergic inflammation (63) as well as attract inflammatory cells. Mast cells appear to be critical during acute asthma episodes, and the release of histamine and other vasoactive mediators elicits acute bronchoconstriction, edema, and secretion of mucus. However, the role of mast cells is not confined to acute asthma because they also release Th2-like cytokines (64).

Basophils are probably important cells of the late-phase reaction following allergen challenge (65), but their role in asthma is still far from being confirmed. Basophils are also able to release Th2 cytokines.

The regulation of IgE production by metachromatic cells has been proposed. Isolated mast cells and basophils can be induced to express CD40L, and IgE synthesis can be induced by the interaction of B cells with mast cells in the presence of exogenous IL-4, whereas basophil-mediated IgE synthesis can take place even in the absence of exogenous IL-4 or IL-13 (66). Although in vivo evidence is still lacking, these results suggest that mast cells and basophils can induce the induction of IgE, independently of T cells, which is emphasized by the capacity of these cells to produce IL-4 (64,67).

E. Other Cell Types

Polymorphonuclear neutrophils may be involved in acute asthma (68), in nocturnal asthma (69), and in some patients with long-standing or corticosteroid-dependent asthma (70).

The importance of *platelets* in asthma still remains to be confirmed, although they are activated in aspirin-induced asthma (71).

V. Importance of Inflammation in Asthma

Inflammation can be demonstrated in allergic (2), nonallergic (3), occupational (4,72–74), and aspirin-induced asthma (75–77) The profile of inflammatory cells and cytokine gene expression appears to be similar in allergic and nonallergic asthma, although the presence or absence of IL-4 protein has been debated in the nonallergic form (3,78–80). Chronic inflammation may be sharply increased by exposure to allergens (81), pollutants (5,6), or a virus infection (7,8).

Inflammation occurs early in the course of the disease (82), in patients with mild intermittent asthma (Bousquet, J; unpublished data), and during remissions (83). The severity of asthma is correlated with many inflammatory indices, such as epithelial denudation (33) and activation (23,35,38), eosinophil number and activation (42,84,85), T-cell activation (3), or cytokine expression (86).

In nocturnal asthma, several studies have shown an increase in airway eosinophil and neutrophil numbers (69,87,88), and superoxide (89) and cytokine levels (90), as well as lymphocyte and macrophage activation (91) when bronchoscopy with BAL or mucosal biopsies were performed during the night. Histamine (92,93) and ECP levels (94) are increased in the peripheral blood during the night. These findings are important because asthma is an inflammatory process that worsens at night in some patients (95,96). However, other mechanisms may also be responsible for nocturnal asthma. The Gly-16 polymorphism of the β_2-adrenergic receptor (AR), which imparts an enhanced downregulation of receptor number, is overrepresented in nocturnal asthma and appears to be an important genetic factor in the expression of this asthmatic phenotype (97).

VI. Airway Remodeling

Inflammation is a beneficial, nonspecific response of tissues to injury, generally leading to repair. Asthma is a chronic inflammatory disease of the airways, the evolution of which follows the natural course of inflammation. It is invariably associated with healing, which begins very early in the inflammation process and results in repair and the replacement of dead or damaged cells by viable cells. Repair usually involves two distinct processes: regeneration, which is the replacement of injured tissue by parenchymal cells of the same type; and replacement by connective tissue and its eventual maturation into scar tissue. In many instances both processes contribute to the healing response, and inflammation in asthma can be followed by a wide variety of consequences, from complete or partial restitution of airways structure and function to fibrosis (98).

A. Cellular and Molecular Criteria of Airway Remodeling in Asthma

Several criteria have been proposed for the repair processes: (1) activation of macrophages, (2) release of growth factors and fibrogenic cytokines, (3) activation of fibroblasts and myofibroblasts, (4) elastolysis and elastosynthesis, (5) increased collagen synthesis, (6) deposition of collagen, and (7) increased synthesis and release of ECM components.

Connective tissue cells produce and secrete an array of macromolecules forming a complex network filling the extracellular space of the submoca, called the ECM. The macromolecules that constitute the ECM are secreted locally by all cells present. The composition of the secreted matrix depends on the cell types, their state of differentiation, and their metabolic status. The molecules that compose the ECM consist of fibrous proteins (collagen and elastin), structural or adhesive proteins (fibronectin and laminin) embedded in a hydrated polysaccharide gel that contains several glycosaminoglycans, including hyaluronic acid (HA). The glucosaminoglycans, proteoglycans, and structural proteins trap water molecules to form a highly hydrated gel-like “ground substance” in which the insoluble fibrous proteins are embedded, giving the matrix strength, rigidity, and resilience. Until recently, the ECM was thought to be an inert scaffolding having a mechanical role in supporting and maintaining tissue structure. However, it has been recently shown that ECM also modulates a multitude of cell functions, such as development, migration, and proliferation. The ECM abnormalities in asthma are still poorly understood, but may be of major importance.

There is pseudothickening of the basement membrane from collagen, fibronectin, and laminin deposition (99). The size of the basement membrane has been correlated with the number of myofibroblasts present beneath it (100) and the number of TGF-β-positive cells (Vignola AM, et al., unpublished data).

Superficial elastic fibers of the airways are fragmented. In the deeper layer, fibers are often patchy, tangled, and thickened, suggesting that fibers from asthmatics have the appearance of solar elastolysis in skin (101).

Fibronectin, laminin, and tenascin (102) deposition in the submucosa was found in the biopsies of asthmatics, but not in those of normal subjects. Hyaluronic acid is also increased in the airways of asthmatics, as shown by its levels in the BAL fluid (103).

Growth factors, such as TGF-β, are increased in asthma epithelium, and its expression is correlated with the fibroblast number and the thickness of the basement membrane (104). On the other hand, platelet-derived growth factor (PDGF) does not seem to be increased in asthma (105).

B. Hypertrophy and Hyperplasia of Airway Smooth Muscle

Smooth muscle mass is usually increased in large and small airways in both fatal and nonfatal cases of asthma (106–110). This increase in muscle mass is usually not seen in chronic bronchitis and chronic obstructive pulmonary disease (COPD), although some studies have found an increase (107,108). There is a three- to four-fold increase in muscle volume in asthmatic airways by comparison with normal subjects (111). In some patients the muscle may occupy up to 20% of the bronchial wall (106). However, whereas Dunnill et al. (106) reported an increase in smooth muscle in the major bronchi of asthmatic subjects, others (109,110) showed that increased smooth-muscle thickness was also present in the peripheral airways. However, the importance of these findings are not completely clear because a study in asthmatic patients who died of other causes did not reveal any hyperplasy or hypertrophy (112). More recent studies pointed out some degree of heterogeneity of the smooth-muscle thickening (113,114). They morphometrically studied cross sections of the airways taken from the segmental bronchi to the terminal bronchioles. In most patients, muscle hypertrophy was most pronounced in larger bronchi, but some patients had hypertrophy involving the entire range of the airways, including bronchioles. There may be some heterogeneity in the smooth muscle distribution in the airways of asthmatics, and the increased thickness is primarily due to hyperplasia, rather than smooth muscle hypertrophy (108).

C. Increase in Mucous Glands

Mucous glands are distributed throughout the airways in asthma and are even present in peripheral bronchioles where normally they are absent. The mucous glands in the segmental bronchi of asthmatics are considerably enlarged, and Dunnill et al. (106) showed that in asthmatics their volume was twice that of normal subjects. These values overlap those found in chronic bronchitis. However, in asthma, hypertrophy of mucous glands appears to be the cause of increased volume, whereas hyperplasia of the mucus-secreting cells is usually observed in chronic bronchitis. The hypercriny measured by the Reid index is a feature of chronic bronchitis, but is inconstantly found in asthma. Pathological changes in bronchi caused by smoking (115–117) show enlargement of the submucosal glands, with dilation of their ducts and moderate infiltration with neutrophils and lymphocytes.

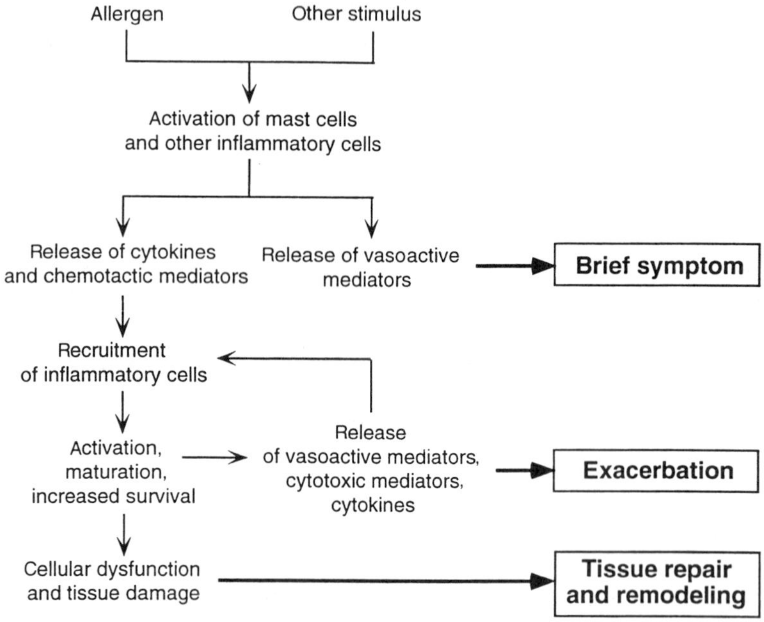

Figure 1 Acute and chronic inflammation in asthma.

VII. Conclusions

Asthma is a chronic inflammatory disease of the airways involving the activation of many different cell types. A process of healing and repair follows inflammation, and this leads to a variable degree of remodeling of the airways (Fig. 1).

References

1. Huber H, Koessler K. The pathology of bronchial asthma. Arch Intern Med 1922; 30:689–696.
2. Bradley BL, Azzawi M, Jacobson M, et al. Eosinophils, T-lymphocytes, mast cells, neutrophils, and macrophages in bronchial biopsy specimens from atopic subjects with asthma: comparison with biopsy specimens from atopic subjects without asthma and normal control subjects and relationship to bronchial hyperresponsiveness. J Allergy Clin Immunol 1991; 88:661–674.
3. Bentley AM, Menz G, Storz C, et al. Identification of T lymphocytes, macrophages, and activated eosinophils in the bronchial mucosa in intrinsic asthma. Relationship to symptoms and bronchial responsiveness. Am Rev Respir Dis 1992; 146:500–506.
4. Saetta M, Di-Stefano A, Maestrelli P, et al. Airway mucosal inflammation in occupational asthma induced by toluene diisocyanate. Am Rev Respir Dis 1992; 145:160–168.
5. Devalia JL, Rusznak C, Herdman MJ, Trigg CJ, Tarraf H, Davies RJ. Effect of nitrogen dioxide and sulphur dioxide on airway response of mild asthmatic patients to allergen inhalation. Lancet 1994; 344:1668–1671.

6. Arsalane K, Gosset P, Vanhée D, Voisin C, Tonnel A. Ozone stimulates synthesis of inflammatory cytokines by alveolar macrophages in vitro. Am J Respir Cell Mol Biol 1995; 1995; 13(1):60–68.
7. Fraenkel DJ, Bardin PG, Sanderson G, Lampe F, Johnston SL, Holgate ST. Lower airways inflammation during rhinovirus colds in normal and in asthmatic subjects. Am J Respir Crit Care Med 1995; 151:879–886.
8. Busse WW. The role of respiratory infections in airway hyperresponsiveness and asthma. Am J Respir Crit Care Med 1994; 150:S77–S79.
9. Georas SN, Liu MC, Newman W, Beall LD, Stealey BA, Bochner BS. Altered adhesion molecular expression and endothelial cell activation accompany the recruitment of human granulocytes to the lung after segmental antigen challenge. Am J Respir Cell Mol Biol 1992; 7:261–269.
10. Montefort S, Roche WR, Howarth PH, et al. Intercellular adhesion molecule-1 (ICAM)-1 and endothelial leucocyte adhesion molecule-1 (ELAM-1) expression in the bronchial mucosa of normal and asthmatic subjects. Eur Respir J 1992; 5:815–823.
11. Tonnel AB, Lassalle P, Delneste Y. Role of endothelial cells in the pathogenesis of bronchial asthma. Ann Allergy 1993; 71:306–311.
12. Chanez P, Vago P, Demoly P, et al. Airway macrophages from patients with asthma do not proliferate. J Allergy Clin Immunol 1993; 92:869–877.
13. Demoly P, Simony-Lafontaine J, Chanez P, et al. Cell proliferation in the bronchial mucosa of asthmatics and chronic bronchitics. Am J Respir Crit Care Med 1994; 150:214–217.
14. Granger DN, Kubes P. The microcirculation and inflammation: modulation of leukocyte–endothelial cell adhesion. J Leukoc Biol 1994; 55:662–675.
15. Tedder TF, Steeber DA, Chen A, Engel P. The selectins: vascular adhesion molecules. FASEB J 1995; 9:866–873.
16. Weller PF, Rand TH, Golez SE, Chi-Rosso G, Lobb RR. Human eosinophil adherence to vascular endothelium mediated by binding to vascular cell adhesion molecule 1 and endothelial leukocyte adhesion molecule 1. Proc Natl Acad Sci USA 1991; 88:7430–7433.
17. Bochner B, Schleimer R. The role of adhesion molecules in human eosinophil and basophil recruitment. J Allergy Clin Immunol 1994; 94:427–439.
18. Sur S, Kita H, Gleich GJ, Chenier TC, Hunt LW. Eosinophil recruitment is associated with IL-5, but not with RANTES, twenty-four hours after allergen challenge. J Allergy Clin Immunol 1996; 97:1272–1278.
19. Lopez AF, Sanderson CJ, Gamble JR, Campbell HD, Young IG, Vadas MA. Recombinant human interleukin 5 is a selective activator of human eosinophil function. J Exp Med 1988; 167:219–224.
20. Yamaguchi Y, Hayashi Y, Sugama Y, et al. Highly purified murine interleukin 5 (IL-5) stimulates eosinophil function and prolongs in vitro survival. IL-5 as an eosinophil chemotactic factor. J Exp Med 1988; 167:1737–1742.
21. Alam R, Stafford S, Forsythe P, et al. RANTES is a chemotactic and activating factor for human eosinophils. J Immunol 1993; 150:3442–3448.
22. Simon HU, Blaser K. Inhibition of programmed eosinophil death: a key pathogenic event for eosinophilia? Immunol Today 1995; 16:53–55.
23. Vignola AM, Campbell AM, Chanez P, et al. HLA-DR and ICAM-1 expression on bronchial epithelial cells in asthma and chronic bronchitis. Am Rev Respir Dis 1993; 148:689–694.
24. Wallaert B, Desreumaux P, Copin MC, et al. Immunoreactivity for interleukin 3 and 5 and granulocyte/macrophage colony-stimulating factor of intestinal mucosa in bronchial asthma. J Exp Med 1995; 182:1897–1904.
25. Benard A, Desreumeaux P, Huglo D, Hoorelbeke A, Tonnel AB, Wallaert B. Increased intestinal permeability in bronchial asthma. J Allergy Clin Immunol 1996; 97:1173–1178.
26. Wallaert B, Janin A, Lassalle P, et al. Airway-like inflammation of minor salivary gland in bronchial asthma. Am J Respir Crit Care Med 1994; 150:802–809.

27. Onorato J, Merland N, Terral C, Michel FB, Bousquet J. Placebo-controlled double-blind food challenge in asthma. J Allergy Clin Immunol 1986; 78:1139–1146.
28. Kraft M, Djukanovic R, Wilson S, Holgate S, Martin R. Alveolar tissue inflammation in asthma. Am J Respir Crit Care Med 1996; 154:1505–1511.
29. Carroll N, Cooke C, James A. The distribution of eosinophils and lymphocytes in the large and small airways of asthmatics. Eur Respir J 1997; 10:292–300.
30. Faul J, Thorney V, Leonard C, et al. The distribution of eosinophils and lymphocytes in the large and small airways of asthmatics. Eur Respir J 1997; 10:301–308.
31. Jeffery PK. Pathology of asthma. Br Med Bull 1992; 48:23–39.
32. Laitinen A, Partanen M, Hervonen A, Laitinen LA. Electron microscopic study on the innervation of the human lower respiratory tract: evidence of adrenergic nerves. Eur J Respir Dis 1985; 67:209–215.
33. Jeffery PK, Wardlaw AJ, Nelson FC, Collins JV, Kay AB. Bronchial biopsies in asthma. An ultrastructural, quantitative study and correlation with hyperreactivity. Am Rev Respir Dis 1989; 140:1745–1753.
34. Poston RN, Chanez P, Lacoste JY, Litchfield T, Lee TH, Bousquet J. Immunohistochemical characterization of the cellular infiltration in asthmatic bronchitis. Am Rev Respir Dis 1992; 145:918–921.
35. Campbell AM, Chanez P, Vignola AM, et al. Functional characteristics of bronchial epithelium obtained by brushing from asthmatic and normal subjects. Am Rev Respir Dis 1993; 147:529–534.
36. Springall DR, Howarth PH, Counihan H, Djukanovic R, Holgate ST, Polak JM. Endothelin immunoreactivity of airway epithelium in asthmatic patients. Lancet 1991; 337:697–701.
37. Campbell AM, Vignola AM, Chanez P, Godard P, Bousquet J. Low-affinity receptor for IgE on human bronchial epithelial cells in asthma. Immunology 1994; 82:506–508.
38. Demoly P, Basset-Seguin N, Chanez P, et al. c-*fos* proto-oncogene expression in bronchial biopsies of asthmatics. Am J Respir Cell Mol Biol 1992; 7:128–133.
39. Devalia JL, Campbell AM, Sapsford RJ, et al. Effect of nitrogen dioxide on synthesis of inflammatory cytokines expressed by human bronchial epithelial cells in vitro. Am J Respir Cell Mol Biol 1993; 9:271–278.
40. Vignola AM, Campbell AM, Chanez P, et al. Activation by histamine of bronchial epithelial cells from nonasthmatic subjects. Am J Respir Cell Mol Biol 1993; 9:411–417.
41. Rossi GA, Sacco O, Balbi B, et al. Human ciliated bronchial epithelial cells: expression of the HLA-DR antigens and of the HLA-DR alpha gene, modulation of the HLA-DR antigens by gamma-interferon and antigen-presenting function in the mixed leukocyte reaction. Am J Respir Cell Mol Biol 1990; 3:431–439.
42. Bousquet J, Chanez P, Lacoste JY, et al. Eosinophilic inflammation in asthma. N Engl J Med 1990; 323:1033–1039.
43. Lacoste JY, Bousquet J, Chanez P, et al. Eosinophilic and neutrophilic inflammation in asthma, chronic bronchitis, and chronic obstructive pulmonary disease. J Allergy Clin Immunol 1993; 92:537–548.
44. Gleich GJ, Adolphson CR, Leiferman KC. The biology of the eosinophilic leukocyte. Annu Rev Med 1993; 44:85–101.
45. Busse WW, Coffman RL, Gelfand EW, Kay AB, Rosenwasser LJ. Mechanisms of persistent airway inflammation in asthma. A role for T cells and T-cell products. Am J Respir Crit Care Med 1995; 152:388–393.
46. Broide DH, Paine MM, Firestein GS. Eosinophils express interleukin 5 and granulocyte–macrophage colony-stimulating factor mRNA at sites of allergic inflammation in asthmatics. J Clin Invest 1992; 90:1414–1424.
47. Ohno I, Nitta Y, Yamauchi K, et al. Eosinophils as a potential source of platelet-derived growth factor β-chain (PDGF-β) in nasal polyposis and bronchial asthma. Am J Respir Cell Mol Biol 1995; 13:639–647.
48. Corrigan CJ, Kay AB. Asthma. Role of T-lymphocytes and lymphokines. Br Med Bull 1992; 48:72–84.

49. Saetta M, Di-Stefano A, Maestrelli P, et al. Activated T-lymphocytes and macrophages in bronchial mucosa of subjects with chronic bronchitis. Am Rev Respir Dis 1993; 147:301–306.
50. Robinson DS, Hamid Q, Jacobson M, Ying S, Kay AB, Durham SR. Evidence for Th2-type T helper cell control of allergic disease in vivo. Springer Semin Immunopathol 1993; 15:17–27.
51. Pene J, Lagier B, Rivier A, Chanez P, Vendrell JP, Bousquet J. Phenotype of T cell clones obtained from bronchial biopsies and peripheral blood from three asthmatics. Cell Biol Int 1993; 17:353–357.
52. Walker C, Bode E, Boer L, Hansel TT, Blaser K, Virchow J Jr. Allergic and nonallergic asthmatics have distinct patterns of T-cell activation and cytokine production in peripheral blood and bronchoalveolar lavage. Am Rev Respir Dis 1992; 146:109–115.
53. Godard P, Chaintreuil J, Damon M, et al. Functional assessment of alveolar macrophages: comparison of cells from asthmatics and normal subjects. J Allergy Clin Immunol 1982; 70:88–93.
54. Cluzel M, Damon M, Chanez P, et al. Enhanced alveolar cell luminol-dependent chemiluminescence in asthma. J Allergy Clin Immunol 1987; 80:195–201.
55. Tonnel AB, Joseph M, Gosset P, Fournier E, Capron A. Stimulation of alveolar macrophages in asthmatic patients after local provocation test. Lancet 1983; 1:1406–1408.
56. Joseph M, Tonnel AB, Torpier G, Capron A, Arnoux B, Benveniste J. Involvement of immunoglobulin E in the secretory processes of alveolar macrophages from asthmatic patients. J Clin Invest 1983; 71:221–230.
57. Vignola A, Chanez P, Chiappara G, et al. Transforming growth factor-β expression in mucosal biopsies in asthma and chronic bronchitis. Am J Respir Crit Care Med 1997; 156:591–599.
58. Vignola AM, Chanez P, Chiappara G, et al. Release of transforming growth factor-beta (TGF-beta) and fibronectin by alveolar macrophages in airway diseases. Clin Exp Immunol 1996; 106:114–119.
59. Howell CJ, Pujol JL, Crea AE, et al. Identification of an alveolar macrophage-derived activity in bronchial asthma that enhances leukotriene C_4 generation by human eosinophils stimulated by ionophore A23187 as a granulocyte–macrophage colony-stimulating factor. Am Rev Respir Dis 1989; 140:1340–1347.
60. Aubas P, Cosso B, Godard P, Michel FB, Clot J. Decreased suppressor cell activity of alveolar macrophages in bronchial asthma. Am Rev Respir Dis 1984; 130:875–878.
61. Poulter LW, Janossy G, Power C, Sreenan S, Burke C. Immunological/physiological relationships in asthma: potential regulation by lung macrophages. Immunol Today 1994; 15:256–261.
62. Pesci A, Foresi A, Bertorelli G, Chetta A, Oliveri D. Histochemical characteristics and degranulation of mast cells in epithelium and lamina propria of bronchial biopsies from asthmatic and normal subjects. Am Rev Respir Dis 1993; 147:684–689.
63. Bradding P, Feather IH, Howarth PH, et al. Interleukin 4 is localized to and released by human mast cells. J Exp Med 1992; 176:1381–1386.
64. Bradding P, Roberts JA, Britten KM, et al. Interleukin-4, -5, and -6 and tumor necrosis factor-alpha in normal and asthmatic airways: evidence for the human mast cell as a source of these cytokines. Am J Respir Cell Mol Biol 1994; 10:471–480.
65. Liu MC, Hubbard WC, Proud D, et al. Immediate and late inflammatory responses to ragweed antigen challenge of the peripheral airways in allergic asthmatics. Cellular, mediator, and permeability changes. Am Rev Respir Dis 1991; 144:51–58.
66. Gauchat JF, Herchoz S, Mazzei G, et al. Induction of human IgE synthesis in B cells by mast cells and basophils. Nature 1993; 365:340–343.
67. Brunner T, Heusser CH, Dahinden CA. Human peripheral blood basophils primed by interleukin 3 (IL-3) produce IL-4 in response to immunoglobulin E receptor stimulation. J Exp Med 1993; 177:605–611.
68. Sur S, Hunt LW, Crotty TB, Gleich GJ. Sudden-onset fatal asthma [editorial]. Mayo Clin Proc 1994; 69:495–496.

69. Martin RJ, Cicutto LC, Smith HR, Ballard RD, Szefler SJ. Airways inflammation in nocturnal asthma. Am Rev Respir Dis 1991; 143:351–357.
70. Tanizaki Y, Kitani H, Mifune T, Mitsunobu F, Kajimoto K, Sugimoto K. Effects of glucocorticoids on humoral and cellular immunity and on airway inflammation in patients with steroid-dependent intractable asthma. J Asthma 1993; 30:485–492.
71. Joseph M, Capron A, Tsicopoulos A, Ameisen JC, Martinot JB, Tonnel AB. Platelet activation by IgE and aspirin. Agents Actions Suppl 1987; 21:169–177.
72. Di-Stefano A, Saetta M, Maestrelli P, et al. Mast cells in the airway mucosa and rapid development of occupational asthma induced by toluene diisocyanate. Am Rev Respir Dis 1993; 147:1005–1009.
73. Boulet LP, Milot J, Boutet M, St-Georges F, Laviolette M. Airway inflammation in nonasthmatic subjects with chronic cough. Am J Respir Crit Care Med 1994; 149:482–489.
74. Fabbri LM. Airway inflammation in occupational asthma. Am J Respir Crit Care Med 1994; 150:S80–S82.
75. Sladek K, Dworski R, Soja J, et al. Eicosanoids in bronchoalveolar lavage fluid of aspirin-tolerant patients with asthma after aspirin challenge. Am J Respir Crit Care Med 1994; 149:940–946.
76. Szczeklik A. Aspirin-induced asthma: an update and novel findings. Adv Prostaglandin Thromboxane Leukot Res 1994; 22:185–198.
77. Nasser SM, Pfister R, Christie PE, et al. Inflammatory cell populations in bronchial biopsies from aspirin-sensitive asthmatic subjects. Am J Respir Crit Care Med 1996; 153:90–96.
78. Bentley AM, Maestrelli P, Saetta M, et al. Activated T-lymphocytes and eosinophils in the bronchial mucosa in isocyanate-induced asthma. J Allergy Clin Immunol 1992; 89:821–829.
79. Walker C, Virchow J Jr, Bruijnzeel PL, Blaser K. T cell subsets and their soluble products regulate eosinophilia in allergic and nonallergic asthma. J Immunol 1991; 146:1829–1835.
80. Humbert M, Durham S, Ying S, et al. IL-4 and IL-5 mRNA and protein in bronchial biopsies from atopic and nonatopic asthma: evidence against "intrinsic" asthma being a distinct immunopathological entity. Am J Respir Crit Care Med 1996; 154:1490–1496.
81. Djukanovic R, Feather I, Gratziou C, et al. Effect of natural allergen exposure during the grass pollen season on airways inflammation cells and asthma symptoms. Thorax 1996; 51:575–581.
82. Laitinen LA, Laitinen A, Haahtela T. Airway mucosal inflammation even in patients with newly diagnosed asthma. Am Rev Respir Dis 1993; 147:697–704.
83. Foresi A, Bertorelli G, Pesci A, Chetta A, Oliveri D. Inflammatory markers in bronchoalveolar lavage and in bronchial biopsy in asthma during remission. Chest 1990; 98:528–535.
84. Walker C, Kaegi MK, Braun P, Blaser K. Activated T cells and eosinophilia in bronchoalveolar lavages from subjects with asthma correlated with disease severity. J Allergy Clin Immunol 1991; 88:935–942.
85. Roisman GL, Peiffer C, Lacronique JG, Le-Cae A, Dusser DJ. Perception of bronchial obstruction in asthmatic patients. Relationship with bronchial eosinophilic inflammation and epithelial damage and effect of corticosteroid treatment. J Clin Invest 1995; 96:12–21.
86. Wang JH, Trigg CJ, Devalia JL, Jordan S, Davies RJ. Effect of inhaled beclomethasone dipropionate on expression of proinflammatory cytokines and activated eosinophils in the bronchial epithelium of patients with mild asthma. J Allergy Clin Immunol 1994; 94:1025–1034.
87. Kraft M, Djukanovic R, Torvik J, et al. Evaluation of airway inflammation by endobronchial and transbronchial biopsy in nocturnal and nonnocturnal asthma. Chest 1995; 107:(3 Suppl.):162S.

88. Oosterhoff Y, Timens W, Postma DS. The role of airway inflammation in the pathophysiology of nocturnal asthma. Clin Exp Allergy 1995; 25:915–921.
89. Jarjour NN, Busse WW, Calhoun WJ. Enhanced production of oxygen radicals in nocturnal asthma. Am Rev Respir Dis 1992; 146:905–911.
90. Jarjour NN, Busse WW. Cytokines in bronchoalveolar lavage fluid of patients with nocturnal asthma. Am J Respir Crit Care Med 1995; 152:1474–1477.
91. Oosterhoff Y, Hoogsteden HC, Rutgers B, Kauffman HF, Postma DS. Lymphocyte and macrophage activation in bronchoalveolar lavage fluid in nocturnal asthma. Am J Respir Crit Care Med 1995; 151:75–81.
92. Barnes P, FitzGerald G, Brown M, Dollery C. Nocturnal asthma and changes in circulating epinephrine, histamine, and cortisol. N Engl J Med 1980; 303:263–267.
93. Szefler SJ, Ando R, Cicutto LC, Surs W, Hill MR, Martin RJ. Plasma histamine, epinephrine, cortisol, and leukocyte beta-adrenergic receptors in nocturnal asthma. Clin Pharmacol Ther 1991; 49:59–68.
94. Fitzpatrick MF, Mackay T, Walters C, et al. Circulating histamine and eosinophils cationic protein levels in nocturnal asthma. Clin Sci 1992; 83:227–232.
95. Mackay TW, Wallace WA, Howie SE, et al. Role of inflammation in nocturnal asthma. Thorax 1994; 49:257–262.
96. Oosterhoff Y, Kauffman HF, Rutgers B, Zijlstra JF, Koeter GH, Postma DS. Inflammatory cell number and mediators in bronchoalveolar lavage fluid and peripheral blood in subjects with asthma with increased nocturnal airways narrowing. J Allergy Clin Immunol 1995; 96:219–229.
97. Turki J, Pak J, Green SA, Martin RJ, Liggett SB. Genetic polymorphisms of the beta 2-adrenergic receptor in nocturnal and nonnocturnal asthma. Evidence that Gly 16 correlates with the nocturnal phenotype. J Clin Invest 1995; 95:1635–1641.
98. Bousquet J, Chanez P, Lacoste JY, et al. Asthma: a disease remodeling the airways. Allergy 1992; 47:3–11.
99. Roche WR, Beasley R, Williams JH, Holgate ST. Subepithelial fibrosis in the bronchi of asthmatics. Lancet 1989; 1:520–524.
100. Brewster CE, Howarth PH, Djukanovic R, Wilson J, Holgate ST, Roche WR. Myofibroblasts and subepithelial fibrosis in bronchial asthma. Am J Respir Cell Mol Biol 1990; 3:507–511.
101. Bousquet J, Lacoste JY, Chanez P, Vic P, Godard P, Michel FB. Bronchial elastic fibers in normal subjects and asthmatic patients. Am J Respir Crit Care Med 1996; 153:1648–1654.
102. Laitinen LA, Laitinen A. Remodeling of asthmatic airways by glucocorticosteroids. J Allergy Clin Immunol 1996; 97:153–158.
103. Bousquet J, Chanez P, Lacoste JY, et al. Indirect evidence of bronchial inflammation assessed by titration of inflammatory mediators in BAL fluid of patients with asthma. J Allergy Clin Immunol 1991; 88:649–660.
104. Bousquet J, Vignola AM, Chanez P, Campbell AM, Bonsignore G, Michel FB. Airways remodelling in asthma: no doubt, no more? Int Arch Allergy Immunol 1995; 107:211–214.
105. Chanez P, Vignola M, Steinger R, Vic P, Michel F, Bousquet J. Platelet-derived growth factor in asthma. Allergy 1995; 50:878–883.
106. Dunnill M, Massarella G, Anderson J. Comparaison of the quantitative anatomy of the bronchi in normal subjects, in status asthmaticus, in chronic bronchitis, and in emphysema. Thorax 1969; 24:176–179.
107. Hossain S, Heard BE. Hyperplasia of bronchial muscle in chronic bronchitis. J Pathol 1970; 101:171–184.
108. Heard BE, Hossain S. Hyperplasia of bronchial muscle in asthma. J Pathol 1973; 110:319–331.
109. Saetta M, Di-Stefano A, Rosina C, Thiene G, Fabbri LM. Quantitative structural analysis of peripheral airways and arteries in sudden fatal asthma. Am Rev Respir Dis 1991; 143:138–143.

110. Carroll N, Elliot J, Morton A, James A. The structure of large and small airways in nonfatal and fatal asthma. Am Rev Respir Dis 1993; 147:405–410.
111. Hogg JC. Pathology of asthma. J Allergy Clin Immunol 1993; 92:1–5.
112. Sobonya RE. Quantitative structural alterations in long-standing allergic asthma. Am Rev Respir Dis 1984; 130:289–292.
113. Ebina M, Yaegashi H, Takahashi T, Motomiya M, Tanemura M. Distribution of smooth muscles along the bronchial tree. A morphometric study of ordinary autopsy lungs. Am Rev Respir Dis 1990; 141:1322–1326.
114. Ebina M, Takahashi T, Chiba T, Motomiya M. Cellular hypertrophy and hyperplasia of airway smooth muscles underlying bronchial asthma. A 3-D morphometric study. Am Rev Respir Dis 1993; 148:720–726.
115. Wright JL, Hobson J, Wiggs BR, Pare PD, Hogg JC. Effect of cigarette smoking on structure of the small airways. Lung 1987; 165:91–100.
116. Mullen JB, Wright JL, Wiggs PR, Pare PD, Hogg JC. Structure of central airways in current smokers and ex-smokers with and without mucus hypersecretion: relationship to lung function. Thorax 1987; 42:843–848.
117. Thurlbeck W. Chronic airflow obstruction. In: WM T, ed. Pathology of the Lung. New York: Thieme Medical Publishers, 1988:519–577.

5

The Prognosis and Natural History of Asthma

JORRIT GERRITSEN and MARION H. GROL

Beatrix Children's Hospital
University Hospital Groningen
Groningen, The Netherlands

JAN P. SCHOUTEN

University of Groningen and
University Hospital Groningen
Groningen, The Netherlands

DIRKJE S. POSTMA

University Hospital Groningen
Groningen, The Netherlands

I. Introduction

Asthma is one of the most common chronic diseases throughout life and has an enormous influence on socioeconomics. Therefore, studies on the onset, short-term and long-term course, and prognosis of asthma remain relevant topics for health professionals, patients, and parents, both from a clinical and public health perspective. Although many follow-up studies have been performed and recent advances have been made in understanding the pathophysiology of asthma, numerous gaps exist in our knowledge of the factors that affect the long-term prognosis of asthma. In allergic families, future parents often have questions about the chance for the newborn to develop allergy or asthma and how to prevent this. And when the child has developed allergic phenomena or asthma, they wish to hear whether their child will outgrow the disease or remain affected. Furthermore, limited knowledge is available about the chances of subsequent development into a chronic, more serious, condition in adults of working age and after retirement. Thus, it is important to gain insight into the foregoing factors.

Many influences contribute to the complexity of solving the questions about the natural history of asthma. For instance, wheezing in young children has often been labeled as asthma, but the proportion of all wheezing illnesses labeled as asthma has varied considerably over time (1–5). Thus, one of the main problems is the definition of the diagnosis of asthma, which has not been clearly defined in many studies, a fact that makes it difficult to interpret the conclusions (6). Terms used are "asthma," "asthmatic bronchitis," "wheezy bronchitis," "allergic asthma," "bacterial asthma," and "wheezing," and chronic asthma in an advanced, irreversible state is frequently difficult to differentiate from chronic obstructive pulmonary disease (COPD), and chronic obstructive lung disease. Consequently, we have defined *asthma*, as published previously, as a syndrome characterized by variable and often reversible airway obstruction, airway inflammation, and bronchial responsiveness.

Persons with asthma have episodes of wheezing or breathlessness, with intervals of relative or complete freedom from symptoms. These attacks of breathlessness can be elicited by several stimuli, such as exercise, viral infection, and specific (allergic) and nonspecific irritants (e.g., cold, fog, perfume, and smoke).

A serious problem in defining asthma starting at different ages (infancy, childhood, puberty, or young and advanced adulthood) is the uncertainty that identical meanings for asthma in all age groups are used, both in population- and in patient-based studies (7). In studies focused on the outcome of asthma, remarkable differences are found in patient selection and study design. Differences in the outcome of asthma might be expected between epidemiological and clinical studies, and when patients with different severity of the disease are being studied. Furthermore, the age of the population at the onset of the study may also affect the outcome. Where possible, we will try to alert the reader to this point in the studies reviewed in this chapter. In addition, we will focus on factors that precede wheezing asthma, and next to factors that influence the outcome of the disease, because asthma may have originated soon after birth (8,9).

II. Asthma Symptoms

The onset of asthma is generally based on the occurrence of repeated episodes of wheezing, bronchial obstruction, dyspnea, and asthma attacks (9). Nevertheless, a high percentage of children who do not develop subsequent asthma frequently suffer from these symptoms early in life. Therefore, first episodes of asthma are often skewed because many infants have episodes of wheezing associated with a viral upper or lower respiratory illnesses (10). Neither the pathogenesis of these episodes nor their relation to asthma has been completely elucidated (11). Recent data suggest that two groups of children can be distinguished. A group of children who have self-limited illness, which peaks in incidence during the first year of life and then disappears. The incidence of asthma, on the other hand, peaks between the age of 3 and 5 years, but begins at an earlier age in many children. Therefore, owing to overlap during preschool years and the nonspecific wheezing illness at that time, these children are indistinguishable from the transient wheezers. In a prospectively designed study, 1246 newborns were enrolled, and complete follow-up was obtained at the ages of 1, 3, and 6 years in 826 (66.3%) (12). Of the 277 who had wheezing before the age of 3, 164 (59.2%) had not wheezed during the previous year when they were evaluated at 6 years of age. This indicates that wheezing before the age of 3 is not predictive of the subsequent development of asthma and that wheezing illness and asthma can become manifest in about 40% after that age. On the other hand, almost all children who wheezed at the age of 3 had wheezing and asthma at the age of 6. In this study, maternal asthma was highly associated with late-onset wheezing (3 years, or older) and persistent wheezing. Further follow-up of the same cohort until the age of 11 years confirmed these findings (13). Whether this will also be true for persistence into adulthood is an important issue, and we hope that this cohort will be followed for a longer time. Onset of childhood wheeze generally occurs in infancy, and it has been suggested that in utero and early life exposures are important in the development and persistence of wheeze and the occurrence of reduced lung function and even chronic irreversible airway obstruction later in life (14). Wheezing, furthermore, is strongly associated with maternal smoking continuously during pregnancy, and with low birth weight (15,16).

Initial reports raised enthusiasm that elevated neonatal IgE level and diminished T-lymphocyte subsets could predict allergic disease (17–19). However, recent studies have been unable to confirm the level of prediction of these earlier findings (20–23).

III. Factors Affecting the Outcome or Onset of Asthma

A. Symptoms and Outcome

The outcome of childhood asthma has been related to the age at onset of respiratory symptoms. Some studies have shown that onset of wheeze before the age of 2 years was a predictor of persistence of respiratory symptoms in adulthood (24–26). Others, however, could not find any relation or even found a favorable effect between an early age at onset of wheeze and the persistence of respiratory symptoms into adulthood (27–34). An important factor in whether or not early age at onset of symptoms of asthma is predictive for a worse outcome is that most follow-up studies recruited their subjects from the age of 6 or 7 onward. Therefore, these studies are susceptible to "recall bias." Furthermore, it is difficult in early childhood to discriminate between transient wheezing and asthma (27,29,35–38).

The severity of symptoms early in life is largely determined by the perception and interpretation of the parents. Differences in the combination of symptoms used in the analysis for prediction of prognosis and the structure of the questionnaire may strongly influence the results (39,40). Many studies have suggested that more severe symptoms at the time of onset correlate with a negative outcome (29,31,36,41,42). Severity of symptoms is to only a small extent associated with the perception of the degree of bronchial obstruction. Some asthmatic subjects report only minor discomfort in combination with severe (induced) airway obstruction, and others experience marked discomfort with small increases in airway obstruction (43–45). For parents, it may be expected that the perception of airway obstruction in their child is even more difficult and almost impossible. Age at onset of respiratory symptoms may be even less reliable when follow-up starts at an adult age (34). Strachan et al. recently published results of a study in adult individuals followed from birth onward to ages 7, 11, 16, 23, and 33 years. Among 763 subjects selected for a history of asthma at age 16, 41% denied ever having asthma or wheeze and 28% reported onset of symptoms to be later than that recorded prospectively (46).

Another principal question is whether the asthma diagnosed in early infancy is etiologically and pathophysiologically comparable with asthma diagnosed at an early or a late-adult age. This must be taken into account when follow-up studies both in children and in adults are interpreted, and it restricts the use of severity of respiratory symptoms for outcome assessment of asthma. Even less is known about which respiratory and other factors lead to the subsequent development of chronic asthma and persistent chronic obstructive pulmonary disease and even of emphysema. One prospective study showed that wheeze in adulthood was related to lower 1-sec forced expiratory volume (FEV_1) values and, even more importantly, that the earlier wheezing had started, the more explicit and larger this difference was (46). These individuals with onset of wheeze at younger than 7 years old, who wheezed at age 34–35 had a mean FEV_1 of 90.1%, whereas those who did not wheeze had an FEV_1 of 97.5%. In contrast, values for those who started wheezing at ages between 17 and 23 years and between 24 and 35 years were 97.4 and 96.2% and 92.8 and 97.4%, respectively (Fig. 1). This study may suggest that the early-life occurrence of wheezing may result in lower lung function in later life.

B. Infections in Relation to Onset

Infants and young children frequently present with symptoms when they have viral infections. Viral infections appear to constitute a high risk for the development of asthma in childhood (47,48). Furthermore, several studies have shown that subjects who had a history of recurrent or severe lower respiratory tract illnesses as infants have significantly lower levels of lung function later in life (11). Strachan et al. performed a long-term follow-up in a cohort of 11,765 children aged 11–16 years for whom a positive history of neonatal infectious illness had been recorded systematically at 1 month of age (49). In this study, allergic sensitization and hay fever in adolescence were neither consistent with nor protected by, neonatal infection, whereas in the retrospective study of 212 Finnish 7-year-old children, the opposite results were obtained (50). In this study, a significant two- to threefold excess of physician-diagnosed atopic disease or positive skin-prick tests among children with a history of fever, gastrointestinal illness, or otitis media in infancy was observed. An important limitation of the latter study was the distant recall by

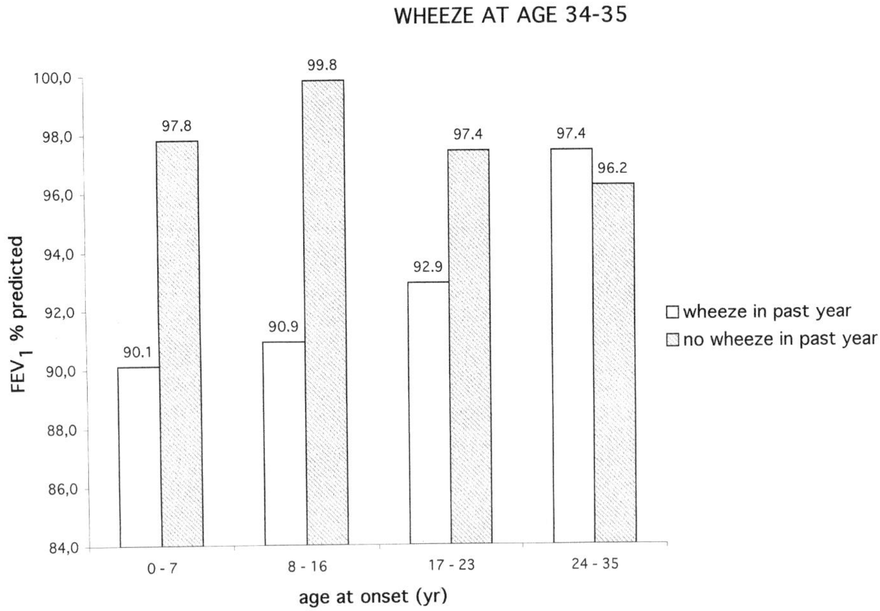

Figure 1 Mean spirometric values before albuterol (salbutamol) administration by age at onset and wheeze in the past year. (From Ref. 49.)

parents of illnesses in the first year of life. From the differences in prevalence of atopy and respiratory tract infections between East and West Germany, another hypothesis has been put forward, in that frequent bacterial infections protect against the development of allergy and asthma and that allergen load and viral infections may have an opposite effect (51).

In the last years, attention has been focused on the importance of respiratory syncytial virus (RSV) infection in the development of aeroallergen sensitization during the first 2 years of life (52). Of a birth cohort of 7609 full-term newborns, 609 were followed until their first birth date and 265 until 24 months. At the first year, a significant positive relation was found between RSV-infection and sensitization against at least one aeroallergen. No correlation of RSV seropositivity to allergic manifestation at the age of 24 months could be found. However, recently, it was stated that 1 month after RSV-infection, lymphocytes acquire specific susceptibility to *Dermatophagoides farinae* and food allergens, specifically ovalbumin. Positive interleukin (IL)-2 responsiveness to allergens was more frequently present in those individuals who developed atopic symptoms (n = 16) than in asymptomatic children (n = 9) during a follow-up of 3 years (Fig. 2; 53,54).

The question whether viral and bacterial infections facilitate the development of allergy in children who are prone to this disease remains open and has to be elu-

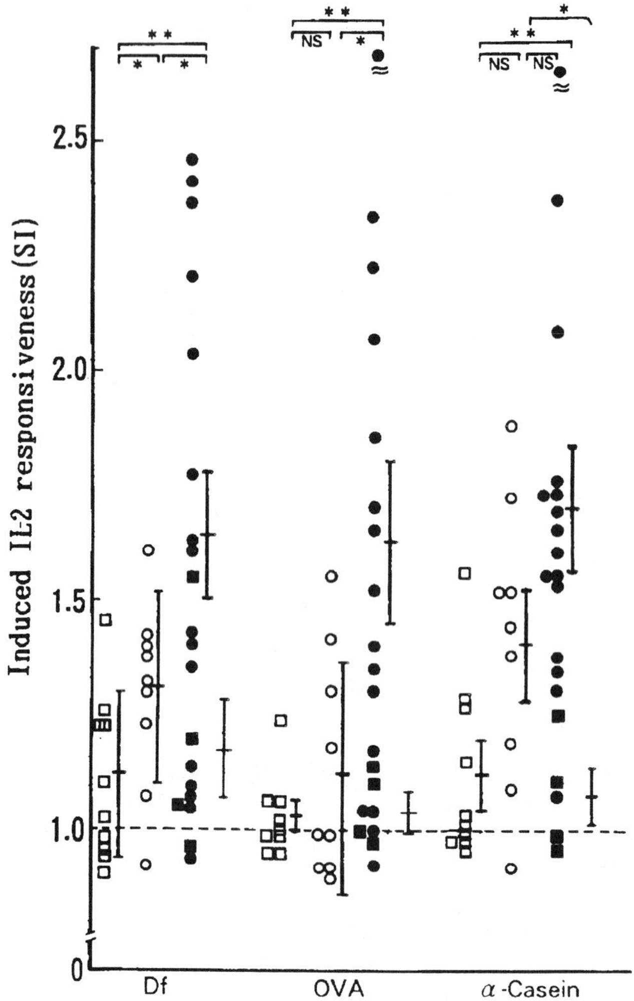

Figure 2 Infants after RSV infection, showing allergen-induced IL-2 responsiveness after stimulation with ovalbumin, *Dermatophagoides farinae*, and α-casein, had recurrent wheezing or bronchial asthma within a few years. Filled circles, wheezing group after RSV infection; open circles, healthy group after RSV infection; filled squares, wheezing group after non-RSV infection; open squares, healthy group after non-RSV infection. Data are expressed as means ± SEM. $*p < 0.05$, $**p < 0.01$. (From Ref. 53.)

cidated in future prospective studies. Also, a link has been reported from a prospectively designed study in 618 adults between pneumonia documented in the first 2 years of life and low lung function at age 70, probably associated with a slower rate of growth of lung function, adjusted for age and height (55,56). In men, the difference was –0.65 L, and this estimate did not diminish after adjustment for smoking and asthma. In women, the effect of pneumonia before the age of 2 years on lung function was smaller and nonsignificant. More information must be obtained about the long-term effects into adulthood and later life and the possible relation between respiratory tract infection in early life and the development of irreversible airway obstruction.

C. Genetics in Relation to Onset

It is generally accepted that 30–40% of the population have a risk for atopy or asthma (57,58). Linkage studies have found a couple of candidate regions that have been reported to be associated with onset of atopy, bronchial hyperresponsiveness, and asthma. First is the human homologue region of the mouse β-chain of the IgE receptor on chromosome 11q, and the region at chromosome 5q with multiple candidate genes that directly or indirectly regulate IgE production. This latter region includes the IL-4 group of cytokines (IL-4, IL-5, IL-3, granulocyte–macrophage colony-stimulating factor [GM-CSF]), IL-9, IL-13, and other factors (59–61). Recently, chromosome 14 has also been reported to be associated with manifestations of atopy and asthma (62). From all these studies it becomes evident that no single genetic factor is responsible for the inheritance of atopy and asthma. Future studies must not only unravel which combination of genetic loci and environmental factors will contribute to the development of atopy and asthma, but also how they are related to the severity of disease and progression.

D. Gender in Relation to Onset and Outcome

A consistent finding in all epidemiological studies is that the prevalence of atopy and asthma is higher in boys than in girls; male/female ratios of about 1.5:1 have been reported (24,39,41,63). Boys also have lower flow rates such as $V_{\text{max FRC}}$, from birth to early adolescence, and increased muscle tone in the airways compared with girls (64). Despite these differences in expression of atopy, asthma, lung function, and bronchial responsiveness between boys and girls, most studies do not show any effect of gender on the outcome of the disease (8,24–26,30,37,61). Other studies have found a better prognosis for either men (27,37) or for women (41,65).

Near puberty and young adolescence the prevalences change, and an equalization of asthma in men and women appears (27,41). A suitable explanation for this phenomenon is not available, but it has been assumed that differences in hormonal changes between both sexes at about this time play a role. In children with Turner's syndrome, treated for 6 months with estrogen, an increase in bronchial responsiveness was observed. Given this effect on bronchial responsiveness, it might be hypothesized that hormonal changes could partly be responsible for the changes seen in epidemiological studies (66). Further studies are required to unravel these changes in prevalence of atopy, hyperresponsiveness, and asthma.

E. Atopy in Relation to Onset and Outcome

Exposure to allergens plays an important and crucial role in the development and persistence of asthma, especially in children and, probably also, in adults. Atopy can express itself in many ways; early in life, it can manifest itself as infantile eczema or cow's milk allergy. Later on, atopic dermatitis, allergic rhinitis, and allergy of the airways on exposure to inhalant allergens become more prominent. These allergic phenomena can be the first sign of atopy in infancy and childhood, and they may precede the development of subsequent asthma. One of the problems in studying these risk factors is that, in the follow-up studies, different definitions are used for the atopic manifestations, which makes comparison of these surveys less reliable and even almost impossible. A study in West and East Germany in adults showed that both childhood factors and exposure to indoor allergens and irritants are likely to be more important for the development of atopy and asthma than the potential long-term exposure to high concentrations of sulfur dioxide and particulate matter (67).

The studies that have shown an effect on the prognosis of childhood asthma all point to a negative association of atopy (33,41,68–72). However, many studies did not find any or only a slight effect of atopy on the natural history of asthma (27,73–76). Because almost all population-based follow-up studies did find a relation between childhood atopy and outcome of asthma, it might be expected that the severity of atopy is a risk factor. The presence of atopy and decline in lung function has also been associated, independently of the presence of clinical asthma (77–81). However, these studies performed in adults have different age ranges in atopic and nonatopic subjects. This may have influenced the degree of decline in lung function, and also, because the expression of atopy declines with age, it can be questioned whether the investigated groups are comparable (60,82,83). To solve the question of whether atopy plays a role in the long-term prognosis of childhood and adult asthma, large population-based cohort studies, starting at infancy, are necessary.

F. Bronchial Responsiveness in Relation to Onset and Outcome

Increased bronchial responsiveness is known to constitute a risk factor for the development of airway symptoms. It may precede the development of asthma, not only in children but also in young adults, as well as in middle-aged men with asthma, when chronic bronchitis and sinusitis were excluded (84–86). The inflammatory process of the airways is considered to be the most important primary component in asthma, but there is no certainty of when in early life this inflammatory process begins (87). Indications of early inflammatory changes within the airways at birth include abnormal T-cell maturation, increased IgE levels, and elevated IL-4 and decreased IL-2 and interferon-γ (IFN-γ) levels in those at risk for atopy (88–90). The exact influence of these findings on the development of asthma is uncertain, for no information is available in these infants and young children relative to the structure and the degree of inflammation of the airways and the degree of bronchial responsiveness. Measurement of bronchial responsiveness in infants and young children in birth cohorts is hardly possible, which accounts for the gap in the knowledge on the predictive value of these measurements for the long-term prognosis of childhood asthma. Several studies in which measurements of bronchial responsiveness were performed in school-aged children show that increased bronchial responsiveness in childhood predicted the outcome of disease in adulthood (29,36,69,91–93). Especially the combination of wheeze and bronchial responsiveness characterizes asthmatic subjects who will have ongoing respiratory symptoms (92). This has been demonstrated in the East Boston childhood respiratory disease study among 770 children aged 5–9 years at entry. Changes in airway responsiveness in relation to onset of wheeze and recurrent asthma episodes were followed into young adulthood (94). Bronchial responsiveness was assessed by cold air challenge. An elevated risk for onset of wheeze and recurrent asthma in young adulthood in this study was associated with more severe bronchial responsiveness in childhood (94).

Van Schayck et al. studied 71 adult patients with asthma, who completed a 2-year, randomized controlled intervention study with bronchodilators. In this study group, with a mean age of 51 years, bronchial hyperresponsiveness was related to a more pronounced annual decline in FEV_1 in atopic subjects, but not in nonatopic patients (95). This is in contrast with Panhuysen et al., who did not find this effect over a period of 25 years (34). However, ages of these individuals ranged from 13 to 34 years (mean 24 years) at baseline, considerably younger than those in the former study. It may well be that the presence or persistence of atopy into an older age interferes with hyperresponsiveness in different ways, or it may merely signify a different type of patient. Here again prospective studies are needed; comparing two studies that start at different ages most likely gives a misleading interpretation.

No information is available on the link between childhood bronchial responsiveness and the development of irreversible airway obstruction later in life nor on the course of airway obstruction. Even in the ongoing studies, it may be difficult, or nearly impossible, to find such a relationship because with time, almost all circumstances have changed, such as the introduction of inhaled corticosteroid therapy, the improvement of the social standards, prosperity, vaccination of children, early treatment of respiratory infection, which leads to less damage of the lungs, and so on. This makes it uncertain to what extent control of bronchial responsiveness by allergen avoidance and by medication may affect the long-term outcome of the disease.

G. Smoking in Relation to Onset and Outcome

Maternal smoking during pregnancy leads to decreased birth weight, abnormal lung function, and elevated IgE levels in cord blood, and appears to be associated with an increased frequency of atopy or asthma (96,97). Maternal smoking during pregnancy has consistently been associated with reduced $V_{max\ FRC}$ during the first year of life, which may persist throughout life (98). These findings are more marked in females, who normally have a higher V_{max} than males (12). It is supposed that maternal smoking affects the fetal lung by hypoxia, CO, and nicotine, which all are vasoactive agents, thereby affecting placental function or the developing pulmonary or systemic vasculature. Besides, maternal smoking is responsible for increased hospitalization for respiratory illness, especially bronchiolitis, in the first year of life. It might be expected that, in these cases, the persistence of exposure postnatally also plays an important role. Meyer et al. showed that even in children who have developed asthma, parental smoking is a risk factor for instability of disease, as assessed by a large circadian peak expiratory flow (PEF) variation (99). Smoking also has a long-term effect on lung function and wheezing. Parental smoking was associated with persistent impairment of lung function in both wheezing adolescents and nonwheezing subjects in a longitudinal study in New Zealand (100). Similar findings were shown in a cross-sectional population-based study in China (101).

The analysis of the effects of active smoking in adolescents can be obscured by the fact that many of these subjects were already exposed to passive smoking during childhood. In follow-up studies in subjects with asthma, aged 20 to 30 years, no effect or even a better lung function was observed in smokers, which is generally considered to be a "healthy smoker effect" (i.e., only those with less severe asthma are able to take up smoking; 29,36) Others did find that active smoking during adolescence is associated with shortening of the plateau phase of FEV_1, generally occurring between 20 and 35 years of age (102). It suggests that an overall negative effect of (passive) smoking in adolescence is present, and that this also might be present in asthmatic subjects. The importance of passive smoking has been further demonstrated by Corbo et al. who reported a negative effect on lung function, even when parents of these children were nonsmokers (103). Whether cessation of smoking during adolescence has a positive influence on lung growth, as suggested by Selroos et al., is still questionable, and must be confirmed by other studies (104).

H. Lung Function and the Onset and Outcome of Asthma

In analyzing the course of lung function from childhood to adulthood and later life, some important facts have to be appreciated. Lung function develops throughout life with a high tracking correlation, and asthmatic subjects progres in a way similar to normal subjects. Lung function increases with age until early adolescence, stabilizes until the mid-30s and then starts to decline (105).

The degree of bronchial obstruction, as measured by FEV_1, has been reported to be predictive for the continuation of symptoms from childhood to adulthood as well as an increased decline of lung function later in life (5,29,36,77,80,95,105). On the other hand, about 30% of the children with severe bronchial obstruction, measured without medication, have normal FEV_1 values as adults and do not report ongoing respiratory symptoms (29,36). In the Australian cohort study, many children tended to have an elevated forced vital capacity (FVC), which was interpreted as a sign of hyperinflation of the lung (77). Borsboom et al. found that lung function in adolescents with a positive history of prepubertal respiratory symptoms was lower than in healthy controls, even if they lose their symptoms (106). Given these findings and those of the study by Greenough et al. showing an increased hyperinflation in young asthmatics, there is growing concern that some children have a persistently high functional residual, capacity (FRC), and this is associated with increased risk of developing irreversible lung function impairment later in life (107). Panhuysen et al. investigated 181 young adults with asthma (ages 13–44; median 24 years), who were followed for 25 years. Twenty subjects (11%) were asymptomatic after 25 years, had no bronchial hyperresponsiveness, and an FEV_1 higher than the 90% predicted. This group had a younger age at baseline testing and better FEV_1. Thus, low lung function, whatever its cause, appears to be an important risk factor for symptomatic disease both in childhood and adulthood (34).

I. The Role of Intervention in Relation to Onset and Outcome

Early exposure to house dust mite allergens has been proposed as one of the major risk factors for the development of atopy and asthma in childhood (108). It has been demonstrated that house dust mite exposure precedes the development of symptoms and that avoidance reverses the effect (109–111). With this knowledge, studies on prevention of early sensitization to house dust mite and other aeroallergens are presently being developed in many countries. How rigourously allergen avoidance measurements must be instituted is uncertain, because low-level exposure to house dust mites already stimulates allergen-specific T-cell responses during early childhood (112). This stimulation is supposed to be a normal part of the education of the immune system in early childhood. Priming per se does not imply clinically significant sensitivity, however (113).

In both children and adults, anti-inflammatory therapy with inhaled corticosteroids results in a decrease in respiratory symptoms, asthma attacks, and the use of additional medication. It also improves lung function and bronchial responsiveness and diminishes signs of inflammation in the airways. Therefore, the idea has been put forward that early initiation of anti-inflammatory therapy may prevent long-term (irreversible) changes of the airways both in children and adults, based on prospective studies with a relatively short duration of follow-up (114,115).

Van Essen-Zandvliet et al. showed that 22 months of follow-up with the use of 400 μg of inhaled steroids reduced clinical severity of asthma (115). However, only a minority (20/58) reached remission, as defined by absence of symptoms and use of additional β_2-agonist and prednisolone courses or absence from school during an 8-month period. Of these 20 individuals, only 8 had a normal level of airway responsiveness. Furthermore, the results of studies on cessation of regular treatment after 1 and 2.5 years of regular treatment showed that the effects have already disappeared within 3 months after cessation (116,117). Thus, it may be interpreted

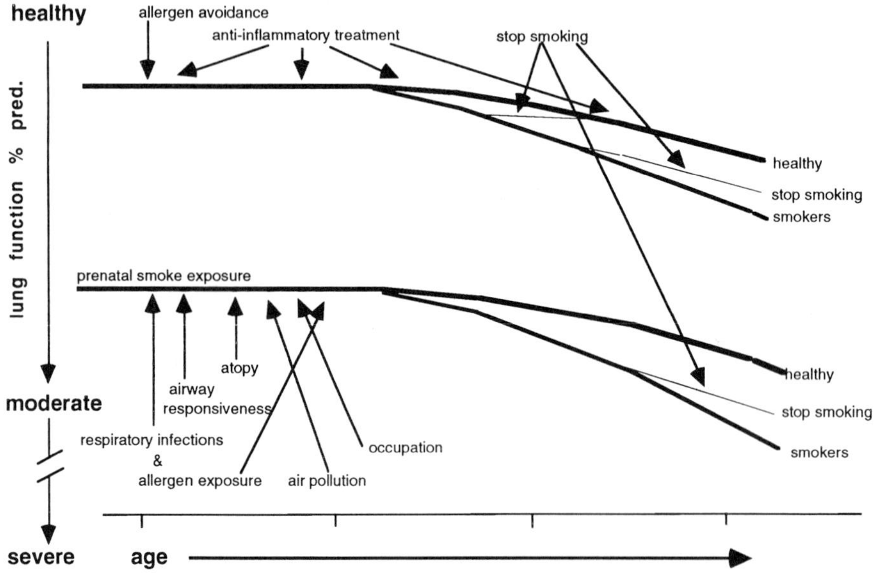

Figure 3 Schematic presentation of slopes of lung function and the influences of different factors.

that treatment with the now available anti-inflammatory drugs results only in modulations of asthma, but does not cure the disease. A retrospective study in young adults with asthma, however, suggested that earlier institution of therapy is important for a beneficial outcome in asthma. Other intervention studies have also suggested that delayed treatment by inhaled corticosteroids leads to smaller effects on improvement of bronchial hyperresponsiveness (115–117).

Whether prolonged treatment following early institution (but at which time is best?) may "cure" some individuals remains to be established.

IV. Conclusion

Although many studies have focused on short-term and long-term outcome of asthma, its natural history is still unclear, nor is it apparent which risk factors determine the ultimate prognosis. No certainty exists whether severe asthma in infancy and childhood is a risk factor for development of irreversible airway obstruction later in life.

How treatment of asthma interferes with the natural history and whether it has to be introduced during an early stage of the disease, and at what dose, has to be unraveled. It becomes more and more evident that environmental factors and passive and active smoking are major risk factors in both the onset and the course of the disease (Fig. 3).

References

1. Broder I, Higgins MW, Matthews KP, Keller JB. Epidemiology of asthma and allergic rhinitis in a total community, Tecumseh, Michigan IV. Natural history. J Allergy Clin Immunol 1974; 54:100–110.
2. Bronnimann S, Burrows B. A prospective study of the natural history of asthma. Chest 1986; 90:480–484.
3. Anderson HR. Is asthma really increasing. Paediatr Respir Med 1993; 1:6–10.
4. Lenney W, Wells NEJ, O'Neill BA. The burden of paediatric asthma. Eur Respir Rev 1994; 4:49–62.
5. Strachan D, Gerritsen J. Long-term outcome of early childhood wheezing: population data. Eur Respir J 1996; 9:S42–47.
6. Fagerberg E. Studies in bronchial asthma. II. A comparative examination between patients with endogenous and exogenous bronchial asthma respectively, with regard to age when taken ill. Acta Allergol 1957; 11:327–342.
7. Martinez FD. The origins of asthma in early life. In: Postma DS, Gerritsen J, eds. Proceedings of the Bronchitis V International Syposium, Groningen, The Netherlands. Assen, The Netherlands: Van Gorcum 1994; 161–169.
8. Grol MH, Gerritsen J, Postma DS. Asthma: from childhood to adulthood. Allergy 1996; 51:855–869.
9. Bronnimann S, Burrows B. A prospective study of the natural history of asthma. Chest 1986; 90:480–484.
10. Wright AL, Taussig LM, Ray CG, Harrison HR, Holberg CJ. The Tuscon Children's Respiratory Study II. Lower respiratory tract illness in the first year of life. Am J Epidemiol 1989; 129:1232–1246.
11. Samet JM, Tager IB, Speizer FE. The relationship between respiratory illness in childhood and chronic airflow obstruction in adulthood. Am Rev Respir Dis 1983; 127:508–523.
12. Martinez FD, Wright AL, Taussig LM, Holberg CJ, Halonen M, Morgan WJ. Asthma and wheezing in the first six years of life. N Engl J Med 1995; 332:133–138.
13. Dodge R, Martinez FD, Cline MG, Lebowitz MD, Burrows B. Early childhood respiratory symptoms and the subsequent diagnosis of asthma. J Allergy Clin Immunol 1996; 98:48–54.
14. Barker DJP, Godfrey KM, Fall C, Osmond C, Winter PD, Shaheen SO. Relation of birth weight and childhood infection to adult lung function and death from chronic airways disease. Br Med J 1991; 303:671–675.
15. Seidman DS, Laor A, Gale R, Stevenson DK, Danon YL. Is low birth weight a risk factor for asthma during adolescence Arch Dis Child 1991; 66:584–587.
16. Lewis S, Richards D, Bynner J, Butler N, Britton J. The aetiology of wheezing illness in childhood and adolescence: a prospective study of the independent effects of passive smoking, birth weight, maternal age, and socio-economic status. Eur Respir J 1995;8:349–356.
17. Croner S, Kjellman NIM, Eriksson B, Roth A. IgE screening in 1701 newborn infants and the development of atopic disease during infancy. Arch Dis Child 1982; 57:374–378.
18. Kjellman NIM, Croner S. Cord blood IgE determination for allergy prediction—a follow-up to seven years of age in 1651 children. Ann Allergy 1984; 53:167–171.
19. Zeiger RS. Devolopment and prevention of allergic disease in childhood. In: Middleton E Jr, Reed CE, Ellis EF, Adkinson NF Jr, Yunginger JW, Busse WW, eds. Allergy: Principles and Practice, 4th ed. St Louis: CV Mosby, 1993: 1137–1171.
20. Kjellman NIM. IgE in neonates is not suitable for general allergy risk screening. Pediatr Allergy Immunol 1994; 5:1–4.
21. Hattevig G, Kjellman NIM, Björkstén B. Clinical symptoms and IgE responses to common food proteins and inhalants in the first 7 years of life. Clin Allergy 1987; 17:571–578.

22. Lilja G, Oman H. Prediction of atopic disease in infancy by determination of immunological parameters: IgE, IgE- and IgG-antibodies to food allergens, skin prick tests and T-lymphocyte subsets. Pediatr Allergy Immunol 1991; 2:6–13.
23. Zeiger RS, Heller S. The development and prediction of atopy in high-risk children: follow-up at age seven years in a prospective randomized study of combined maternal and infant food allergen avoidance. J Allergy Clin Immunol 1995; 95:1179–1190.
24. Williams HB, McNicol KN. Prevalence, natural history, and relationship of wheezy bronchitis and asthma in children. Br Med J 1969; 4:321–325.
25. Croner S, Kjellman N. Natural history of bronchial asthma in childhood. Allergy 1992; 47:150–157.
26. Godden DJ, Ross S, Adalla M, et al. Outcome of wheeze in childhood. Symptoms and pulmonary function 25 years later. Am J Respir Crit Care Med 1994; 149:106–112.
27. Martin AJ, McLennan LA, Landau LI, Phelan PD. The natural history of childhood asthma to adult life. Br J Med 1980; 280:1397–1400.
28. Foucard T, Sjöberg O. A prospective 12-year follow-up study of children with wheezy bronchitis. Acta Paediatr Scand 1984; 73:577–583.
29. Gerritsen J, Koëter GH, Postma DS, Schouten JP, Knol K. Prognosis of asthma from childhood to adulthood. Am Rev Respir Dis 1989; 140:1325–1330.
30. Sporik R, Holgate ST, Cogswell JJ. Natural history of asthma in childhood—a birth cohort study. Arch Dis Child 1991; 66:1050–1053.
31. Kokkonen J, Linna O. The state of childhood asthma in young adulthood. Eur Respir J 1993; 6:657–661.
32. Gergen PJ, Turkeltaub PC, Kramer RA. Age of onset in childhood asthma: data from a national cohort. Ann Allergy 1992; 68:507–514.
33. Giles G, Lickiss N, Gibson HB, Shaw K. Respiratory symptoms in Tasmanian adolescents: a follow-up of the 1961 birth cohort. Aust NZ J Med 1984; 14:631–637.
34. Panhuysen CIM, Vonk JM, Koëter GH, et al. Adult patients may outgrow their asthma; a 25 year follow-up study. Am J Respir Crit Care Med 1997; 155:1267–1272.
35. Friberg S, Bevegård S. Graff-Lonnevig V. Asthma from childhood to adult age. Acta Paediatr Scand 1988; 77:424–431.
36. Roorda RJ, Gerritsen J, van Aalderen WMC, et al. Risk factors for the persistence of respiratory symptoms in childhood asthma. Am Rev Respir Dis 1993; 148:1490–1495.
37. Kjellman B, Hesselmar B. Prognosis of asthma in children: a cohort study into adulthood. Acta Paediatr 1994; 83:854–861.
38. Carey VJ, Weiss ST, Tager IB, Leeder SR, Speizer FE. Airways responsiveness, wheeze onset and recurrent asthma episodes in young adolescents. The East Boston childhood respiratory disease cohort. Am J Respir Crit Care Med 1996; 153:356-361.
39. Knol K. A clinical and epidemiological study of the significance of bronchial hyperreactivity in children with chronic non-specific lung disease (CNSLD). Dissertation, Groningen, 1965.
40. Kerrebijn KF, Hoogeveen-Schroot HCA, van der Wal MC. Chronic non-specific respiratory disease in children: a five year follow-up study. Acta Paediatr Scand 1969; 261:S1–S72.
41. Kelly WJW, Hudson I, Phelan PD, Pain MCF, Olinsky A. Childhood asthma in adult life: a further study at 28 years of age. Br Med J 1987; 294:1059–1062.
42. Anderson HR, Bland JM, Patel S, Peckham C. The natural history of asthma in childhood. J Epidemiol Community Health 1986; 40:121–129.
43. Brand PLP, Rijcken B, Schouten J, Koëter GH, Weiss ST, Postma DS. Perception of airway obstruction in a random population sample: relationship to airway hyperresponsiveness in the absence of respiratory symptoms. Am Rev Respir Dis 1992; 146:396–401.
44. Barnes PJ. Poorly perceived asthma. Thorax 1992; 47:408–409.
45. Rubinfield AR, Pain MCF. Perception of asthma. Lancet 1976; 1:882–884.
46. Strachan DP, Griffiths JM, Johnston IDA, Anderson HR. Ventilatory function in British adults after asthma or wheezing illness at ages 0–35. Am J Respir Crit Care Med 1996; 154:1629–1635.

47. Yarnell JW, St Leger AS. Respiratory infections and their influence on lung function in children: a multiple regression analysis. Thorax 1981; 36:847–851.
48. Sigurs N, Bjarnason R, Sigurbergsson F, Kjellman B, Björkstén B. Asthma and immunoglobulin after respiratory syncytial virus bronchiolitis: a prospective cohort study with matched controls. Pediatrics 1995; 95:500–505.
49. Strachan DP, Taylor EM, Carpenter RG. Family structure, neonatal infection, and hay fever in adolescence. Arch Dis Child 1996; 74:422–426.
50. Backman A, Björksten F, Ilmonen S, Juntonen K, Suoniemi I. Do infections in infancy affect sensitization to airborne allergens and development of allergic disease? Allergy 1984; 309–315.
51. Wichmann HE. Possible explanation for the different trends of asthma and allergy in East and West Germany. Clin Exp Allergy 1996; 26:621–623.
52. Forster J, Tacke U, Krebs H, et al. Respiratory syncytial virus infection: its role in aeroallergen sensitization during the first two years of life. Pediatr Allergy Immunol 1996; 7:55–60.
53. Noma T, Mori A, Yoshizawa I. Induction of allergen-specific IL-2 responsiveness of lymphocytes after respiratory syncytial virus infection and prediction of onset of recurrent wheezing and bronchial asthma. J Allergy Clin Immunol 1996; 98:1–26.
54. Pullan CR, Hey EN. Wheezing, asthma and pulmonary dysfunction, 10-years after infection with respiratory syncytial virus in infancy. Br Med J 1982; 284:1665–1669.
55. Shaheen SO, Barker DJP, Shiell AW, Crocker FJ, Wield GA, Holgate ST. The relationship between pneumonia in early childhood and impaired lung function in late adult life. Am J Respir Crit Care Med 1994; 149:616–619.
56. Gold DR, Tager IB, Weiss ST, Tosteson TD, Speizer FE. Acute lower respiratory illness in childhood as a predictor of lung function and chronic respiratory symptoms. Am Rev Respir Dis 1989; 140:877–884.
57. Haahtela TMK. The prevalence of allergic conditions and immediate skin test reactions among Finnish adolescents. Clin Allergy 1979; 9:53–60.
58. Hattevig G, Kjellman B, Björkstén B, Johansson SGO. The prevalence of allergy and IgE antibodies to inhalant allergens in Swedish school children. Acta Paediatr Scand 1987; 76:349–355.
59. Cookson WOCM, Young RP, Sandalford AJ, et al. Maternal inheritance of atopic IgE responsiveness and chromosome 11q. Lancet 1992; 340:381–384.
60. Postma DS, Bleecker ER, Amelung PJ, et al. Genetic susceptibility to asthma—bronchial hyper-responsiveness is coinherited with a major gene for atopy. N Engl J Med 1995; 333:894–900.
61. Panhuysen CI. Genetics and natural history of asthma. Dissertation; Groningen, The Netherlands, 1996.
62. VanHerwerden L, Harrap SB, Wong ZYH, et al. Linkage of high affinity IgE receptor gene with bronchial hyperreactivity, even in absence of atopy. Lancet 1995; 356:1262–1265.
63. Dawson B, Horobin G, Illsley R, Mitchell R. A survey of childhood asthma in Aberdeen. Lancet 1969; 1:827–830.
64. Landau LI, Morgan W, McCoy KS, Taussig LM. Gender related differences in airway tone in children. Pediatr Pulmonol 1993; 16:31–35.
65. Barr LW, Logan GB. Prognosis of children having asthma. Paediatrics 1964; 34:856–860.
66. Villa MP, Bernardi F, Burnaccini M, et al. Bronchial reactivity and sex hormones: study in a Turner's population. Pediatr Pulmonol 1990; 9:199–205.
67. Nowak D, Heinrich J, Jörres R, et al. Prevalence of respiratory symptoms, bronchial hyperresponsiveness and atopy among adults: West and East Germany. Eur Respir J 1996; 9:2541–2552.
68. Kelly WJW, Hudson J, Phelan PD, Pain MCF, Olinsky A. Atopy in subjects with asthma followed to the age of 28 years. J Allergy Clin Immunol 1990; 85:548–557.
69. de Gooijer A, Brand PLP, Gerritsen J, Koëter GH, Postma DS, Knol K. Changes in res-

piratory symptoms and airway hyperresponsiveness after 27 years in a population-based sample of schoolchildren. Eur Respir J 1993; 6:848–854.

70. Peat JK, Salome CM, Woolcock AJ. Longitudinal changes in atopy during a 4-year period; relation to bronchial hyperresponsiveness and respiratory symptoms in a population sample of Australian schoolchildren. J Allergy Clin Immunol 1990; 85:65–74.
71. Clough JB, Williams JD, Holgate ST. Effect of atopy on the natural history of symptoms, peak expiratory flow, and bronchial responsiveness in 7- and 8-year-old children with cough and wheeze. Am Rev Respir Dis 1991; 143:755–760.
72. Peat JK, Toelle BG, van den Berg DJ, Britton WJ, Woolcock AJ. Serum IgE levels, atopy, and asthma in young adults: results from a longitudinal cohort study. Allergy 1996; 51:804–810.
73. Conolly CK, Chan NS, Prescott RJ. The relationship between age and duration of asthma and the presence of persistent obstruction in asthma. Postgrad Med J 1988; 64:422–425.
74. Gerritsen J, Koëter GH, de Monchy JG, Knol K. Allergy in subjects with asthma from childhood to adulthood. J Allergy Clin Immunol 1990; 85:116–125.
75. Roorda RJ, Gerritsen J, van Aalderen WMC, Knol K. Influence of a positive family history and associated allergic diseases on the natural course of asthma. Clin Exp Allergy 1991; 22:627–634.
76. Kagamimori S, Naruse Y, Kakiuchi H, et al. Does an allergy skin test on school-children predict respiratory symptoms in adulthood? Clin Exp Allergy 1996; 26:262–269.
77. Kelly WJW, Hudson J, Raven J, Phelan PD, Pain MCF, Olinsky A. Childhood asthma and lung function. Am Rev Respir Dis 1988; 138:26-30.
78. Burrows B, Halonen M, Lebowitz MD, Knudson RJ, Barbee RA. The relationship of serum immunoglobulin E, allergy skin test and smoking to respiratory disorders. J Allergy Clin Immunol 1982; 70:199–204.
79. Almind M, Viskum K, Evald T, Dirksen A, Kok-Jensen A. A seven year follow-up study of 343 adults with bronchial asthma. Dan Med Bull 1992; 39:561-565.
80. Ulrik CS, Backer V, Dirksen A. Mortality and decline in lung function in 213 adults with bronchial asthma: a ten-year follow-up. J Asthma 1992; 47:14–18.
81. Gottlieb DJ, Sparrow D, O'Connor GT, Weiss ST. Skin test reactivity to common aeroallergens and decline of lung function. Am J Respir Crit Care Med 1996; 153:561–566.
82. Barbee RA, Kaltenborn WT, Lebowitz MD, Burrows B. Longitudinal changes in allergic skin test reactivity in a community population sample. J Allergy Clin Immunol 1987; 79:16–24.
83. van Schayk CP, Dompeling E, van Herwaarden CLA, van Wever AMJ, van Weel C. Interacting effects of atopy and bronchial hyperresponsiveness on the annual decline in lung function and the exacerbation rate in asthma, Am Rev Respir Dis 1991; 144:1297–1301.
84. Hopp RJ, Townley RG, Biven RE, Bewtra AK, Nair NM. The presence of airway reactivity before the development of asthma. Am Rev Respir Dis 1990; 141:2–8.
85. Zhong NS, Chen RC, O-Yang M, Wu JY, Fu WX, Shi LJ. Bronchial responsiveness in young students of southern China: relation to respiratory symptoms, diagnosed asthma, and risk factors. Thorax 1990; 45:860–865.
86. Sparrow D, O'Connor G, Colton T, Barry CL, Weiss ST. The relationship of nonspecific bronchial responsiveness to the occurrence of respiratory symptoms and decreased level of pulmonary function. Am Rev Respir Dis 1987; 135:1255–1260.
87. Forastiere F, Corbo GM, Dell'Orco V, Pistelli R, Agabiti N, Kriebel D. A longitudinal evaluation of bronchial responsiveness to methacholine in children: role of baseline lung function, gender, and change in atopic status. Am J Respir Crit Care Med 1996; 153:1098–1104.
88. Holt PG, Clough JB, Holt BJ, et al. Genetic risk for atopy is associated with delayed postnatal maturation of T cell competence. Clin Exp Allergy 1992; 22:1093–1097.
89. Croner S, Kjellman NIM, Development of atopic disease in relation to family history and

cord blood IgE levels: eleven year follow-up in 1654 children. Pediatr Allergy Immunol 1990; 1:14–20.

90. Warner JA, Miles EA, Jones AC, Quint DJ, Colwell BM, Warner JO. Is deficiency of interferon gamma production by allergen triggered blood cells a predictor of atopic eczema? Clin Exp Allergy 1994; 24:423–430.
91. Peat JK, Salome CM, Woolcock AJ. Factors associated with bronchial hyperresponsiveness in Australian adults and children. Eur Respir J 1992; 5:921–929.
92. Peat JK, Toelle BG, Salome CM, Woolcock AJ. Predictive nature of bronchial responsiveness and respiratory symptoms in one year cohort study of Sydney schoolchildren. Eur Respir J 1993; 6:662–669.
93. Britton JR, Burney PGJ, Chinn S, Papacosta AO, Tattersfield AE. The relation between change in airway reactivity and change in respiratory symptoms and medication in a community study. Am Rev Respir Dis 1988; 135:530–534.
94. Carey VJ, Weiss ST, Tager IB, Leeder SR, Speizer FE. Airways responsiveness, wheeze onset, and recurrent asthma in young adolescents. The East Boston childhood respiratory disease cohort. Am J Respir Crit Care Med 1996; 153:356–361.
95. van Schayck CP, Dompeling E, van Herwaarden CLA, van Wever AMJ, van Weel C. Interacting effects of atopy and bronchial hyperresponsiveness on the annual decline in lung function and the exacerbation rate in asthma. Am Rev Respir Dis 1991; 144:1297–1301.
96. Hanrahan JP, Tager IB, Segal MR, et al. The effect of maternal smoking during pregnancy on early lung function. Am Rev Respir Dis 1992; 145:1129-1135.
97. Søyseth V, Kongerud J, Boe J. Postnatal maternal smoking increases the prevalence of asthma but not of bronchial hyperresponsiveness or atopy in their children. Chest 1995; 107:389–394.
98. Landau LI. Risks of developing asthma. Pediatr Pulmonol 1996; 22:314-318.
99. Meyer GG, Postma DS, van der Heide S, de Reus DM, Roorda RJ, Koëter GH, van Aalderen, WMC. Am J Respir Crit Med 1996.
100. Sherill DL, Martinez FD, Lebowitz MD, et al. Longitudinal effects of passive smoking on pulmonary function in New Zealand children. Am Rev Respir Dis 1992; 145:1136–1141.
101. Xu X, Li B. Exposure–response relationship between passive smoking and adult pulmonary function. Am J Respir Crit Care Med 1995; 151:41–46.
102. Tager IB, Segal MR, Speizer FE, Weiss ST. The natural history of expiratory volumes. Effects of cigarette smoking and respiratory symptoms. Am Rev Respir Dis 1988; 138:837–849.
103. Corbo GM, Agabiti N, Forastiere F, et al. Lung function in children and adolescence with occasional exposure to environmental tobacco smoke. Am J Respir Crit Care Med 1996; 154:695–700.
104. Selroos O, Pietinalho A, Löfroos AB, Riska H. Effect of early vs late intervention with inhaled corticosteroids in asthma. Chest 1995; 108:1228–1234.
105. Postma DS, Vries K de, Koëter GH, Sluiter HJ. Independent influence of reversibility of air-flow obstruction and nonspecific hyperreactivity on the long-term course of lung function in the chronic air-flow obstruction. Am Rev Respir Dis 1986; 134:276–280.
106. Borsboom GJJ, van Pelt W, Quanjer PH. Pubertal growth curves of ventilatory function: relationship with childhood respiratory symptoms. Am Rev Respir Dis 1993; 147:372–378.
107. Greenough A, Everett L, Pool J, Price JF. A 2-year longitudinal study of lung hyperinflation in young asthmatics. Respir Med 1991; 85:379–382.
108. Peat JK, Tovey E, Toelle BG, et al. House dust mite allergens: a major risk factor for childhood asthma in Australia. Am J Respir Crit Care Med 1996; 153:141–146.
109. Sporik S, Holgate ST, Platt-Mills TAE, Cogswell JJ. Exposure to house-dust mite allergen (Der p I) and the development of asthma in childhood. A prospective study. N Engl J Med 1990; 323:502–507.
110. Warner JO, Boner AL. Allergy and childhood asthma. Clin Immunol Allergy 1988; 2:217–229.

111. Platt-Mills TAE, Tovey ER, Mitchell EB, Moszoro H, Nock P, Wilkins SR. Reduction of bronchial hyperreactivity during prolonged allergen avoidance. Lancet 1982; 2:675–677.
112. Björkstén B, Holt BJ, Baron-Hay MJ, Munir AKM, Holt PG. Low-level exposure to house dust mites stimulates T-cell responses during early childhood independent of atopy. Clin Exp Allergy 1996; 26:775–779.
113. Agertoft L, Pedersen S. Effects of long-term treatment with an inhaled corticosteroid on growth and pulmonary function in asthmatic children. Respir Med 1994; 88:373–381.
114. Overbeek SE, Kerstjens HAM, Bogaard JM, Mulder PGH, Postma DS. Is delayed introduction of inhaled corticosteroids harmful in patients with obstructive airways disease (asthma and COPD)? Chest 1996; 110:35–41.
115. van Essen-Zandvliet EEM, Hughes MD, Wallkens HJ, Duiverman EJ, Kerrebijn KF. Remission of childhood asthma after long-term treatment with an inhaled corticosteroid (budesonide): can it be achieved? Eur Respir J 1994; 7:63–68.
116. Waalkens HJ, van Essen-Zandvliet EE, Hughes MD, et al. Cessation of long-term treatment with inhaled corticosteroid (budesonide) in children with asthma results in deterioration. Am Rev Respir Dis 1993; 148:1252–1257.
117. Haahtela T, Järvinen M, Kava T, et al. Effects of reducing or discontinuing inhaled budesonide in patients with mild asthma. N Engl J Med 1994; 331:700–705.

Part Two

ALLERGEN-SPECIFIC IMMUNOTHERAPY

CURRENT KNOWLEDGE

6

Allergen Immunotherapy

Therapeutic Vaccines for Allergic Diseases

JEAN BOUSQUET

Montpellier University and
Service des Maladies Respiratoires–
INSERM U454
Montpellier University Hospital
Montpellier, France

RICHARD F. LOCKEY

University of South Florida
College of Medicine
Tampa, Florida

HANS-JØRGEN MALLING

National University Hospital
Copenhagen, Denmark

WHO Position Paper, Executive Summary

Chairmen: J. Bousquet, R. Lockey, H.-J. Malling
Panel members: E. Alvarez-Cuesta, G. W. Canonica, M. D. Chapman, P. J. Creticos, J. M. Dayer, S. R. Durham, P. Demoly, R. J. Goldstein, T. Ishikawa, K. Ito, D. Kraft, P. H. Lambert, H. Løwenstein, U. Müller, P. S. Norman, R. E. Reisman, R. Valenta, E. Valovirta, H. Yssel

Cosponsored by

American Academy of Allergy, Asthma, and Immunology (AAAAI)
European Academy of Allergology and Clinical Immunology (EAACI)
European Society of Pediatric Allergy and Clinical Immunology (ESPACI)
IUIS/IAACI Subcommittee on Allergen Standardization
Japanese Society of Allergology
National Institute of Allergy and Infectious Diseases (NIAID)
World Health Organization (WHO)

and endorsed by The American College of Allergy, Asthma, and Immunology (ACAAI) and Interasma.

I. Introduction

Allergen immunotherapy is the practice of administering gradually increasing quantities of an allergen extract to an allergic subject to ameliorate the symptoms associated with the subsequent exposure to the causative allergen. Allergen immunotherapy was introduced to treat "pollinosis" or allergic rhinitis by Noon and Freeman in 1911 (1). For the past 80 years, immunotherapy has been used to treat allergic diseases caused by inhalant allergens and Hymenoptera venoms. Venom immunotherapy is accepted as the standard of care for Hymenoptera-induced systemic allergic reactions. There is good evidence that immunotherapy using inhalant allergens to treat seasonal or perennial allergic rhinitis and asthma is clinically effective.

Guidelines and indications for immunotherapy with inhalant allergens or venoms were proposed in 1987 (2) and have been published within the past years by the World Health Organization (WHO; 3,4) the European Academy of Allergy and Clinical Immunology (EAACI; 2,5,6), the International Consensus Report on Asthma (7), the Global Strategy for Asthma Management and Prevention (8), the International Consensus Report on Rhinitis (9), the British Society for Allergy and Clinical Immunology (10), the American Academy of Allergy, Asthma, and Immunology (AAAAI), and the American College of Allergy, Asthma, and Immunology (ACAAI; 11).

These reports provide guidelines for a better understanding of the use of allergen immunotherapy. However, none of them represent a consensus report of experts from various parts of the world where such therapy is used (3,5,10–12), and some address only specific issues on one of the target organs in relation to asthma (7,8) or to rhinitis (9).

Physicians and scientists from several countries convened at WHO headquarters in Geneva, January 27–29, 1997, to review the science of, and indications for, allergen immunotherapy to treat allergic diseases. New forms of therapy, currently under development, that may prove to be safer and more effective than conventional treatments were also discussed.

Vaccines are used in medicine as immune modifiers. So, too, is allergen immunotherapy. Knowledge gained from studies of allergic mechanisms, such as the importance of T helper (Th)1 and Th2 cells, cytokine regulation of the immune responses, and specific inhibition or ablation of pathogenic immune responses by means of tolerance induction, may be applicable to a variety of allergic and other immunological diseases. This is especially true for autoimmune diseases, such as juvenile diabetes mellitus and multiple sclerosis. Thus, the concepts used and the scientific data that support the use of allergen immunotherapy to treat allergic diseases are now being applied scientifically for other immunological diseases. Therefore, the panel entitled this position statement *Allergen Immunotherapy: Therapeutic Vaccines for Allergic Diseases* to indicate that vaccines (allergen extracts) that modify or downregulate the immune response for allergic diseases are part of this broad-based category of therapies presently employed and being developed to treat other immunological and infectious diseases.

II. Allergen Standardization

The quality of the allergen vaccine is critical for both diagnosis and treatment. Where possible, standardized vaccines of known potency and shelf life should be used. The most common vaccines used in clinical allergy practice are now available as standardized products or are pending standardization. However, there are many vaccines currently being marketed (many of which are used only occasionally), and it is neither feasible nor economic to standardize all of them. The measurement of major allergens for standardization is now a realistic and desirable goal that should be encouraged (13,14). Allergen vaccines should be distributed, provided their potency, composition, and stability have been documented as (1) vaccines from a single-source material; (2) mixtures of related, cross-reacting allergen vaccines, such as grass pollen vaccines; deciduous tree pollen vaccines; related ragweed pollen vaccines and related mite vaccines; or (3) mixtures of other allergen vaccines, provided that stability data (15) and data on clinical efficacy are available. Where mixtures are marketed, the relative amounts of each component of the mixture should be indicated.

III. Mechanisms

Immunotherapy is specific to the antigen administered (16). The mechanisms of immunotherapy are complex and may differ, depending on the allergen (venoms or inhalant allergens) and the route of immunization. Whereas earlier work focused on circulating antibody (17,18), newer studies suggest that immunotherapy acts by modifying T-cell responses, either by immune deviation (increase in Th0/Th1) or T-cell anergy (decrease in Th2/Th0), or more likely both (19–21). Systemic and local increases in $CD8^+$ cells have also been observed. Immunotherapy also reduces inflammatory cell recruitment and activation, and mediator secretion (22,23).

IV. Subcutaneous Immunotherapy

A. Efficacy

Controlled studies demonstrate that allergen immunotherapy is effective for patients with stinging insect hypersensitivity (for review, see Ref. 24), allergic rhinitis or conjunctivitis, and allergic asthma. Immunotherapy is effective treatment for many pollen species, including grasses, ragweed, *Parietaria*, and mountain cedar (for review see Ref. 5). Immunotherapy with house dust mite vaccines is effective for treatment of asthma (25) and rhinitis. Fewer studies indicate that immunotherapy is effective for patients allergic to cat (26), *Alternaria* (27), and *Cladosporium* (28). A metanalysis of clinical trials of allergen immunotherapy demonstrated that it is effective for treatment of asthma (29).

Immunotherapy dosing raises contrasting efficacy and safety issues. Low-dose immunotherapy is ineffective (30), and high doses of allergen vaccines may induce a high and unacceptable rate of systemic reactions. Thus, optimal doses using vaccines labeled either in biological units (BU) (31) or in mass of major allergens (allergy unit; AU) (32) have been proposed. The *optimal dose* is defined as the dose of allergen vaccine inducing a clinically relevant effect in the majority of patients without causing unacceptable side effects (33,34). The optimal dose should be the maintenance target dose for all patients (31). Doses of 5–20 μg of the major allergen are optimal doses for domestic mites (31,34,35), cat dander (26,36), ragweed pollen (37–39), and Hymenoptera venoms (6,40). Most patients with allergic diseases can tolerate this target dose without difficulty. However, in selected individuals who have experienced reactions during their build-up treatment phase, a lower maintenance dose may be necessary. As with any therapeutic approach, the benefit/risk ratio must be carefully considered to determine whether immunotherapy should be continued.

Immunotherapy is the only treatment that may affect the natural course of allergic diseases. The use of allergen immunotherapy requires specialist assessment, especially in children, because there are special problems and questions in this age group. Immunotherapy started early in the disease process may modify the spontaneous long-term progress of the allergic inflammation and disease (5,41). Immunotherapy is rarely started before the age of 5 years.

B. Safety

The major risk of allergen immunotherapy is anaphylaxis (42–45). Asthma appears to be a significant risk factor for systemic reactions (46,47). Therefore, allergen immunotherapy should be administered by or under the close supervision of a trained physician who can recognize early symptoms and signs of anaphylaxis and administer emergency treatment.

C. Indications

The treatment of allergic diseases is based on allergen avoidance, pharmacotherapy, allergen immunotherapy, and patient education. Physicians should know the local and regional aerobiology and be aware of the potential allergens in the patient's indoor and outdoor environments. Only physicians with a training in allergology can select the clinically relevant allergen vaccines for therapy. Immunotherapy, where appropriate, should be used in combination with other forms of therapy, with the hope that the patient will become as symptom-free as medically possible.

Allergen immunotherapy is indicated for patients who have demonstrable evidence of specific IgE antibodies to clinically relevant allergens and whose allergic symptoms warrant the time and risk of allergen immunotherapy. Contraindications for inhalant allergen and venom immunotherapy may be absolute or relative (5). Patient selection is important, and efficacy must always be balanced against the risk of side effects. The necessity for initiating allergen immunotherapy depends on the degree to which symptoms can be reduced by medication, the amount and type of medication required to control symptoms, and whether effective allergen avoidance is possible.

The indications for venom immunotherapy are provided in the position paper of EAACI (6). An absolute indication is a history of severe allergic systemic reactions with respiratory or cardiovascular symptoms and positive diagnostic tests (skin tests or serum-specific IgE).

The indications for immunotherapy in asthma and rhinitis have been separated in some guidelines (7–9), and this artificial separation has led to unresolved questions (48,49), possibly because the IgE-mediated reaction has not been considered to be a multiple organ involvement. Therefore, it is important to consider immunotherapy based on the allergen sensitization, rather than on a particular disease manifestation.

Immunotherapy for treatment of allergic rhinitis–conjunctivitis is indicated (1) when antihistamines and topical drugs insufficiently control symptoms, (2) in patients who do not wish to receive pharmacotherapy, (3) when pharmacotherapy produces undesirable side effects, (4) when the patient is concerned about long-term pharmacological therapy, or (5) if the season is prolonged or polysensitized patients are exposed to several subsequent pollen seasons (i.e., tree, grass, and weed pollen sensitivity; 3,5). The risk/benefit ratio should be considered in every patient.

Although efficacy of immunotherapy has been shown for treatment of allergic asthma, the increased risk of systemic reactions in patients with asthma has been considered a contraindication in the United Kingdom guidelines (10), although not in the other published national or international guidelines (7–9).

Patients allergic to mites are candidates for mite allergen immunotherapy if they have significant symptoms of rhinitis or asthma when they are exposed to domestic mite allergens.

Avoidance is the treatment of choice for animal dander–induced allergic diseases. However, complete avoidance is often impossible, sometimes because of exposure to animal allergens in environments in which animals are not present (50). Immunotherapy may be prescribed for patients in whom avoidance of animal allergens is not fully effective, such as occupational exposure or refusal to evict an animal from the home.

For mold allergy, avoidance, where possible, of indoor mold allergens is the treatment of choice. Some studies have demonstrated clinical improvement when well-characterized vaccines of *Cladosporium* or *Alternaria* have been used in the treatment of mold-induced allergy. Patients with positive skin tests and symptoms when exposed to other relevant mold allergens may be considered for immunotherapy.

Immunotherapy with vaccines of undefined allergens, such as house dust, bacteria, *Candida albicans*, and *Trichophyton*, should not be used (5).

The duration of immunotherapy required to maintain improvement in clinical symptoms is still unknown. For those patients who respond to treatment, many clinicians advise 3–5 years of therapy. However, a decision on when to discontinue allergen immunotherapy should be individualized. Several studies suggest that venom immunotherapy may be discontinued after 3–5 years in most patients.

V. Other Routes of Immunotherapy

New routes of administration of immunotherapy are currently being explored: nasal, sublingual–swallow or oral immunotherapy using high allergen doses (for review, see Ref 51). Given the results of current studies, immunotherapy by the oral or bronchial route cannot be recommended. Properly controlled, well-designed studies employing high-dose sublingual–swallow and intranasal immunotherapy provide evidence that this form of therapy may be a viable alternative to parenteral injection therapy in the treatment of allergic airways disease. Sublingual without swallowing is still questionable. Further studies need to be performed to fully characterize the most appropriate patients, the optimal therapeutic target dose, and the degree of effectiveness when compared with conventional injection immunotherapy.

VI. Future Vaccines

In the future, new technologies and the improvement of our knowledge of the basic mechanisms of allergic diseases may completely alter the way allergen immunotherapy is used. These advances should result in new, safer, and substantially more effective methods of manipulating the human immune response. These new approaches will be directed at every disease induced by antigen, such as asthma, as well as autoimmune diseases, such as type I diabetes and multiple sclerosis. For allergic diseases, several approaches may be used such as the development of nonanaphylactic allergens, or allergen fragments or peptides for active immunotherapy (52,53), IgE-binding haptens of major allergens for passive saturation of effector cells and induction of blocking antibodies (54), allergen-specific antibodies, and antibody fragments for passive therapy in the allergic effector organs (55,56), plasmid DNA immunization (57), and anti-IgE humanized monoclonal antibodies (58).

VII. Research Needs

Future studies of immunotherapy are needed in the following areas:

1. Cost-effectiveness
2. Quality of life and patient's satisfaction

3. Comparison with pharmacological treatment
4. "Add-on" studies (e.g., effect of immunotherapy added to treatment with topical therapy)
5. Optimal duration
6. Reduction of the severity of asthma in terms of hospital admissions and emergency room visits
7. Decrease of the incidence of asthma in patients suffering from allergic rhinitis and no asthma
8. Altering the natural course of the allergic rhinoconjunctivitis or asthma
9. Decreasing the long-term sequellae associated with allergic rhinitis or asthma
10. Long-term effects after cessation
11. Efficacy and safety for animal allergy (dogs, horses)
12. Efficacy and safety for occupational allergy (e.g., laboratory animal allergy)
13. Efficacy and safety in children younger than 5 years of age

Abbreviations

AAAAI: American Academy of Allergy, Asthma, and Immunology
AU: allergy unit
*BAU: Bioequivalent allergy unit
BU: biologic unit
CBER: Center for Biologic Evaluation and Research
EAACI: European Academy of Allergy and Clinical Immunology
EU: European Union
IAACI: International Association of Allergy and Clinical Immunology
*IU: international unit
IUIS: International Union of Immunological Societies
*PNU: protein nitrogen unit

References

1. Noon L. Prophylactic inoculation against hay fever. Lancet 1911; 1:1572–1573.
2. Bousquet J, Muller UR, Dreborg S, et al. Immunotherapy with Hymenoptera venoms. Position paper of the Working Group on Immunotherapy of the European Academy of Allergy and Clinical Immunology. Allergy 1987; 42;401–413.
3. The current status of allergen immunotherapy (hyposensitisation). Report of a WHO/IUIS working group. Allergy 1989; 44:369–379.
4. Current status of allergen immunotherapy. Shortened version of a World Health Oganisation/ International Union of Immunological Societies working group report. Lancet 1989; 1:259–261.
5. Malling H, Weeke B. Immunotherapy. Position paper of the European Academy of Allergy and Clinical Immunology. Allergy 1993; 48 (suppl 14):9–35.
6. Muller U, Mosbech H. Position paper: immunotherapy with Hymenoptera venoms. Allergy 1993; 48(suppl 14):37–46.

7. International Consensus report on diagnosis and management of asthma. International Asthma Management Project. Allergy 1992; 47:1–61.
8. Global strategy for asthma management and prevention. WHO/NHLBI workshop report. In: National Institutes of Health, National Heart, Lung and Blood Institute, Publication 95-3659, 1995.
9. International Consensus report on the diagnosis and management of rhinitis. Allergy 1994; 49(suppl 19):1–33.
10. Frew AJ. Injection immunotherapy. British Society for Allergy and Clinical Immunology working party. Br Med J 1993; 307:919–923.
11. Nicklas R, Bernstein I, Blessing-Moore J, et al. Practice parameters for allergen immunotherapy. J Allergy Clin Immunol 1996; 6:1001–1011.
12. Creticos P, Lockey R. Immunotherapy practice. Guide to current procedures. American Academy of Allergy, Asthma, and Immunology, Milwaukee, WI, 1994; 1–77.
13. Dreborg S, Frew A. Allergen standardization and skin tests. EAACI position paper. Allergy 1993; 48(suppl 14).
14. The use of standardized allergen extracts. Position statement. American Academy of Allergy, Asthma and Immunology (AAAAI). J Allergy Clin Immunol 1997; 99:583-586.
15. Nelson HS, Ikle D, Buchmeier A. Studies of allergen extract stability: the effects of dilution and mixing. J Allergy Clin Immunol 1996; 98:382–388.
16. Norman PS, Lichtenstein LM. The clinical and immunologic specificity of immunotherapy. J Allergy Clin Immunol 1978; 61:370–377.
17. Golden DB, Meyers DA, Kagey-Sobotka A, Valentine MD, Lichtenstein LM. Clinical relevance of the venom-specific immunoglobulin G antibody level during immunotherapy. J Allergy Clin Immunol 1982; 69:489–493.
18. Van der Zee JS, Aalberse RC. The role of IgG in immediate-type hypersensitivity. Eur Respir J Suppl 1991; 13:91s–96s.
19. Varney VA, Hamid QA, Gaga M, et al. Influence of grass pollen immunotherapy on cellular infiltration and cytokine mRNA expression during allergen-induced late-phase cutaneous responses. J Clin Invest 1993; 92:644–651.
20. Secrist H, Chelen CJ, Wen Y, Marshall JD, Umetsu DT. Allergen immunotherapy decreases interleukin 4 production in $CD4^+$ T cells from allergic individuals. J Exp Med 1993; 178:2123–2130.
21. Jutel M, Pichler WJ, Skrbic D, Urwyler A, Dahinden C, Muller UR. Bee venom immunotherapy results in decrease of IL-4 and IL-5 and increase of IFN-gamma secretion in specific allergen-stimulated T cell cultures. J Immunol 1995; 154:4187–4194.
22. Hedlin G, Silber G, Naclerio R, et al. Comparison of the in-vivo and in-vitro response to ragweed immunotherapy in children and adults with ragweed-induced rhinitis. Clin Exp Allergy 1990; 20:491–500.
23. Bousquet J, Becker WM, Hejjaoui A, et al. Differences in clinical and immunologic reactivity of patients allergic to grass pollens and to multiple-pollen species. II. Efficacy of a double-blind, placebo-controlled, specific immunotherapy with standardized extracts. J Allergy Clin Immunol 1991; 88:43–53.
24. Muller U, Helbling A, Berchtold E . Immunotherapy with honeybee venom and yellow jacket venom is different regarding efficacy and safety. J Allergy Clin Immunol 1992; 89:529–535.
25. Bousquet J, Michel FB. Specific immunotherapy in asthma: is it effective? J Allergy Clin Immunol 1994; 94:1–11.
26. Alvarez-Cuesta E, Cuesta-Herranz J, Puyana-Ruiz J, Cuesta-Herranz C, Blanco-Quiros A. Monoclonal antibody-standardized cat extract immunotherapy: risk-benefit effects from a double-blind placebo study. J Allergy Clin Immunol 1994; 93:556–566.
27. Horst M, Hejjaoui A, Horst V, Michel FB, Bousquet J. Double-blind, placebo-controlled rush immunotherapy with a standardized *Alternaria* extract. J Allergy Clin Immunol 1990; 85:460–472.
28. Malling HJ, Dreborg S, Weeke B. Diagnosis and immunotherapy of mould allergy. V. Clini-

cal efficacy and side effects of immunotherapy with *Cladosporium herbarum*. Allergy 1986; 41:507–519.

29. Abramson MJ, Puy RM, Weiner JM. Is allergen immunotherapy effective in asthma? A meta-analysis of randomized controlled trials [see comments]. Am J Respir Crit Care Med 1995; 151:969-974.
30. van Metre TEJ, Adkinson N Jr, Lichtenstein LM, et al. A controlled study of the effectiveness of the Rinkel method of immunotherapy for ragweed pollen hay fever. J Allergy Clin Immunol 1980; 65:288–297.
31. Bousquet J, Des-Roches A, Paradis L, Dhivert H, Michel FB. Specific immunotherapy in house dust mite allergy. Clin Rev Allergy Immunol 1995; 13:151–159.
32. Carreira J, Lombardero M, Ventas P. New developments in in vitro methods. Quantification of clinically relevant allergens in mass units. Arb Paul Ehrlich Inst Bundesamt Sera Impfstoffe Frankf A M 1994; 87:155–164.
33. Creticos PS, van Metre TE, Mardiney MR, Rosenberg GL, Norman PS, Adkinson N Jr. Dose response of IgE and IgG antibodies during ragweed immunotherapy. J Allergy Clin Immunol 1984; 73:94–104.
34. Haugaard L, Dahl R, Jacobsen L. A controlled dose–response study of immunotherapy with standardized, partially purified extract of house dust mite: clinical efficacy and side effects. J Allergy Clin Immunol 1993; 91:709–722.
35. Olaguibel J, Tabar A, Garcia-Figueroa B, Cortes C. Immunotherapy with standardized extract of *Dermatophagoides pteronyssinus* in bronchial asthma: a dose–titration study. Allergy 1997; 52:68–72.
36. van Metre TE J, Marsh DG, Adkinson N Jr, et al. Immunotherapy for cat asthma. J Allergy Clin Immunol 1988; 82:1055–1068.
37. Creticos PS, Marsh DG, Proud D, et al. Responses to ragweed-pollen nasal challenge before and after immunotherapy. J Allergy Clin Immunol 1989; 84:197–205.
38. van Metre TEJ, Adkinson N Jr, Amodio FJ, et al. A comparison of immunotherapy schedules for injection treatment of ragweed pollen hay fever. J Allergy Clin Immunol 1982; 69:181–193.
39. Creticos PS, Reed CE, Norman PS, et al. Ragweed immunotherapy in adult asthma [see comments]. N Engl J Med 1996; 334:501–506.
40. Hunt KJ, Valentine MD, Sobotka AK, Benton AW, Amodio FJ, Lichtenstein LM. A controlled trial of immunotherapy in insect hypersensitivity. N Engl J Med 1978; 299:157–161.
41. Ownby DR, Adinoff AD. The appropriate use of skin testing and allergen immunotherapy in young children [see comments]. J Allergy Clin Immunol 1994; 94:662–665.
42. Lockey RF, Benedict LM, Turkeltaub PC, Bukantz SC. Fatalities from immunotherapy (IT) and skin testing (ST). J Allergy Clin Immunol 1987; 79:660–677.
43. Lockey RF, Turkeltaub PC, Olive ES, Hubbard JM, Baird-Warren IA, Bukantz SC. The Hymenoptera venom study. III: Safety of venom immunotherapy. J Allergy Clin Immunol 1990; 86:775–780.
44. Stewart GD, Lockey RF. Systemic reactions from allergen immunotherapy [editorial]. J Allergy Clin Immunol 1992; 90:567–578.
45. Lüderitz-Püchel U, May S, Haustein D. Zwischenfälle nach Hyposensibilisierung. Münch Med Wochenschr 1996; 138:129–132.
46. Committee on Safety of Medicines. Desensitizing vaccines. Br Med J 1986; 293:948.
47. Bousquet J, Hejjaoui A, Dhivert H, Clauzel AM, Michel FB. Immunotherapy with a standardized *Dermatophagoides pteronyssinus* extract. III. Systemic reactions during the rush protocol in patients suffering from asthma. J Allergy Clin Immunol 1989; 83:797–802.
48. Norman P. Is there a role for immunotherapy in the treatment of asthma? Yes. Am J Respir Crit Care Med 1996; 154:1225–1228.
49. Barnes P. Is there a role for immunotherapy in the treatment of asthma? No. Am J Respir Crit Care Med 1996; 154:1227–1228.
50. Munir AK, Bjorksten B, Einarsson R, et al. Cat (Fel d 1), dog (Can f 1), and cockroach

allergens in homes of asthmatic children from three climatic zones in Sweden. Allergy 1994; 49:508-516.

51. Malling H. Local immunotherapy. EAACI–ESPACI position paper. Allergy 1998.
52. Ferreira F, Hirthenlehner K, Briza P, et al. Isoforms of atopic allergens with reduced allergenicity but conserved T cell antigenicity: possible use for specific immunotherapy. Int Arch Allergy Immunol 1997; 113:125–127.
53. Yssel H, Fasler S, Lamb J, de Vries JE. Induction of non-responsiveness in human allergen-specific type 2 T helper cells. Curr Opin Immunol 1994; 6:847–852.
54. Ball T, Vrtala S, Sperr WR, et al. Isolation of an immunodominant IgE hapten from an epitope expression cDNA library. Dissection of the allergic effector reaction. J Biol Chem 1994; 269:28323–28328.
55. Visco V, Dolecek C, Denepoux S, et al. Human IgG monoclonal antibodies that modulate the binding of specific IgE to birch pollen Bet v 1. J Immunol 1996; 157:956-962.
56. Lebecque S, Dolecek C, Laffler S, et al. Immunologic characteristization of monoclonal antibodies which modulate human immunoglobulin E binding to the major birch pollen allergen Bet v 1. J Allergy Clin Immunol 1997; 99:374–384.
57. Raz E, Tighe H, Sato Y, et al. Preferential induction of a Thl immune response and inhibition of specific IgE antibody formation by plasmid DNA immunization. Proc Natl Acad Sci USA 1996; 93:5141–5145.
58. Fahy J, Fleming H, Wong H, et al. The effect of an anti-IgE monoclonal antibody on the early and late phase responses to allergen inhalation in asthmatic subjects. Am J Respir Crit Care Med 1997; 1828–1834.

7

Allergen-Specific Immunotherapy

New Strategies Using Recombinant Allergens

ALISA M. SMITH and MARTIN D. CHAPMAN

Asthma and Allergic Diseases Center
University of Virginia School of Medicine
Charlottesville, Virginia

I. Introduction

Over the past 10 years, epidemiological studies have demonstrated a strong relationship between sensitization to indoor allergens (development of IgE) and asthma. Among the potential risk factors, such as air pollution, passive smoking, or viral infections, indoor allergens from dust mites, cat, dog, and cockroach consistently demonstrate the strongest association with asthma (odds ratio > 10). A variety of study designs, including population studies, emergency room studies, and prospective studies, as well as studies from different geographic regions of the world, have conclusively shown that sensitization to indoor allergens is the strongest risk factor for asthma. In particular, up to 85% of patients with asthma have IgE antibodies to house dust mite allergens (1–10). Development of IgE-type antibodies is dependent on allergen exposure. Recently, studies have confirmed that, in communities with high levels of dust mites, such as the southeastern United States, coastal Australia, Germany, and the United Kingdom, there is a dose-response relationship between mite allergen exposure and prevalence of sensitization among asthmatics (5,11–13). In areas with low mite levels, such as arid regions of the United States (Arizona) and Australia (Moree/Narrabri) or regions of high altitude (New Mexico, the French Alps), other indoor allergens become more important (8,14). For example, among middle-school children living in Los Alamos, New Mexico, cat and dog allergens are strongly associated with symptomatic bronchial hyperreactivity, whereas in Arizona, *Alternaria* is most important (15,16). Cockroach allergens are a strong risk factor for asthma in those communities where cockroach infestation is common, such as crowded urban apartment buildings and low-income housing projects (e.g., Atlanta, Georgia, Wilmington, Delaware, and Strasbourg, France; 11,17,18). Thus, indoor allergens are the most important source of allergens associated with asthma worldwide (Table l; 19–35).

In parallel with epidemiological studies, molecular cloning techniques have become established for the identification and analysis of allergen molecules. More than 20 indoor allergens, as well as many pollen and venom allergens, have been cloned and sequenced, and allergens now constitute a large, well-defined group of proteins for biomedical research (36–39). Strategies for improving diagnosis of allergic disease and asthma therapy, based on recombinant allergens, have become feasible now that major allergens can be produced in large quantities, purified to homogeneity, and modified using genetic engineering. Recombinant allergens can also be used for the development of sensitive immunoassays that are useful for studies of allergen exposure and the characterization of the aerodynamic properties of allergens.

In spite of the advances in characterization and standardization of allergen extracts, immunotherapy for allergic disease is practiced today much the same as it has been over the course of this century. In 1911, Noon and Freeman established the fundamental approach of administering allergen-derived extracts, in their case pollen, for the treatment of seasonal hay fever (40,41). The effectiveness of immunotherapy was initially attributed to the development of IgG-type antibodies that were thought to block the interaction of IgE and allergen, but by the mid-1970s, several studies had failed to establish a correlation between IgG titers and improvement of symptoms (42,43). Subsequently, allergen immunotherapy was proposed to stimulate suppressor T cells that downregulated IgE production (44). Today, the regulation of T-cell responses to allergens is thought to be the key to successful immunotherapy; however, the precise mechanisms remain obscure (45). It is clear that the dose, the quality of the allergen extract, and the length of the therapy are key to achieving effective treatment (46). However, there are problems associated with conventional immunotherapy, including side effects ranging from swelling at the site of injection to systemic reactions that may result in anaphylaxis. Currently, research is focused on improving allergen-specific immunotherapy by using recombinant DNA technology. The aims of this chapter are to review the current knowledge of the molecular biology of the principal indoor allergens associated with asthma and to outline different strategies for the use of recombinant allergens in immunotherapy.

Date; Ref.	Geographic location	Allergens	Odds ratio	Significance
Population studies				
1991; 19	Sao Paulo, Brazil	Mite	nd	$p < 0.001$[a]
1991–1996; 5,8–10,20	Coastal and inland Australia	Mite, cat, dog	2.7–20.9[a], 2.4–4[a]	
1989; 21	Germany	Mite	5–11[c]	
1990; 22	London, England	Mite	nd	$p < 0.01$[c]
1991, 1993; 23,24	Stockholm, Sweden	Mite	4.9[a], 25.7[a]	
1992–1995; 25–27	Southwestern Germany	Mite, "animal dander"	2.2–4[a], 2.6–3.6[a], 2.8[b]	
1996; 28	Manchester, England	Mite	nd	$p < 0.01$[b]
Emergency room studies				
1996; 29	Florida	Mite	nd	$p < 0.001$
1996; 29	Florida	Cockroach	nd	$p < 0.05$
1993; 17	Wilmington, DE	Mite, cat, cockroach	6.2–16.3[a]	$p < 0.001$[a]
1992; 11	Atlanta, GA	Mite, cat, cockroach	9.5[b]	$p < 0.001$[a]
1993; 30	Charlottesville, VA	Mite	4.5[a]	
1993; 31	Poole, England	Mite, cat	nd	$p < 0.001$[a]
1989; 12	Charlottesville, VA	Mite, cat, cockroach	nd	$p < 0.001$[a]
Prospective studies				
1992; 32	Isle of Wight, England	Mite, cat	6.1[c]	$p < 0.01$[c]
1992; 34	Isle of Wight, England	Mite, cat	3.2[a]	$p = 0.002$[a]
1994; 33	Isle of Wight, England	Mite, cat	16.1[c]	
1990; 13	Poole, England	Mite	19.7[a], 4.8[b]	
1989; 4	Dunedin, NZ	Mite, cat, dog	6.7, 4.2, 3.7[a]	
High-altitude studies				
1995; 15	Los Alamos, NM	Cat, dog	6.2[b]	$p < 0.001$[a]
1995; 16	Los Alamos, NM	Cat, dog	nd	$p < 0.001$[a]
1988, 1991; 6,7	Martigues and Briancon, France	Mite	nd	$p < 0.001$[a]

[a]Sensitization (IgE antibodies) alone.
[b]Sensitization and exposure.
[c]Exposure as a risk factor for sensitization.
nd, not determined.

II. Molecular Biology of Indoor Allergens

A. Identification and Cloning

The first inhaled allergen to be cloned was Der p 1, by Chua and Thomas in 1988 (47,48). This was followed by Der p 2 and the group 1 and group 2 homologues from *Dermatophagoides farinae* (49–52). The group 1 and group 2 mite allergens had previously been identified by protein purification from extracts of mite culture media and were shown to be important, based on their reactivity with IgE from most dust mite allergic patients. Today, cDNA cloning has defined the primary amino acid sequence of at least ten different groups of allergens from *Dermatophagoides* spp., as well as several homologous allergens from *Euroglyphus*, *Lepidoglyphus*, and *Blomia* spp. (36,37). The prevalence of IgE binding to these proteins may vary, depending on the patient population; however, as many as six of these allergens react with IgE from more than 50% of mite allergic patients and are considered to be important allergens.

The major cat allergen Fel d 1 and the cockroach allergen Bla g 2, also originally identified by immunochemical techniques, have been cloned and sequenced (53,54). cDNA cloning has identified additional cockroach allergens: Bla g 4 and Bla g 5 (55,56). These proteins had not previously been identified by classic protein purification approaches, and this provides a good example of the strength of cloning studies for the identification and characterization of allergens. Most recently, sensitization to fungal allergens has been associated with asthma, and allergens from *Aspergillus*, *Alternaria*, and *Cladosporium* have been cloned (57–59).

The biological function of several allergens has been determined by sequence homology searches. Der p 1, Der p 3, and Der p 4 are cysteine or serine proteases, and Der p 4 is an amylase. Given the proteolytic activity of these allergens, Stewart and others have postulated that the enzyme activity of allergens influences the IgE response, perhaps by facilitating allergen uptake by the respiratory mucosa or by cleavage of cell surface CD23, which causes an upregulation of this IgE receptor (60,61). Many allergens also belong to the ligand-binding family or calycins; these include Bla g 4, rat and mouse urinary proteins, and the dog allergen Can f 1. Homology with proteins of known structure has been used to model the tertiary structure of allergens; for example, Der p 1 has been modeled on the papain structure, and Bla g 4 has been modeled on the calycin, bilin-binding protein (55,62). Not only does this provide information about the biological function of these allergens but structural models provide a picture of the antigenic surface recognized by antibodies; information that is important for identifying antigenic determinants for IgE and T cells. Table 2 lists characteristics of the major indoor allergens.

B. Expression of Recombinant Allergens

High-level in vitro expression systems have been developed as a consequence of cloning studies. This has provided larger quantities and more pure preparations of

Table 2 Structural and Functional Properties of Indoor Allergens

Source	Allergen[a]	MW	Function/homology
House dust mite			
Dermatophagoides	Group 1	23 kDa	Cysteine protease
	Group 2	14 kDa	Unknown[a]
	Group 3	25 kDa	Serine protease[b]
	Der p 4	60 kDa	Amylase
	Der p 5	14 kDa	Unknown
	Der p 6	25 kDa	Chymotrypsin
	Group 7	22–28 kDa	Unknown
	Der p 8	26 kDa	Glutathione transferase
	Der p 9	24 kDa	Serine protease[b]
	Der p 10	36 kDa	Tropomyosin
Euroglyphus maynei	Eur m 1	25 kDa	Cysteine protease
Blomia tropicalis	Blo t 5	14 kDa	Unknown
Lepidoglyphus destructor	Lep d 2	14 kDa	Unknown
Mammals			
Felis domesticus	Fel d 1	36 kDa	Uteroglobin
Canis familiaris	Can f 1	25 kDa	Calycin[c]
Mus musculus	Mus m 1	19 kDa	Calycin[d]
Rattus norvegicus	Rat n 1	19 kDa	Calycin[d]
Cockroach			
Blattella germanica	Bla g 1	20–25 kDa	Unknown
	Bla g 2	36 kDa	Aspartic protease
	Bla g 4	21 kDa	Calycin[e]
	Bla g 5	22 kDa	Glutathione transferase
	Bla g 6	18 kDa	Troponin
Periplaneta americana	Per a 1	20–25 kDa	Unknown
	Per a 3	72–78 kDa	Unknown
Fungi			
Aspergillus fumigatus	Asp f 1	18 kDa	Cytotoxin (mitogillin)
	Asp f 2	34 kDa	Unknown
Alternaria	Alt a 1	30 kDa	Unknown
	Alt a 2	23 kDa	Unknown
Cladosporium	Cla h 1	13 kDa	Unknown
	Cla h 2	23 kDa	Unknown
	Cla h 3	53 kDa	Aldehyde dehydrogenase
	Cla h 4	11 kDa	P2 ribosomal protein

[a]Group 2 allergens show sequence homology to a mammalian epididymal cDNA sequence.
[b]Group 3 allergens have trypsin-like substrate specificity; Der p 9 is a collagenolytic protease.
[c]Ligand-binding protein involved in taste recognition.
[d]Pheromone-binding protein.
[e]Member of the ligand-binding protein family; ligand has not been identified.

allergens than was previously possible using conventional protein purification techniques. Most commonly, recombinant allergens have been expressed in *Escherichia coli* or in the yeasts *Saccharomyces* and *Pichia*. For example, recombinant Der p 2 has been produced in bacteria with a final yield of 15 mg/L and recombinant Bla g 4 has been expressed in *P. pastoris* at 30 mg/L (63,64). Many of the recombinant allergens show immunoreactivity comparable with the native allergens, measured using the radioallergosorbent test (RAST), in vitro T-cell proliferation responses, and skin testing. Recombinant group 2, 5, and 7 allergens show an excellent correlation with native allergen for IgE binding using serum from patients with asthma, atopic dermatitis, and rhinitis, and quantitative skin testing has also confirmed this correlation (36). The group 1 mite allergens have been an exception; recombinant Der p 1 (rDer p 1) produced in bacteria or yeast showed only 50% reactivity (IgE binding) compared with the native allergen. However, Shoji et al. recently demonstrated that rDer f 1, with immunoreactivity and enzyme activity similar to the native allergen, could be produced in insect cells using a baculovirus expression system (65). Recombinant allergen expression systems have provided material for the development of sensitive immunoassays for detecting picogram quantities of allergen in house dust (39). In addition, high-level expression systems have provided material for structural studies of pollen (Bet v 1, Amb a 5) and dust mite (Der p 2) allergens using nuclear magnetic resonance and X-ray crystallography (66–68). This is especially important for those allergens for which primary amino acid analysis has failed to define the structure or function, such as the group 2 and group 5 mite allergens.

Recombinant allergens can be produced in unlimited supply, as pure preparations, and can be readily standardized in mass units, thereby providing well-defined reagents.

III. New Strategies for Immunotherapy

A. Rationale

Conventional immunotherapy using increasing doses of standardized extracts can be associated with adverse reactions, including swelling and discomfort at the site of injection, local edema, itching of the eyes or nose, generalized hives, and more serious systemic reactions that may lead to anaphylaxis. It is possible that the frequency of adverse reactions associated with immunotherapy might decrease using recombinant allergens. This might occur because preparations would lack the nonallergenic components found in extracts, and dosing could be better controlled. However, immunotherapy with recombinant allergens may produce side effects similar to those seen with the natural allergens, thus the rationale behind new strategies is to reduce IgE reactivity, with the aim of decreasing side effects, while providing effective treatment (Table 3).

Table 3 New Forms of Immunotherapy for Asthma

Recombinant allergens
Allergen variants (do not bind IgE)
Allergen peptides[a]
Allergens linked to adjuvants
Plasmid DNA vaccines
Anti-IgE therapy[a]
Antisense DNA

[a]Currently in phase 2 and phase 3 clinical trials.

B. T-Cell–Targeted Therapies

Advances in our knowledge of T-cell immunology, including the characterization of the T-cell receptor, major histocompatibility complex (MHC), and peptide interactions; antigen processing; and cytokine production, have focused attention on the T-cell compartment of immediate hypersensitivity as a prime target for intervention strategies (69). In addition, synthetic peptide chemistry has made it possible to evaluate the T-cell epitopes for any allergen of known primary amino acid sequence. The allergic response is dominated by T cells of the T helper type 2 (Th2) phenotype, secreting primarily interleukin (IL)-4 and IL-5, which are required for IgE production and eosinophilia. Downregulating this Th2 response, or redirecting the response to the Th1 phenotype, is the focus of several studies.

Peptide Therapy

The notion of downregulating allergic responses by using peptides corresponding to T-cell epitopes was supported by studies in murine systems demonstrating that T-cells could be rendered nonresponsive by immunization with high doses of a peptide representing an immunodominant T-cell epitope (70,71). This T-cell anergy was characterized by functional changes, including decreased IL-4 production, as well as changes in cell surface molecules, such as downregulation of the T-cell receptor (TCR) and upregulation of the IL-2 receptor, and increased turnover of CD28 transcripts (71,72). Usually, peptides from allergens react poorly with IgE, and thus peptide immunotherapy would be associated with fewer side effects. Peptides can be produced in large quantities, and this strategy does not depend on in vitro protein expression and purification systems.

Detailed studies on the use of T-cell peptides have been carried out using the cat allergen Fel d 1. Stimulatory T-cell epitopes are found throughout both chain 1 and chain 2 (Fig. 1; 73,74). However, two large peptides from chain 1 were identified that stimulated T cells from most cat allergic subjects and an immunotherapy

Primary structure and T cell epitopes of Fel d 1

```
                *-----IPC-1-------------------*
Chain 1:   EICPAVKRDVDLFLTGTPDEYVEQVAQYKALPVVLENARILKNCV45
           *-----------------*          *-------IPC-2-----
                *-------------------*

           DAKMTEEDKENALSLLDKIYTSPLC70
           ----------**---------------*

Chain 2:   VKMAETCPIFYDVFFAVANGNELLLDLSLTKVNATEPERTAMKKI45
           *--------------------------**-------------------
                  *------------------------**------------

           QDCYVENGLISRVLDGLVMTTISSSKDCMGEAVQNTVEDLKLNTLGR92
           --**--------------------IAIN*-EY *------------------*
           ----------------**---------------------------*
```

Figure 1 Primary amino acid sequence of Fel d1: Fel d 1 consists of two chains (70 and 92 amino acids) linked by two disulfide bonds. Stimulatory T-cell peptides were identified throughout both chains; representative epitopes are indicated by *——*. IPC-1 and IPC-2, from chain 1, are the peptides selected for an immunotherapy trial in cat-allergic subjects.

trial has been conducted using these peptides: IPC-1 represents residues 7–33 and IPC-2 represents residues 29–55 (see Fig. 1). The design and outcome of this trial have recently been published (75). Briefly, cat allergic patients received one of four dosing regimens: placebo, 7.5 μg, 75 μg, or 750 μg. Patients received subcutaneous injections weekly for 4 weeks and were evaluated for symptoms (on exposure to cats) before treatment and at 6 weeks after treatment. Those patients receiving the highest dose of peptide showed significantly fewer symptoms after exposure than the placebo group ($p < 0.05$). The 75-μg–dose group showed an intermediate decrease in symptoms, and there was no difference between the 7.5-μg group and the placebo controls. Figure 2 shows the symptom scores over time for the four patient groups.

Importantly, although the peptides did not induce skin test reactivity before beginning the study, there were side effects in 16 of 24 patients receiving the 750-μg dose. The side effects included chest tightness, runny nose, and itching without hives, and these symptoms decreased with subsequent doses. It is also important that the challenge used in this study was more rigorous than natural exposure conditions, making it difficult to equate the symptom improvement seen in this study with improvement seen during conventional immunotherapy. This strategy appears promising, partly because the injections were given over 4 weeks; as opposed to standard immunotherapy, which requires a much longer period to reach a maintenance dose. Recently, the results of a similar trial using three peptides from the rag-

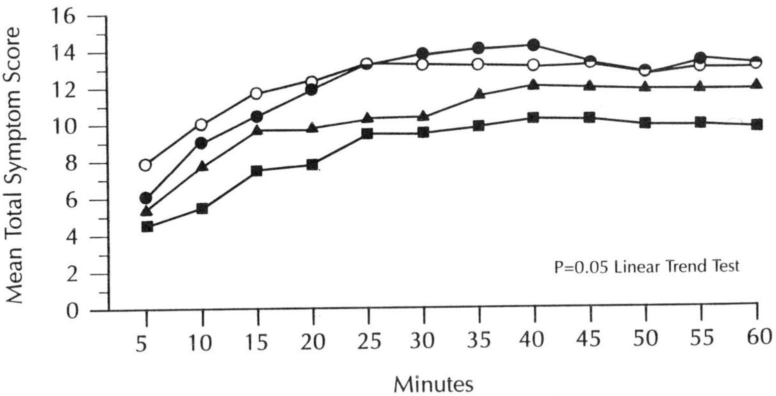

Figure 2 Clinical efficacy of Fel d 1 T-cell peptide vaccine; symptom scores following exposure in the cat room: Mean total symptom scores after exposure up to 1 hr in the cat room are shown for the four treatment groups: placebo (○); 7.5 μg of peptide (●); 75 μg of peptide (▲); and 750 μg peptide (■). The 750-μg group showed significantly lower symptom scores than did the placebo group, $p = 0.05$. (From Ref. 75.)

weed allergen Amb a 1 have been reported (76). The treatment group, receiving eight doses of 250 μg of peptide, showed a statistically significant improvement in symptom and medication scores, compared with the placebo group. Thus, peptide-based immunotherapy appears to be partially effective for the treatment of cat and ragweed allergy, for which one major allergen is responsible for inducing symptoms. These results raise the question: "Can such a strategy be applied to treatment of dust mite allergy?" for which three or more allergens stimulate IgE responses.

The T-cell response to Der p 1 and Der p 2 has been studied using population responses of peripheral blood lymphocytes as well as T-cell clones from atopic and nonatopic subjects (77–83). These studies have demonstrated that T-cell epitopes can be found throughout the entire coding sequence of Der p 1 and Der p 2 (Fig. 3). However, regions of Der p 1, for example, recognized by most allergic individuals were localized to three overlapping peptides, spanning amino acids 107–131 (78). Similarly, immunodominant Der p 2 peptides were mapped to amino acids 11–35 and 61–104 (79,80). Studies by Hoyne and colleagues showed that Der p 1 sensitized mice treated intranasally with the peptide 111–139 were unresponsive to parenteral challenge with Der p 1 (71,72). An important conclusion from these studies was that the T-cell response to the entire Der p 1 could be downregulated using a single peptide. It may thus be possible to prepare a mixture of peptides representing T-cell epitopes of three or four mite allergens, for evaluation in clinical trials. A test of this hypothesis awaits further in vitro T-cell studies to identify immunodominant T-cell epitopes from additional mite allergens other than group 1 and group 2.

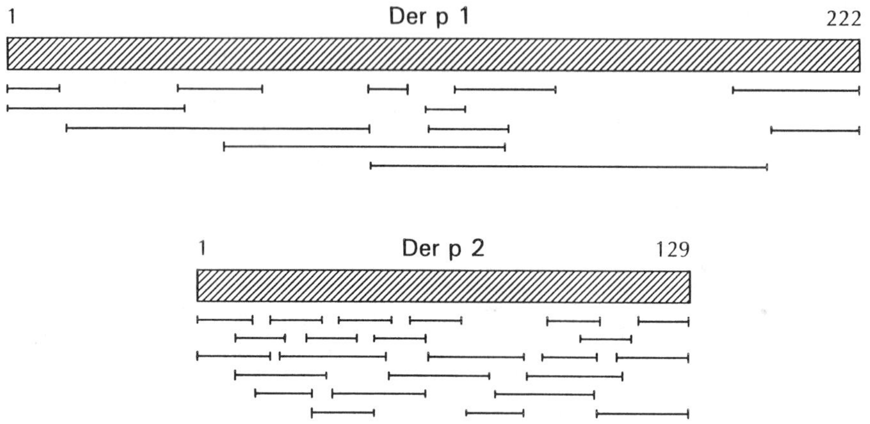

Figure 3 T-cell epitopes of the *Dermatophagoides* allergens Der p 1 and Der p 2. The primary amino acid sequence of Der p 1 (222 amino acids) and Der p 2 (129 amino acids) are represented by the hatched lines. Stimulatory T-cell epitopes were identified using synthetic peptides corresponding to the regions indicated by the solid lines. T-cell epitopes are found throughout the sequence for both allergens. (From Ref. 83.)

Allergen Variants

One drawback to peptide-based immunotherapy is the requirement for identifying immunogenic epitopes of a particular allergen that are recognized by T cells from the diverse HLA haplotypes of the allergic population. No clear correlation exists between response to a major allergen and a specific HLA type (83). An alternative strategy involves using the entire allergen molecule containing a more complete repertoire of T-cell epitopes, but in a form with reduced IgE reactivity. Michael and colleagues produced peptic digests of Amb a 1 and compared the fragmented allergen preparation with a conventional extract in an immunotherapy trial. The digested allergen was well tolerated, and the group of subjects receiving this form of the allergen showed greater improvement in symptom scores and IgG levels, compared with the group receiving the conventional treatment (84). Other strategies for modifying allergens include polymerization with gluteraldehyde or formaldehyde, or coating the allergen with a polymer, such as polyethylene glycol (PEG) (81,85,86). These treatments are effective in reducing IgE reactivity of the allergens, and murine studies have shown that gluteraldehyde-aggregated allergen can preferentially induce interferon gamma (IFN)-γ (87). However, the difficulty in controlling the extent of modification from batch to batch made these reagents not readily acceptable to regulatory agencies. Most recently, this idea has been approached using genetically engineered allergen variants. Site-specific mutagenesis in vitro of allergen cDNA can be used to change the amino acid sequence to produce precisely defined variants. For example, one or two amino acid substitutions in Der p 2 were produced using oligonucleotide-directed mutagenesis; these substitutions were targeted to alter cysteine residues, thereby selectively disrupting one or two disulfide bonds. These variants showed reduced IgE reactivity on skin testing by up to 100-fold (88). In vitro T-cell proliferative responses to these variants were similar to proliferation using unmodified Der p 2, suggesting that these variants retain T-cell epitopes (Table 4; 89). Such modified allergens could be given in doses similar to those used for conventional immunotherapy, and patients would be expected to reach a maintenance dose more rapidly and with fewer side effects because of the decreased IgE reactivity of the variants.

In a parallel study, Der p 2 variants, generated at predicted surface residues, also showed significant loss in IgE reactivity (89). Thus, structural information is important for targeting amino acids for mutagenesis and extending this strategy to other allergens, such as the group 1 proteins. Occasionally, naturally occurring variants have been identified that show decreased IgE binding (e.g., Bet v 1), and this suggests an additional source of allergen variants suitable for immunotherapy (91).

C. Plasmid DNA-Based Therapy

Another approach to reducing the probability of adverse reactions is to provide the allergen gene, rather than the protein. Such DNA-based vaccine strategies have been investigated in animal model systems. In murine models, scarification or intramuscular injection of a cytomegalovirus expression vector (pCMV) carrying the coding sequences for β-galactosidase induced a specific IgG2a response, but not an IgE response, and was also able to inhibit an ongoing secondary IgE response (92,93). Similar studies in rats sensitized to Der p 5 and administered an intramuscular injection of pCMV–Der p 5 DNA showed a decrease in airway hyperresponsiveness, suppression of the IgE response, and reduction in histamine levels in bronchoalveolar lavage (BAL) fluid following challenge (94). It is thought that plasmid DNA exists extrachromasomally within the host cell, and the expressed protein is processed into

Table 4 Immune Responses to Der p 2 Variants

	Quantitative intradermal skin test endpoint (μg/mL)[a]			T-cell response[b] (cpm; SI)	
Patient	r Der p 2	C73R	C21/C73	r Der p	C73R
1	10^{-2}	10^{0}	$>10^{0}$	12,999 (6)	36,410 (16)
2	10^{-2}	10^{-1}	$>10^{0}$	9,324 (20)	9,188 (20)
3	10^{-2}	$>10^{0}$	$>10^{0}$	2,100 (4)	3,008 (5)
4	10^{-2}	10^{-1}	$>10^{0}$	1,479 (4)	1,001 (3)

[a]Values represent the endpoint dilution that gave a larger than 8 × 8 mm wheal at 15 min. Negative skin tests are recorded as $> 10^{0}$.

[b]Proliferative responses were measured on day 7 in PBMC cultures stimulated with 10 μg/mL of antigen.

the MHC class I pathway (i.e., presented to $CD8^+$ T cells which, in turn, influence the development of Th1 lymphocytes by IFN-γ). In addition, plasmid DNA sequences outside the allergen-coding region preferentially induce T cells with the Thl cytokine phenotype (95). Although preliminary, these studies suggest a strategy for immunization that does not require high-level expression vectors. The adverse effects of DNA vaccines have not been investigated. It may be that cells harboring plasmids will become targets for cytotoxic T lymphocytes or natural killer cells, similar to vitally infected cells. This might result in the elimination of the allergen expressing cells, thereby removing the immunogenic stimulus for the "protective" response. Further studies in the mouse and rat models will help address the long-term effectiveness and risks associated with plasmid DNA-based immunotherapy.

Adjuvants

Adjuvants have historically been included in conventional vaccine strategies, although the mechanism by which they promote an immune response is poorly understood. Adjuvants are thought to slow the release of antigen, to target antigen to particular subsets of antigen-presenting cells (macrophages), and perhaps, to specifically activate macrophages through IL-12. Studies of Th2-mediated diseases, such as murine leishmaniasis have shown that IL-12 can be used in place of conventional bacterial adjuvants in promoting a cell-mediated immune response to *Leishmania* antigens (96). In another murine model, IgE antibody to ovalbumin could be suppressed in mice initially immunized with OVA-linked to IL-12 (97).

The idea of a prophylactic vaccine composed of allergen with a Thl adjuvant has recently been put forward by Holt (98,99). This vaccine would be targeted to children of atopic parents, who are at risk for developing allergic disease. This type of immunization would be expected to promote a Th1–IgG response that would be protective and would steer the immune system away from subsequent Th2–IgE responses. There still have been no clinical studies of immunization of infants at risk of developing allergic disease, but there are parallels with other pediatric vaccines such as *Haemophilus influenzae* conjugate vaccines. These consist of the bacterial capsular polysaccharide antigen coupled with a carrier protein, either diphtheria toxoid, tetanus toxoid, or a meningiococcal protein. These conjugate vaccines have been successful in preventing *H. influenzae* disease by converting a T-independent antigen into a T-dependent antigen that produces high levels of protective antibody. This technology is now being applied to other bacterial diseases of children including those caused by *Neisseria meningitidis* and pneumococcus (100). It may be possible to formulate conjugate vaccines that contain allergens or modified allergens, to prophylactically immunize at-risk children. Some support for the idea of steering the immune system toward a Thl-type response has come from the observation by Shirakawa and colleagues that Japanese school children with delayed hypersensitivity to *Mycobacterium* (developed as a result of BCG vaccination) have a lower incidence of asthma (101).

D. Allergen-Nonspecific Therapy

Anti-IgE

Two groups have independently developed a monoclonal antibody (MAb) that binds to the IgE heavy-chain domain recognized by the high-affinity IgE receptor, and thus blocks antibody–receptor interactions (102,103). In addition, this MAb binds to membrane IgE and downregulates IgE synthesis from B cells. The combining site from the MAb has been substituted onto a human IgG1 framework to produce an antibody that has only 5% murine sequence. This humanized MAb appears to be well tolerated and is currently in clinical trials. Subjects show a significant drop in serum IgE levels, and the duration of the decrease is dependent on the dose of anti-IgE as well as the baseline serum IgE titer. In addition, subjects enrolled in a phase 2 allergic rhinitis trial show improved symptoms and lower medication scores (104).

Anticytokine Therapy

Another nonspecific approach to downregulating the IgE response is to block the primary cytokines responsible for IgE class switching (IL-4 and IL-13) and eosinophil differentiation and recruitment (IL-5) (105). A human IL-4 variant (IL-4.Y124D) blocks IL-4 and IL-13 binding to the IL-4R and IL-13R, respectively. In the SCID-Hu mouse model, this variant was effective in reducing IgE levels by more than 90%, and these results suggest that cytokine antagonists may be useful in therapy (106).

Murine and monkey models of airway hyperresponsiveness have been used to demonstrate that anti-IL-5 antibody can block airway eosinophilia and bronchial hyperreactivity (107,108). In the monkey model, this effect lasted up to 3 months after treatment. Although there are as yet no clinical data on cytokine-targeted immunotherapy for asthma, these animal models suggest that such strategies warrant further investigation.

Transcription Inhibitors

Selectively interfering with transcription or translation of cytokines or mast cell mediators is another strategy for nonspecific therapy. In particular, Okudaira and colleagues have developed a new immunosuppressive agent, OM-01, that acts specifically on IL-5 transcription (109). By using in vitro T-cell cultures, these investigators demonstrated, that OM-01 selectively inhibited IL-5 gene transcription, but not that of IL-2 or IL-4. In a murine experimental asthma model, OM-01 was able to inhibit the late-phase pulmonary eosinophilia, suggesting that this agent, or similar gene-specific transcription inhibitors, may be useful for the management of asthma.

Antisense oligodeoxynucleotide-based therapy has been proposed for many diseases including human immunodeficiency virus (HIV) infection, cancer, and connective tissue disorders. Antisense oligodeoxynucleotides inhibit protein production by binding to mRNA in a sequence-specific fashion and blocking translation.

Recently, Nyce and Metzger reported on their study of a rabbit model of asthma and the use of antisense oligodeoxynucleotides to downregulate the adenosine A_1 receptor (110). Asthmatics demonstrate bronchial hyperresponsiveness to adenosine, which may be due to an upregulation of adenosine receptors on mast cells in the asthmatic lung. In the rabbit model, adenosine A_1 receptors were selectively downregulated by a specific oligodeoxynucleotide (A_1AS), and the treated animals showed a 61% reduction in bronchial hyperresponsive to histamine challenge. The lung may be an ideal target for antisense DNA therapy owing to its natural surfactant properties that favor uptake of antisense oligodeoxynucleotides.

It may be that a combination of allergen-nonspecific treatment, such as anti-IgE or anticytokine therapy, could be used initially to reduce IgE titers and that this could then be followed by allergen-specific treatment that might be safer and more effective under such conditions.

IV. Conclusions

Advances in the molecular biology of important indoor allergens, including mite, cat, cockroach, and fungal proteins, have supported extensive research studies aimed at standardizing allergen extracts, developing new diagnostic tests, and developing new forms of immunotherapy. It is clear that recombinant allergens can be produced in large quantities, purified to homogeneity, and these products show immunoreactivity comparable with the native counterparts; thus, they can be used for standardization of allergen extracts or for diagnosis, especially for allergens for which good extracts are not commercially available, such as *Blomia*. New forms of allergen-specific immunotherapy, based on recombinant allergens and in particular, peptides, have progressed to phase 2 and 3 clinical trials, after phase 1 trials of peptide immunotherapy for cat and ragweed allergy showed promising results. Whether this strategy can be used for allergy to complex mixtures, for example, dust mites that are a source of at least ten allergens, needs further evaluation of T-cell responses in large populations. Alternatives to peptide immunotherapy, such as allergen variants with reduced IgE reactivity, may be more appropriate for dust mite immunotherapy, or other multiallergen systems. Such allergen-specific treatments may be combined with nonspecific approaches, such as anti-IgE therapy, and this type of dual therapy may prove more efficacious. It is also possible that a preventive vaccine can be formulated to promote a protective response to common indoor allergens. These new strategies require further studies, but clearly, the use of recombinant allergens and peptides shows great promise for downregulating T-cell responses and providing safer and more effective immunotherapies for asthma.

Acknowledgments

Supported in part by National Institutes of Health grants AI 34607 and AI 32557.

References

1. Platts-Mills TAE, Thomas WR, Aalberse RC, et al., Co-chairmen. Indoor allergens and asthma: report of a 3rd International Workshop. J Allergy Clin Immunol 1997; 100:S1–924.
2. Burrows B, Martinez FD, Halonen M, Barbec RA, Cline MG. Association of asthma with serum IgE levels and skin test reactivity to allergens. N Engl J Med 1989; 320:271–277.
3. Di Bernadino L, Angrisano A, Gorli L, Catlaneo M, Lodi A. Allergy to house dust and storage mites in children: epidemiologic observation. Ann Allergy 1987; 59:104–106.
4. Sears MR, Herbison GP, Holdaway MD, Hewitt CJ, Flannery EM, Silva PA. The relative resk of sensitivity to grass pollen, house dust mite and cat dander in the development of childhood asthma. Clin Exp Allergy 1989; 19:419–424.
5. Peat JK, Tovey E, Gray EJ, Mellis CM, Woolcock AJ. Asthma severity and morbidity in a population sample of Sydney schoolchildren: part II—importance of house dust mite allergen. Aust NZ J Med 1994; 24:270–276.
6. Charpin D, Kleisbauer JP, Lanteaume A, Razzouk H, Vervloet D, Toumi M, Faraj F, Charpin, J. Asthma and allergy to house dust mites in population living in high altitudes. Chest 1988; 93:758–761.
7. Charpin D, Birnbaum J, Haddi E, Genard G, Lanteaume A, Toumi M, Faraj F, Van der Brempt X, Vervloet D. Altitude and allergy to house dust mites. *Am Rev Respir Dis* 1991; 143:983–986.
8. Peat JK, Tovey E, Mellis CM, Leeder SR, Woolcock AJ. Importance of house dust mite and *Alternaria* allergens in childhood asthma: an epidemiological study in two climatic regions of Australia. Clin Exp Allergy 1993; 23:812–820.
9. Peat JK,Toelle BG, Gray EJ, Haby MM, Belousova E, Mellis CM, Woolcock AJ. Prevalence and severity of childhood asthma and allergic sensitization in seven climatic regions of New South Wales. Med J Aust 1995; 163:22–26.
10. Peat JK, Tovey ER, Toelle BG, Haby MM, Gray EL, Mahmic A, Woolcock AJ. House-dust mite allergens: a major risk factor for childhood asthma in Australia. Am J Respir Crit Care Med 1996; 153:141–146.
11. Call RS, Smith TF, Morris E, Chapman MD, Platts-Mills TAE. Risk factors for asthma in inner city children. J Pediatr 1992; 121:862–866.
12. Pollart SM, Chapman MD, Riocco GP, Rose G, Platts Mills TAE. Epidemiology of acute asthma: IgE antibodies to common inhalant allergens as a risk factor for emergency room visits. J Allergy Clin Immunol 1989; 83:875–882.
13. Sporik R, Holgate S, Platts-Mills TAE, Cogswell J. Exposure to house dust mite allergen (Der p 1) and the development of asthma in childhood. *N Engl J Med* 1990; 323:502–507.
14. Halonen M, Stern DA, Wright AL, Tussig LM, Martinez F. *Alternaria* as a major allergen for asthma in a desert environment. Am J Respir Crit Care Med 1997; 155:1356–1361.
15. Sporik R, Ingram JM, Price W, Sussman JH, Honsinger RW, Platts-Mills TAE. Association of asthma with serum IgE and skin test reactivity to allergens among children living at high altitude; tickling the dragon's breath. Am J Respir Crit Care Med 1995; 151:1388–1392.
16. Ingram JM, Sporik R, Rose G, Honsinger R, Chapman MD, Platts-Mills TAE. Quantitative assessment of exposure to dog (Can f 1) and cat (Fel d 1) allergens: relation to sensitisation and asthma among children living in Los Alamos, New Mexico. J Allergy Clin Immunol 1995; 96:449–456.
17. Gelber LE, Seltzer LH, Bouzoukis JK, Pollart SM, Chapman MD, Platts-Mills TAE. Sensitisation and exposure to indoor allergens as risk factor for asthma among patients presenting to hospital with asthma. Clin Exp Allergy 1993; 91:844–849.
18. DeBlay F, Sanchez J, Hedelin G, Perez-Infante A, Verot A, Chapman M, Pauli G. Dust and airborne exposure to allergens derived from cockroach (*Blatella germanica*) in low-cost public housing in Strasbourg (France). J Allergy Clin Immunol 1997; 99:107–112.

19. Arruda LK, Rizzo MC, Chapman MD, Naspitz CK, Platts-Mills TAE. Exposure and sensitisation to dust mite allergens among asthmatic children in Sao Paulo, Brazil. Clin Exp Allergy 1991; 21:433–439.
20. Peat JK, van der Berg RH, Green WF, Mellis CM, Leeder SR, Woolcock AJ. Changing prevalence of asthma in Australian children. Br Med J 1994; 308:1591–1596.
21. Lau S, Falkenhorst G, Weber A, Werthmann I, Lind P, Buettner-Goetz P, Wahn U. High mite-allergen exposure increases the risk of sensitization in atopic children and young adults. J Allergy Clin Immunol 1989; 84:718–725.
22. Price JA, Pollock I, Little SA, Longbottom JL, Warner JO. Measurement of airborne mite antigen in homes of asthmatic children. Lancet 1990; 336:895–897.
23. Wickmann M, Nordvall SL, Pershagen G, Sundell J, Schwartz B. House dust mite sensitisation in children and residential characteristics in a temperate region. J Allergy Clin Immunol 1991:88:89-95.
24. Wickmann M, Nordvall SL, Pershagen G, Korsgaard J, Johansen N. Sensitisation to domestic mites in a cold temperate region. Am Rev Respir Dis 1993; 148:58–62.
25. Kuehr J, Frischer T, Karmaus W, Meinert R, Barth R, Herrmann-Kung E. Early childhood risk factors for sensitisation at school age. J Allergy Clin Immunol 1992; 90:358–363.
26. Kuehr J, Fisher T, Meinert R, Barth R, Schraub S, Urbanek R, Karnaus W, Forster J. Sensitisation to mite allergens is a risk factor for early and late onset of asthma and for persistence of asthmatic signs in children. J Allergy Clin Immunol 1995; 95:655–662.
27. Kuehr J, Fischer T, Meinert R, Barth R, Forster V, Schraub S, Urbanek R, Karmaus W. Mite allergen exposure is a risk for the incidence of specific sensitization. J Allergy Clin Immunol 1994; 94:44–52.
28. Custovic A, Taggart SCO, Francis HC, Chapman MD, Woolcock A. Exposure to house dust mite allergens and the clinical activity of asthma. J Allergy Clin Immunol 1996; 98:67–72.
29. Nelson RP, DiNicolo R, Fernandez-Caldez E, Seleznick MJ, Lockey R, Good R. Allergen-specific IgE levels and mite allergen exposure in children with acute asthma first seen in an emergency department and in nonasthmatic control subjects. J Allergy Clin Immunol 1996;98:258-263.
30. Duff AL, Pomeranz ES, Gelber LE, Price GW, Farris H, Hayden F, Platts-Mills TAE. Risk factors for acute wheezing in infants and children: viruses, passive smoke, and IgE antibodies to inhalant allergens. *Pediatrics* 1993; 92:535–540.
31. Sporik R, Platts Mills TAE, Cogswell JJ. Exposure to house dust mite allergen of children admitted to hospital with asthma. Clin Exp Allergy 1993; 23:740–746.
32. Arshad SH, Matthews S, Gant C, Hide DW. Effect of allergen avoidance on development of allergic disorder in infancy. Lancet 1992; 339:1493–1497.
33. Hide DW, Matthews S, Matthews L, Stevens M, Ridout S, Twiselton R, Gant C, Arshad SH. Effect of allergen avoidance in infancy on allergic manifestation at age two years. J Allergy Clin Immunol 1994; 93:842–846.
34. Arshad SH, Hide DW. Effect of environmental factors on the development of allergic disorders in infancy. J Allergy Clin Immunol 1992; 90:235–241.
35. Piacentini G, Martinati L, Mingoni S, Boner A. Influence of allergen avoidance on the eosinophil phase of airway inflammation in children with allergic asthma. J Allergy Clin Immunol 1996; 97:1079–1084.
36. Thomas WR. Molecular analysis of house dust mite allergens. In: Walker MR, Roberts AM eds. Molecular Analysis of Immediate Hypersensitivity and Strategies for Immunologic Intervention. John Wiley and Sons, Chichester, 1996.
37. Chapman MD, Smith AM, Vailes LD, Arruda LK. Recombinant mite allergens: new technologies for the management of patients with asthma. Allergy 1997; 52:374–379.
38. Scheiner O, Kraft D. Basic and practical aspects of recombinant allergens. Allergy 1995; 50:384-391.
39. Chapman MD, Smith AM, Slunt JB, Vailes LD, Arruda LK. Immunochemical and mo-

lecular methods for defining and measuring indoor allergens: in dust and air. Pediatr Allergy Immunol 1995; 6:8–12.
40. Noon L. Prophylactic inoculation for hay fever Lancet 1911; 1:1572–1573.
41. Freeman J. Further observations on the treatment of hayfever by hypodermic inoculation of pollen vaccine. Lancet 1911; 2:814–817.
42. McHugh SM, Lavelle B, Kemeny DM, Patel S, Ewan PW. A placebo-controlled trial of immunotherapy with two extracts of *D. pteronyssinus* in allergic rhinitis comparing clinical outcome with changes in antigen-specific IgE, IgG and IgG subclasses. J Allergy Clin Immunol 1990; 86:521–531.
43. Norman PS. An overview of immunotherapy: implications for the future. J Allergy Clin Immunol 1980; 65:87–96.
44. Rocklin RE, Sheffer AL, Greineder DK, Melmon KL. Generation of antigen-specific suppressor cells during allergy desensitization. N Engl J Med 1980; 302:1213–1219.
45. Wallner BP, Gefter ML. Immunotherapy with T-cell–reactive peptides derived from allergens. Allergy 1994; 49:302–308.
46. Creticos PS, Marsh DG, Proud D. Responses to ragweed-pollen nasal challenge before and after immunotherapy. J Allergy Clin Immunol 1989; 84:197–205.
47. Chua KY, Stewart GA, Thomas WR, Simpson RJ, Dilworth RJ, Plozza TM, Turner KJ. Sequence analysis of cDNA coding for a major house dust mite allergen, Der p 1. Homology with cysteine proteases. J Exp Med 1988; 167:175–182.
48. Thomas WR, Stewart GA, Simpson RJ, Chua KY, Plozza TM, Dilworth RJ, Nisbet A, Turner KJ. Cloning and expression of DNA coding for the major house dust mite allergen Der p 1 in *Escherichia coli.* Int Arch Allergy Appl Immunol 1988; 85:127–129.
49. Chua KY, Doyle CR, Simpson RJ, Turner KJ, Stewart GA, Thomas WR. Isolation of cDNA coding for the major mite allergen Der p 2 by IgE plaque immunoassay. *Int Arch Allergy Appl Immunol* 1990; 91:118–123.
50. Dilworth RJ, Chua KY, Thomas WR. Sequence analysis of cDNA coding for a major house dust mite allergen, Der f 1. *Clin Exp Allergy* 1991; 21:25–32.
51. Yuuki T, Okumura Y, Ando T, Yamakawa H, Suko M, Haida M, Okudaira H. Cloning and sequencing of cDNAs corresponding to mite major allergen Der f 2. Averugi Jpn J Allergol 1990; 39:557–561.
52. Trudinger M, Chua KY, Thomas WR. cDNA encoding the major mite allergy Der f 2. Clin Exp Allergy 1991; 21:33–37.
53. Morgenstern JP, Griffith IJ, Brauer AW, Rogers BL, Bond JF, Chapman MD, Kuo MC. Amino acid sequence of Fel d 1, the major allergen of the domestic cat; protein sequence analysis and cDNA cloning. Proc Natl Acad Sci USA 1991; 88:9690–9694.
54. Arruda LK, Vailes LD, Mann BJ, Shannon J, Fox JW, Vedvick TS, Hayden ML, Chapman MD. Molecular cloning of a major cockroach (*Blatella germanica*) allergen, Bla g 2. J Biol Chem 1995; 270:19563–19568.
55. Arruda LK, Vailes LD, Hayden ML, Benjamin DC, Chapman MD. Cloning of cockroach allergen, Bla g 4, identifies ligand binding proteins (or calycins) as a cause of IgE antibody responses. J. Biol Chem 1995; 270:31196–31201.
56. Arruda LK, Vailes LD, Platts-Mills TAE, Hayden ML, Chapman MD. Induction of IgE antibody responses by glutathione *S*-transferase from the German cockroach (*Blatella germanica*). J Biol Chem 1997; 272:20907–20912.
57. Arruda LK, Platts-Mills TAE, Fox JW, Chapman MD. *Aspergillus fumigatus* allergen 1, a major IgE-binding protein, is a member of the mitogillin family of cytotoxins. J Exp Med 1990; 172:1529–1532.
58. Achatz G, Oberkofler H, Lechenauer E, Simon B, Unger A, Kandler D, Ebner C, Prillinger H, Kraft D, Breitenbach M. Molecular cloning of major and minor allergens of *Alternaria alternata* and *Cladosporium herbarum.* Mol Immunol 1995; 32:213–227.
59. Banerjee B, Kurup V, Phadnis S, Greenberger P, Fink J. Molecular cloning and expression of a recombinant *Aspergillus fumigatus* protein Asp f 2 with significant immunoglobulin E reactivity in allergic bronchopulmonary aspergillosis. J Lab Clin Med 1996; 127:253–262.

60. Robinson C, Kalsheker NA, Srinivasan N, King CM, Garrod DR, Thompson PJ, Stewart GA. On the potential significance of the enzymatic activity of mite allergens to immunogenicity. Clues to structure and function revealed by molecular characterization. Clin Exp Allergy 1997; 27:10–21.
61. Hewitt CRA, Brown AP, Hart BJ, Pritchard DI. A major house dust mite allergen disrupts the immunoglobulin E network by selectively cleaving CD23; innate protection by antiproteases. J Exp Med 1995; 182:1537–1544.
62. Topham C, Srinivasan N, Thorpe C, Overington J, Kalsheker N. Comparative modelling of major house dust mite allergen Der p 1: structure validation using an extended environmental amino acid propensity table. Protein Eng 1994; 7:869–894.
63. Mueller GA, Smith AM, Hakkaart G, Aalberse R, Chapman MD, Benjamin DC, Rule GS. Bacterial expression and NMR structure of Der p 2. J Allergy Clin Immunol 1997; 99 (1, p 2):abstr 536.
64. Vailes LD, Arruda LK, Chapman MD. High level expression of German cockroach calycin allergen Bla g 4 in the yeast *Pichia pastoris*. J Allergy Clin Immunol 1997; 99 (1, p 2):abstr 2027.
65. Shoji H, Hanawa M, Shibuya I, Hirai M, Yasukara T, Okumura Y, Yamakawa H. Production of recombinant mite allergen Der f 1 in insect cells and characterization of products—removal of pro-sequences is essential to IgE-binding activity. Biosci Biotechnol Biochem 1996; 60:621–625.
66. Gajhede M, Osmark P, Poulsen R, Ipsen H, Larsen J, van Neerven RJJ, Schou C, Lowenstein H, Spangfort M. X-ray and NMR structure of Bet v 1, the origin of birch pollen allergy. Nature Struct Biol 1996; 3:1040–1045.
67. Metzler W, Valentine K, Roebber M, Briedrichs M, Marsh D, Mueller L. Determination of the three dimensional solution structure of ragweed allergen Amb t 5 by nuclear magnetic resonance spectroscopy. Biochemistry 1992; 31:5117–5127.
68. Metzler W, Valentine K, Roebber M, Marsh D, Mueller L. Proton resonance assignments and three-dimensional solution structure of the ragweed allergen Amb a 5 by nuclear magnetic resonance spectroscopy. Biochemistry 1992; 31:8697–8705.
69. O'Hehir RE, Garman RD, Greenstein JL, Lamb JR. The specificity and regulation of T-cell responsiveness to allergens. Annu Rev Immunol 1991; 9:67–95.
70. Lamb JR, Skidmore BJ, Green N, Chiller JM, Feldmann M. Induction of tolerance in influenza-virus immune T lymphocyte clones with synthetic peptides of influenza haemaglutinin. J Exp Med 1983; 157:1434–1447.
71. Hoyne GF, O'Hehir RE, Wraith DC, Thomas WR, Lamb JR. Inhibition of T-cell and antibody responses to house dust mite allergen by inhalation of the dominant epitope in naive and sensitized mice. J Exp Med 1993; 178:1783–1788.
72. Lake RA, O'Hehir RE, Verhoef A, Lamb JR. CD28 mRNA decays when activiated T-cells are functionally anergized with specific peptide. Int Immunol 1993; 5:461–466.
73. van Neerven RJJ, van de Pol MM, van Milligen FJ, Jansen HM, Aalberse RC, Kapsenberg ML. Characterization of cat dander specific T lymphocytes from atopic patients. J Immunol 1994; 153:4203–4210.
74. Counsell CM, Bond JF, Ohman JL, Greenstein JL, Garman RD. Definition of the human T-cell epitopes of Fel d1, the major allergen of the domestic cat. J Allergy Clin Immunol 1996; 98:884–894.
75. Norman PS, Ohman JL, Long AA, Creticos RS, Gefter MA, Shaked Z, Wood RA, Eggleston PA, Hafner KB, Rao P, Lichtenstein LM, Jones NH, Nicodemus CF. Treatment of cat allergen with T-cell reactive peptides. Am J Respir Crit Care Med 1996; 154:1623–1628.
76. Creticos PS, Hebert J, Philip G, Allervax Ragweed Study Group. Efficacy of Allervax ragweed peptides in the treatment of ragweed-induced allergy. J Allergy Clin Immunol 1997; 99(1 p 2):abstr 1631.
77. Yssel H, Johnson KE, Schneider PV, Wideman J, Terr A, Kastelein R, de Vries JE. T cell activation-inducing epitopes of the house dust mite allergen Der p 1. Proliferation and lym-

phokine production patterns by Der p 1-specific CD4+ T cell clones. J Immunol 1992; 148:738–745.
78. Higgins JA, Thorpe CJ, Hayball JD, O'Hehir RE, Lamb JR. Overlapping T cell epitopes in the group 1 allergen of *Dermatophagoides* spp. (house dust mite) restricted by HLA-DP and HLA-DR class II molecules. J Allergy Clin Immunol 1994; 93:891–899.
79. O'Brien RM, Thomas WR, Tait BD. An immunogenic analysis of T cell reactive regions on the major allergen from the house dust mite, Der p 1, with recombinant truncated fragments. J Allergy Clin Immunol 1994; 93:628–634.
80. van Neerven RJJ, van't Hof W, Ringrose J, Jansen H, Aalberse R, Wierenga E, Kapsenberg M. T cell epitopes of house dust mite major allergen Der p 2. J Immunol 1993; 151:4203–4210.
81. O'Hehir R, Verhoef A, Panagiotopoilou E, Keswani S, Hayball J, Thomas WR, Lamb JR. Analysis of human T cell responses to the group II allergen of *Dermatophagoides* species: localization of major antigenic sites. J Allergy Clin Immunol 1993; 92:105–113.
82. Verhoef A, Higgins JA, Thorpe CJ, Marsh SG, Hayball JO, Lamb JR, O'Hehir RE. Clonal analysis of the atopic immune response to the group 2 allergen of *Dermatophagoides* spp.: identification of HLA-DR and DQ restricted T cell epitopes. Int Immunol 1993; 5:1589–1597.
83. van Neerven RJJ, Ebner C, Yssel H, Kapsenberg ML, Lamb JR. T cell responses to allergens: epitope specificity and clinical relevance. Immunol Today 1996: 17:526–532.
84. Litwin A, Pesce AJ, Fisher T, Michael M, Michael JG. Regulation of the human immune response to ragweed pollen by immunotherapy. A controlled trial comparing the effects of immunosuppressive peptic fragments of short ragweed with standard treatment. Clin Exp Allergy 1992; 21:457–465.
85. Ishizaka K, Kishimoto T, Delespesse G, King TP. Immunogenic properties of modified antigen E. I. Presence of specific determinants for T cells in denatured antigen and polypeptide chains. J Immunol 1974; 113:70–77.
86. Guerra F, Moreno C, Daza JC, Miguel R, Garcia M, Sanchez Guijo P. Linear monitoring of patients sensitive to *Olea* and grass pollens treated with immunotherapy based on glutaraldehyde-modified (allergoid) extracts. J Invest Allergol Clin Immunol 1993; 3:182–190.
87. Yang X, Gieni RS, Mosmann TR, HayGlass KT. Chemically modified antigen preferentially elicits induction of Thl-like cytokine synthesis patterns *in vivo.* J Exp Med 1993; 178:349–353.
88. Smith AM, Chapman MD. Reduction in IgE binding to allergen variants generated by site-directed mutagenesis: contribution of disulfide bonds to the antigenic structure of the major house dust mite allergen Der p 2. Mol Immunol 1996; 33:399–405.
89. Smith AM, Taketomi EA, Mueller GA, Rule GS, Benjamin DC, Chapman MD. Antigenic and molecular structure of the mite allergen Der p 2. Int Arch Allergy Immunol 1997; 113:99–101.
90. Smith AM, Chapman MD. Localization of antigenic sites on Der p 2 using oligonucleotide-directed mutagenesis targeted to predicted surface residues. Clin Exp Allergy 1997; 27:593–599.
91. Ferreira F, Hirtenlehner K, Jilek A, Godnik-Cvar J, Breiteneder H, Grimm R, Hoffman-Sommergruber K, Scheiner O, Kraft D, Breitenbach M, Rheinberger HJ, Ebner C. Dissection of immunoglobulin E and T lymphocyte reactivity of isoforms of the major birch pollen allergen Bet v 1: potential use of hypoallergenic isoforms for immunotherapy. J Exp Med 1996; 183:599–609.
92. Raz E, Carson DA, Parker SE, Parr TB, Abai AM, Aichinger G, Gromkowski SH, Shing M, Lew D, Yankauckas MA, Baird SM, Rhodes GH. Intradermal gene immunization: the possible role of DNA uptake in the induction of cellular immunity to viruses. Proc Natl Acad Sci USA 1994: 9:9519–9523.
93. Raz E, Tighe H, Sato Y, Corr M, Dudler J, Roman M, Swain S, Spiegelberg H, Carson D. Preferential induction of a Thl immune response and inhibition of specific IgE anti-

body formation by plasmid DNA immunization. Proc Natl Acad Sci. USA 1996; 93:5141–5145.

94. Hsu C-H, Chua KW, Tao MH, Lai YL, Wu HD, Huang SK, Hsieh KH . Immunoprophylaxis of allergen-induced immunoglobulin E synthesis and airway hyperresponsiveness in vivo by genetic immunization. Nature Med 1996; 2:540–544.
95. Sato Y, Roman M, Tighe H, Lee D, Corr M, Nguyen M-D, Silverman J, Lotz M, Carson D, Raz E. Immunostimulatory DNA sequences necessary for effective intradermal gene immunization. Science 1996; 273:352–354.
96. Julia V, Rassoulzadegan M, Glaichenhaus N. Resistance to *Leishmania major* induced by tolerance to a single antigen. Science 1996; 274:421–423.
97. Manetti R, Parronchi P, Giudizi MG, Piccinni MP, Maggi E, Trinchieri G, Romagnani S. Natural killer cell stimulatory factor (interleukin 12, IL-12) induces T helper type 1 (Th1) specific immune responses and inhibits the development of IL-4 producing Th cells. J Exp Med 1993; 177:1199–1204.
98. Holt PG. Immunoprophylaxis of atopy: light at the end of the tunnel? Immunol Today 1994; 15:484–489.
99. Brown MA, Halonen MJ, Martinez FD. Cutting the cord: is birth already too late for primary prevention of allergy? Clin Exp Allergy 1997; 27:4–6.
100. Frasch CE. *Haemophilus influenzae* type b conjugate and combination vaccines. Clin Immunother 1995; 4(5):376–386.
101. Shirakawa T, Enomoto T, Shimazu S-I, Hopkin JM. The inverse association between tuberculin responses and atopic disorder. Science 1997; 275:77–79.
102. Shields RL, Whether WR, Zioncheck K, O'Connell L, Fendly B, Presta LG, Thomas D, Saban R, Jardieu P. Inhibition of allergic reactions with antibodies to IgE. Int Arch Allergy Immunol. 1995; 107:308–312.
103. Chang TW, Davis FM, Sun CRY, MacGlashan DW, Hamilton RG. Monoclonal antibodies specific for human IgE-producing B cells: a potential therapeutic for IgE-mediated allergic diseases. *Biotechnology* 1990; 8:122–126.
104. Davis, F. Anti-IgE therapy: non-specific immunotherapy. AAAAI/AAI/CIS Joint Meeting, San Francisco, CA, Feb 21–26, 1997.
105. Renz H, Enssle K, Lauffer L, Kurrle R, Gelfand EW. Inhibition of allergen-induced IgE and IgGl production by soluble IL-4 receptor (sIL-4R). Int Arch Allergy Immunol 1995; 106:46–54.
106. Kruse N, Tony HP, Sebald W. Conversion of human IL-4 into a high affinity antagonist by a single amino acid replacement. EMBO J 1992; 11:3237–3244.
107. Egan RW, Athwahl D, Chou CC, Emtage S, Jehn DH, Kung TT, Mauser PJ, Murgolo NJ, Bodmer MW. Inhibition of pulmonary eosinophilia and hyperreactivity by antibodies to interleukin-5. Int Arch Allergy Immunol 1995; 107:321–322.
108. Kung TT, Stelts DM, Zurcher JA, Adams GK, Egan RW, Kreutner W, Watnick AS, Jones H, Chapman RW. Involvement of IL-5 in the murine model of allergic pulmonary inflammation: prophylactic and therapeutic effect of an anti-IL-5 antibody. Am J Respir Cell Mol Biol 1995; 13:360–365.
109. Okudaira H, Mori A, Kaminuma O, Suko M. IL-5 regulation—a new approach to allergy therapy. ACI Int 1996; 8/5 + 6:172–179.
110. Nyce JW, Metzger WJ. DNA antisense therapy for asthma in an animal model. Nature 1997; 385:721–725.

8

Elimination of Allergens

FRÉDÉRIC DE BLAY, FRANÇOIS SPIRLET, MARTINE OTT, JEAN-CLAUDE BESSOT, and GABRIELLE PAULI

Hôpitaux Universitaires de Strasbourg
Strasbourg, France

I. Introduction

Numerous studies have demonstrated an increasing prevalence and severity of asthma in certain countries (1,2). Reasons for this increase are not fully known, but an increased allergen load could be partially responsible. For genetically predisposed persons (3), allergen exposure is a risk factor for sensitization. House dust mite and domestic animal allergens are an important documented risk factor for airway hyperresponsiveness (AHR) and asthmatic symptoms (4–6). Recognition of this risk is essential. The therapeutic implication is that allergen avoidance may prevent the onset of asthma in some atopic children and thus play an important role in the management of asthma. The development of new means of detecting allergens (i.e., immunochemical assays involving monoclonal antibodies, and quantitative and semiquantitative guanine measurements for mite allergens; 7,8) has made it possible to identify allergen sources and reservoirs more precisely. Consequently, the effects of a reduction in allergen exposure could be better evaluated. The problem of allergen avoidance involves mainly dust mites, domestic animals, and fungi.

II. Dust Mites

A. Allergen Reservoirs

Usually, major mite allergens measured in domestic environments are group 1 major allergens (i.e., Der p 1; *Dermatophagoïdes pteronyssinus* 1, and Der f 1; *D. farinae* 1; 9). Mattresses have been described as one of the major reservoirs of mite allergens (10–12). However, recently we have pointed out the role of upholstered mattress base as another major reservoir; the allergen content in those bases was statistically higher than in mattresses ($p < 8 \times 10^{-5}$, $N = 50$) (12). In the same study, we were able to confirm that the amount of group 1 mite allergen in house dust samples from carpeted floors was greater (geometric mean = 2.4 μg/g of group 1 mite allergens) than in house dust samples from floors covered with linoleum or a wood product (i.e., geometric mean = 0.15 μg/g of group 1 mite allergens). Early in 1981, Tovey et al. reported the presence of house dust mite allergens in carpet rugs, chairs, sofas, and clothing (10). Recently, a study has demonstrated the presence of mite allergens on soft toys (13). Mite allergens have also been found in dust from day care centers (14) and different various public places (15).

B. Elimination Methods

Mite infestation in a given house is related to the presence of textile objects and also to indoor relative humidity. Mite growth requires humidity (> 50% relative humidity) and warmth (> 25°C) (11). These conditions are very close to those sought by humans. The question arises of how we can use limiting factors for long-term decrease of mite population growth and allergen exposure. Removal of all suitable niches is a possibility. Bedding is considered essential for healthy living in Western countries; moreover, upholstered furnishings and carpets are still widely used. Therefore, a total removal of textiles is unrealistic.

Physical Methods

Reduction of Indoor Relative Humidity

House-dust mites do not tolerate a low humidity in the surrounding air; at a relative humidity of 45% at an indoor temperature of 20–22°C (= 8–9 g water vapor/ per cubic meter of air), or at a lower humidity, in winter they will desiccate and die out (9). The relevance of outdoor humidity to mite development is at variance within Europe (16). Harving et al. (17); in Scandinavia, created a dry indoor winter climate to halt mite population growth using mechanical ventilation with an air-exchange rate of 1.5 ACH in new flats. These authors showed that it had been possible to completely remove the house dust mite population in 11 of 16 mattresses within a year. Other studies have confirmed such data (18–20). In the same experiment, Harving et al. (16) found a clinical benefit in symptoms and an increase in respiratory function and medication scores. In contrast, in warmer climates, such as in Marseille and northwest England, two studies showed that increasing air exchange did not lead to any decrease in mite allergen levels (21,22). Moreover, in the United Kingdom, Custovic et al. (23) did not obtain any mite allergen reduction using dehumidifiers. In the United States, air-conditioning has lowered temperature and humidity sufficiently to reduce seasonal mite allergen levels up to fivefold, depending on the month, and the mite levels up to 17-fold (24). These data were not confirmed by an Australian epidemiological study (25). These results suggest that a reduction of indoor relative humidity (45% at 20–22°C) can be achieved in countries with a dry and cold winter. Mechanical ventilation with heat exchange is usually needed to ensure a stable ventilation level in combination with thermal comfort and low energy costs.

Other Physical Methods

Vacuuming. Intensive dry vacuum-cleaning can partially remove a mite allergen reservoir. In one study, 5–10% of mites were removed after two consecutive vacuumings, and in another one, up to 20% after 40 min (26). Kalra et al. (27) showed that a high-efficiency particulate air (HEPA) filter vacuum cleaner vented less respirable, aerosolized allergens than conventional vacuum cleaners. These data were confirmed by Hegarty et al. (28). Wassenaar showed that wet vacuum-cleaning of a carpet was associated with a subsequent increase in population density of *D. pteronyssinus* probably owing to elevated humidity (29). By using a wet vacuum cleaner, Fell et al. (30) obtained a 66% reduction in Der p 1 levels per square meter, and a 37% reduction in Der p 1 levels per gram of dust. In another study, simple shampooing was no more effective than intensive dry vacuuming (31). Colloff showed, after steam treatment of standardized areas of carpet in a home, a mean reduction in Der p 1 concentrations of 87% in treated areas, compared with only 5% in untreated control areas (32).

Changing. This method seems to be very effective. However, it took 2 months for a new mattress to be reinfested if it was set on an infested mattress base (de Blay F, unpublished data).

Washing. This method can remove allergens from soft furnishings and bedding, but only hot water (> 58°C) will kill mites (33). A cold cycle of laundry washing, with or without laundry powder, did not remove most live mites from bedding; however the allergen concentration (Der p 1/g of dust) was reduced by more than 90%. The effect of dry cleaning on group 1 mite allergen levels is controversed (34,35). Recently, it has been shown that mite control by low-temperature washing is possible with a mite control additive, provided that a concentration of benzyl benzoate of about 0.03% is achieved in the washing suds (36).

Heating. Mite densities were successfully reduced by the use of electric blankets to decrease mattress humidity (37).

Freezing. Large reductions in mite densities in beds and carpets were also achieved in a controlled clinical trial with adult asthmatics using liquid nitrogen and vacuum cleaning (38). However, the method is not widely applicable.

Air Cleaners. The use of HEPA filters fitted to bed headboards was associated with clinical improvement in a 4-week crossover study with house dust–sensitive children with asthma (39). Another very similar study (40) also reported significant improvement. Mitchell et al. (41) used electroprecipitators in homes of ten mite-sensitive children, but reported no clinical improvement. More recently, a double-blind crossover study using ionizers in 20 mite-allergic children with asthma during 6 weeks did not show any clinical or functional improvement. However, a significant decrease in airborne Der p 1 was found (42). A committee consulted about the use of air-cleaning devices concluded that air cleaners (HEPA filters, electrostatic filters, electroprecipitators) could not be recommended in the absence of other forms of environmental control (43).

Barrier Methods. Several studies have demonstrated the efficiency of mattress covers to reduce group 1 allergen levels in dust collected at the surface (44–46). A multicenter double-blind controlled study with dust and air monitoring of group 1 mite allergen levels in mite-allergic children and adults with asthma did not find any improvement in clinical or medication scores, in nonspecific bronchial hyperrresponsiveness, or in cost effectiveness, when the only reduction methods used were mattress, pillow, and duvet covers (46). However, four control studies found clinical improvement, as well as a decrease in nonspecific hyperresponsiveness (45,47–49), when other reduction methods were associated with mattress covers. By using liquid nitrogen on the mattress and other eviction methods, one study found clinical and functional improvement and a decrease in medication score and in airway hyperresponsiveness (38). Recently, a controlled study of mite allergen avoidance showed clinical improvement in atopic dermatitis (50). In contrast, five controlled studies, including mattress covers and very intensive allergen eviction, did not find any improvement in mite allergic children or adults (51–55). Except for the study performed by Marks et al. (54), it should be underlined that the negative studies were short-term of 3 months or less (Tables 1 and 2).

Chemical Methods

Acaricides

It has long been accepted that pest infestation, affecting both the environment and humans, may be successfully treated by means of killing agents. Killing of house dust mites under laboratory condition is a relatively simple task (56,57). Most acaricides reduced the number of live mites by 65–100%. However, the application of such substances in the home has raised a number of as yet unanswered questions and has clearly indicated that the high degree of mite mortality achieved in the laboratory cannot be reproduced simply in the home. Several considerations are very important for acaricide efficacy:

The delivery method
The allergen concentration and the quantity of dust recovered
The role of local factors, such as type of carpeting or furnishings

Table 1 Controlled Studies of Global Mite Elimination Methods with Positive Results: Main Characteristics

Ref.	Patients	n	Time (mo)	Mite monitoring	Mattress cover	Other methods	Clinical results	Functional status	Medication scores	Airway responsiveness
48	Children A	20 T = 10 C = 9	1	No	Vinyl cover	Cover for pillow and box spring Washed blankets and mattress every 2 wk Cleaned drawer and closets Electric radiators	Improvement	Improvement	Improvement	T: improved (less than one doubling dose)
49	Adults A	41 T = 21 C = 19	12	T: significant decrease C : no significant decrease	Yes	Changed duvet, quilts, and blanket. Bedding washed weekly Vacuumed regularly	T: improvement C: NS	T: improvement C: NS	T : improvement C: NS	Increase PC_{20} histamine (more than 1 doubling dose)
45	Children 7–15 yr A	24 8 P 8 T1:MC+ A 8 T2: A	12	Der p 1 T1: significant decrease T2: no difference C : no difference	T1: yes	T1: tannic acid: carpet T2: Acarosan: mattress and carpet	ND	ND	ND	T1: increase PC_{20} histamine (more than 2 doubling doses)
38	Adults A	18 T = 9 C = 9	2	T: significant decrease C: nonsignificant decrease mites/m^2	Liquid nitrogen	Box spring vacuumed weekly Bedding washed; soft furnishings removed	T: improvement C: NS	PEFR: T: improvement C: NS	T: improvement C: NS	T: significant increase PC_{20} histamine (~2 doubling doses) C: NS
47	Children	21 crossover	2 T = 1 C = 1	ND	Yes	New sleeping bag and pillow Vacuuming once a week	ND	T: improvement in PEFR	ND	ND
50	Adults (24) Children (24)	48 T = 28 C = 20	6	Der p 1 T: significant decrease C: no decrease	Yes Goretex	Benzyltannate (carpet) High-filtration vacuum cleaner	T: improvement > C	ND	ND	ND
17	Adults	25 T = 14 C = 11	15	Mite count : T = significant decrease %C	No	Increase air exchange per hour from 0.4 to 1.5 ACH	T : improvement (intragroup) NS compared with C	T : improvement in FEV_1%C	T : improvement compared with baseline	T : increase in PC_{20} but NS

NS, not significant; ND, not done.
T, treated; C, control, A: asthmatic.

Table 2 Controlled Studies of Global Mite Elimination Methods with Negative Results: Main Characteristics

Ref.	Patients	*n*	Time (mo)	Mite monitoring	Mattress cover	Other methods	Clinical results	Functional status	Medication scores	Airway responsiveness
52	Children A	53 T = 26 C = 27	24	Mite counts: NS	ND	Bedding washed New sleeping bag Quilts and sofa removed Vacuuming; once per week		NDPEFR: NS	ND	ND
53	Adults A	46 T = 23 C = 23	3	Mite counts: NS	Yes	Carpet removed Bedding washed Vacuuming; once per week	NS	PEFR: NS	ND	ND
54	Adults A	35 T = 17 C = 18	6	Der p 1 T = NS C = NS	Yes	Covered duvet and pillow Tannic acid: bedding, carpet, and furniture	NS	PEFR: NS	NS	NS
55	Children A	12 cross-over	1 T = 0.5 C = 0.5	ND	Yes	New pillow: 1st wk Air cleaners: 2nd wk	NS	PEFR: NS	ND	ND
51	Children A	26 T = 14 C = 12	1.5	Mite count T: significant decrease C: significant decrease	Yes	Enclosed pillow Vacuuming the room	NS	PEFR: NS	ND	NS
60	Adults A	23 T = 11 C = 12	12	Der p 1 + Der f 1 carpet. T: significant decrease (intragroup) C: significant decrease (intragroup) Mattress: NS	No	Acaricide: Acarosan powder: Carpet Upholstered furniture Acarosan Foam, mattress Every 6 months	T: improvement intragroup C: improvement T % C: NS	T: improvement C: improvement T %: NS	NS	ND
64	Adults A	12 T = 6 C = 6	12	Der p 1 = Der f 1 T = NS C = NS	Yes	Acaricide: Acarosan powder (carpet)	ND	NS	NS	ND

The intensive vacuuming of treated surfaces after acaricide treatment
The assessment of efficacy
The toxicity of acaricides

Delivery Methods. Hayden et al. (58) have demonstrated that Acarosan powder was efficient only if left in the carpet for 24 hr before extensive vacuuming. Tovey et al. (59) showed that tannic acid sprays were only temporarily effective when applied at the manufacturers' recommended volumes.

Allergen Concentration and Quantity of Dust Recovered. Two controlled studies have clearly shown that mite infestation in mattresses cannot be significantly reduced with acaricides (45,60).

Assessment of Efficacy. According to the Third International Workshop on dust mite allergy, measurement of acaricide efficacy should be based on the quantity of allergen recovered per unit area and not on concentration per unit weight (61).

Toxicity. There is no acaricidal product available for domestic use that is nontoxic to humans. Almost all are considered to have low or very low toxicity (56,57). Indeed, the use of acaricides in a clinical circumstance necessitates that rigorous safety (toxicity) studies with continuous long-term exposure be undertaken.,

Controlled studies have found a clinical efficacy on mite allergic rhinitis with Acarosan powder and foam (62). However, in three studies of adult mite-asthmatic patients, no significant clinical improvement was found in the study group compared with the control (60,63,64) when using Acarosan and Natamycin. In contrast, two clinical studies found a decrease in Der p 1 levels and peak expiratory flow rate (PEFR) improvement using Natamycin and Acardust, respectively (65,66). However, the authors did not find any clinical improvement in the study using Acardust (66).

III. Animals

There is a widespread impression that allergies related to animals have become more common during the past 15–20 years (67). In Western countries, during the same period, the houses have become tighter, the number of furred pets (particularly cats and dogs) have increased, and animals have been more often kept inside the house.

A. Cat

In Western countries, cat allergen is the most important indoor aeroallergen after mite allergen. In the general population, about one of four dwellings houses a cat. Exposures to cats is very important, and varied from 21.8 to 30.8% (68,69). Barbee et al. (70) have found that 25% of the general population was sensitized to cat allergen. In a non-mite–exposed population, 68% of asthmatic children were sensitized to cat allergens (71). There is no precise cat allergen risk level for sensitization or asthma symptoms. Skin Fel d 1 levels are under hormonal control, and are related to the volume of sebaceous cells and glands. The highest Fel d 1 levels have been found in anal sac secretions, with a geometric mean of 41 U/g of secretion and a range of 2–339 U/g, with a high cat-to-cat variability (72). There is a relation between airborne cat allergen and sensitization to cat (73). Recently, we have found a correlation between dust and airborne Fel d 1 levels ($r = 0.49$; $p < 0.003$; $n = 50$) using a portable sampler (74). It seems clear that the absolute amounts of Fel d 1 inducing a positive response during a bronchial challenge test were significantly higher than those that provoked symptoms at home (75). Fel d 1 has been measured in dust, and the highest levels were found in dust from carpet or upholstered furniture, up to 5000 μ/g. In mattresses, the levels were lower, ranging from 0.1 to 1000 μg/g (76). One study measured Fel d 1 in hospital dust (0.4–0.8 μg/g) and allergists offices (0.02–4.4 μg/g) (77). Fel d 1 was measured in dust in Swedish classrooms from various sources (chair; 1 μg/g; tables, 0.1–1 μg/g; floor, 0.05–1 μg/g) (78). More recently, low Fel d 1 levels have been found in floor dust of day care centers (79,80). In the air, Fel d 1 is carried by particles with a wide-range of sizes, including smaller than 2.5 μm. In the absence of the cat and under undisturbed conditions, a mean value of 14 ng/m^3 was obtained, and 40% of airborne Fel d 1 was associated with particles smaller than 5 μm (81,82). The best elimination method is to have the animal removed; however, after the cat's removal, it took 6 months to obtain a reduction in dust Fel d 1 to levels comparable with those of a house without a cat (83). Despite the occurrence of allergic respiratory disease, certain patients remained exposed to animal allergens, only 15% of these subjects with bronchial and ear, nose, or throat (ENT) symptoms of allergy were aware of the animal's responsibility (84). Ohman et al. (85) found that close to a third of cat allergic asthmatics had at least one cat in their homes. Thus, removal of the "family pet" is not as simple as it seems. Evoking the possible departure of the animal may often be the cause of conflict within the family and of a deterioration in the doctor–patient relationship (86). Hering et al. (86) consider the presence of an animal next to an allergic child to be an example of the family's inability adapting to the presence of a child with a chronic disease. Moreover, 55% of parents with an allergic child refuse to recognize the risk of aggravation caused by the animal. Thus, we were initially led to perform an experimental study that showed that it was possible to reduce airborne concentrations of the major cat allergen (i.e., Fel d 1) even when the animal still resided at home (87). Different factors influence airborne Fel d 1 levels, one factor is the cat itself. It has been demonstrated that there are "high-producer" and "low-producer" cats, with an eightfold difference (88). To reduce airborne allergen exposure in dwellings of patients who refused to get rid of their cats, it has been proposed that the cat be washed weekly and that carpets and upholstered furniture be removed, as much as possible, and that vacuum cleaners and air cleaners with HEPA filters be used (87). Ohman et al. (89) have shown that Fel d 1 production by three male cats decreased as a result of washing the cat weekly. Glinert et al. (90) have confirmed these results in seven cats after washing the, cat monthly. Conflicting data have been obtained by Klucka et al. (91), who did not find significant differences in airborne Fel d 1 concentrations produced by washed or unwashed cats, or cats treated with Allerpet.

These experimental data lacked clinical confirmation of their efficacy. Therefore, we selected 13 monosensitized patients who had one or more cats at home. Nine among them have employed methods aimed at reducing airborne Fel d 1 concentrations (i.e., polyurethane–cotton mattress covers). Patients were also encouraged to reduce their carpets as much as possible, and washed their cats once a week. Four other patients did not employ these measures and served as controls. Clinical, medication, and functional respiratory evaluations were performed during a 1-month run-in period, and then every month during the 3 months of study. In both groups, bronchial hyperreactivity was assessed before and at the end of 3 months. Similarly, airborne Fel d 1 levels were measured twice a month, before and during the elimination measures, by a glass fiber filter connected to a portable pump. In the group employing elimination measures, there was a decrease in clinical and medication scores, however; there was no decrease in bronchial hyperreactivity. A significant decrease ($p = 0.03$) in the geometric mean of airborne Fel d 1 levels from 13.5 to 6.2 ng/m^3 was observed. Although the patient series was limited, these results suggest that it is possible to reduce exposure to airborne cat allergens in the homes of patients housing a cat, and also to obtain clinical benefits in very selected cat-allergic patients (92).

B. Dog

A study showed that over 50% of households in the United States contained dog allergens (93). The prevalence of sensitization varied from 3 to 14% in a nonselected population and 40% in asthmatic children (94,95). The main source is the pelt, but Can f 1 was also measured in saliva and in dander. The highest levels of Can f 1 were found in carpet or sofas, ranging from 10 to 10,000 μg/g (96). Classroom levels have ranged from 10 to 50 μg/g (78). In Japanese dwellings, airborne levels have varied from 1 to 10 ng/m^3 (97). Twenty percent of airborne Can f 1 is carried on particles smaller 5 μm. Airborne Can f 1 levels could be reduced by the use of HEPA air cleaners (98).

C. Rodents

Rodents allergens are found mostly in laboratory facilities, but more people (particularly children) like to keep rabbits, guinea pigs, or mice at home.

Rat

Rat allergens were detected using a radioallergosorbent technique (RAST) or RAST-inhibition methods in the dust taken from the ventilation grill of a rat room (99), but also in the shelf dust (99). Of the airborne rat allergens, 28.7% appeared to be associated with particles smaller than 5 μm (100). Feeding and cleaning were responsible for the highest increase of airborne rat allergen, 21 ng/m^3 (101). In contrast, sacrifice of the rat provoked a lower increase 3.1 ng/m^3. Allergic symptoms were found in 30% of laboratory workers (102). Reduction of airborne rat allergens has been achieved using a filtration system on the rat cage (103). In a prospective study, improved work practices and the use of approved paper masks could effect a progressive reduction in disease incidence to about one-third of the initial rate (from about 30% to about 10%) (104).

IV. Fungal Allergens

There is no question that molds grow in domestic houses and that many patients with asthma give positive immediate skin tests to fungal extracts (105). In addition, there is striking evidence that exposure to outdoor fungi may play an important role in severe asthma (106). However, information about the role of indoor fungal allergens in asthma is very incomplete. Thus, there is little epidemiological evidence connecting asthma to sensitization by indoor fungi (with or without exposure). Indeed, there are no simple assays for indoor fungal allergens, and we do not even know whether fungal spores or some other part of the organism are the major form in which these allergens become airborne. Thus, most advice given about reducing fungal allergens in houses is based on basic knowledge about their growth conditions, rather than any objective measurements of the relationship between exposure and disease. Fungal growth can occur on any surface and is primarily dependent on humidity plus a source of organic matter. Fungi can grow under much colder conditions than mites and are a common contaminant of unheated basements. These organisms commonly grow on food, stored wood, wicker baskets, and household plants, as well as kitchen or bathroom surfaces. Normal recommendations include reducing organic matter in the house to the minimum and controlling humidity by structural maintenance, and ventilation or dehumidification. In addition, surfaces that tend to grow molds, particularly in the kitchen or bathrooms, should be cleaned with chemicals, designed to kill molds (e.g., chlorine bleach). The use of room (or house) humidifiers presents a special hazard for mold growth, and if used, they should be washed with chlorine solution at least twice weekly.

V. Other Allergens

Many other allergens can be important in house dust (i.e., cockroaches or pollen). High levels of cockroach allergens accumulated in kitchen dust, and airborne cockroach allergens are carried on large particles (> 10 μm) (107). There is no controlled clinical study on avoidance of these allergens; thus, most advice is based simply on knowledge of the biology of the source. Nonetheless, specific advice about avoidance is appropriated to exterminate cockroaches and reduce pollen entry in the house,

Table 3 Advice Given to Patient for Reducing Exposure to House Dust Mites (University of Strasbourg, Chest Diseases and Allergy Department)

Immediately Applicable Methods	Procedures for reducing dust mite should first focus on bedroom, because more time is spent there than in any other room. Concerning mattresses, mattress bases, carpets, or upholstered furniture: the elimination methods will depend on the Acarex-test results. If the Acarex-test is positive, *elimination methods should be performed with individual counseling provided by an indoor environmental technician.*
Mattresses	Should be encased in a cover (vapor-permeable allergen-proof fabric). Upholstered mattress bases: change to a slatted mattress base cleaned every 2 wk.
Carpets	Not all are infested by mites. Carpets should be vacuum-cleaned weekly using a vacuum cleaner with an effective filter. The patient should either avoid vacuuming or wear a mask while doing so: If Acarex-test is negative, no treatment, but verify every year the absence of mite infestation. If Acarex-test is positive: if the removal of the carpet is not possible, use an acaricide treatment (Acarosan powder, Tannic acid, acardust) and check the efficacy of the treatment every 3 mo. If Acarex-test is ++: remove the carpet if possible.
Bedding	Use synthetic pillow and duvet washed at the hottest temperature possible (usually 40–50°C) every 2 mo, or covered with vapor-permeable covers. Wash all bedding, including mattress pad, pillowcases, and sheets weekly,

(*continued*)

Table 3 Continued

	using hottest cycle possible.
Small objects	Small objects that accumulate dust, such as books, should be placed in drawers or closed cabinets. Stuffed animals should be washed every 2 mo.
	Clothing should be stored in closed cupboard or closet.
	Unused clothing should be stored away from the bedroom.
Control humidity in the home	This can be achieved by increasing ventilation if the outdoor conditions are cold or dry, using mechanical ventilation, or by opening the window. Alternatively, reducing humidity seems to be achieved with central air conditioning. The objective is to keep relative humidity below 50%.
	If there is faulty construction, consult a building expert.
Eventual Methods	
Choice of house and apartments	Basements are not recommended for any allergic patients.
	Bedrooms should be upstairs.
Choice of ventilation system	Air filters on central air-conditioning should be cleaned regularly, use mechanical ventilation when outdoor conditions are cold or dry.
Choice of flooring and furnishings	Carpets fitted to a concrete slab either in a basement or on the ground floor tend to become damp and remain damp. All floors should have a primary polished layer and carpets should be movable.
Choice of bedding	See recommendations above.

VI. Conclusion

Early allergenic exposure is a risk factor for sensitization in predisposed subjects. Indeed, it seems logical that early reduction of exposure could decrease the onset of sensitization to aeroallergens. An English prospective control study of primary prevention in babies at risk for atopy showed a significant decrease in the frequency of atopy, 1, 2, and 4 years after starting allergen avoidance methods at birth (108). Similar studies need to be performed to determine the responsibility of indoor aeroallergens in the pathophysiology of allergic asthma. In addition to primary prevention, allergen removal is a logical treatment for allergic asthma. However, these measures should be applied for patients with symptoms that can be attributed to allergy. Therefore, for mite allergens, the first step is to document exposure to the house dust mite by environmental tests. There is good evidence that mite allergic patients with very low mite exposure or in mite-free environments have significant clinical improvement, decreases in medication scores, specific and nonspecific bronchial hyperresponsiveness, and in bronchial inflammation (109). At sealevels or in usual domestic environments combined reduction methods must be used to obtain the lowest mite exposure (Table 3). Clinical improvement has been observed in most controlled clinical studies when using global avoidance measures, but one of the main problems in allergen avoidance is the patient acceptability of the methods. Given the trend away from heavily furnished interiors, patients seem to be more prone to follow advice for exposure reduction, as has been shown by a Canadian study (110) and one from our group (111). In these two studies over 50% of the patients applied the indicated measures. In our study, over 70% of patients did not have the impression that their bedroom differed greatly from any other. The acceptability of an avoidance plan dramatically increased when a technician or nurse who specialized in indoor environments gave advice tailored to the individual situation in the patient's home. The individual clinical improvement resulting from such global avoidance studies varies from one patient to another. In the future, it would be interesting to develop biological markers to identify more accurately patients who have a clinical improvement after allergen elimination.

References

1. Britton J. Asthma's changing prevalence: establishing the true figure is difficult. Br Med J 1992; 304:857–589.
2. Burr M, Butland B, King S, Waughan-Williams E. Changes in asthma prevalence: two surveys 15 years apart. Arch Dis Child 1989; 64:1452–1456.
3. Woolcock A, Peat J, Trevillion L. Is the increase in asthma prevalence linked to increase in allergen load? Allergy 1995; 50:935–940.
4. Custovic A, Simon CO, Taggart H, Chapman M, Woodcock A. Exposure to house dust mite allergens and the clinical activity of asthma. J Allergy Clin Immunol 1996; 98:64–72.
5. Peat J, Woolcock A. Sensitivity to common allergens: relation to respiratory symptoms

and bronchial hyperresponsiveness in children from three different climatic areas of Australia. Clin Exp Allergy 1991; 21:573–581.
6. Sears HR, Herbison GP, Holdaway MD, Hewitt CJ, Flannery EM, Silva PA. The relative risks of sensitivity to grass pollen, house dust mite and cat dander in the development of childhood asthma. Clin Exp Allergy 1989; 19:412–424.
7. Chapman M. Monoclonal antibodies as structural probes for mite, cat and cockroach allergens. In: Said El Shami A, Meretts T, eds. Advances in the Biosciences. Allergy and Molecular Biology. Oxford: Pergamon Press, 1989; 281–285.
8. Pauli G, Hoyet C, Tenabene A, Le Mao J, Thierry R, Bessot JC. Guanine and mite allergenicity in house dust. Clin Allergy 1988; 18:383–392.
9. Platts-Mills TAE, Thomas WR, Aalberse RC, Vervloet D, Chapman MD. Dust mite allergens and asthma: report of a second international workshop. J Allergy Clin Immunol 1992; 89:1046–1060.
10. Tovey E, Chapman M, Wells C, Platts-Mills T. The distribution of dust mite allergen in the houses of patients with asthma. Am Rev Respir Dis 1981; 124:630–635.
11. van Bronswijk J. *Dermatophagoides pteronyssinus* (Trouessard, 1897) in mattress and floor dust in a temperate climate (Acari: Pyroglyphidae). J Med Entomol 1973; 10:63–70.
12. Pauli G, de Blay F, Bessot JC, Ott M, Gries P. The role of mattress bases in the mite infestation of dwellings. J Allergy Clin Immunol 1997; 99:261–263.
13. Nagakura T, Yasueda H, Obata T, Kanmuri M, Masaki T, Ihara N, Maekawa K. Major *Dermatophagoides* mite allergen, Der 1, in soft toys. Clin Exp Allergy 1996; 26:585–589.
14. Munir AKM, Einarsson R, Dreborg SKG. Mite (Der p 1, Der f 1), cat (Fel d 1) and dog (Can f 1) allergens in dust from Swedish day-care centres. Clin Exp Allergy 1995; 25:119–126.
15. Custovic A, Taggart S, Woodcock A. House dust mite and cat allergen in different indoor environments. Clin Exp Allergy 1994; 24:1164–1168.
16. van Nes A, Kort H, Koren L, Pernot C, Schellen H, van Boven F, van Bronswijk J. The abundance of house dust mites (Pyroglyphidae) in different home textiles in Europe, in relation to outdoor climates, heating and ventilation. In: Wildey KB, Robinson WH, eds. Proceedings of the First International Conference on Insect Pests in the Urban Environment. Exeter, Wheatons, 1993:229–239.
17. Harving H, Korsgaard J, Dahl R. Clinical efficacy of reduction in house-dust mite exposure in specially designed, mechanically ventilated, healthy homes. Allergy 1994; 49: 866–870.
18. Van Strien RT, Verhoeff AP, Brunekreef B, Van Wijnen JH. Mite antigen in house dust: relationship with different housing characteristics in the Netherlands. Clin Exp Allergy 1994; 24:843–853.
19. Kuehr J, Frischer T, Karmamus W, Meinert R, Barth R, Schraub S, Daschner A, Urbanek R, Forster J. Natural variation in mite antigen density in house dust and relationship to residential factors. Clin Exp Allergy 1994; 24:229–237.
20. Wickman M, Emenius G, Egmar A, Axelsson G, Pershagen G. Reduced mite allergen levels in dwellings with mechanical exhaust and supply ventilation. Clin Exp Allergy 1994; 24:109–114.
21. Dornelas de Andrade A, Birnbaum J, Lanteaume A, Izard JL, Corget P, Artillan MF, Toumi M, Vervloet D, Charpin D. Housing and house-dust mites. Allergy 1995; 50:142–146.
22. Fletcher A, Pickering C, Custovic A, Simpson J, Kennaugh J, Woodcock A. Reduction in humidity as a method of controlling mites and mite allergens: the use of mechanical ventilation in British domestic dwellings. Clin Exp Allergy 1996; 26:1051–1056.
23. Custovic A, Taggart S, Kennaugh J, Woodcock A. Portable dehumidifiers in the control of house dust mites and mite allergens. Clin Exp Allergy 1995; 25:312–316.
24. Lintner TJ, Brame KA. The effects of season, climate, and air-conditioning on the prevalence of *Dermatophagoides* mite allergens in household dust. J Allergy Clin Immunol 1993; 91:862–867.

25. Tovey E, Mahmic A. Special problems in cooling climates. In: van Bronswijk J, Pauli G, eds. An Update on Long-Lasting Mite Avoidance. Aachen: GUT 1996:32–42.
26. Van Bronswijk J. Neues zur Okologie der Wohnungsmilben. Allergologie 1984; 11:438–445.
27. Kalra S, Owen SJ, Hepworth J, Woodcock A. Airborne house dust mite antigen after vacuum cleaning. Lancet 1990; 336:449.
28. Hegarty J, Rouhbakhsh S, Warner JA, Warner JO. A comparison of the effect of conventional and filter vacuum cleaners on airborne house dust mite allergen. Respir Med 1995; 89:1–6.
29. Wassenaar DPJ. Effectiveness of vacuum cleaning and wet cleaning in reducing house-dust mites, fungi and mite allergen in a cotton carpet: a case study. Exp Appl Acarol 1988; 4:53–62.
30. Fell P, Mitchell B, Brostoff J. Wet vacuum-cleaning and house dust-mite allergen. Lancet 1992; 340:788–789.
31. de Boer R. The control of house dust mite allergens in rugs. J Allergy Clin Immunol 1990; 86:808–814.
32. Colloff MJ, Taylor C, Merrett T. The use of domestic steam cleaning for the control of house dust mites. Clin Exp Allergy 1995; 25:1061–1066.
33. Andersen A, Rosen J. House dust mite *Dermatophagoides pteronyssinus* and its allergens: effects of washing. Allergy 1989; 44:496–500.
34. Van den Hove T, Soler M, Birnbaum J, Charpin D, Vervloet D. Effect of dry cleaning on mite allergen levels in blankets. Allergy 1993; 48:264–266.
35. Mc Donald L, Tovey E. The role of water temperature and laundry procedures in reducing house dust-mite populations and allergen content of bedding. J Allergy Clin Immunol 1992; 90:599–608.
36. Bischoff E, Fisher A, Liebenberg B, Kniest F. Mite control with low temperature washing. I. Elimination of living mites on carpet pieces. Clin Exp Allergy 1996; 26:945–952.
37. Mosbech H, Korsgaard J, Lind P. Control of house dust mites by electrical heating blankets. J Allergy Clin Immunol 1988; 81:706–710.
38. Dorward A, Colloff M, Mc Kay N, Mc Sharry C, Thompson N. Effect of house dust mite avoidance measures in adult atopic asthma. Thorax 1988, 43:98–102.
39. Zwemer R, Karibo J. Use of laminar control device as adjunct to standard environmental control measures in symptomatic asthmatic children. Ann Allergy 1973; 31:284–290.
40. Villaveces J, Rosengren H, Evan J. Use of laminar flow portable filter in asthmatic children. Ann Allergy 1977; 38:400–404.
41. Mitchell E, Elliott R. Controlled trial of an electrostatic precipitator in childhood asthma. Lancet 1980; 2:559–561.
42. Warner JA, Marchant JL, Warner JO. Double blind trial of ionizers in children with asthma sensitive to the house dust mite. Thorax 1993; 48:330–333.
43. Nelson H, Hirsch R, Ohman J, Platts-Mills T, Reed C, Solomon W. Recommendations for the use of residential air-cleaning devices in the treatment of allergic respiratory diseases. J Allergy Clin Immunol 1988; 82:661–669
44. Owen S, Morgenstern M, Hepworth J, Woodcock A. Control of house dust mite antigen in bedding. Lancet 1990; 335:396–397.
45. Ehnert B, Lau-Schadendorf S, Weber A, Buettner P, Schou C, Wahn U. Reducing domestic exposure to dust mite allergen reduces bronchial hypereactivity in sensitive children with asthma. J Allergy Clin Immunol 1992; 90:135–138.
46. Birnbaum J, de Blay F, Paty E, Just J, Pauli G, Vervloet D, Charpin D. Clinical study of bedding covers in mite-allergic asthmatic patients [abstr]. J Allergy Clin Immunol 1996; 97:223.
47. Burr M, Dean B, Verrier Jones E. Effect of change to mite free bedding on children with mite-sensitive asthma: a controlled trial. Thorax 1980; 35:513–514.
48. Murray A, Ferguson A. Dust free bedrooms in the treatment of asthmatic children with house dust mite allergy: a controlled trial. Pediatrics 1983; 71:418–422

49. Walshaw M, Evans C. Allergen avoidance in house dust mite sensitive adult asthma. Q J Med 1986; 58:199–215.
50. Tan B, Weald D, Strickland I, Friedmann P.Double-blind controlled trial of effect of house dust mite allergen avoidance on atopic dermatitis. Lancet 1996; 347:15–18.
51. Gillies D, Littlewood J, Sarsfield J. Controlled trial of house dust mite avoidance in children with mild to moderate asthma. Clin Allergy 1987; 17:105–111.
52. Burr M, Neale E, Dean B, Verrier-Jones E. Effect of a change to mite-free bedding on children with mite-sensitive asthma: a controlled trial. Thorax 1980; 35:506–512.
53. Korsgaard J. Preventive measures in mite asthma. Allergy 1983; 38:93–102.
54. Marks G, Tovey E, Green W, Shearer M, Salome C, Woolcock AS. House dust mite allergen avoidance: a randomized controlled trial of surface chemical treatment and encasement of bedding. Clin Exp Allergy 1994; 24:1078–1083.
55. Bowler S, Mitchell C, Miles J. House dust mite control and asthma: a placebo control trial of cleaning air filtration. Ann Allergy 1985; 55:498–500.
56. de Saint Georges-Gridelet D, Kniest FM, Schober G, Penaud A, Van Bronswijk JEMH. Lutte chimique contre les acariens de la poussière de maison. Rev Fr Allergol 1988; 28:131–138.
57. Colloff MJ. House dust mites—Part II. Chemical control. Pestic Outlook 1990; 1:3–8.
58. Hayden ML, Rose G, Diduch KB, Domson P, Chapman M, Heymann P, Platts-Mills T. Benzyl benzoate moist powder: investigation of acaricidal activity in cultures and reduction of dust mite allergens in carpets. J Allergy Clin Immunol 1992; 89:536–545.
59. Tovey E, Marks G, Matthews M, Green W, Woolcock A. Changes in mite allergen Der p 1 in house dust following spraying with a tannic acid/acaricide solution. Clin Exp Allergy 1992; 22:67–74.
60. Dietemann A, Bessot JC, Hoyet C, Ott M, Vérot A, Pauli G. A double-blind, placebo controlled trial of solidified benzyl benzoate applied in dwellings of asthmatic patients sensitive to mites: clinical efficacy and effect on mite allergens. J Allergy Clin Immunol 1993; 91:738–746.
61. Third International Workshop on indoor allergens and asthma. Cuenca. Spain, June 30–July 2, 1995.
62. Kniest F,Young E, Van Praag M, Vos H, Kort H, Koers W, De Maat-Bleecker F, Van Bronswijk J. Clinical evaluation of a double-blind dust-mite avoidance trial with mite-allergic rhinitic patients. Clin Exp Allergy 1991, 21:39–47.
63. Rieser J, Ingram D, Mitchell EB, Warner JO. House dust mite allergen levels and an anti-mite mattress spray (natamycin) in the treatment of childhood asthma. Clin Exp Allergy 1990; 20:561–567.
64. Huss R, Huss K, Squire E, Carpenter G, Smith L, Salata K, Hershey J. Mite allergen control with acaricide fails. J Allergy Clin Immunol 1994; 94:27–32.
65. Leclercq-Foucart J, de Saint Georges-Guidelet D, de Geubelle F, Lebrun P. Contrôle de l'acarien des poussières (*Dermatophagoides pteronyssinus*) par utilisation d'un fongicide. Observations expérimentales. Essai clinique chez l'enfant allergique au *Dermatophagoides*. Rev Med Liège 1985; 40:91–99.
66. Charpin D, Birnbaum J, Haddi E, N'Guyen Fondarai J, Vervloet D. Evaluation de l'efficacité d'un acaricide Acardust dans le traitement de l'allergie aux acariens. Rev Fr Allergol 1990; 30:149–155.
67. Blumenthal M, Blumenthal M, Bousquet J, Burney P, Burr M, Bryan S, Charpin D, Kaslow RA, Kay B, Kjellman N, Mapp C, Miyamoto T, Paoletti P, Pollock J, Ronchetti R, Rung-Weelce E, Svendsen UG, Szeuer P, Troix C, Wahn U, Weiss K, Zweiman B. Evidence for an increase in atopic disease and possible causes. Clin Exp Allergy 1993; 23:484–492.
68. Kjellman B, Petterson R. The problem of furred pets in childhood atopic disease. Allergy 1983; 38: 65–73.
69. Popp W, Rauscher H, Sertl K, Wanke T, Zwick H. Risk factor for sensitization to furred pets. Allergy 1990; 45:75–79.

70. Barbee R, Brown W, Kaltenborn W, Halonen M. Allergen skin-test-reactivity in community population sample: correlation with age, histamine, skin reactions and total serum immunoglobulin E. J Allergy Clin Immunol 1981; 68: 15–19.
71. Sporik R, Ingram JM, Price W, Sussman J, Honsinger R, Platts-Mills T. Association of asthma with serum IgE and skin test reactivity to allergens among children living at high altitude. Am J Respir Crit Care Med 1995; 151:1388–1392
72. Vervloet D, Charpin D, Birnbaum J. Origine des allergènes du chat. Rev Fr Allergol 1995; 35:533–538.
73. Warner J, Little S, Pollock I, Longbottom J, Warner J. The influence of exposure to house dust mite, cat, pollen and fungal allergens in home on primary sensitization in asthma. Pediatr Allergy Immunol 1991; 1:79–86
74. Ott M, de Blay F,Gries P, Pauli G. Cat major allergen (Fel d 1): correlation between dust and airborne exposure using a portable air sampler (abstr). J Allergy Clin Immunol 1996; 97:215.
75. deBlay F, Kopferschmitt MC, Gries P, Frey F, Linder J, Mahr L, Vérot A, Pauli G. Comparison between Fel d 1 levels provoking respiratory symptoms at home and during bronchial challenge tests (abstr). J Allergy Clin Immunol 1995; 95:262.
76. van der Brempt X, Charpin D, Haddi E, Da Mata P, Vervloet D. Cat removal and Fel d 1 levels in mattresses. J Allergy Clin Immunol 1991; 87:595–596.
77. Shamie S, Enberg R, Terry L, Ownby D. The consistent presence of cat allergen (Fel d 1) in various types of public places (abstr). J Allergy Clin Immunol 1990; 85:331.
78. Munir A, Einarsson R, Schou C, Dreborg S. The amount of the major cat (Fel d 1) and dog (Can f I) allergens in dust from Swedish schools is high enough to probably cause perennial symptoms in most children with asthma who are sensitized to cat and dog. J Allergy Clin Immunol 1993; 91:1067–1071.
79. Munir AKM, Einarsson R, Dreborg SKG. Mite (Der p 1, Der f 1), cat (Fel d 1) and dog (Can f 1) allergens in dust from Swedish day-care centres. Clin Exp Allergy 1995; 25:119–126.
80. Dornelas de Andrade A, Charpin D, Birnbaum J, Lanteaume A, Chapman M, Vervloet D. Indoor allergen levels in day nurseries. J Allergy Clin Immunol 1995; 95:1158–1163.
81. Luczynska C, Li Y, Chapman M, Platts-Mills T. Airborne concentrations and particle size distribution of allergen derived from domestic cats (*Felis domesticus*): measurements using cascade impactor, liquid impinger and a two site monoclonal antibody assay for Fel d 1. Am Rev Respir Dis 1990; 141:361–367.
82. de Blay F, Heymann P, Chapman M, Platts-Mills T. Airborne dust mite allergens: comparison of group II allergens with group I mite and cat allergen Fel d 1. J Allergy Clin Immunol 1991; 88:919–926.
83. Wood RA, Chapman M, Adkinson N, Eggleston P. The effect of cat removal on allergen content in household dust samples. J Allergy Clin Immunol 1989; 83:730–734.
84. Charpin D, Vervloet D, Lanteaume A, Kleisbauer JP, Kulling G. Allergie respiratoire et animaux domestiques. Rev Mal Respir 1989; 6:325–328.
85. Ohman J. Allergy in man caused by exposure to mammals. J Am Vet Med Assoc 1978; 172:1403–1406.
86. Hering S, McGeady S, Jones J, Mansmann A. The maintenance of pets in allergic families. I. A survey of health beliefs. Ann Allergy 1981; 46:24–27.
87. de Blay F, Chapman M, Platts-Mills T. Environmental control with the cat in situ. Am Rev Respir Dis 1991; 143:1334–1339.
88. Wentz PE, Swanson MC, Reed OE. Variability of cat-allergen shedding. J Allergy Clin Immunol 1990; 85:94–98.
89. Ohman JL, Baer H, Anderson MC, Leitermann K, Brown P. Surface washes of living cats: an improved method of obtaining clinically relevant allergen. J Allergy Clin Immunol 1983; 72:288–293.

90. Glinert R, Wilson P, Wedner HJ. Fel d 1 is markedly reduced following sequential washing of cats (abstr). J Allergy Clin Immunol 1990; 87:327.
91. Klucka CV, Ownby DR, Green J, Zoratti E. Cat shedding of Fel d 1 is not reduced by washings, Allerpet-C spray, or acepromazine. J Allergy Clin Immunol 1995; 95:1164–1171.
92. Soldatov D, de Blay F, Gries P, Charles P, Charpentier C, Ott M, Pauli G. Effects of environmental control measures on patient status and airborne Fel d 1 levels with a cat in situ (abstr). J Allergy Clin Immunol 1995; 95:263.
93. Lind P, Norm P, Newton M, Lowenstein H, Schwartz B. The prevalence of indoor allergens in Baltimore area: house-dust mite and animal dander antigens measured by immunochemical techniques. J Allergy Clin Immunol 1987; 80:541–547.
94. Haahtela T, Jaakonmaki I. Relationship of allergen specific IgE antibodies, skin prick tests and allergic disorders in unselected adolescents. Allergy 1981; 36:251–256.
95. Vanto T, Koivikko A. Dog hypersensitivity in asthmatic children. Acta Paediatr Scand 1983; 72:571–575.
96. Wood R, Eggleston P, Lind P, Ingemann L, Schwartz B, Graveson S, Terry D, Wheeler B, Adkinson NF. Antigenic analysis of household dust samples. Am Rev Respir Dis 1988; 137:358–363.
97. Sakaguchi M, Inouye S, Irie T, Miyazawa H, Watanabe M, Yasueda H, Shida T, Nitta H, Chapman M, Schou C, Aalberse R. Airborne cat (Fel d 1), dog (Can f 1) and mite (Der 1 and Der 2) allergen levels in the homes of Japan. J Allergy Clin Immunol 1993; 92:797–802.
98. Custovic A, Green R, Fletcher A, Smith A, Anthony C, Pickering C, Chapman M, Woodcock A. Aerodynamic properties of the major dog allergen, Can f 1 distribution in homes, concentration and particle size of allergen in the air. Am J Respir Crit Care Med. 1997; 155:94–98.
99. Walls A, Longbottom J. Comparison of rat fur, urine, saliva and other rat allergen extracts by skin testing, RAST and RAST inhibition. J Allergy Clin Immunol 1985; 75:242–251.
100. Platts-Mills T, Heyman P, Longbottom J, Wilkins S. Airborne allergens associated with asthma: particle size carrying dust mite and rat allergens measured with a cascade impactor. J. Allergy Clin Immunol 1987; 79:781–791
101. Eggleston P, Newill C, Ansari A, Pustelnik A, Lou S, Evans R, Marsh D, Longbottom JL, Corn M. Task-related variation in airborne concentrations of laboratory animal allergens: studies with Rat n 1. J Allergy Clin Immunol 1989; 84:347–352.
102. Venables K, Tee R, Howkins E. Laboratory animal allergy in a pharmaceutical company. Br J Ind 1988; 45:660–666.
103. Swanson M, Campbell A, O'Hallaren M, Reed C. Role of ventilation, air filtration and allergen production rate in determining concentrations of rat allergens in the air of animal quarters. Am Rev Respir Dis 1990; 141:1578–1581.
104. Botham P, Teasdale E. Allergy to laboratory animals. Biologist 1987; 34:162–163.
105. Lehrer S, Lopez M, Butcher B, Olson J, Reed M, Salvaggio J. Basidiomycete mycelia and spore-allergen extracts: skin test activity in adults with symptoms of respiratory allergy. J Allergy Clin Immunol 1986; 78:478–485.
106. O'Hallaren M,Yunginger J, Offord K, Somers M, O'Connell E, Ballard D, Sachs M. Exposure to an aeroallergen as a possible precipitating factor in respiratory arrest in young patients with asthma. N Engl J Med 1991; 324:359–363.
107. de Blay F, Sanchez J, Hedelin G, Perez-Infante A, Verot A, Chapman M, Pauli G. Dust and airborne exposure to allergens derived from cockroach (*Blattella germanica*) in low cost public housing of Strasbourg (France). J Allergy Clin Immunol 1997; 99:107–112.
108. Hide D, Matthews S, Tariq S, Arshad S. Allergen avoidance in infancy and allergy at 4 years of age. Allergy 1996; 51:89–93.
109. Peroni D, Boner A, Vallone G, Antolini I, Warner J. Effective allergen avoidance at high altitude reduces allergen-induced bronchial hyperresponsiveness. Am J Respir Crit Care Med 1994; 143:1442–1446.

110. Côte J, Robichaud P, Boutin H, Filion A, Lavallée M, Krausky M, Rouleau M, Malo JL, Cartier A, Boulet P. Impact of an individual teaching program on environmental control in moderate to severe asthmatics (abstr). J Allergy Clin Immunol 1995; 97:223.
111. Krieger P, Spirlet F, Strauss N, Ott M, Pauli G, de Blay F. Evaluation de la faisabilité de l'éviction des allergènes des acariens chez des patients asthmatiques, allergiques aux acariens (abstr). Rev Mal Respir 1996; 13:81.

9

Standardization of Allergens

JEAN BOUSQUET and FRANCOIS-BERNARD MICHEL

Montpellier University and
Service des Maladies Respiratoires–INSERM U454
Montpellier University Hospital
Montpellier, France

I. Introduction

Allergen extracts prepared from biological materials are very complex, heterogeneous, and particularly unstable. They are composed of a mixture of proteins, carbohydrates, enzymes, and other substances, some of them having a biological or a toxic activity. In most extracts, allergens represent only a small fraction of the total mixture. For a given allergen, the quality and shelf life of the extract varies according to the nature of the raw material, preparation, and storage.

Allergenic extracts and products have been defined as follows. *Allergenic extract* means a preparation of an allergen obtained by extraction of the active constituents from animal or vegetable substances with a suitable menstruum. *Allergenic product* means a biological product, including allergenic extracts and others, that is administered to humans for diagnosis, prevention, and treatment of allergy and allergenic diseases (1). In the *European Pharmacopoeia*, “allergen products are pharmaceutical preparations which are derived from vaccines of naturally occurring source materials containing allergens, which are substances that cause and/or provoke allergic (hypersensitivity) disease. The allergenic compounds are most often of a proteinaceous nature. Allergen products are intended for in vivo diagnosis and/or treatment of allergic hypersensitivity diseases attributed to these allergens” (2).

Since the introduction of immunotherapy in 1911, allergen extracts have been used in millions of subjects throughout the world for the diagnosis and treatment of allergic patients. The production of allergens has been strongly influenced by the fundamental work of pioneers of allergy. Noon (3) proposed to define extracts in units of weight to volume (w/v) and Stull and Cooke (4) devised protein nitrogen units (PNU). These two units are completely independent of the biological activity of the extract, and when the Panel on Review of Allergenic extracts (1) published its report in 1985 (the report was submitted to FDA in 1981), most extracts were labeled in these allergen-independent units, and their quality was often not optimal. It is only within the past 20 years that the introduction of in vitro techniques based on IgE have made it possible, at least, for the main allergenic materials, to characterize and quantify the major allergens in the extracts and to quantitate the total allergenic potency. These methods have permitted the definition and preparation, under the aegis of the International Union of Immunological Societies (IUIS), of extracts of reference called *standards*, of which six have been accepted by the World Health Organization (WHO). The Bureau of Biologics (now known as the Center for Biologics Evaluation and Research; CBER) in the United States has prepared, for this country, a range of national extracts of reference. Since 1980, new technologies, based on monoclonal antibodies (MAbs) and recombinant allergens, have been made available, they are increasingly used in the standardization of allergenic extracts and are significantly improving the labeling of allergen extracts (5).

In 1998, many allergen extracts are standardized throughout the world, and the overall quality of these extracts has been considerably improved. It is proposed that most if not all allergens should be standardized to improve allergy practice, both for the diagnosis and the treatment of allergic diseases (6,7).

II. Control of Allergen Extracts

The composition of the allergen extracts which, because of the nature of the raw material, is more heterogeneous than that of other biological products, does not make it possible to conceive a system of control based only on a definition of analytical normal values. It requires the definition and production of reference extracts that may be compared, batch-to-batch, with routine production extracts, using methods that have been well established.

The potency of allergen extracts is defined by U.S. Code CRF 21 600.3 (1) as follows: "The word potency is interpreted to mean the specific ability or capacity of the products, as initiated by appropriate laboratory tests or by adequately controlled clinical data obtained through the administration of the product in the manner intended, to effect a given result." The control of an allergen extract requires several methods to assay its total potency and composition by comparison with reference standards.

New recombinant cDNA technology has considerably modified the standardization of allergens; it is a potent tool for their characterization and could provide large amounts of identical cloned allergens for diagnosis and standardization purposes. The cDNAs of several important human allergens have been isolated and sequenced, including house dust mites (8,9), insect venoms, cat (10), various pollens (11–16), and some molds (17,18). Some of the recombinant allergens (RA) are able to react with human IgE in solid-phase assays and to stimulate allergen-specific T cells (16,19). The RAs used for in vitro diagnosis should have the same IgE-binding activity as their natural counterparts, but this is rarely obtained. Rafnar et al. (20) compared Amb a 5 and Amb t 5 RA with native proteins by immunologic assays and nuclear magnetic resonance (NMR) spectroscopy and found that, although RAs may be effective in stimulating T cells, they have different three-dimensional structures. Moreover, the strategy of cDNA cloning requires that IgE epitopes be mainly proteins and that the carbohydrate moiety of the allergen participates to only a minor extent in IgE binding. Moreover, they should possess all IgE-binding epitopes relevant to standardize a given native allergen (21). The production in unlimited amounts of perfectly characterized proteins bearing an identical structure makes their use in standardization very attractive.

A. Allergen Extracts Used for Diagnosis

Allergen extracts used for the diagnosis of allergic disorders include those for skin tests and provocative challenges. To measure allergenic potency and composition both in vivo and in vitro tests have been proposed (Table 1).

Skin Tests

In vivo methods carried out directly in allergic individuals are widely used for the standardization of allergenic extracts. They measure the biological reaction of sensitized individuals to allergens, and their results are given in biological units. The only in vivo tests available are based on skin tests.

Several methods for performing skin tests have been proposed (Table 2), but there is no general agreement on methods for performing quantitative skin tests. Variable parameters include the selection of the allergic patients (unselected to highly allergic), the method of skin testing (prick test or intradermal reaction), the analysis of the wheal or the flare, or both, the comparison of the allergen-induced skin test with a reference standard preparation (histamine, codeine phosphate, or compound 48/80) or not, the statistical analysis, and finally the unitage. There are two methods that are more commonly accepted: the United States (22,23) and the Nordic methods (24–26). However, other methods are also used (27). Unitage systems have been modified within the past 15 years because of our evolving knowledge. Finally, the three main units (IU, AU or BAU, and BU) have not yet been compared.

Skin testing is of paramount importance because it represents the only feasible method to obtain extracts standardized biologically in sensitive individuals. These extracts give skin reactions of a comparable size whatever the allergen spe-

Table 1 Methods for Analysis of Allergen Extracts Used in Standardization

1. In vivo techniques
Skin test titration
2. In vitro techniques
Physical methods
Characterization using molecular size
Ultracentrifuge analysis
Gel filtration
Sodium dodecyl sulfate–polyacrylamide gel electrophoresis (SDS–PAGE)
Chromatographic methods
Characterization using electrical charge
Isoelectric focusing (IEF)
Electrophoresis (starch gel, agarose gel)
Chemical methods
Protein analysis (PNU, total protein content, amino acid analysis)
Carbohydrate analysis
Enzyme assays
Immunological methods
Inhibition immunoassays including RAST and ELISA-based techniques
Monoclonal antibody-based assays (measurement of major allergens)
Immunodiffusion
Quantitative immunoelectrophoresis
Cross-immunoelectrophoresis
Rocket immunoelectrophoresis
Cross-radioimmunoelectrophoresis
Immunoprecipitation and laser nephelometry
Electroimmunodiffusion
Radioimmunoprecipitation
Histamine release
Complement consumption
Combined methods
Allergenic profiles of isoelectric focusing
Allergenic profiles of chromatographic fractions including CRIE

cies tested (Fig. 1), whereas those only standardized by radioallergosorbent technique (RAST)-inhibition do not. Usually, manufacturers standardize their reference extracts in biological units and then compare their in-house reference preparations with freshly prepared extracts by means of allergen-related in vitro assays.

In Vitro Assays Unrelated to Allergens

For decades, allergen extracts have been standardized either by the weight/volume (w/v) method proposed in 1911 (3), or by their content in proteins, such as the total nitrogen unit proposed in the 1920s by Cooke et al. (4) and the protein nitrogen unit (PNU; 28), because most allergens are of protein origin. More recently, the

Table 2 Comparison Between Skin Test Methods to Standardize Allergens

	U.S. method	Nordic Council method
Skin test method	intradermal	prick test
Dosage increment	threefold	tenfold
Number of patients tested	15	20
Selection of patients	highly allergic	no selection
Reaction analyzed	erythema	wheal
Histamine reference	no	yes
Calculation	means	geometric means
Units	allergy unit (AU) and bioequivalent allergy unit (BAU)	biological unit (BU)

analysis of amino acids has also been used. Some allergens are glycoproteins, and the carbohydrate content of allergens may be measured by techniques, such as gas–liquid chromatography. Studies examining the correlation between these units and allergen-related in vitro assays found no significant correlation, even for pollen extracts. It is, therefore, desirable to avoid labeling extracts in such units only.

In Vitro Assays Measuring Total Allergenic Potency

RAST Inhibition and Inhibition Immunoassays

The direct RAST titration (5) has been replaced by inhibition immunoassays, such as RAST inhibition, and derived techniques, such as the CAP System, other tech-

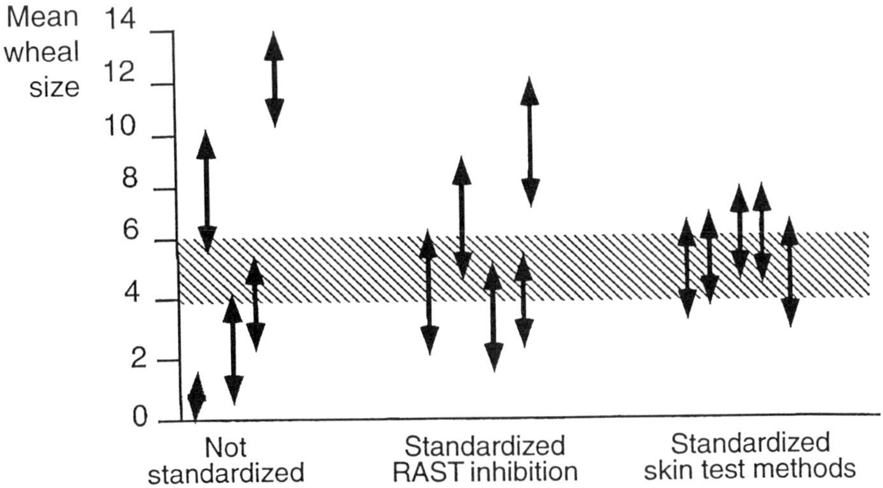

Figure 1 Mean wheal sizes induced by unstandardized and standardized allergen extracts.

niques of solid-phase immunoassays, or enzyme-linked immunosorbent assay (ELISA) tests (29). Inhibition immunoassays are the most widely used for the control of the total allergenic potency of an extract. These assays should follow precise procedures, and they require (1) a solid-phase allergen, prepared from a high-quality source material, in which all major and minor allergens are represented; (2) a pool of serum prepared from multiple individuals sensitive to the allergen tested; and (3) a high-quality reference extract to be used as a standard. These inhibition immunoassays express only the sum of the total allergenic activity, but do not give any information on individual allergenic components. Moreover, a single, purified major allergen, such as Amb a 1 can totally inhibit the RAST (to short ragweed pollen). The parallelism of the different curves has to be examined because extracts that give nonparallel curves may not have the same antigenic composition. The concentration of extract required to induce a 50% inhibition represents a measure of the potency (Fig. 2). The technique has been standardized and is now suitable for allergen standardization.

Measurement of Individual Allergenic Components Without Enzymatic Activity

The rapid development of new technologies for both DNA and protein analysis offers opportunities for improved standardization. Many important allergens from pollen, dust mites, animal danders, insects, and foods have been cloned and are being expressed as homogeneous recombinant proteins that, in several cases, have allergenic activity comparable with the natural protein allergens (reviewed in Ref. 30). With these new technologies, an allergen extract can be characterized in terms of

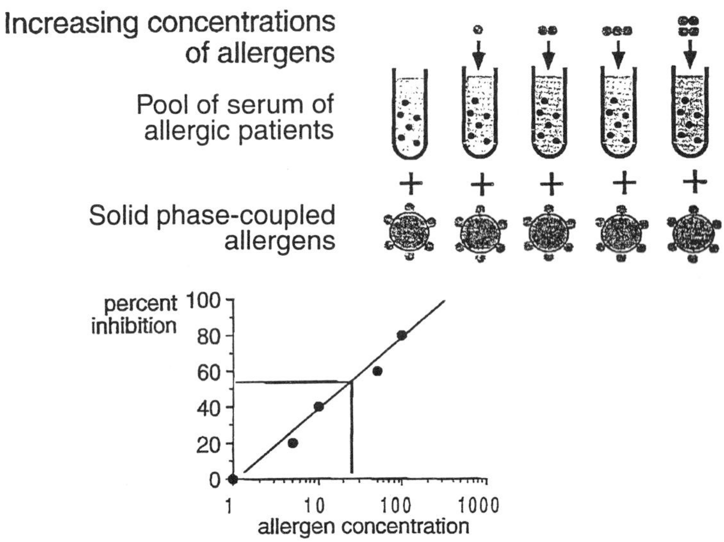

Figure 2 RAST inhibition assay.

major allergen content (nanograms or micrograms), and the consistency of each lot can be accurately monitored. It has been observed that the major allergen content of allergenic preparations reflects their biological activity measured by skin tests, and that, for birch, *Dermatophagoides pteronyssinus,* cat, *Alternaria*, and ragweed pollen 1 biological unit (BU) was equivalent to 1 ng of the major allergen (31). Such measurements will facilitate objective comparisons of allergen extracts (32–36). They should focus on proteins of established allergenic importance, which fulfill criteria for inclusion in the WHO/IUIS nomenclature (e.g. Fel d 1, Der p 1, Lol p 1, Amb a 1, Bet v 1, and others, (37,38). It is important that there should be a consistent relationship between the amount of allergen measured and the amounts of other allergens present in the extract (39). Although monoclonal antibody-based assays are preferred because the reagents are available in perpetuity and have defined specificity (40), tests using polyclonal antibodies may be equally valid, provided the antibodies are monospecific, or the major allergen activity can be quantified separately. At present, for example, measurements of Fel d 1 form the basis of assigning a bioequivalent allergy unit (BAU) to cat hair and cat extracts by the US Food and Drug Administration (FDA). Major allergen measurements have been shown to correlate with estimates of biological potency (31,39).

The measurement of major allergens for standardization is now a realistic and desirable goal that should be encouraged. A key element in this process is the maintenance of reference standards containing known amounts of relevant allergens. Standards for several vaccines have been produced as part of the WHO/IUIS/IAACI allergen standardization program (41–45). Several of these standards (e.g., short ragweed, mite [*D. pteronyssinus*], and dog) contain known amounts of the major allergens from these sources (32,34). The allergen content of some CBER reference preparations has also been determined. It is vital that standards with defined allergen content are maintained under stable conditions, in approved repositories, such as the FDA, WHO, Central Bureau for Schimmelsvampes (CBS), or the American Type Culture Collection (ATCC) facilities. In the future, it is likely that recombinant allergens will provide primary standards for allergen analysis and form the basis for development of new diagnostic and therapeutic products to diagnose and treat allergic disorders (21,46,47).

Measurement of Individual Allergenic Components with Enzymatic Activity

Phospholipase A (48) and hyaluronidase are allergens of Hymenoptera venoms with enzymatic activity. This activity is used for the standardization of the venoms.

Study of the Composition of Allergen Extracts

Besides the total allergenic potency, it is necessary to measure the composition of the allergen extract.

Physicochemical Techniques

Proteins in an allergenic extract can be separated by isoelectric point or molecular size using isoelectric focusing (IEF; 49), polyacrylamide gel electrophoresis (PAGE), gel chromatography, isotachophoresis, or high-performance liquid chromatography (HPLC). These are relatively simple techniques separating proteins without taking into account the antigenic and allergenic composition. They are, however, widely used for the batch-to-batch quality control of allergenic extracts.

Immunochemical Techniques

Cross-radioimmunoelectrophoresis (CRIE; 50,51), immunoblotting (52,53), and the titration of purified antigens using monoclonal antibodies are preferred because they give the composition of one or all allergens present in the extract.

B. Allergen Extracts Used for Treatment

It is now recognized that efficacy of specific immunotherapy requires relatively large doses of allergens that are close to the dose that can elicit anaphylactic reactions. Thus, for safety, it is important that the amount of allergen be accurately known and be consistent lot-to-lot (6). Although assays of potency of therapeutic extracts can be made only by controlled clinical trials in humans, it is absolutely impossible to do so with sequential production batches. It is not yet possible to assay potency in the accepted sense of efficacy, but it is possible to assay the composition of the vaccines. Aqueous extracts present few problems because they can be directly assayed by the methods described for extracts used in diagnosis. However, skin test titration may not always be possible owing to the lower potency of the extracts used for treatment.

For adsorbed vaccines, it is necessary either to release the allergen or to use a modified RAST assay (54). When the allergenic components have been chemically modified, it is more difficult to assay the final product except if there is a marker that is easy to titrate, such as Amb a 1 (if not modified). Some of these extracts can be standardized by means of skin test titration (55).

For adsorbed or modified extracts, the composition of the finished product cannot be extrapolated from the initial composition of the standardized extracts, for even simple adsorption on gel introduces selection to the molecules that have been insolubilized.

III. Units of Standardized Extracts

A. Arbitrary Units

Each allergen extract, once standardized, is assigned a potency unit. Several approaches to the choice of potency have been suggested. The "old" allergen-independent units are still in use, but they tend to be replaced by "allergen-related" units. These are either assigned an arbitrary unitage (i.e., 100,000 allergy units [AU] to the reference), or units are based on the quantity of allergen in the extract (i.e., amount of antigen Amb a 1), or finally, the quantity of protein with defined allergenic activity (i.e., micrograms of hyaluronidase).

The international units (IU) labeling, the international reference preparations, and the international standardized preparations (ISP) are "an arbitrary measure adopted in the absence of any absolute measurement that can be invariably related to allergic activity" (56). By way of example, the *D. pteronyssinus* ISP of 100,000 IU/mL has been standardized by skin testing, RAST-inhibition, and the measurement of Der p 1 and Der p 2 using monoclonal antibody-based assays (57,58). They are of relevant importance because it is hoped that in the future all extracts will be labeled in IU; and this will end much of the confusion that makes communication difficult between physicians and researchers who are using an extract.

B. Biological Units

Several biological units have been proposed since the introduction of the histamine equivalent prick (HEP), in 1978 by Aas et al. (24–26). The HEP (1 HEP = 1000 BU/mL) is a biological unit based on the skin sensitivity of the patients by comparison with that of histamine. Other biological units in current use do not include a reference test with histamine or codeine (59). Some of the AUs and all the bioequivalent allergy units (BAUs) are based on the $ID_{50}EAL$ skin test procedure (22,23,60).

IV. Standardized Extracts

Standardized extracts should contain measured quantities of allergenic activity and are produced with lot-to-lot consistency. Such extracts should at best contain all the relevant allergens from a source in the relative proportion found in the raw material. Their use should help improve the reliability of in vivo and in vitro tests, as well as that of specific immunotherapy.

A. International Reference Standards

In 1980, allergen extracts were rarely standardized; and international standards were not available. The Allergen Standardization Subcommittee of the International Unions of Immunological Societies (IUIS) decided to prepare international allergen standards. This subcommittee included members of regulatory agencies; scientists in the field of allergy, chemistry, immunology biology, and molecular biology; clinical allergists; and members of research laboratories of various manufacturers. These members were distributed throughout the world and met regularly several times a year. They first devised steps to prepare a reliable standard:

1. Review of the published data, which makes possible the production of a technical dossier for the intended extract
2. Definition of norms and selection of raw materials
3. Preparation of a pool of serum from subjects who are clinically allergic and sensitive to the substance under consideration

4. Preparation of specific reagents that are necessary for the specific techniques (sera from immunized animals, monoclonal antibodies . . .)
5. An appeal to manufacturing companies or public institutions for production of batches of the future reference material
6. Analysis of several proposed batches and selection of an ad hoc committee for the product that will be the reference extract
7. Organization of a multicenter study for validation, using all available methods of control of allergenic extracts
8. Adoption by the members of the ad hoc committee and then by the members of the Allergen Subcommittee of IUIS of the preparation and unitage (IU: international units)
9. Conduct a program of stability studies
10. Definitive adoption as an IUIS standard, a WHO standard, or a reference preparation
11. Storage of batches on behalf of IUIS or WHO
12. Distribution of laboratories and institutions wishing to define their reference or control their commercial products

Several allergens have been studied and reference preparations are available for some of them. To complete the system of standardization, the subcommittee has started the preparation of a manual of analytical procedures specifying the protocols and reagents that should be used, inspired by the techniques proposed by the Bureau of Biologics in the United States, the National Institute for Biological Standardization and Control in the United Kingdom and the Nordic countries guidelines for allergen standardization. These guidelines have thus incredibly improved the quality and standardization of the techniques of control and of the allergens used in clinical practice because the manufacturers applied their improved knowledge not only for preparing a "good" standard extract that might be accepted as an international standard but also in the preparation of routine extracts.

Each vial distributed by WHO as a standard (and possibly by other agencies because some extracts may not be accepted by WHO as an ISP) is accompanied by a leaflet defining the major and sometimes the minor allergens, together with reagents required and methods that are appropriate for the measurements (61). For some allergens there are still unsolved problems. The Fel d 1 and albumin content of the cat standard allergen is still a matter of discussion. For the *D. pteronyssinus* ISP the problem is even more complicated because it is made from a spent culture, including metabolic and somatic antigens (62), whereas some regulatory agencies specify that extracts should be made from "pure" mites. This is the reason for the preparation of a *D. pteronyssinus* U.S. national standard different from the ISP.

There are five standards that are accepted as being ISP (international standard preparations) of WHO: *D. pteronyssinus* (57,58), short ragweed (44), timothy grass (42), birch pollen, and dog hair and dander extracts (43). One extract is accepted as being IRP (international reference preparation): Bermuda grass.

The Allergen Standardization Subcommittee of IUIS, in general recommendations, has emphasized that these international standards should be used as calibrators (i.e., standards for measurement of relative potency) and are not recommended for use as prototypes (i.e., materials to which an extract is to be matched in all respects). The ampules of standards are available only as reference materials to calibrate national or internal laboratory standards, but are not to be used in day-to-day work.

B. National Reference Extracts

National reference extracts have been prepared in the United States by the CEBR (former Bureau of Biologics), in the United Kingdom by the National Institute for Biological Standardization and Control, and in Denmark for several allergens, including pollens, mites, molds, foods, and venoms. The preparation and control of these extracts usually meet the criteria of the international reference preparations and the short ragweed ISP is in fact the U.S. national reference extract.

C. Clinical Importance of Standardized Extracts with Common Unitage

Standardized allergens of reproducible potency are not prepared for use in laboratories and research institutes, but represent a major improvement in allergy clinical practice. Standardized extracts from different manufacturers are less variable in potency, whereas they are not interchangeable. The batch-to-batch variability of standardized extracts from the same company is now acceptable, and this leads to an increased safety of immunotherapy when vials are changed. However, standardized extracts are more expensive and more potent than older extracts. Therefore, they are more difficult to use for nonspecialists.

Hymenoptera venoms were the first standardized and lyophilized extracts. Owing to their remarkable activity, specific immunotherapy with venoms is highly effective. The importance of venoms was emphasized by Yunginger (63), estimating that the availability of standardized Hymenoptera venoms represented one of the major improvements of allergy in the 1970s.

As stated by Norman (64), former chairman of the Subcommittee on Allergen Standardization of IUIS, standardization of allergenic extracts led to labeling them in IU so that physicians and investigators will be able to communicate more easily about the sensitivity of their patients as well as about specific immunotherapy protocols. It was observed that extracts labeled in biological units gave a similar mean wheal size whatever allergen species used when tested by skin tests. Several protocols to study standardized extracts have been proposed (65).

Standardized extracts are essential to ensure safety (66) because it is important that the amount of allergen is accurately known and consistent from time-to-time. Low-dose immunotherapy is ineffective (67–69) and high doses of allergen vaccines induce a high and unacceptable rate of systemic reactions. Thus, optimal doses using vaccines labeled either in biological units (70,71) or in mass of major allergens (39) have been proposed. The *optimal dose* may be defined as the dose of allergen vaccine inducing a clinically relevant effect in most patients, without causing unacceptable side effects (72,73). The optimal dose should be target for maintenance dose for all patients (70): a dose of 5–15 μg of major allergen is required for domestic mites (70,73,74), cat dander (75,76), ragweed pollen (77–79), or Hymenoptera venoms (80,81). Systemic side effects in some patients will require adjustment of this goal.

V. Allergen Nomenclature

To bring some order into the rather chaotic situation created by the use of multiple systems of identification of allergens that have been progressively isolated and described in the main allergenic extracts by different investigators, a common and unique nomenclature has been proposed (82) and revised (38).

1. The source of the allergen is clearly defined, including its accepted taxonomic name and any further identification.
2. Highly purified allergens are designed by the first three letters of the genus (italicized); space; first letter of the species name also in italics; and a Roman numeral. For example, Lol p 1 refers to *Lolium perenne* allergen number one (perennial rye group I—rye 1). In the rare event that two species have identical designations, they are discriminated from another one by adding one or more letters to each species designation.
3. The allergens are usually numbered in the order they were isolated, or by general agreement of the IUIS Nomenclature Subcommittee. Some exceptions have been proposed to solve, for example, the problems of isoallergens, of chemically defined allergens, or of fungal allergens isolated in certain strains.

References

1. Biological products: allergenic extracts: implementation of efficacy review. Federal Register, Food and Drug Administration 1985; 21 CRF Parts 600, 610 and 680 [Docket 81N-0096].
2. Allergen products (*Producta allergenica*). European Pharmacopeia 1997; 1063–1068.
3. Noon L. Prophylactic inoculation against hay fever. Lancet 1911; 1:1572–1573.
4. Stull A, Cooke R, Tennant J. The allergen content of pollen extracts. Its determination and its deterioration. J Allergy 1933; 4:455–460.
5. Bousquet J, Michel F. Standardization of allergens. In: Spector S, ed. Provocation Testing in Clinical Practice. New York: Marcel Dekker, 1994: 15–50. (Kaliner M, ed. Clinical Allergy and Immunology.
6. Reed CE, Yunginger JW, Evans R. Quality assurance and standardization of allergy extracts in allergy practice. J Allergy Clin Immunol 1989; 84:4–8.
7. Chapman N. Allergen standardization. J Allergy Clin Immunol 1998.
8. Chua KY, Kehal PK, Thomas WR, Vaughan PR, Macreadie IG. High-frequency binding of IgE to the Der p allergen expressed in yeast. J Allergy Clin Immunol 1992; 89:95–102.

9. Chua KY, Dilworth RJ, Thomas WR. Expression of *Dermatophagoides pteronyssinus* allergen, Der p 2, in *Escherichia coli* and the binding studies with human IgE. Int Arch Allergy Appl Immunol 1990; 91:124–129.
10. Morgenstern JP, Griffith IJ, Brauer AW, et al. Amino acid sequence of Fel d 1, the major allergen of the domestic cat: protein sequence analysis and cDNA cloning. Proc Natl Acad Sci USA 1991; 88:9690–9694.
11. Rafnar T, Griffith IJ, Kuo MC, Bond JF, Rogers BL, Klapper DG. Cloning of Amb a 1 (antigen E), the major allergen family of short ragweed pollen. J Biol Chem 1991; 266:1229–1236.
12. Silvanovich A, Astwood J, Zhang L, et al. Nucleotide sequence analysis of three cDNAs coding for Poa p 9 isoallergens of Kentucky bluegrass pollen. J Biol Chem 1991; 266:1204–1210.
13. Breiteneder H, Pettenburger K, Bito A, et al. The gene coding for the major birch pollen allergen Bet v 1, is highly homologous to a pea disease resistance response gene. EMBO J 1989; 8:1935–1938.
14. Breiteneder H, Hoffmann-Sommergruber K, O'Riordain G, et al. Molecular characterization of Api g 1, the major allergen of celery (*Apium graveolens*), and its immunological and structural relationships to a group of 17-kDa tree pollen allergens. Eur J Biochem 1995; 233:484–489.
15. Breiteneder H, Ferreira F, Hoffmann-Sommergruber K, et al. Four recombinant isoforms of Cor a 1, the major allergen of hazel pollen, show different IgE-binding properties. Eur J Biochem 1993; 212:355–362.
16. Valenta R, Duchene M, Vrtala S, et al. Recombinant allergens for immunoblot diagnosis of tree-pollen allergy. J Allergy Clin Immunol 1991; 88:889–894.
17. Moser M, Crameri R, Menz G, et al. Cloning and expression of recombinant *Aspergillus fumigatus* allergen I/a (rAsp f I/a) with IgE binding and type I skin test activity. J Immunol 1992; 149:454–460.
18. Moser M, Crameri R, Menz G, Suter M. Recombinant *Aspergillus fumigatus* allergen I/a (rAsp f I/a) in the diagnosis of *Aspergillus* related diseases. Agents Actions Suppl 1993; 43:131–137.
19. Yang M, Olsen E, Dolovich J, Sehon AH, Mohapatra SS. Immunologic characterization of a recombinant Kentucky bluegrass (*Poa pratensis*) allergenic peptide. J Allergy Clin Immunol 1991; 87:1096–1104.
20. Rafnar T, Ghosh B, Metzler WJ, et al. Expression and analysis of recombinant Amb a V and Amb t V allergens. Comparison with native proteins by immunological assays and NMR spectroscopy. J Biol Chem 1992; 267:21119–21123.
21. Bousquet J. Clinical use of recombinant allergens and epitopes. Arb Paul Ehrlich Inst Bundesamt Sera Impfstoffe Frankf A M 1994; 87:257–262.
22. Turkeltaub PC, Rastogi SC, Baer H, Anderson MC, Norman PS. A standardized quantitative skin-test assay of allergen potency and stability: studies on the allergen dose–response curve and effect of wheal, erythema, and patient selection on assay results. J Allergy Clin Immunol 1982; 70:343–352.
23. Turkeltaub PC. Biological standardization of allergenic extracts. Allergol Immunopathol Madr 1989; 17:53–65.
24. Aas K, Backman A, Belin L, Weeke B. Standardization of allergen extracts with appropriate methods. The combined use of skin prick testing and radioallergosorbent tests. Allergy 1978; 33:130–137.
25. Belin L. Biologic standardization—the HEP unit. Arb Paul Ehrlich Inst Georg Speyer Haus Ferdinand Blum Inst Frankf A M 1987; 80:145–153.
26. Nordic Council on Medicines. Registration of Allergen Preparations, 2nd ed. Uppsala: Nordiska Läkemedelsnämnden. NLN Publication 23, 1989.
27. Bousquet J, Guerin B, Michel FB. Units of allergen extracts. Arb Paul Ehrlich Inst Bundesamt Sera Impfstoffe Frankf A M 1992; 85:105–116.
28. Stull A, Cooke R, Chobot R. The allergenically active substance in pollen. A chemical and biologic study of *Phleum pratense* (timothy) pollen. J Allergy 1931; 3:341–357.

29. Gleich G, Larson J, Jones R, Baer H. Measurement of the potency of allergy extracts by their inhibitory capacities in the radioallergosorbent test. J Allergy Clin Allergol 1974; 53:158–169.
30. Scheiner O, Kraft D. Basic and practical aspects of recombinant aspects. Allergy 1995; 50:384–391.
31. Dreborg S, Einarsson R. The major allergen content of allergenic preparations reflect their biological activity. Allergy 1992; 47:418–423.
32. Platts-Mills TA, Chapman MD. Allergen standardization. J Allergy Clin Immunol 1991; 87:621–625.
33. Liu DT. Regulation of allergenic products in the USA; CBER initiatives. Arb Paul Ehrlich Inst Bundesamt Sera Impfstoffe Frankf A M 1994; 87:8–12.
34. Norman PS. WHO-IUIS International Standards: advantages of these extracts. Arb Paul Ehrlich Inst Bundesamt Sera Impfstoffe Frankf A M 1994; 87:59–64.
35. Chapman M. Monoclonal antibody immunoassays: quantitative methods for allergen standardization. Arb Paul Ehrlich Inst Bundesamt Sera Impfstoffe Frankf A M 1994; 87:120–124.
36. van-Ree R. Analytical aspects of standardization of allergenic extracts. Allergy 1997; 52:785–806.
37. Allergen nomenclature. WHO/IUS Allergen Nomenclature Subcommittee World Health Organization, Geneva, Switzerland. Clin Exp Allergy 1995; 25:27–37.
38. King TP, Hoffman D, Lowenstein H, Marsh DG, Platts-Mills TA, Thomas W. Allergen nomenclature. Allergy 1995; 50:765–774.
39. Carreira J, Lombardero M, Ventas P. New developments in in vitro methods. Quantification of clinically relevant allergens in mass units. Arb Paul Ehrlich Inst Bundesamt Sera Impfstoffe Frankf A M 1994; 87:155–164.
40. Afferni C, Pini C, Tinghino R, et al. Use of monoclonal antibodies in the standardization of *Parietaria judaica* allergenic extracts. Biologicals 1995; 23:239–247.
41. Lowenstein H. Report on behalf of the International Union of Immunological Societies (IUIS) Allergen Standardization Subcommittee. Arb Paul Ehrlich Inst Georg Speyer Haus Ferdinand Blum Inst Frankf A M 1983; 78:41–48.
42. Gjesing B, Jager L, Marsh DG, Lowenstein H. The international collaborative study establishing the first international standard for timothy (*Phleum pratense*) grass pollen allergenic extract. J Allergy Clin Immunol 1985; 75:258–267.
43. Larsen JN, Ford A, Gjesing B, et al. The collaborative study of the international standard of dog, *Canis domesticus*, hair/dander extract. J Allergy Clin Immunol 1988; 82:318–330.
44. Helm RM, Gauerke MB, Baer H, et al. Production and testing of an international reference standard of short ragweed pollen extract. J Allergy Clin Immunol 1984; 73:790–800.
45. Helm RM, Squillace DL, Aukrust L, et al. Production of an international reference standard *Alternaria* extract. I. Testing of candidate extracts. Int Arch Allergy Appl Immunol 1987; 82:178–189.
46. Mohapatra SS. Recombinant allergens and allergen standardization. J Allergy Clin Immunol 1992; 89:921–922.
47. Kraft D, Sehon A. Molecular Biology and Immunology or Allergens. Boca Raton, Fl: CRC Press, 1992.
48. Haberman E. Bee and wasp venoms. Science 1972; 177:314–316.
49. Topping MD, Brostoff J, Brighton WD, Danks J, Minnis M. Allergenic activity of fractions of cocksfoot (*Dacylis glomerata*) pollen. Clin Allergy 1978; 8:33–38.
50. Løwenstein H. Quantitative immunoelectrophoretic methods: a tool for the analysis and isolation of allergens. Prog Allergy 1978; 25:1–60.
51. Einarsson R. Biochemical and immunochemical methods for purification, characterization and standardization of allergen extracts. Allergy 1985; 4:35–49.
52. Peltre G, Lapeyre J, David B. Heterogeneity of grass pollen allergens (*Dactylis glomerata*) recognized by IgE antibodies in human patients sera by a new nitrocellulose immunoprint technique. Immunol Lett 1982; 5:127–131.

53. Bengtsson A, Rolfsen W, Einarsson R. Characterization of allergens and patient sera by a nitrocellulose immunoprint technique. Int Arch Allergy Appl Immunol 1985; 78:139–144.
54. Weeke B. Standardization of allergen preparations. Allergy 1980; 35:172–176.
55. Maasch HJ, Marsh DG. Standardized extracts modified allergens—allergoids. Clin Rev Allergy 1987; 5:89–106.
56. Norman PS. International units. Arb Paul Ehrlich Inst Bundesamt Sera Impfstoffe Frankf A M 1988; 82:45–49.
57. Ford A, Seagroatt V, Platts-Mills TA, Lowenstein H. A collaborative study on the first international standard of *Dermatophagoides pteronyssinus* (house dust mite) extract. J Allergy Clin Immunol 1985; 75:676–686.
58. Ford AW, Rawle FC, Lind P, Spieksma FT, Lowenstein H, Platts-Mills TA. Standardization of *Dermatophagoides pteronyssinus*: assessment of potency and allergen content in ten coded extracts. Int Arch Allergy Appl Immunol 1987; 76:58–67.
59. Carreira J, Rubio M, Herrero T, et al. Collaborative clinical assay of the biological potency of allergen skin-test extracts. Clin Allergy 1984; 14:503–507.
60. Baer H. Potency units for allergenic extracts in the USA. Arb Paul Ehrlich Inst Georg Speyer Haus Ferdinand Blum Inst Frankf A M 1987; 80:167–168.
61. Seagroatt V, Ford A. RAST inhibition: a collaborative study on its suitability and reproducibility for the assay of cocksfoot pollen extracts. Clin Allergy 1986; 16:213–220.
62. Tovey ER, Baldo BA. Comparison by electroblotting of IgE-binding components in extracts of house dust mite bodies and spent mite culture. J Allergy Clin Immunol 1987; 79:93–102.
63. Yunginger JW. Standardization of allergenic extracts. Ann Allergy 1991; 66:107–111.
64. Norman PS. Why standardized extracts? [editorial]. J Allergy Clin Immunol 1986; 77:405–406.
65. Bousquet J, Guerin B, Michel FB. Design of protocols to evaluate the safety and efficacy of allergenic extracts. Arb Paul Ehrlich Inst Georg Speyer Haus Ferdinand Blum Inst Frankf A M 1987; 80:213–228.
66. Lockey BF, Benedict LM, Turkeltaub PC, Bukantz SC. Fatalities from immunotherapy (IT) and skin testing (ST). J Allergy Clin Immunol 1987; 79:660–677.
67. Van-Metre Te J, Adkinson N Jr, Lichtenstein LM, et al. A controlled study of the effectiveness of the Rinkel method of immunotherapy for ragweed pollen hay fever. J Allergy Clin Immunol 1980; 65:288–297.
68. Hirsch SR, Kalbfleisch JH, Golbert TM, et al. Rinkel injection therapy: a multicenter controlled study. J Allergy Clin Immunol 1981; 68:133–155.
69. Hirsch SR, Kalbfleisch JH, Cohen SH. Comparison of Rinkel injection therapy with standard immunotherapy. J Allergy Clin Immunol 1982; 70:183–190.
70. Bousquet J, Des-Roches A, Paradis L, Dhivert H, Michel FB. Specific immunotherapy in house dust mite allergy. Clin Rev Allergy Immunol 1995; 13:151–159.
71. Turkeltaub PC, Campbell G, Mosimann JE. Comparative safety and efficacy of short ragweed extracts differing in potency and composition in the treatment of fall hay fever. Use of allergenically bioequivalent doses by parallel line bioassay to evaluate comparative safety and efficacy. Allergy 1990; 45:528–546.
72. Creticos PS, Van-Metre TE, Mardinay MR, Rosenberg GL, Norman PS, Adkinson N Jr. Dose response of IgE and IgG antibodies during ragweed immunotherapy. J Allergy Clin Immunol 1984; 73:94–104.
73. Haugaard L, Dahl R, Jacobsen L. A controlled dose–response study of immunotherapy with standardized, partially purified extract of house dust mite: clinical efficacy and side effects. J Allergy Clin Immunol 1993; 91:709–722.
74. Olaguibel J, Tabar A, Garcia-Figueroa B, Cortes C. Immunotherapy with standardized extract of *Dermatophagoides pteronyssinus* in bronchial asthma: a dose–titration study. Allergy 1997; 52:168–179.
75. Van-Metre Te J, Marsh DG, Adkinson N Jr, et al. Immunotherapy for cat asthma. J Allergy Clin Immunol 1988; 82:1055–1068.

76. Alvarez-Cuesta E, Cuesta-Herranz J, Puyana-Ruiz J, Cuesta-Herranz C, Blanco-Quiros A. Monoclonal antibody-standardized cat extract immunotherapy: risk–benefit effects from a double-blind placebo study. J Allergy Clin Immunol 1994; 93:556–566.
77. Creticos PS, Marsh DG, Proud D, et al. Responses to ragweed-pollen nasal challenge before and after immunotherapy. J Allergy Clin Immunol 1989; 84:197–205.
78. Van-Metre Te J, Adkinson N Jr, Amodio FJ, et al. A comparison of immunotherapy schedules for injection treatment of ragweed pollen hay fever. J Allergy Clin Immunol 1982; 69:181–193.
79. Creticos PS, Reed CE, Norman PS, et al. Ragweed immunotherapy in adult asthma. N Engl J Med 1996; 334:501–506.
80. Hunt KJ, Valentine MD, Sobotka AK, Benton AW, Amodio FJ, Lichtenstein LM. A controlled trial of immunotherapy in insect hypersensitivity. N Engl J Med 1978; 299:157–161.
81. Muller U, Mosbech H. Position paper: Immunotherapy with Hymenoptera venoms. Allergy 1993; 48 (suppl 14):37–46.
82. Marsh DG, Goodfriend L, King TP, Lowenstein H, Platts-Mills TA. Allergen nomenclature. Bull WHO 1986; 64:767–774.

10

Allergen-Specific Immunotherapy
Past and Present

PHILIP S. NORMAN

Johns Hopkins University School of Medicine
Baltimore, Maryland

I. Introduction

Although originally developed 75 years ago as a treatment for summer hay fever and asthma, immunotherapy for allergies has become widely applied to a variety of conditions and provides the principal basis for a major subspecialty of medicine and pediatrics. As originally studied by Noon in 1911, injections of boiled water extract of grass pollens were given in gradually increasing doses weekly over several months, with the goal of inducing immunity to a supposed toxin contained in the pollen. Noon demonstrated that the strength of the extract that was required to elicit an immediate conjunctival reaction in the eye gradually increased during the injection series, and his patients told him their symptoms were less severe during the natural season of grass pollination (1). The work was continued by Freeman, who formed the opinion that asthmatic symptoms during the grass pollination season were helped more completely than nasal symptoms (2).

By 1918, Cooke considered the mechanism of action to be "desensitization and not a true immunity," which made it necessary to continue injections at weekly intervals for maintenance (3). In 1922, Cooke proposed revising the term as applied to treating allergic patients to "hyposensitization" because protection was less than complete (4). "Immunotherapy" has been considered a better term, because it was suggested by Lichtenstein and Norman that a number of potentially protective immunological responses were elicited by injections of an allergenic extract.

II. Clinical Changes

The thorough study of a small number of respiratory (inhaled) allergens that cause hay fever and asthma symptoms provides a persuasive demonstration of the efficacy of immunotherapy when applied appropriately. Although grass hay fever was studied first, ragweed hay fever in the United States has been the subject of the most thoroughgoing exploration of the several aspects of optimum usage of immunotherapy. These studies have been aided considerably by the identification and isolation of the principal allergenic protein of ragweed, referred to as Amb a 1. Controlled clinical studies of immunotherapy in ragweed hay fever demonstrate that (1) clinical results depend on an adequate dose, with small doses having a poor rate of success or being totally ineffective (5,6); (2) relapse may occur once booster injections are discontinued (7); and (3) results are specific, being effective only for the allergen(s) being administered, and ineffective for excluded allergens (8,9). These results depended on performing studies that compare a treatment regimen with either placebo treatment or another regimen as controls. Groups of patients large enough to obtain statistically valid comparisons of the results from symptom diaries collected during natural exposure were required.

A. Challenge Techniques

Both bronchial and nasal challenges have been used in the study of immunotherapy and to demonstrate efficacy. Bronchial challenges are carried out by inhalations of aerosols of allergen solutions, given in graded increases in concentration. Each increase in concentration is followed by physiological measurements of airway function. When a measure such as 1-sec forced expiratory volume (FEV_1) declines by 20%, the challenge is stopped. The initial decline in pulmonary function usually recovers rapidly, but often is followed by a secondary and more long-lasting decline or *late-phase* response several hours later. A nasal challenge method, developed by Naclerio et al., employs mucosal exposure to either whole pollen or pollen extracts, followed by measurement of mediators appearing in nasal secretions (10).

Immediate Allergic Responses

To determine whether specific immunotherapy alters in vivo mediator release, Creticos et al. compared 27 untreated, highly sensitive ragweed allergic subjects with 12 similarly sensitive patients receiving long-term immunotherapy with ragweed extract (median dose = 6 μg Amb a 1). The two groups were equally sensitive by skin tests and basophil histamine release. Patients receiving immunotherapy required larger-threshold pollen doses not only to provoke sneezing, but also to elicit release of the mediators tosyl anginine methly esterase, (TAME), prostaglandin D_2 (PgD_2), and histamine. At any given dose, the treated groups released less mediator. In most treated patients, the thresholds for both mediator release and sneezing required a pollen challenge dose higher than that typically encountered in natural exposure. Although the pollen challenges are in excess of natural exposure, they do demonstrate that reactivity has not been completely ablated (11). In a prospective study, patients starting immunotherapy were challenged serially over many months and showed increasing thresholds for mediator release as the therapeutic dose was raised. At a dose equivalent to 0.6 μg Amb a 1, there was little change in the response, but at 12.4 μg, there was a significant reduction in mediator release. A further increase of the treatment dose to 24.8 μg produced little additional change (12).

Several studies of immunotherapy of asthma show that the threshold for the immediate airways constriction response to aerosol challenge with extracts is increased after immunotherapy with extracts of house dust (13), cat pelt (14), and ragweed pollen (15). Mediator measurement in bronchial secretions has yet to be done.

Late-Phase Allergic Responses

In humans several studies indicate that immunotherapy changes the late-phase reaction to bronchial challenge more than it changes the immediate reaction. By using *Alternaria*, a common mold allergen, Metzger challenged sensitive asthmatic patients before and after high-dose immunotherapy (> 100,000 PNU). After immunotherapy, the acute response was not changed, but the late reaction was decreased by about 70% (16). In a controlled trial of immunotherapy with extract of the house dust mite, *Dermatophagoides pteronyssinus*, Warner found that the immediate response to antigen challenge was unchanged, whereas the late response was lost in half of the patients. Furthermore, the children who lost the delayed response had the best clinical outcome (17).

In addition, patients who have received immunotherapy for allergic rhinitis have much smaller late skin responses to antigen than untreated control patients, even though the early skin responses are the same (18). This has been confirmed in patients whose late-phase skin responses were studied before and after immunotherapy for ragweed (19). In mountain cedar pollinosis, suppression of the late cutaneous response correlated significantly with dose of extract, post-seasonal levels of IgG1 and IgG2 antibodies, and improvement in symptoms (20). With ragweed pollinosis, although not everyone has a late-phase mediator response to nasal challenge, as it is usually carried out, in those individuals who did have a late response, it was suppressed after immunotherapy (19). In another study, the numbers of eosinophils found in secretions 24 h after challenge no longer rose in two groups of ragweed extract-treated patients (21).

Priming and Nonspecific Hyperreactivity

Priming is a phenomenon originally described in hay fever patients challenged when no natural allergic exposures were occurring. Connell exposed ragweed-sensitive patients on successive days to pollen in sufficient amounts to invoke symptoms and found that comparable reactions could be induced with less pollen each day. The priming effect was nonspecific and local: repeated exposures to one pollen induced overreactivity to another immunologically unrelated pollen; if only one nostril was exposed, the unexposed nostril did not become primed. Biopsies of the mucosa after such repeated exposures showed eosinophil infiltration and basement membrane changes (22,23). Naclerio et al. found that a single challenge with pollen extract large enough to elicit a late-phase reaction with release of mediators, also enhanced immediate reactivity to a second low-level challenge 11 hr after the original challenge. Late-phase responses in this system are also accompanied by increased eosinophils and neutrophils in secretions (24).

Hyperreactivity of the bronchi in asthmatic patients appears to be associated with eosinophilic inflammation. In seasonal allergic asthmatics, hyperreactivity is enhanced during exposure and tends to improve after exposure is over (25). Isolation of allergic asthmatic children from their principal allergen results in improvement of hyperreactivity (26). Two studies suggest that immunotherapy might be useful not only to ablate allergic reactions, but to diminish nonspecific hyperreactivity. In cat-sensitive patients who had received immunotherapy with cat dander extract for 3 years, bronchial reactivity to inhaled histamine was reduced (27). Untreated ragweed hay fever patients show increased responses to simple saline challenges to the nasal mucosa during the season. Patients given immunotherapy no longer have this hyperreactivity (28).

III. Immunological Changes

Immunologically, a variety of changes have been demonstrated that may partly be responsible for the relief of allergic symptoms. Among these changes are (1) a rise in serum IgG "blocking" antibodies (29–31); (2) a suppression in the usual seasonal rise in IgE antibodies that follows environmental exposure and a slow decline during several years in the level of specific IgE antibodies, although complete disappearance is rare (32,33); (3) increase in blocking IgA and IgG antibodies in secretions (34,35); (4) reduced basophil reactivity and sensitivity to allergens, as determined by in vitro leukocyte histamine release studies (31,36); (5) changes in lymphocyte responses attributable to T cells (described later).

Correlations between antibody change and clinical results have been difficult to establish. The serum IgG response has at times shown a relationship to clinical improvement (6,37). In general, those patients who have higher titers of specific antiragweed IgG have more favorable clinical responses, and those who have low levels of IgG antibody have less favorable clinical responses, but there are clear exceptions to such a general rule. Studies of IgG subclass show that the initial response is usually a combination of IgG1 and IgG4, but with continued immunotherapy, after 1 year, circulating antibodies are almost entirely IgG4 (38,39). The

IgG4 antibodies are functionally monovalent and do not make precipitates with antigen or fix complement (40); hence, they appear to be the appropriate class of antibodies for blocking. Nevertheless, no clear relationship between the development of IgG4 antibodies and the success or failure of immunotherapy has emerged (40).

Antibodies in secretions may be ideally placed to interfere with mucosal reactions between allergens and mediator-containing cells, but are present in vanishingly small amounts, and so far they have shown little correlation with clinical improvement (34,35).

Immunotherapy by the usual regimen raises serum IgE before IgG begins to rise. This may be associated with the higher incidence of untoward reactions while the dose of allergen is being raised. Eventually, IgE declines to levels below baseline after a year or more (41). With allergens such as ragweed that involve seasonal exposure, the usual postseasonal rise in IgE levels no longer occurs (32,42). At best, however, the specific IgE levels remain in the range found in sensitive patients; consequently, it is difficult to attribute improvement to these modest changes.

Basophil reactivity to in vitro antigen challenge may decline dramatically in some patients and become almost nil. This change has no relationship to serum IgE and may represent a nonspecific change in cell reactivity (36). Although this change may have significance for the patients who develop it, it is not induced in many patients and cannot account for the effects of immunotherapy in most persons.

A variety of indirect measures of lymphocyte activity in the presence of allergen are reduced in patients undergoing immunotherapy, in comparison with untreated controls (43,44). These activities are now attributed to T cells. Proliferation of short-term cultures of peripheral blood mononuclear cells (PBMC) in the presence of allergen (driven by T cells) is reduced in treated patients. Cytokine production in these cultures is reduced. This effect is more readily observed in T-cell lines grown in the presence of allergen. If these lines are rested and then recultured with allergen and suitable antigen-presenting cells (APC), the proliferation is largely abrogated in lines from patients undergoing immunotherapy. Production of interleukin (IL)-4 and IL-5 is much less (45). Another study in patients receiving immunotherapy, the PBMC cultured in the presence of allergen showed decreased production of IL-4 protein after treatment, but no change in production of IL-2 and interferon (IFN)-γ, in comparison with untreated allergic control patients (46).

In patients treated successfully for grass pollen hay fever with a commercial grass pollen extract, out of season skin challenges were performed, and biopsies of the late-phase reaction were taken 24 hr after challenge. Placebo-treated control patients had an increase in $CD4^+$ helper T cells and activated eosinophils, as identified by a monoclonal antibody (EG2) that recognizes eosinophil cationic protein (ECP). In the treated patients, the total number of inflammatory cells ($CD45^+$) remained unchanged, but the number of $CD4^+$ (helper) cells was reduced. Eosinophils were also reduced, but not enough to meet a test of significance. Cells labeled for the CD45 activation marker were increased in the treated group, but not the placebo group. This is a general activation marker that may be found on macrophages and other cell types, as well as on lymphocytes. Unlike the findings in PBMC after immunotherapy, in the biopsy material there was no change in expression of IL-4 and IL-5. Indeed, although there was little expression of IL-2 and IFN-γ before treatment, after treatment a significant number of patients (8/16 and 616, respectively) expressed these inflammation-promoting cytokines (47). In a further study of these patients, biopsies of the nasal mucosa after allergen challenge have been taken. Inhibition of late nasal responses was associated with a decrease in allergen-induced increases in $CD4^+$ cells and total and "activated" eosinophils, a nonsignificant decrease in IL-4 and IL-5 $mRNA^+$ cells, and an increase in cells positive for IFN-γ mRNA (48).

Patients treated for mountain cedar pollinosis were studied by collecting cells and fluid from skin blisters stimulated by allergen to produce a late-phase reaction. There was a significant decrease in eosinophil viability in blister fluid from the first to the ninth hour after challenge. There was indirect evidence of a reduced appearance of IL-3, IL-5, and granulocyte–macrophage colony-stimulating factor (GM-CSF) in the blister fluid (49).

The data from examination of cells from the peripheral blood, on one hand, and from tissues after an induced allergic reaction thus seem to give quite different answers for cytokine production. Peripheral blood cells appear to show a down-regulation of type-2 T helper cell (Th2) proinflammatory cytokines that also encourage IgE production. Examination of tissues tends, on the other hand, to show an upregulation of the inflammation-promoting cytokines that encourage IgG production. These two processes are not mutually exclusive; but which one is more important will require more investigation.

IV. Studies with Specific Allergens

A. Plants

Grasses

Although the considerations discussed in the foregoing should lead to studies to test hypotheses about mechanism of action under controlled conditions, practical evaluations of immunotherapy in hay fever and asthma caused by a variety of allergens indicate some of the allergens for which the method should be considered. Frankland and Augustin carried out a study of 200 patients who had grass pollen hay fever, asthma, or both. Seventy-nine percent of the patients with hay fever had either good or excellent results following pollen treatment, whereas only 33% reported good results after inactive materials. Results with asthma were more striking: 94% of those receiving the active materials had good or excellent results, whereas only 30% of those who received inactive treatments reported good or excellent results (50). Subsequent studies of immunological response in grass pollen immunotherapy have confirmed that IgG-blocking antibodies increase, and IgE, as measured by RAST, decreases (51). The blocking antibodies are principally of the IgG4 subclass (52).

Ragweed

In the United States shortly after the foregoing studies, three controlled studies in hay fever and asthma caused by ragweed pollen showed convincing symptomatic improvement in both children and adults (8,53,54). These and other studies on mechanisms were described earlier. A multicenter study, specifically directed toward asthma exacerbation during the pollen season, showed that the seasonal decrease in peak expiratory flow rate (PEFR) occurred regularly in a ragweed-sensitive asthmatic population and was largely ablated after immunotherapy, when compared with placebo-treated patients. After one preseasonal course, medication was decreased in the treated group versus the placebo group. In the face of the medication use, reported symptoms were not changed by immunotherapy (55).

Mountain Cedar

Seasonal symptoms caused by the pollen of mountain cedar trees in the North American Southwest are also reduced by immunotherapy, as shown in a controlled study that also found a reduction in IgE titers (56).

Birch

In birch tree pollinosis, several studies show significant improvement in symptoms during the birch pollen season in Scandinavia (57,58). Immunotherapy leads to an increase in antigen-binding activity in serum (presumably caused by IgG), an initial increase in IgE, and an eventual decline (59).

B. House Dust

In house dust sensitivity, results are mixed. Some of the conflicting results may arise out of differences in dosage. For instance, in house dust asthma, a cooperative study of treatment with house dust extract, in rather modest doses, revealed no relief after 15 weekly injections (60), whereas a study by Åas of house dust-sensitive children, treated with house dust extract for 2 1/2 to 3 years in large doses, showed not only symptomatic improvement in comparison with controls, but also a reduction in reactivity on bronchial challenge (13). This difference may be explained by the observations of May et al. that unusually large amounts of house dust extract, in terms of protein nitrogen, are necessary to obtain a blocking antibody response (61). It appears likely that the large doses employed over a long period by Åas were necessary to demonstrate efficacy. As individual sources of allergens in house dust have become identified, emphasis has shifted from the use of crude house dust extracts to identification of and treatment with the specific allergens from indoor environments to which a patient is sensitive. The principal indoor sources of sensitization are house dust mites, animal pets, cockroaches, rodents, and molds.

House Dust Mite

House dust mite extracts appear to be a more effective material in areas where the mites are the major allergen in dust. Several double-blind trials demonstrate efficacy in controlling symptoms, a decrease in responsiveness to allergen on nasal challenge, a rise in specific IgG antibodies, and a decline in IgE antibodies (62–64).

Animal Danders

A study of immunization with cat pelt extract showed that the response to bronchial challenge by an aerosol of extract was reduced (14). Subsequent study of sera taken from treated patients showed rises in IgG to cat allergen (Fel d 1) and cat albumin (65) challenge. A double-blind study employing a purified fraction of cat pelt extract again demonstrated significant reductions in bronchial sensitivity along with increases in IgG to Fel d 1. These changes were accompanied by significant delays in ocular and pulmonary symptoms on exposure to living cats, although nonspecific reactivity to methacholine was unchanged (66). Dog allergy has been less completely studied, but a study in children with allergy to cat or dog or both showed significant improvement in asthma symptoms when the patients were treated with the hair and dander extracts that were positive by skin test (67). Another study found favorable immunological and challenge responses to a dog hair and dander extract in children with dog allergy. There was not much change in the course of asthma symptoms when this one extract was employed (68).

Molds

Therapeutic study with mold extracts is more recent. Two preliminary reports have appeared concerning molds that grow seasonally on decaying vegetation: one with *Cladosporium herbarum* (*Hormodendrum*) extract in children reports a decrease in bronchial and ocular sensitivity, but little change in reported symptoms presumably because the patients were sensitive to other allergens (69). A study in adult asthmatics with *Cladosporium* sensitivity showed significant improvement in symptoms related to seasonal exposure (70). Asthmatic patients with *Alternaria* sensitivity showed decreased severity of the late-phase response to challenge, but no change in the early-phase response, after treatment with *Alternaria* extract (16). Study of extracts of *Alternaria* and *Cladosporium* indicates that most, if not all, commercial extracts of these two species are seriously deficient in the proteins that induce the allergic response in patients (71–73). Therefore, immunotherapy with these extracts is difficult to evaluate unless the extract chosen for study has sufficient biological activity. The therapeutic studies cited appear to have been performed with adequate extracts. Nevertheless, the problem with mold extracts illustrates that the analogy created by study of a few well-defined allergenic extracts does not automatically extend to every extract of every allergen.

C. Others

The use of all other pollen, mold, dander, and inhalant materials for immunotherapy depends on uncontrolled clinical observation, without the support of any evidence of immunological response. To what extent the well-established information available from the study of such a small list of allergens can be extrapolated to hundreds of other allergens is a matter for judgment by the individual physician.

V. Problem Areas

A. Incomplete Relief

Despite the considerable number of facts developed about clinical responses to immunotherapy with extracts of airborne allergens and the immunological changes invoked, significant problems remain that limit widespread application to the millions of patients with respiratory allergy. For instance, patients in controlled studies of treatment with a single allergen usually report significant residual symptoms, despite doses of extract that appear to be the optimum required to provide maximum immunological and clinical response. Although it might be thought that a practical limit to the efficacy of immunotherapy has been reached, other explanations should be considered. Even patients selected who have simple seasonal hay fever, rarely have sensitivity to a single allergen (74). No study has yet examined whether treatment with all significant allergens will produce greater relief of symptoms than treatment with the dominant allergen.

B. Extract Adequacy

Another possible explanation for less than complete relief is that extracts may not contain all significant individual allergenic proteins in sufficient quantity. For ragweed pollen, for example, patients with continuing symptoms, despite adequate responses to Amb a 1 could still be reacting symptomatically to other allergens in ragweed. This point is further emphasized by the finding that Amb a 1 is slowly released from ragweed pollen suspended in water, whereas several basic allergens are rapidly released (75). On the other hand, increasing the pH to 8.0 or more leads to ten times more rapid release of Amb a 1. Because the pH of nasal secretions is normally low and rises during an attack of rhinitis, rapidly released basic allergens may initiate the attack, and Amb a 1 subsequently becomes important as the rhinitis develops. Platts-Mills et al. have examined immunological responses to the minor allergen of ragweed Amb a 3 in sensitive patients treated with standard unpurified extract of pollen. All patients with a pretreatment IgE sensitivity and IgG antibody to Ra3 had a rise in blocking antibody (75). Although this single study does not close the subject, preliminary results indicate that responses to at least one minor allergen are adequate. The other possibility that has been raised is that patients receiving crude extracts may become sensitized de novo to one or more components. The Platts-Mills study with Amb a 3 did not detect such an occurrence in patients not already sensitive to it (75), but the topic deserves more study.

C. Efficacy for Allergic Asthma

Despite continued use by specialists in allergy and immunology worldwide, immunotherapy for asthma is a perennial target for criticism by nonallergists who also care for asthma patients. Immunotherapy for hay fever, on the other hand, generates little controversy even though the immunological pathogenesis of hay fever is essentially identical. The reasons for this difference are not apparent from the evidence collected in the two diseases. Similar numbers of studies may be found; both find similar clinical improvement and the immunological changes are not different.

Placebo-controlled studies carried out over 40 years demonstrate both objective and subjective improvement of asthma in patients undertaking immunotherapy for specific allergies. Abramson et al. summarized these findings in metanalysis covering 20 studies that found improved odds for symptomatic improvement, decreased medication use, and improvement in pulmonary function (76). Not included in that analysis was a recently published multicenter ragweed immunotherapy study headed by Creticos. After starting treatment in the spring, the same three parameters improved during the fall season of ragweed pollination (55).

Any discussion of the use of immunotherapy should include a comparison of its risks and benefits with those of other methods of treatment. Unfortunately, neither prospective nor organized comparisons are available. Immunotherapy, however, continues to offer benefits to certain patients with asthma and can reduce the burden of repeated medications for control of their disease. Selection of patients is paramount. Patients with no apparent allergies are not candidates; nor are patients whose pulmonary function is continuously compromised. Rather, it is the patient with proved IgE-mediated allergies, who finds environmental controls unhelpful and drug treatment either burdensome or less than satisfactory. Such patients are often children or young adults with recent onset of disease. Indeed, a recent study confirmed previous observations that early immunotherapy of hay fever in children can prevent eventual onset of asthma (77).

VI. Untoward Reactions

There are three types of allergic reactions to pollen extracts administered subcutaneously. Early in treatment there is usually a wheal and erythema at the site of injection, which resembles a positive reaction to a skin test, appears in 10–30 min, and subsides in a few hours. A second type of local reaction appears as an itching, erythematous swelling of the subcutaneous tissues without wheal formation, beginning 2–4 h after the injection. These reactions commonly reach a maximum in 18–24 h, without necrosis, subside in 1 or 2 days, and represent the late-phase reaction discussed earlier. These local reactions are ordinarily a minor problem unless a too rapid progression in dosage leads to a large uncomfortable swelling at the injection site.

"Constitutional" reactions, on the other hand, although relatively uncommon and usually mild, are a potentially serious consequence of therapy, because they represent anaphylaxis and, if severe, require prompt management with epinephrine. Administration of corticosteroids for several days after a severe constitutional reaction will prevent a series of recurrences of hives and angioedematous swellings, but these drugs have no effect on the immediate anaphylactic response itself. Immunological correlates with the tendency to have either constitutional or local reactions have not been described except for one study in 1962, which indicated that patients who had one or more systemic reactions to ragweed had skin-sensitizing antibody (now known to be IgE) titers higher than those found in other groups of ragweed-sensitive patients. The reacting patients did not have lower blocking antibody titers than other patients similarly treated who went without such reactions (78).

A retrospective survey, by Lockey et al., of fatal misadventures from both skin tests and immunotherapy uncovered 46 deaths in the United States between 1945 and 1985, which averages little more than 1 per year. Considering that probably several million people receive immunotherapy, this is an extremely low rate. Examination of the circumstances of these deaths identified several risk factors: (1) mistakes in dosage (6 of 17 instances for which mistakes were commented on); (2) asthma (16 of 30 fatalities for which there were data); (3) patients symptomatic during a season of exposure; and (4) sensitivity greater than average by skin test or RAST (79). Attention to these factors could further lower the number of deaths associated with immunotherapy. The rate of systemic reactions depends not only on the dose of extract employed, but also on the program of escalation of dose. A survey in an actual practice found a rate of 1 systemic reaction per 1600 visits or 1 per 47 patients (80). On the other hand, a specific research study of dose and reactions in ragweed extract immunotherapy noted 13 systemic reactions (405 injections) in 7 of the 15 patients under treatment with a standard regimen, based on common practice (81).

Guidelines prepared by the American Academy of Allergy and Immunology recommend that patients who have received an immunotherapy injection be observed for at least 20 min for signs of a systemic reaction before being dismissed.

> Personnel who are expert in the following procedures should be immediately available: (1) adjustment of dose of allergenic extract for skin testing and immunotherapy in order to minimize reaction, (2) recognition and treatment of local reactions to allergenic extract, (3) recognition and treatment of systemic reactions to allergenic extracts, and (4) basic cardiopulmonary resuscitation.

> The following equipment and reagents should be available: (1) stethoscope and sphygmomanometer; (2) tourniquets, syringes, hypodermic needles, and large-bore (14-gauge) needles; (3) aqueous epinephrine HC1 1:1000; (4) equipment for administering oxygen; (5) equipment for administering fluids; (6) oral airway; (7) diphenhydramine or similar antihistamine for injection: (8) aminophylline for intravenous administration; (9) corticosteroids for intravenous injection; and (10) vasopressor (82).

Side effects of immunotherapy beyond the well-known local and constitutional allergic reactions are exceedingly rare. Two groups have investigated the occurrence of circulating immune complexes in patients undergoing immunotherapy with various mixes of allergens. The frequency of circulating complexes, as detected by several sensitive methods, was no greater in allergic patients undergoing immunotherapy than in untreated allergic individuals (83,84).

VII. Depot Methods

Because of the large number of injections required to build up the immunotherapeutic dose slowly enough to minimize allergic reactions, methods have been sought to obtain the slow release of allergenic extract from a depot injection. The only method that has met any acceptance in the United States is precipitation of pollen extracts with alum. In a controlled study, alum-precipitated ragweed extract gave therapeutic results equal to those obtained with aqueous extract. Although immunological responses with the two types of extract were similar, about half the number of injections of alum precipitate were required for an adequate dose. Fewer systemic reactions, but larger local reactions, were noted with alum precipitate (85).

VIII. Cross-Linked or Polymerized Antigens

Marsh et al. introduced formaldehyde treatment under mild conditions to prepare "allergoids" from grass and ragweed pollen extracts. Allergoid proteins have an average molecular weight increase from 30,000 daltons before modification to 1 million after modification owing to extensive cross-linking. Allergenicity (ability to elicit allergic reactions in skin tests or histamine release) is reduced several hundredfold (86), but immunogenicity is reduced only about twofold, as indicated by IgG antibody responses in animals, normal humans (87), and allergic humans. Allergoids of several pollen extracts can be administered in courses abbreviated to about ten visits with satisfactory clinical and immunological results. IgG levels rise more rapidly to higher levels than with aqueous extract. Relief of symptoms is similar after an initial series, but patients receiving perennial boosters of allergoid have fewer severe seasonal symptoms than patients receiving aqueous boosters (88). Boosters of allergoids may be given at 6-week or 3-month intervals with equal clinical results. Allergoids of ragweed, grass, plantain, and oak pollens have been safely given to sensitive patients singly or in mixes.

Glutaraldehyde also modifies allergens to produce "polymerized" antigens. When remaining low molecular weight materials are removed, the resulting product has an average molecular size of 10 million daltons (range 200,000–20 million). Allergenicity measured by skin test is reduced 10^5–10^8 times. Such altered allergens also demonstrate retained or even heightened antigenicity for IgG in animals and humans. Clinical studies show a reduced rate of systemic allergic reaction, stimulation of IgG similar to that found with aqueous extracts, and similar relief of hay fever symptoms (89,90).

Grass pollen extract has also been reacted with glutaraldehyde and adsorbed to suspensions of L-tyrosine (91). A double-blind trial of four injections of ragweed extract modified in this fashion showed that treated patients achieved the same symptoms score with half of the symptomatic medication used by placebo-treated patients (92). Although these methods have met considerable acceptance outside the United States, they have yet to gain acceptance by the FDA and are not available to U.S. physicians.

IX. How Long to Continue Immunotherapy?

One of the first studies on the efficacy of ragweed immunotherapy for hay fever compared matched groups of patients who had been on immunotherapy, one group with ragweed, but not other allergens, discontinued, and the other group continued on treatment. After less than 1 year off ragweed treatment, seasonal symptoms were greater in the discontinued group (8). An uncontrolled study indicated a relapse of symptoms when a preseasonal course of ragweed injections was omitted after 5 years of successful therapy (7).

With venom immunotherapy patients on treatment for an average of 14 months and then discontinued had a rate of systemic reactions of 22% from stings in the field. This clearly indicated a relapse in at least some people when compared with the rate of less than 1% systemic reactions from stings in patients receiving continuing immunotherapy (93). On the other hand, patients who stopped venom immunotherapy after 5–6 years had no systemic reactions when stung in the laboratory. Furthermore, a sting did not sensitize any patient to the point at which a sting 1 month later caused systemic symptoms (94).

Further studies of the consequences of discontinuation of immunotherapy are clearly needed. It does appear that sufficient treatment (such as 5 years) does result in a change that does not relapse readily when injections are stopped.

X. Standardization of Allergens

The methods most commonly used for labeling are weight/volume (w/v; dry weight of starting material/volume of extracting fluid) and PNU (1 protein nitrogen unit = 0.00001 mg protein nitrogen, as determined by precipitating protein with phosphotungstic acid and performing a Kjeldahl nitrogen analysis on the precipitate; 95). Neither is necessarily related to allergenic activity or immunizing activity in immunotherapy and, in practice, fail to provide adequate information to the physician (96,97).

The essential problem in assigning units to allergenic extracts has three aspects. The first is that the active principals are found in crude extracts mixed with variable amounts of inert materials, so that isolation of the active material for measurement is too time-consuming to be practical. Therefore, one has to resort to biological assay which, no matter how accurate, cannot usually be referred back to some absolute or purified material quantifiable in terms of weight. Not only are few active principals isolated and characterized, but there is a second aspect to the problem: namely, the crude material contains multiple active principals, all of which are important to disease, and should be present in materials prepared for diagnostic testing or immunization (98). In the present state of our technology, only a biological assay offers a way of making a measurement of the overall activity that results from multiple immunological systems acting simultaneously. In the presence of such a number of active materials, it seems best to describe the overall resultant of their separate activities in a biological term with a single number.

The third aspect of the problem is probably unique to allergens. Patients vary greatly in their response to allergens. For instance, the threshold of reactivity to antigen E of ragweed varies from 10^{-6} to 10^{-14} g (i.e., 100-millionfold; 99). It is also apparent from studies using purified materials for skin or RAST testing and crossed radioimmunoelectrophoresis studies of sera from several patients, that each patient has a unique pattern of the substances he reacts to, some reacting to only a few allergens, and others reacting to many (100).

The problem is to assign unitage to a complex mixture of materials with highly variable activities that can ordinarily be measured only by indirect biological methods. Furthermore, the unit must be something that can be measured many times over in a variety of commercial establishments in a fashion that is not so complicated that it makes the whole enterprise unendurably expensive. The unit must be usable by physicians to develop diagnostic information about their patients and to describe immunizing doses used in therapy.

An Allergen Standardization Subcommittee of the International Union of Immunologic Societies has developed standard extracts of short ragweed (101), timothy grass (102), *D. pteronyssinus* (103), dog (104), and birch (105), and prepared large batches of glass-sealed ampules labeled in arbitrary units. These materials have been extensively tested for biological activity and the content of specific allergens by immunological methods and have been accepted by WHO as International Standard Preparations (ISP).

A. RAST Inhibition for Standardization

Radioallergosorbent technique inhibition seemed to be the most feasible of current in vitro assays for comparing an unknown with a yardstick standard (106,107).

Reagents to carry out the technique are readily available, the method is well understood in many laboratories, and reproducibility has already been demonstrated. A standard extract, properly prepared, can be expected to be stable for a long period, and human serum containing IgE can also be stored and exchanged readily for comparison. Pooling serum from many patients would increase the change that all the potential allergens in a particular species of allergen would be represented, and variability from patient to patient would be minimized, for the pool would represent the average of several subjects. Products to be sold in the medical marketplace may require other tests to establish that a single species of allergen is present and that the mix of proteins does not vary greatly from the norm. Employment of a yardstick standard leaves the way open to adapt newer, and perhaps better, techniques when they arise with a transition that does not overturn clinical usage.

The development of actual standards has tended to prove the usefulness of this general approach. In each case, with the four standards submitted to the WHO, candidate standards have been studied cooperatively in many laboratories by various biological techniques. The agreement among techniques has been good, showing that a variety of biological and in vitro methods can give similar, results and the agreement among laboratories using the same technique, notably RAST inhibition, has also been excellent (101–103).

B. Skin Testing for Standardization

Direct skin testing can also be employed for comparison of unknown extracts with standardized materials. Two methods have achieved acceptance: (1) in the histamine equivalent in prick testing (HEP) system, the concentration of allergen extract is adjusted to elicit a wheal in the skin-prick test equivalent to that produced by a histamine hydrochloride solution of 1 mg/mL. A preparation of this strength is said to contain 1000 biological units (BU)/mL (108). The HEP system is employed in Scandinavia (2). An intradermal bioassay employs testing of allergic patients with threefold dilutions and establishes a best-fit linear regression line from four serial dilutions. In each subject the dilution producing a 50-mm sum of erythema response (D_{50}) is calculated. The mean D_{50} in a population of 15 maximally sensitive subjects defines the potency of a reference. Potency is denominated in bioequivalent allergy units (BAU). The Center for Biologics Evaluation and Research (CBER) of the U.S. Food and Drug Administration (FDA) is introducing this system in the United States. Short ragweed pollen extracts are likely to have a potency of 10,000 BAU/mL, whereas grass pollen extracts are likely to have a potency of 100,000 BAU/mL (109).

The CBER provides standards labeled in BAU, and IgE-containing serum pools for comparisons of commercial extracts by RAST inhibition or enzyme-linked immunosorbent assay (ELISA). Mite and cat extracts are currently standardized in this way, with ragweed and grass pollen soon to follow. For short ragweed and cat, where major allergens have been identified and isolated, reference standards and antiserum are furnished for a radial immunodiffusion assay of the allergen. Short ragweed extracts are labeled based on their Amb a 1 content and cat extracts are labeled on their Fel d 1 content. Isoelectric focusing and crossed-immunoelectrophoresis also serve as laboratory controls for allergenic products.

The use of recombinant DNA technology to make virtually pure examples of the active proteins in several allergens, combined with the development of monoclonal antibodies (MAbs) specific to allergenic proteins, offers the opportunity to assay extracts for these "marker" proteins. Such assays could be quickly accomplished accurately. Although the ability of an MAb reagent to assay biologically active allergen needs to be established in each case, once that is done, an unlimited supply of a reliable reagent becomes available. Labeling in mass units of one or more active proteins thereby becomes possible. CBER has proposed moving forward the labeling by content of marker proteins (110). Such labeling might allow a more rational approach to developing the optimum dosage for immunotherapy as described in the following section.

XI. Optimum Doses

A certain number of efficacy studies have employed extracts standardized in a way that allows comparison. Because international, biological, and allergy units have been introduced only recently, the only method that offers a common denominator in a sufficient number of studies is the content in mass units of one or more major allergens in the extract. Table 1 summarizes data on five classes of allergens, showing (when available) both the largest single dose and the cumulative annual dose in terms of micrograms of major allergen. In several early studies only the cumulative dose was available.

From both clinical and immunological evidence, it seems likely that the maximum or the final dose is more meaningful than a cumulative annual dose. From the data in this table, the maximum dose is remarkably similar for a variety of allergens, lying somewhere between just under 5 up to 20 μg. It should be noted that most of these studies have been designed to describe the maximum tolerated dose; hence, the lower figures may be more appropriate as a guide to a safe, but effective, dose. Two studies with ragweed indicate that doses of less than 1 μg Amb a 1 equivalent are not measurably effective by present clinical or challenge methods (12,111). Because any of the biologically determined units can usually be estimated by determination of a major allergen, these numbers provide a rough guide to the target dosage in an immunotherapy regimen. As the relation between biologically determined units and the content of major allergen is worked out, it should be possible to accurately describe a target dose that is likely to be effective for various allergens.

Table 1 Effective Immunotherapy Doses in Micrograms of Major Allergen: Final Injection

Dose (μg)	Range	Antigen	Ref.
Ragweed			
9.4	1.7–18.8	Amb a 1	81
4.7	0.4–28.1	Amb a 1	81
11.1	3.7–46.8	Amb a 1	111
6	1.2–18.6	Amb a 1 (challenge study)	11
12.4	No range	Amb a 1 (challenge study)	11
Grass			
18.6	Not given	Lol p 1	119
18	12.9–20.4	Phl p 6 } Two major allergens in one extract	120
36	25.8–40.8	Phl p 5	
Cat			
15.1	9.0–23	Fel d 1	121
Dust Mite			
24	3–24	Der p 1	122
No mean	0.5–11.5	Der p 1	123
No mean	0.6–6.5	Der p 1	123
7	No range	Der p 1	124
21	No range	Der p 1	124

XII. Dosage Programs

In 1930, Freeman described three different protocols according the frequency of allergen injections, weekly, daily, and rush, the latter calling for five or six injections in a day (112). The most commonly used schedule, however, has traditionally been injections once or twice a week. Interest in more rapid schedules revived when a relatively short "clustered" program, calling for an initial series of two or three injections in 1 day, followed by additional clusters a week apart was successful in insect venom immunization. In immunotherapy for ragweed allergy, the clustered regimen produced immunological and clinical responses similar to those of a more conventional weekly program (81). When better-standardized extracts became available, interest in rush immunotherapy revived because dosages would presumably be more reproducible. Rush protocols have been studied by Bousquet and colleagues with grass pollen (113), *D. pteronyssinus* (114–117), and *Alternaria* (118) extracts. Immune responses (rise in IgG and decrease in immediate skin tests), were similar to those found with longer regimens, and measures of efficacy (bronchial provocation tests and symptom diary scores) were significantly improved. Systemic reactions occurred more frequently in asthmatic patients, and the authors recommend that a rush program not be used in patients with severe asthma. Safety problems were no different from those observed with more prolonged protocols of immunotherapy.

Note: A thorough review of all aspects of immunotherapy for allergy and allergenic extracts has been developed by the Food and Drug Administration and published in the Federal Register, Wednesday, January 23, 1985, 21 CFR Parts 600, 610, and 680. This 200-page review contains references to the world literature on every allergenic extract for which a report had been made at the time.

References

1. Noon L. Prophylactic inoculation against hay fever. Lancet 1911; 1:1572–1573.
2. Freeman J. Further observations on the treatment of hay fever by hypodermic inoculations of pollen vaccine. Lancet 1911; 2:814.
3. Cooke RA. Hay fever and asthma: the uses and limitations of desensitization. NY Med J 1918; 107:577–583.
4. Cooke RA. Studies in specific hypersensitiveness: III. On constitutional reactions: the dangers of the diagnostic cutaneous test and therapeutic injection of allergens. J Immunol 1922; 7:119–146.
5. Norman PS, Winkenwerder WL, Lichtenstein LM. Immunotherapy of hay fever with ragweed antigen E: comparisons with whole pollen extract and placebos. J Allergy 1968; 42:93–108.
6. Lichtenstein LM, Norman PS, Winkenwerder WL. A single year of immunotherapy for ragweed hay fever. Immunologic and clinical studies. Ann Intern Med 1971; 75:663–671.
7. Norman PS. Specific therapy in allergy. Pro (with reservations). Med Clin North Am 1974; 58:111–125.
8. Lowell FC, Franklin W. A double-blind study of the effectiveness and specificity of injection therapy in ragweed hay fever. N Engl J Med 1965; 273:675–679.
9. Norman PS, Lichtenstein LM. The clinical and immunologic specificity of immunotherapy. J Allergy Clin Immunol 1978; 61:370–377.
10. Naclerio RM, Meier HL, Kagey-Sobotka A, Adkinson NF Jr, Meyers DA, Norman PS, Lichtenstein LM. Mediator release after nasal airway challenge with allergen. Am Rev Respir Dis 1983; 128:597–602.
11. Creticos PS, Adkinson NF Jr, Kagey-Sobotka A, Proud D, Meier HL, Naclerio RM, Lichtenstein LM, Norman PS. Nasal challenge with ragweed pollen in hay fever patients. Effect of immunotherapy. J Clin Invest 1985; 76:2247–2253.
12. Creticos PS, Marsh DG, Proud D, Kagey SA, Adkinson NF Jr, Friedhoff L, Naclerio RM, Lichtenstein LM, Norman PS. Responses to ragweed-pollen nasal challenge before and after immunotherapy. J Allergy Clin Immunol 1989; 84:197–205.
13. Åas K. Hyposensitization in house dust allergy asthma: a double blind controlled study with evaluation of the effect on bronchial sensitivity to house dust. Acta Paediatr Scand 1971; 60:264–268.
14. Taylor WW, Ohman JL, Lowell FC. Immunotherapy in cat-induced asthma. Double- blind trial with evaluation of bronchial responses to cat allergen and histamine. J Allergy Clin Immunol 1978; 61:283–287.
15. Creticos PS, Reed CE, Norman PS. The NIAID cooperative study of the role of immunotherapy in seasonal ragweed-induced adult asthma. J Allergy Clin Immunol 1993; 91:226.
16. Metzger JW, Donnelly BA, Richerson HB. Modification of late asthmatic responses (LAR) during immunotherapy for *Alternaria*-induced asthma. J Allergy Clin Immunol 1983; 71:119.
17. Warner JD, Price JF, Soothill JF, Hey EN. Controlled trial of hyposensitization to *Dermatophagoides pteronyssinus* in children with asthma. Lancet 1978; 2:912.

18. Pienkowski MM, Norman PS, Lichtenstein LM. Suppression of late-phase skin reactions by immunotherapy with ragweed extract. J Allergy Clin Immunol 1985; 76:729–734.
19. Iliopoulos O, Proud D, Adkinson NF Jr, Creticos PS, Norman PS, Kagey-Sobotka A, Lichtenstein LM, Naclerio RM. Effects of immunotherapy on the early, late and rechallenge nasal reaction to provocation with allergen: changes in inflammatory mediators and cells. J Allergy Clin Immunol 1991; 87:855–866.
20. Parker WAJ, Whisman BA, Apaliski SJ, Reid MJ. The relationships between late cutaneous responses and specific antibody responses with outcome of immunotherapy for seasonal allergic rhinitis. J Allergy Clin Immunol 1989; 84:667–677.
21. Furin MJ, Norman PS, Creticos PS, Naclerio RM. Immunotherapy decreases antigen-induced eosinophil cell migration into the nasal cavity. J Allergy Clin Immunol 1991; 88:27–32.
22. Connell JT. Quantitative intranasal pollen challenge: II. Effect of daily pollen challenge, environmental pollen exposure, and placebo challenge on the nasal membrane. J Allergy 1968; 41:123.
23. Connell JT. Quantitative intranasal challenges: III. The priming effect in allergic rhinitis. J Allergy 1969; 43:33.
24. Naclerio RM, Proud D, Togias AG, Adkinson NF Jr, Meyers DA, Kagey-Sobotka A, Plaut M, Norman PS, Lichtenstein LM. Inflammatory mediators in late antigen-induced rhinitis. N Engl J Med 1985; 313:65–70.
25. Cartier A, Bandouvakis J, Ryan G, Dolovich J, Hargreave FE. Asthma and increased nonallergic bronchial responsiveness to methacholine during natural exposure to ragweed pollen. Am Rev Respir Dis 1980; 121(suppl):61.
26. Platts-Mills TE, Tovey ER, Mitchell EB, Maszoro H, Nock P, Wilkens SR. Reduction of bronchial hyperreactivity during prolonged allergen avoidance. Lancet 1982; 2:675–678.
27. Hedlin G, Graft-Lonnevig V, Heilborn H, Lilja G, Norrlind K, Pegelow K, Sundin B, Løwenstein H. Immunotherapy with cat- and dog-dander extracts. J Allergy Clin Immunol 1991; 87:955–964.
28. Majchel AM, Proud D, Friedhoff L, Creticos PS, Norman PS, Naclerio RM. The nasal response to histamine challenge—effect of the pollen season and immunotherapy. J Allergy Clin Immunol 1992; 90:85–91.
29. Cooke RA, Barnard JH, Hebald S, Stull A. Serological evidence of immunity with coexisting sensitization in a type of human allergy (hay fever). J Exp Med 1935; 62:733–751.
30. Loveless MH. Immunological studies of pollinosis: IV. The relationship between thermostable antibody in the circulation and clinical immunity. J Immunol 1943; 47:165–180.
31. Lichtenstein LM, Norman PS, Winkenwerder WL, Osler AG. In vitro studies of human ragweed allergy: changes in cellular and humoral activity associated with specific desensitization. J Clin Invest 1966; 45:1126–1136.
32. Lichtenstein LM, Ishizaka K, Norman PS, Sobotka AK, Hill BM. IgE antibody measurements in ragweed hay fever. Relationship to clinical severity and the results of immunotherapy. J Clin Invest 1973; 52:472–482.
33. Gleich GJ, Jacob GL, Yunginger JW, Henderson LL. Measurement of the absolute levels of IgE antibodies in patients with ragweed hay fever: effect of immunotherapy on seasonal changes and relationship to IgG antibodies. J Allergy Clin Immunol 1977; 60:188–198.
34. Platts-Mills TA, von Maur RK, Ishizaka K, Norman PS, Lichtenstein LM. IgA and IgG anti-ragweed antibodies in nasal secretions. Quantitative measurements of antibodies and correlation with inhibition of histamine release. J Clin Invest 1976; 57:1041–1050.
35. Platts-Mills TAE. Local production of IgG, IgA, and IgE antibodies in grass pollen hay fever. J Immunol 1979; 122:2218–2225.
36. Sadan N, Rhyne MB, Mellits ED, Goldstein EO, Levy DA, Lichtenstein LM. Immunotherapy of pollinosis in children. Investigation of the immunologic basis of clinical improvement. N Engl J Med 1969; 280:623–627.

37. Lichtenstein LM, Norman PS, Winkenwerder WL. Clinical and in vitro studies on the role of immunotherapy in ragweed hay fever. Am J Med 1968; 44:514–524.
38. Devey ME, Wilson DV, Wheeler AW. The IgG subclass of antibodies to grass pollen allergens produced in hay fever patients during hyposensitization. Clin Allergy 1976; 6:227–236.
39. Aalberse RC, van der Gaag R, van Leeuwen J. Serologic aspects of IgG4 antibodies. 1. Prolonged immunization results in an IgG4-restricted response. J Immunol 1983; 130:722–726.
40. van der Zee JS, van Swieten P, Aalberse RC. Serologic aspects of IgG4 antibodies. II. IgG4 antibodies form small, nonprecipitating immune complexes due to functional monovalency. J Immunol 1986; 137:3566–3571.
41. Creticos PS, Van Metre TE Jr, Mardiney MR, Rosenberg GL, Norman PS, Adkinson NF Jr. Dose response of IgE and IgG antibodies during ragweed immunotherapy. J Allergy Clin Immunol 1984; 73:94–104.
42. Gleich GJ, Zimmerman BS, Henderson LL, Yunginger JW. Effects of immunotherapy on immunoglobulin E and immunglobulin G antibodies to ragweed antigens: a six year prospective study. J Allergy Clin Immunol 1982; 70:261–271.
43. Rocklin RE, Pence H, Kaplan H, Evans R. Cell-mediated immune response of ragweed-sensitive patients to ragweed antigen E: in vitro lymphocyte transformation and elaboration of lymphocyte mediators. J Clin Invest 1974; 53:735–744.
44. Rocklin RE, Sheffer AL, Greineder DK, Melmon KL. Generation of antigen-specific suppressor cells during allergy desensitization. N Engl J Med 1980; 302:1213–1219.
45. Greenstein JL, Morgenstern JP, LaRaia J, Counsell CM, Goodwin WH, Lussier A, Creticos PS, Norman PS, Barman RD. Ragweed immunotherapy decreases T cell reactivity to recombinant *Amb a* I. J Allergy Clin Immunol 1992; 89:322.
46. Secrist H, Chelen CJ, Wen Y, Marshall JD, Umetsu DT. Allergen immunotherapy decreases interleukin 4 production in CD4+ T cells from allergic individuals. J Exp Med 1993; 178:2123–2130.
47. Varney VA, Hamid QA, Gaga M, Ying S, Jacobson M, Frew AJ, Kay AB, Durham SR. Influence of grass pollen immunotherapy on cellular infiltration and cytokine mRNA expression during allergen-induced late-phase cutaneous responses. J Clin Invest 1993; 92:644–651.
48. Durham SR, Varney VA, Sun Y, Jacobson MR, Sudderick RM, Mackay IS, Kay AB, Hamid Q. Effect of grass pollen immunotherapy on cell infiltration and cytokine mRna expression during allergen-induced late nasal response. J Allergy Clin Immunol 1994; 93:230.
49. Charlesworth EN, Nish WA, Charlesworth MG, Valtier S, George T, Leiferman KM. Standard high dose immunotherapy decreases the production of IL-3, IL-5, and GM-CSF during the cutaneous late-phase response (LPR) to antigen. J Allergy Clin Immunol 1993; 91:252.
50. Frankland AW, Augustin R. Prophylaxis of summer hay-fever and asthma: a controlled trial comparing crude grass-pollen extracts with the isolated main protein component. Lancet 1954; 1:1055–1057.
51. Dieges PH. A prospective study on some immunological changes occurring in the first year of grass pollen desensitization. Acta Allergol 1976; 31:130–140.
52. Van Der Giesen M, Homan WL, Van Kernebeck G, Aalberse RC, Dieges PH. Sibclass typing of IgG antibodies formed by grass pollen-allergic patients during immunotherapy. Int Arch Allergy 1976; 50:625–640.
53. Johnstone DE. Study of the role of antigen dosage in the treatment of pollenosis and pollen asthma. J Dis Child 1957; 94:1–5.
54. Lowell FC, Franklin W. A "double blind" study of treatment with aqueous allergenic extracts in cases of allergic rhinitis. J Allergy 1963; 34:165–182.
55. Creticos PS, Reed CE, Norman PS, Khoury J, Adkinson NF Jr, Buncher CR, Busse WW, Bush RK, Gadde J, Li JT, Richerson HB, Rosenthal RR, Solomon WR, Steinberg P,

Yunginger JW. Ragweed immunotherapy in adult asthma. N Engl J Med 1996; 334:501–506.
56. Pence HL, Mitchell DQ, Greely RL, Updegraff BR, Selfridge HA. Immunotherapy for mountain cedar pollinosis: a double-blind controlled study. J Allergy Clin Immunol 1976; 58:39–50.
57. Viander M, Koivikko A. On seasonal symtoms of hyposensitized and untreated hay fever patients in relation to birch pollen counts: correlation with nasal sensitivity, prick tests and RAST. Clin Allergy 1978; 8:387–396.
58. Petersen RN, Janniche H, Munch EP, Wihl JÄ, Böwadt H, Ipsen H, Løwenstein H. Immunotherapy with partially purified and standardized tree pollen extracts. I. Clinical results from a three-year double-blind study of patients treated with pollen extracts either of birch of combinations of alder, birch and hazel. Allergy 1988; 43:353–362.
59. Ahlstedt S, Eriksson NE. Immunotherapy in atopic allergy—antibody titres and avidities during hyposensitization with birch and timothy pollen allergens. Int Arch Allergy 1977; 55:400–411.
60. Forgacs P, Swan AV. Treatment of house dust allergy. Br Med J 1968; 37:774–777.
61. May CD, Lyman M, Alberto R, Cheng J. Immunochemical evaluation of antigenicity of house dust extract: specificity of dermal wheal reactions and responses to injections for immunotherapy. J Allergy 1970; 46:73–89.
62. Chapman MD, Platts-Mills TAE, Gabriel M, Ng HK, Allan WGL, Hill LE, Nunn AJ. Antibody response following prolonged hyposensitization with *Dermatophagoides pteronyssinus* extract. Int Arch Allergy 1980; 61:431–440.
63. D'Souza MF, Pepys J, Wells ID, Tai E, Palmer F, Overell BG, McGrath T, Megson M. Hyposensitization with *Dermatophagoides pteronyssinus* in house dust allergy: a controlled study of clinical and immunological effects. Clin Allergy 1973; 3:177–193.
64. Smith AP. Hyposensitization with *Dermatophagoides pteronyssinus* antigen: trial in asthma induced by house dust. Br Med J 1971; 4:204–206.
65. Ohman JL Jr, Marsh DG, Goldman M. Antibody responses following immunotherapy with cat pelt extract. J Allergy Clin Immunol 1982; 69:319–326.
66. Ohman JL, Findlay SR, Leitermann KM. Immunotherapy in cat induced asthma. Double-blind trial with evaluation of in vivo and in vitro responses. J Allergy Clin Immunol 1984; 74:230–239.
67. Sundin B, Lilja G, Graff-Lonnevig V, Hedlin G, Heilborn H, Norrlind K, Pegelow K-O, Løwenstein H. Immunotherapy with partially purified and standardized animal dander extracts. I. Clinical results from a double-blind study on patients with animal dander asthma. J Allergy Clin Immunol 1986; 77:478–487.
68. Valovirta E, Viander M, Koivikko A, Vanto T, Ingemann L. Immunotherapy in allergy to dog. Immunologic and clinical findings of a double-blind study. Ann Allergy 1986; 57:173–179.
69. Koivikko A, Agrell B, Dreborg S, Foucard T, Kjellman M, Nilsson S. A double-blind multicenter immunotherapy trial in children with purified and standardized *Cladosporium herbarum* (*Hormodendrum*) preparation. I. Clinical results. J Allergy Clin Immunol 1984; 73:142.
70. Malling H-J. Diagnosis and immunotherapy of mold allergy. V. Clinical efficacy and side effects of immunotherapy with *Cladosporium herbarum*. Allergy 1986; 41:505–519.
71. Aukrust L, Borch SM. Partial purification and characterization of two *Cladosporium herbarum* allergens. Int Arch Allergy Appl Immunol 1979; 60:68.
72. Yunginger JW, Jones RT, Gleich GJ. Studies on *Alternaria* allergens. II. Measurement of the relative potency of commercial *Alternaria* extracts by the direct RAST and by RAST inhibition. J Allergy Clin Immunol 1976; 58:405–413.
73. Yunginger JW, Jones RT, Nesheim ME, Geller M. Studies on *Alternaria* allergens. III. Isolation of a major allergenic fraction (*Alt*-1). J Allergy Clin Immunol 1980; 66:136–147.
74. Norman PS, Lichtenstein LM, Ishizaka K. Diagnostic tests in ragweed hay fever. A com-

parison of direct skin tests, IgE antibody measurements, and basophil histamine release. J Allergy Clin Immunol 1973; 52:210–224.
75. Marsh DG, Belin L, Bruce CA, Lichtenstein LM, Hussain R. Rapidly released allergens from short ragweed pollen: I. Kinetics of release of known allergen in relation to biological activity. J Allergy Clin Immunol 1981; 67:206–216.
76. Abramson MJ, Puy RM, Weiner JM. Is allergen immunotherapy effective in asthma? A meta-analysis of randomized controlled trials. Am J Respir Crit Care Med 1995; 151:969–974.
77. Jacobsen L, Dreborg S, Møller C, Valovirta E, Wahn U, Niggeman B, Koller D, Urbanek R, Halken S, Høst A, Løwenstein H. Immunotherapy as preventive allergy treatment (PAT). J Allergy Clin Immunol 1996; 97:232.
78. Connell JT, Sherman WB, Myers PA. Antibody studies in constitutional reactions resulting from injections of ragweed pollen extract. J Allergy 1962; 33:365–377.
79. Lockey RF, Benedict LM, Turkeltaub PC, Bukantz SC. Fatalities from immunotherapy (IT) and skin testing (ST). J Allergy Clin Immunol 1987; 79:660–677.
80. Tinkelman DG, Cole WQ III, Tunno J. Immunotherapy: a one-year prospective study to evaluate risk factors of systemic reactions. J Allergy Clin Immunol 1995; 95:8–14.
81. Van Metre TE Jr, Adkinson NF Jr, Amodio FJ, Kagey SA, Lichtenstein LM, Mardiney MR Jr, Norman PS, Rosenberg GL. A comparison of immunotherapy schedules for injection treatment of ragweed pollen hay fever. J Allergy Clin Immunol 1982; 69:181–193.
82. Executive Committee American Academy of Allergy and Immunology. Guidelines to minimize the risk from systemic reactions caused by immunotherapy with allergenic extracts. J Allergy Clin Immunol 1994; 93:811–812.
83. Stein MR, Brown GL, Lima JE, Nelson HS, Carr RI. A laboratory evaluation of immune complexes in patients on inhalant immunotherapy. J Allergy Clin Immunol 1978; 62:211–216.
84. Yang WH, Dorval G, Osterland CK, Gilmore NJ. Circulating immune complexes during immunotherapy. J Allergy Clin Immunol 1979; 63:300–307.
85. Norman PS, Winkenwerder WL, Lichtenstein LM. Trials of alum-precipitated pollen extracts in the treatment of hay fever. J Allergy Clin Immunol 1972; 50:31–44.
86. Marsh DG, Lichtenstein LM, Campbell DH. Studies on "allergoids" prepared from naturally occurring allergens: I. Assay of allergenicity and antigenicity of formalinized rye group I component. Immunology 1970; 18:705–722.
87. Marsh DG, Lichtenstein LM, Norman PS. Induction of IgE-mediated immediate hypersensitivity to group I rye grass pollen allergen and allergoids in non-allergic man. Immunology 1972; 22:1013–1028.
88. Norman PS, Marsh DG, Lichtenstein LM, Ishizaka K. Controlled evaluation of allergoid in the immunotherapy of ragweed hay fever. J Allergy Clin Immunol 1982; 70:248–260.
89. Metzger WJ, Patterson R, Zeiss CR, Irons JS, Pruzansky JJ, Suszko IM, Levitz D. Comparison of polymerized and unpolymerized antigen E for immunotherapy of ragweed allergy. N Engl J Med 1976; 295:1160–1164.
90. Bacal E, Zeiss CR, Suszko I, Levitz D, Patterson R. Polymerized whole ragweed: an improved method of immunotherapy. J Allergy Clin Immunol 1978; 62:289–294.
91. Miller ACML, Tees EC. A metabolizable adjuvant: clinical trial of grass pollen–tyrosine adsorbate. Clin Allergy 1974; 4:49–55.
92. Cockroft DW, Cuff MT, Tarlo SM, Dolovich J, Hargreave FE. Allergen injection therapy with glutaraldehyde-modified-ragweed pollen–tyrosine adsorbate. A double-blind trial. J Allergy Clin Immunol 1977; 60:56–62.
93. Gold DBK, Johnson K, Addison BI, Valentine MD, Kagey-Sobotka A, Lichtenstein LM. Clinical and immunologic observations in patients who stop venom immunotherapy. J Allergy Clin Immunol 1986; 77:435–442.
94. Golden DBK, Kwiterovich KA, Kagey-Sobotka A, Valentine MD, Lichtenstein LM. Immunologic response to sequential stings after stopping venom immunotherapy (VIT) in adults. J Allergy Clin Immunol 1988; 81:201.

95. Cooke RA, Stull A. Preparation and standardization of pollen extracts for the treatment of hay fever. J Allergy 1933; 4:87–91.
96. Baer H, Godfrey H, Maloney CJ, Norman PS, Lichtenstein LM. The potency and antigen E content of commercially prepared ragweed extracts. J Allergy 1970; 45:347–354.
97. Baer H, Maloney CJ, Norman PS, Marsh DG. The potency and group I antigen content of six commercially prepared grass pollen extracts. J Allergy Clin Immunol 1974; 54(3):157–164.
98. Platts-Mills TAE. Allergens. In: Frank MM, Austen KF, Claman HN, Unanue ER, eds. Samter's Immunologic Diseases, 5th ed. Boston: Little, Brown & Co, 1994:1231–1256.
99. King TP, Norman PS, Connell JT. Isolation and characterization of allergens from ragweed pollen. II. Biochemistry 1964; 3:458–468.
100. Løwenstein H, Marsh DG. Antigens of *Ambrosia elatior* (short ragweed) pollen. III. Crossed radioimmunoelectrophoresis of ragweed-allergic patient's sera with special attention to quantification of IgE responses. J Immunol 1983; 130:727–731.
101. Helm RM, Gauerke MB, Baer H, Lwenstein H, Ford A, Levy DA, Norman PS, Yunginger JW. Production and testing of an international reference standard of short ragweed pollen extract. J Allergy Clin Immunol 1984; 73:790–800.
102. Gjesing B, Jäger L, Marsh DG, Løwenstein H. The international collaborative study establishing the first international standard for timothy (*Phleum pratense*) grass pollen allergenic extract. J Allergy Clin Immunol 1985; 75:258–267.
103. Ford A, Seagroatt V, Platts-Mills TAE, Løwenstein H. A collaborative study on the first international standard of *Dermatophagoides pteronyssinus* (house dust mite) extract. J Allergy Clin Immunol 1985; 75:676–686.
104. Larsen JN, Ford A, Gjesing B, Levy D, Petrunov B, Silvestri L, Løwenstein H. The collaborative study of the international standard of dog, *Canis domesticus*, hair/dander extract. J Allergy Clin Immunol 1988; 82:318–330.
105. Arntzen FC, Wilhelmsen TW, Løwenstein H, Gjesing B, Maasch H, Strömberg R, Einarsson R, Backman A, Mäkinen-Kiljunen S, Ford A. The international collaborative study on the first international standard of birch (*Betula verrucosa*) pollen extract. J Allergy Clin Immunol 1989; 83:66–82.
106. Foucard T, Johansson SGO, Bennich H, Berg T. In vitro estimation of allergens by a radioimmune antiglobulin technique using human IgE antibodies. Int Arch Allergy Appl Immunol 1972; 43:360–370.
107. Gleich GJ, Larson JB, Jones RT, Baer H. Measurement of the potency of allergy extracts by their inhibitory capacities in the radioallergosorbent test. J Allergy Clin Immunol 1974; 53:158–169.
108. Åas K, Belin L. Suggestion for biologic qualitative testing and standardization of allergen extracts. Acta Allergol 1974; 29:238.
109. Turkeltaub PC. The allergy unit—clinical relevance: issues in allergen standardization. In: Lockey RF, Bukantz SC, eds. Allergen Immunotherapy. New York: Marcel Dekker, 1991: 171–190.
110. Liu DT. Regulation of allergenic products in the USA: CBER initiatives. In: Kurth R, Haustein D, eds. Regulatory Control and Standardization of Allergenic Extracts. New York: Gustave Fischer Verlag, 1994:7–12.
111. Van Metre TE Jr, Adkinson NF Jr, Amodio FJ, Lichtenstein LM, Mardiney MR, Norman PS, Rosenberg GL, Sobotka AK, Valentine MD. A comparative study of the effectiveness of the Rinkel method and the current standard method of immunotherapy for ragweed pollen hay fever. J Allergy Clin Immunol 1980; 66:500–513.
112. Freeman J. "Rush" inoculation with special references to hay fever treatment. Lancet 1930; 1:744–746.
113. Bousquet J, Guerin B, Dotte A, Dhivert H, Djoukader F, Hewitt B, Michel B. Comparison between rush immunotherapy with a standardized allergen and an alum adjuvet pyridine extracted material in grass pollen allergy. Clin Allergy 1985; 15:179–192.
114. Bousquet J, Calvayrac P, Guérin B, Hejjaoui A, Dhivert H, Hewitt B, Michel F-B.

178178Immunotherapy with a standardized *Dermatophagoides pteronyssinus* extract. I. In vivo and in vitro parameters after a short course of treatment. J Allergy Clin Immunol 1985; 76:734–744.

115. Bousquet J, Hejjaoui A, Clauzel A-M, Guérin B, Dhivert H, Skasse-Brociek W, Michel F-B. Immunotherapy with a standardized *Dermatophagoides pteronyssinus* extract. II. Prediction of efficacy of immunotherapy. J Allergy Clin Immunol 1988; 82:971–977.
116. Bousquet J, Hejjauoui A, Dhivert H, Clauzel A-M, Michel F-B. Immunotherapy with a standardized *Dermatophagoides pteronyssinus* extract. III. Systemic reactions during the rush protocol in patients suffering from asthma. J Allergy Clin Immunol 1989; 83:797–802.
117. Hejjaoui A, Dhivert H, Michel F-B, Bousquet J. Immunotherapy with a standardized *Dermatophagoides pteronyssinus* extract. IV. Systemic reactions according to the immunotherapy schedule. J Allergy Clin Immunol 1990; 85:473–479.
118. Horst M, Hejjaoui A, Horst V, Michel F-B, Bousquet J. Double-blind placebo- controlled rush immunotherapy with a standardized *Alternaria* extract. J Allergy Clin Immunol 1990; 85; 460–472.
119. Moss RB, Hsu Y-P, Kwasnicki JM, Sullivan MM, Reid MJ. Isotypic and antigenic restriction of the blocking antibody response to ryegrass pollen: correlation of rye group I antigen-specific IgG1 with clinical response. J Allergy Clin Immunol 1987; 79:387–398.
120. Østerballe O. Immunotherapy with grass pollen allergens. Clinical results from a prospective 3 year double blind study. Allergy 1982; 37:379–388.
121. Van Metre TE Jr, Marsh DG, Adkinson NF Jr, Kagey SA, Khattignavong A, Norman PS, Rosenberg GL. Immunotherapy for cat asthma. J Allergy Clin Immunol 1988; 82:1055–1068.
122. Mosbech H, Dreborg S, Frølund L, Ljungstedt-Påhlman I, Svendsen UG, Søborg M, Taudorf E, Weeke B. Hyposensitization in asthmatics with mPEG modified and unmodified house dust mite extract. I. Clinical effect evaluated by diary cards and a retrospective assessment. Allergy 1989; 44:487–498.
123. Wahn U, Schweter C, Lind P, Løwenstein H. Prospective study on immunologic changes induced by two different *Dermatophagoides pteronyssinus* extracts prepared from whole mite culture and mite bodies. J Allergy Clin Immunol 1988; 82:360–370.
124. Haugaard L, Dahl R, Jacobsen L. A controlled dose–response study of immunotherapy with standardized, partially purified extract of house dust mite: clinical efficacy and side effects. J Allergy Clin Immunol 1993; 91:709–722.

11

Allergen-Specific Immunotherapy

Mechanisms of Immunotherapy

JÉRÔME PÈNE

INSERM U454
Hôpital Arnaud de Villeneuve
Montpellier, France

JEAN BOUSQUET

Montpellier University and
Service des Maladies Respiratoires–
INSERM U454
Montpellier University Hospital
Montpellier, France

I. Introduction

Allergen-specific immunotherapy, which usually involves the subcutaneous administration of increasing amounts of allergens, is highly effective in selected patients with IgE-mediated disease (1) such as allergic rhinitis or asthma. The most common form of administration is the subcutaneous route, but oral or nasal immunotherapy may also be effective. Immunotherapy is highly controversial; most protocols have been decided empirically, many allergens are still poorly defined, the mechanisms of action are not yet clear, properly conducted trials are still sparse, and allergen injections expose the patient to life-threatening reactions. However, specific immunotherapy is one of the most common treatments in children and adolescents in many parts of the world and is effective under optimal conditions, including a demonstrated IgE-mediated disease, a high-quality extract by using standardized allergenic preparations (2), the use of proper doses, and a correct indication. Moreover, immunotherapy cannot be replaced by any other treatment in venom allergy.

Recent studies have provided insight into the mechanisms of this form of treatment. Whereas earlier work focused on circulating antibody and effector cells, recent studies suggest that these changes may be secondary to an influence of immunotherapy on T-cell response to allergen. Indeed, the allergic reaction mediated by IgE manifests itself as an inflammation that develops in several stages. The allergens react, through the membrane-bound IgE molecules, with cells present at the mucosal surfaces. Mast cells are the first cells to be activated, and they start a chain reaction, resulting in an allergic inflammation, and involving several other cell types and factors, including eosinophils, vasoactive mediators (histamine, platelet-activating factor [PAF], leukotrienes, and prostaglandins), cytokines (interleukin [IL]-3, IL-4, IL-5, granulocyte–macrophage colony-stimulating factor [GM-CSF], and others), adhesion molecules, and cytotoxic mediators (in particular those derived from eosinophils). The allergic reaction is initiated by IgE, but rapidly results in a much more widespread inflammation that may last for several days following a single allergic contact. Furthermore, repeated allergic stimulation results in persistent inflammation and is the foundation of nonspecific hyperactivity of the airways. Desensitization mechanisms, therefore, cannot be explained solely on the basis of a reduction in the synthesis of IgE, as has been proposed by some researchers, but must involve various other factors in which modulation of the synthesis of IgE is perhaps not the major mechanism. It is probable that several mechanisms play a sequential role in the process, these mechanisms being perhaps different for specific immunotherapy for pneumoallergens and those for specific immunotherapy for Hymenoptera venoms. Most studies have examined subcutaneous immunotherapy, rather than immunotherapy by alternative routes. However, mechainsms are likely to be heterogeneous, depending on the nature of the allergen; the site of allergy; the route, dose, and duration of immunotherapy; the use of different adjuvants; and last but not least, the genetic status of the host.

II. Serum Antibody Concentrations

For a long time, attempts have been made to demonstrate the clinical advantages of desensitization by measurement of the reduction of IgE and the increase of IgG levels or the variations of IgG subclasses known as "blocking antibodies" (3).

During conventional immunotherapy, serum IgE concentrations initially rise which, curiously, accompanies a clinical improvement. After several months or even years of treatment, the levels of IgE gradually fall to normal, but rarely become lower than their starting value, except in subjects allergic to Hymenoptera venom (4). However, in pollen allergy, one observes no elevation of specific IgE titer in desensitized subjects during the pollen season nor blunting of seasonal increases in IgE (5). Thus, the variation in the levels of specific IgE certainly does not explain the benefits of specific immunotherapy for subjects with allergy to inhaled pneumoallergens.

One of the most common theories underlying the mechanisms of successful immunotherapy, developed over many years, was based on allergen-blocking antibodies (6). This hypothesis was first postulated in the 1930s by Cooke, and

Lichtenstein linked blocking antibodies to IgG. Many studies have confirmed marked rises in allergen-specific IgG, particularly IgG1 and IgG4 subclasses (7). These observations gave rise the so-called blocking antibody theory (8,9) that postulates that IgG, competing with IgE for allergen binding, thereby blocks IgE-dependent activation of mast cells. Recently, it has been shown that human monoclonal IgG antibodies from a hyposensitized birch pollen allergic patient blocked IgE binding to the major birch pollen allergen, Bet v 1, and blocked Bet v 1-induced histamine release (10). An opposed mode of action has been attributed to IgG in immediate-type allergy: a small fraction of IgG may have anaphylactic properties, although this property cannot be attributed to IgG4 (11).

Immunotherapy with Hymenoptera venoms is widely used throughout the world and is accepted as an effective treatment for most patients with Hymenoptera venom allergy. There are, however, still some unresolved problems with this form of treatment. In many patients a strong increase of venom-specific serum IgG antibodies usually parallels clinical protection induced by venom immunotherapy, although many exceptions have been reported. Venom-specific IgG antibodies rise in serum within a few months, then decline, and after some years of treatment the level may not be very different from naturally occurring levels in untreated patients. A protective IgG antibody level after a course of 6–12 months of treatment has been postulated by several authors and estimated by Pharmacia IgG-RAST, to be greater than 5 μg of venom-specific IgG per millitier or 1 ng/ml of phospholipase–IgG. Most individuals with venom-specific IgG levels above these limits, are in fact, protected. However, there are some patients whose serum IgG largely exceeds these limits and who still react to reexposure. Most of these patients are usually highly sensitive with very high IgE titers or have previously experienced a severe anaphylactic reaction. The lack of protection may be related to a heterogeneous IgG response toward some specific venom components or to a very high IgE immune response. On the other hand, many patients with low, or even undetectable, venom IgG are protected. Finally, an early increase in IgG levels was associated with protection against an insect sting in a population of patients, but has no predictive value in individual patients (9,12,13). Moreover, in the long-term follow-up of venom immunotherapy, there appears to be a late-onset, non–IgG-mediated mechanism for suppression of allergic sensitivity (14). Thus, the absolute level of venom IgG may not be the gold standard for predicting the efficacy of venom immunotherapy, nor for the selection of at-risk patients.

The theory of blocking antibodies does not seem to have been demonstrated in allergy to pneumoallergens.

Although immunotherapy to aeroallergens, when optimally administered, has been clinically effective, in at least two independent studies, the changes in IgG antibody concentrations were unrelated to the clinical response to immunotherapy (15,16), suggesting that specific IgG might not be the protective mechanism. In addition, "rush" protocols are effective long before any changes in IgG antibody synthesis could occur. This has led to attempts to explain the efficacy of desensitization by the development of subtypes of IgG (15). However, this hypothesis was not supported by studies in which we examined the predictive value of grass pollen-specific IgG1, IgG2, IgG4, because it was observed that IgG4 increased quickly after the onset of immunotherapy, but that this level was irrelevant to the clinical outcome (17). The efficacy of desensitization has also been explained by increases in IgA or IgG secretion, but no precise correlation with clinical improvement of the patients has yet been found (18). Studies in mite allergy led to similar conclusion, suggesting that IgG levels during inhalant immunotherapy are likely to reflect the amount of injected antigen, rather than a protective effect. However, IgG may modulate the immune reaction through an intermediary of the network idiotype–anti-idiotype (19). The role of IgG in particular tissue antibody or mucosal secretion of antibodies needs to be further studied.

III. Effector Cells

Immunotherapy may act by reducing inflammatory cell recruitment, activation of mediators, or of their secretion by effector cells. When it is effective, specific immunotherapy is accompanied by a reduction in cutaneous (20–22), bronchial (20,23,24), nasal (25–27), or ocular (28,29) reactivity relative to the allergen during skin and provocation tests. In nasal provocation tests, one observes that not only the quantity of allergen necessary to provoke a reaction in the target organ is increased, but also that mediators of anaphylaxis (such as histamine) are released in lower amounts (30,31) and that there is a reduction in cellular recruitment during provocation (32,33). It is a phenomenon, therefore, involving a hyposensitization of the tissue, that is specific to the allergen. At the end of the specific immunotherapy treatment, after a period of several months or a few years, particularly for subjects who have a perennial allergy, the tissue reactivity recurs, often to the same extent as before, suggesting the importance of continuation of the specific immunotherapy.

Immunotherapy in mite-sensitive children has been reported to result in a decrease in mast cells in nasal brushings (34,35). Furthermore, grass pollen immunotherapy in adults was associated with a decrease in cutaneous mast cells numbers, including both "connective tissue" (tryptase- and chymase-containing) and "mucosal" (tryptase only) mast cells (36), as well as a reduction in histamine and prostaglandin (PG)D_2 levels in nasal secretions following allergen challenge (31). In ragweed-sensitive patients, conventional immunotherapy inhibited immedate release of mast cell mediators (30) and eosinophil numbers in nasal lavage in response to allergen provocation in an immunotherapy dose- and time-dependent fashion (32,33). Birch pollen immunotherapy inhibited the seasonal increase in bronchial responsiveness to histamine and an associated increases in eosinophils and eosinophil cationic protein (ECP) concentrations in bronchoalveolar lavage (BAL) fluid during the peak pollen season (37). Several studies have shown a decrease in basophil releasability for histamine, and one recent study demonstrated a reduction in histamine and leukotriene-C_4 production by basophils (only in response to allergen stimulation) following "rush" venom immunotherapy (38).

Tissue hyposensitization appears rapidly when the dose is sufficient, and it does not correlate with levels of immunoglobulins in serum or those secreted that are specific to the allergen (IgE or IgG; 39). On the other hand, it is often correlated with clinical improvements (16). This mechanism seems to occupy an important place in understanding the efficacy of specific immunotherapy to pneumoallergens.

Moreover, a reduction in cellular reactivity to the allergen has been shown in studies involving the degranulation of blood basophils and in those on platelet cytotoxicity (40). Rak et al. have conducted several elegant studies in which they investigated the activation of eosinophils and measured the levels of certain chemotactic factors in serum and in the bronchi during the pollen season (41,42). In patients who had not received specific immunotherapy, an increase in the levels of ECP in the serum (37) as well as chemotactic activity toward eosinophils was observed (43), whereas the appearance of these two mediators was blocked in desensitized subjects. In addition, a reduction of pulmonary inflammation during desensitization to extracts of birch pollen was demonstrated (44). Therefore, an associated cellular hyposensitization is likely to exist.

The mechanisms underlying this cellular and tissue hyposensitization are still poorly understood, but may well involve cytokines and histamine-releasing factors (45), despite that the direct specificity of the reaction tends to suggest another mechanism.

Direct effects of immunotherapy on inflammatory cells seem more likely to be relevant to account for rapid changes, particularly for "systemic" allergens such as venom. However, several recent studies have suggested that immunotherapy may have a prolonged effect, lasting several years following discontinuation (46,47), that is unlikely to be explained by these changes in view of the short half-life of inflammatory cells.

IV. Lymphocyte Response

A. Cytokines Secreted by $CD4^+$ Helper T Cells

The hallmarks of human allergic inflammation are IgE-dependent activation of mast cells and basophils and tissue eosinophilia in which cytokines play a major role. Murine $CD4^+$ T-cell clones were initially divided into three subsets, based on differences between their cytokine production profiles, as well as their functional properties (reviewed in Ref. 48). Although initial reports dealing with human T-cell clones did not demonstrate such a dichotomy—a major proportion of T-cell clones derived in vitro were of the Th0 phenotype (49–51)—it has now been firmly established that human $CD4^+$ T-cell subsets with restricted cytokine production profiles can be demonstrated in vitro and in vivo (reviewed in Ref. 52). Thus, similar to the mouse, three subsets of CD4$^+$ T helper–inducer cells have been identified in humans: CD4$^+$ T helper type 1 (Th1) cells that produce predominantly IL-2 and interferon (IFN)-γ on activation and no IL-4 and IL-5; CD4$^+$ Th2 helper cells that secrete predominantly IL-4 and IL-5, but low amounts of IL-2 and IFN-γ; and a third group called Th0 cells that secrete cytokines of both subsets on activation. Activated human T-cell clones, specific for bacterial antigens (53,54), were reminiscent of murine Th1 cells; whereas T-cell clones, generated from the peripheral blood or skin of atopic patients and specific for various allergens, including house dust and grass pollen (55–57), or *Toxocara canis* antigen (53), have a Th2-like cytokine reduction pattern in that they produce high levels of IL-4 and IL-5, but low or nondetectable levels of IFN-γ on activation (reviewed in Ref. 52).

The Th2 cytokine IL-4 (58–61) and the recently described IL-13 (62–66) play a critical role in allergy by inducing IgE heavy-chain isotype switching by B cells (67–71), whereas this process is inhibitable by the Thl cytokine IFN-γ (58) which, in turn, may be induced by IL-12 (72–75). IL-5 is a major selective growth factor for the differentiation, activation, and persistence of eosinophils (76–78) in tissues (possibly by inhibiting apoptosis of eosinophils). Thus, although in humans a strict dichotomy between T-cell subsets is not as clear as in the murine system (79), an imbalance of Thl and Th2 cells in favor of a polarization of allergen-specific T cells toward an IL-4–producing Th2-dominant phenotype has been proposed to be involved in IgE-mediated allergic disorders and asthma. Many observations made in vitro and in vivo support this notion. T cells secreting IL-4 and IL-5 are recruited and accumulate at the sites of allergic inflammation (52,63,80–86). Allergen-specific T-cell clones isolated from atopic individuals secrete high amounts of IL-4 and IL-5 and low amounts of IFN-γ and give help to B cells for IgE production (51,87,88). Furthermore, increased production of IL-4 by peripheral blood mononuclear cells (PBMC) of allergic patients compared with that of healthy individuals has been reported (89–96). However, the association between increased IL-4 production and atopic allergy has not been observed in several other studies (97–99).

B. Immunotherapy Induces a Shift of the T-Cell Phenotype

Immunotherapy may act by modifying the T-lymphocyte response to that of the subsequent natural allergen. Successful immunotherapy might be associated with a shift in the relative ratio in IL-4 and IFN-γ production, as a consequence of either a downregulation of the functional activity of allergen-specific Th2 cells or of an increased or induced Thl response (100). There is now good evidence that this may indeed occur.

Counsell et al. have shown that cat immunotherapy decreases the T-cell and skin test reactivity to the major allergen Fel d 1 (101). Studies of allergen-induced late responses in the skin (102) and the nose (103) have indicated that immunotherapy results in a decrease in CD4$^+$ cell recruitment and a reduction in local eosinophilia. These changes were accompanied by an increase in a subpopulation of $CD4^+$ cells expressing IFN-γ transcripts after allergen provocation, whereas cells expressing mRNA for IL-4 and IL-5 remained unchanged (102). In the target organ, these late increases in IFN-γ^+ cells out of season correlated closely with the clinical response to immunotherapy, represented by seasonal symptoms and medication requirements, which suggested that these upregulated Thl responses may be "protective," rather than simple bystander events (103). Studies of late cutaneous biopsies suggested that these responses may be amplified or sustained by local production of IL-12, a potent inducer of Thl responses. The cell source of IL-12 was identified as the tissue macrophage ($CD68^+$). A reciprocal association was observed between IL-12^+ cell numbers and IL-4^+ cells and a positive association with IFN-γ cells, which supports that the IFN-γ responses may be IL-12 driven (104). An alternative explanation for these observed increases in IFN-γ^+ cells may be the generation of allergen-specific $CD8^+$ T cells (105). Increases in $CD8^+$ cells have been observed in tissue (102) following conventional immunotherapy.

A series of recent studies on peripheral blood T cells of patients undergoing specific immunotherapy provide further support for a shift in Th cell responses. A decrease in IL-4 and an increase in IFN-γ were demonstrated following immunotherapy in bee venom-sensitive patients in a time-dependent fashion up to 8 weeks following a rush protocol (106). A decrease in IL-4 production by T cells, but no change in proliferative response or IFN-γ production, were observed in grass- and mite-sensitive patients after immunotherapy (107). Increases in IFN-γ and decreases in IL-4 production were found in short-term peripheral blood mononuclear cell cultures following venom immunotherapy (108). From these studies, reporting a modulation of the cytokine profiles by allergen-specific T cells, it has been suggested that a phenotypic switch from a Th2 to a Th0 (102,103) or a Thl cytokine phenotype (106–108) may be the basis of successful immunotherapy. Several other studies sustain this hypothesis. A decrease of serum IL-4 levels in allergic rhinitis patients following immunotherapy has also been reported (109). Moreover, the possibility that T cells are among the targets of immunotherapy is supported by the results of Akoum et al. who reported, when using in situ hybridization, that venom immunotherapy resulted in an altered cytokine mRNA pattern in peripheral blood T cells by decreasing IL-4 mRNA- and increasing IFN-γ mRNA-expressing cells (110), indicating that immunotherapy acts by modifying the phenotype of T cells at the single-cell level. Similarly, Jutel et al. observed that bee venom immunotherapy changed the cytokine secretion patterns of allergen-specific T cells by decreasing IL-4 and IL-5 and increasing IFN-γ production (106).

C. Mechanisms Underlying a Switch of the T-Cell Response by Immunotherapy

The mechanisms underlying this switch in the number of Thl and Th2 populations following immunotherapy are not fully understood, and the conditions of immunization under immunotherapy that could promote the generation of Thl responses instead of Th2, are a matter of current debate (111). Durham et al. reported an increase in the number of cells expressing the transcripts for IFN-γ following grass pollen immunotherapy. They proposed that its mechanisms of action might be the result of inhibition of allergen-induced T-cell and eosinophil recruitment, as well as of eosinophil activation at the sites of allergic inflammation, by increasing local Thl cells (103). Studies in the mouse have demonstrated that various factors can influence the differentiation of a naive T cell into a Th1 or a Th2 cell on activation. Factors determining Thl or Th2 responses include the nature of the antigen (or allergen) and allergen dose and the nature of antigen-presenting cell (APC). A high peptide–major histocompatibility complex (MHC) class I density on the surface of the APC and a strong interaction with the T-cell receptor (TCR) will promote a Thl response, whereas a lower density and a weaker interaction will favor the Th2 phenotype (112,113). High concentrations of allergens administered during immunotherapy would reduce IL-4 synthesis by T cells by altering the type of APC or monokines involved (114–116). The type of APC also influences the outcome of the T-cell response: macrophages tend to favor the induction of Th1 cells, and B cells appear to favor the induction of Th2 cells (117,118). Secrist et al. reported that low-dose allergen presentation by B cells or dendritic cells favors Th2 responses, whereas high-dose allergen processing and presentation by monocytes favors Thl responses by altering the cytokine profile of $CD4^+$ peripheral blood T cells. They have proposed that this mechanism may be responsible for successful immunotherapy (119). In addition, use of different adjuvants and allergen modification may be important.

Whether this shift occurs as a consequence of upregulation of a distinct subset of Th0/Th1 cells ("immune deviation"; 106) or because of induction of an allergen-specific T-cell tolerance of Th2/Th0 cells ("anergy"; 102,120,121) is not known. It has been hypothesized, in animal models, that immunotherapy could induce a state of nonresponsiveness, or clonal anergy, of certain T-cell subsets (allergen-specific Th2 cells), through a mechanism of tolerization in vivo (reviewed in Refs. 122,123). Hoyne et al. reported that intranasally administered high doses of the house dust mite allergen Der p 1-derived peptides might induce the development of T-cell tolerance to this antigen (124). These T cells from the tolerant mice, when restimulated in vitro produce low levels of cytokines and do not provide help for B cells (125). In an other study, allergen-specific Th2 cells could be rendered anergic by incubation with certain allergen T-cell epitopes; these anergic cells failed to produce IL-4 and IL-13 and also failed to give B cells help for IgE synthesis, even in the presence of exogenous IL-4 or IL-13 (123), suggesting that induction of T-cell nonresponsiveness may represent the underlying mechanisms for successful immunotherapy (126). However, approaches geared solely at inhibiting IL-4 synthesis or action may not be sufficient for decreasing persistent IgE levels in allergic patients (127). Higgins et al. have reported that the pretreatment of human T cells with a *Der p* I peptide renders them nonresponsive to a subsequent challenge with the house dust mite allergen, in association with a downregulation of membrane expression of the T-cell antigen receptor (128). Jarman et al. reported an inhibition of human T-cell responses to house dust mite allergens by a TCR peptide seen as a major component of the human house dust mite repertoire, and that this inhibition is mediated by the induction of a $CD8^+$ regulatory T-cell subset (129).

Studies in tissues suggest that immune deviation may be an important component of the mechanisms underlying specific immunotherapy. Although the T-cell surface marker CD28 is downregulated following anergy induction (130), studies of CD28 expression by PBMCs following venom immunotherapy have identified no downregulation of this marker, consistent with immune deviation (131). However, a recent study demonstrated a decrease in bee venom allergen phospholipase A_2 (PLA_2)-specific proliferation and reduced production of both type 2 (IL-4, IL-5, and IL-13), and type 1 (IL-2 and IFN-γ) cytokines in vitro by T-cell lines following bee venom immunotherapy (132). This T-cell tolerization was allergen-specific and partly reversible, because by culturing PBMC with antigen in the presence of IL-2 or IL-15, the specific proliferation and secretion of the type 1 T-cell cytokines could be restored, whereas the type 2 T-cell cytokines remained suppressed. These results provide the first evidence for the induction of anergy following immunotherapy in humans. However, the mechanisms of venom immunotherapy in nonatopic subjects may be different from those involved in immunotherapy for inhalant allergens in atopic patients.

Although the Th2 cytokine IL-4 plays a critical role in allergy by enhancing IgE synthesis, whereas the Thl cytokine IFN-γ has inhibitory properties, the immunotherapy-induced decrease of T-cell reactivity and IL-4 secretion can rarely be correlated with a decrease of serum IgE concentrations. Secrist et al. observed that, although IL-4 secretion was reduced following immunotherapy in allergic rhinitis-sensitive patients, the serum levels of total IgE were not significantly modified (107). Similarly, Jutel et al. showed that the decrease in IL-4 and IL-5 secretion, following bee venom immunotherapy, was not accompanied by a significant decrease in levels of specific IgE antibodies, whereas increased IgG concentrations became significant only after 9 months (106). Counsell et al. also did not find a modification of Fel d 1 IgE and IgG antibodies following immunotherapy (101). In the report of Adkis et al. in vitro produced and serum PLA_2-specific IgE and IgG4 antibodies slightly increased during immunotherapy, whereas the PLA-specific IgE/IgG4 ratio changed in favor of IgG4 (132). However, as discussed previously, a significant correlation between serum antibody levels and the clinical benefits of immunotherapy has rarely been observed (16).

D. Peptide-Mediated Immunotherapy

Because of the presence of B-cell epitopes on the whole molecule of native allergen, which may be recognized by IgE antibodies, the use of allergen extracts for immunotherapy may result in anaphylactic shocks. Recently, the cloning and the characterization of the primary structure of several major allergens made it possible to obtain pure allergen preparations and to generate allergen-derived synthetic peptides that have the linear amino acid sequence of the native allergen. T-cell epitopes have been identified on the sequence of various allergens, and synthetic peptides containing T-cell epitopes have been produced. Of particular interest, is the use of these synthetic peptides for the development of novel approaches in the treatment of allergies by allergen-specific immunotherapy by decreasing the risk and shortening the treatment.

The use of peptides for specific immunotherapy has only recently been investigated and limited data are available in humans. In animals, the effects of peptide immunotherapy have been investigated in allergic responses to the house dust mite Der p 1 (124,133,134), ragweed Amb 5 (135), and cat Fel d 1 allergens (136,137). Effects such as induction of peripheral T-cell tolerance to the entire protein, downregulation, or failure to secrete cytokines by allergen-specific T cells have been described in these studies (reviewed in Ref. 122). Another study has shown that the administration of high doses of the dominant T-cell epitope of Bet v 1 can downregulate the allergen-specific T-cell response by diminishing T-cell proliferation to the peptide and to the whole protein. Skin tests to Bet v 1 were also reduced, but the specific antiboby production was not modified (138). In humans, the exposure of Der p 1-specific Th2-like T-cell clones (139,140) and PLA_2-specific Th2/Th0 T-cell clones (141) to high doses of specific peptides, in a manner providing an incomplete activation of the T cells, induces a state of anergy on antigenic rechallenge. Clinical trials have been performed recently to test the efficacy of two synthetic peptides of 27 amino acids, IPC-1 and IPC-2, derived from the *Felis domesticus* cat allergen Fel d 1 chain I, in the treatment of the clinical symptoms of cat allergic patients. These peptides contain some, but not all, of the T-cell epitopes from the Fel d 1 molecule (136,142). In mice, subcutaneous tolerization with the peptides prevented the T-cell response to nasal challenge with cat allergen by decreasing the T-cell proliferation to the entire recombinant Fel d 1 chain I and suppressing peptide-induced IL-2, IL-4, and IFN-γ in vitro (136). In mice primed with Fel d 1, the peptides also induced a downregulation of the production of specific IgE in vivo (136). In humans, immunotherapy with Fel d 1 peptides resulted in a decrease of clinical symptoms of cat allergic patients and bronchial reactivity following nasal challenge with Fel d 1 in a cat room (143). Simons et al. reported, that immunotherapy with the Fel d 1 peptides did not modify IL-4, IL-10, or IFN-γ production in vitro (144). This result is in contrast to our own study in which immunotherapy with the Fel d 1 peptides of cat allergic individuals resulted in a significant increase of $PD_{20}FEV_1$ and was accompanied by a suppression of the in vitro IL-4 release by PBMC stimulated with a cat allergen extract, whereas the production of IFN-γ was not affected (Pène J; et al, submitted for publication). The differences between the two studies might be related to the fact that, in the study of Simons et al., the Fel d 1 peptides were administered as four weekly injections of 250 μg, whereas we found that IL-4 was significantly reduced only in the group of patients receiving injections of 750 μg. In addition, the optimal dose of Fel d 1 used for the stimulation of the PBMC was much higher than in our study, and we show that for elevated Fel d 1 concentrations, there was strong decrease in IL-4 production in vitro. Another trial has been made by using synthetic peptides, derived from the PLA_2 allergen of the bee venom, to two desensitized bee venom allergic patients (145).

Collectively, these results indicate that a modulation of ongoing immune responses to allergens by treatment with dominant T-cell epitope peptides represents a promising concept for immunotherapy in the future.

References

1. Malling H, Weeke B. Immunotherapy. Position Paper of the European Academy of Allergy and Clinical Immunology. Allergy 1993; 48(suppl 14):9–35.
2. Bousquet J, Michel F-B. Specific immunotherapy in asthma: is it effective? J Allergy Clin Immunol 1994; 94:1–11.
3. Lichtenstein L, Norman P, Kagey-Sobotka A, Adkinson N Jr, Golden D. The immunologic basis for the efficacy of immunotherapy. In: Pepys J, Ganterton MA, eds. Proceedings of the IX International Congress of Allergology and Clinical Immunology. Chester: Mcmillian Press, 1983:285–288.
4. Lichtenstein L, Ishizaka K, Norman P, Sobotka A, Hill B. IgE antibody measurements in ragweed hay fever. Relationship to clinical severity and the results of immunotherapy. J Clin Invest 1973; 52:472–482.
5. Gleich GJ, Zimmermann EM, Henderson LL, Yunginger JW. Effect of immunotherapy on immunoglobulin E and immunoglobulin G antibodies to ragweed antigens: a six-year prospective study. J Allergy Clin Immunol 1982; 70:261–271.
6. Leynadier F, Abuaf N, Halpern GM, Murrieta M, Garcia-Duarte C, Dry J. Blocking IgG antibodies after rush immunotherapy with mites. Ann Allergy 1986; 57:325–359.
7. Djurup R, Malling HJ. High IgG4 antibody level is associated with failure of immunotherapy with inhalant allergens. Clin Allergy 1987; 17:459–468.
8. Star M, Weinstock M. Studies in pollen allergy. The relationship between blocking antibody levels, and symptomatic relief following hyposensitization with Allpyral in hay fever subjects. Int Arch Allergy 1970; 38:514–521.
9. Golden DB, Meyers DA, Kagey-Sobotka A, Valentine MD, Lichtenstein LM. Clinical relevance of the venom-specific immunoglobulin G antibody level during immunotherapy. J Allergy Clin Immunol 1982; 69:489–493.
10. Visco V, Dolecek C, Denépoux S, Le Mao J, Guret C, Rousset F, Guinnepain MT, Kraft D, Valenta R, Weyer A, Banchereau J, Labecque S. Human IgG monoclonal antibodies that modulate the binding of specific IgE to birch pollen Bet v 1. J Immunol 1996; 157:956–962.
11. Van Der Zee JS, Aalberse RC. The role of IgG in immediate-type hypersensitivity. Eur Respir J 1991; 13:91s–96s.
12. Müller U, Helbling A, Bischof M. Predictive value of venom-specific IgE, IgG and IgG subclass antibodies in patients on immunotherapy with honey bee venom. Allergy 1989; 44:412–418.
13. Reisman RE. Should routine measurements of serum venom-specific IgG be a standard of practice in patients receiving venom immunotherapy? [editorial; comment]. J Allergy Clin Immunol 1992; 90:282–284.
14. Golden DB, Kwiterovich KA, Kagey-Sobotka A, Valentine MD, Lichtenstein LM. Discontinuing venom immunotherapy: outcome after five years. J Allergy Clin Immunol 1996; 97:579–587.
15. Djurup R, Osterballe O. IgG subclass antibody response in grass pollen-allergic patients

undergoing specific immunotherapy. Prognostic value of serum IgG subclass antibody levels early in immunotherapy. Allergy 1984; 39:433–441.
16. Bousquet J, Maasch H, Martinot B, Hejjaoui A, Wahl R, Michel FB. Double-blind, placebo-controlled immunotherapy with mixed grass-pollen allergoids. II. Comparison between parameters assessing the efficacy of immunotherapy. J Allergy Clin Immunol 1988; 82:439–446.
17. Bousquet J, Hejjaoui A, Michel F-B. Recent advances in specific immunotherapy for allergic rhinitis. Clin Exp Allergy 1991; 1:259–261.
18. Xia SF, Okuda M, Ohnishi M, Okubo K. Specific IgA and IgG antibodies to house dust mite *Dermatophagoides farinae* in nasal secretions. Aerugi 1994; 43:634–644.
19. Hebert J, Bernier D, Mourad W. Detection of auto-anti-idiotypic antibodies to Lol p 1 (rye I) IgE antibodies in human sera by the use of murine idiotypes: levels in atopic and nonatopic subjects and effects on immunotherapy. Clin Exp Immunol 1990; 80:413–419.
20. Bousquet J, Calvayrac P, Buerin B, Hejjaoui A, Dhivert H, Hewitt B, Michel F-B. Immunotherapy with a standardized *Dermatophagoides pteronyssimus* extract. I. In vivo and in vitro parameters after a short course of treatment. J Allergy Clin Immunol 1985; 76:734–744.
21. Bousquet J, Hejjaoui A, Skassa-Brociek W, Guérin B, Maasch HJ, Dhivert H, Michel F-B. Double-blind, placebo-controlled immunotherapy with mixed grass-pollen allergoids. I. Rush immunotherapy with allergoids and standardized orchard grass-pollen extract. J Allergy Clin Immunol 1987; 80:591–598.
22. Van Metre Te J, Marsh D, Adkinson NJ, Kagey-Sobotka A, Khattignavong A, Norman PSJ, Rosenberg GL. Immunotherapy decreases skin reactivity to cat extract. J Allergy Clin Immunol 1989; 83:888–889.
23. Warner JO, Price JF, Soothill JF, Hey EN. Controlled trial of hyposensitisation to *Dermatophagoides pteronyssinus* in children with asthma. Lancet 1978; 2:912–915.
24. Van Bever HP, Stevens WJ. Effect of hyposensitization upon the immediate and late asthmatic reaction and upon histamine reactivity in patients allergic to house dust mite (*Dermatophagoides pteronyssimus*). Eur Respir J 1992; 5:318–322.
25. Bousquet J, Coulomb Y, Arrendal H, Robinet-Levy M, Michel F-B. Total serum IgE concentrations in adolescents and adults using the phadebas IgE Prist technique. Allergy 1982; 37:397–406.
26. Bousquet J, Lebel B, Dhivert H, Bataille Y, Martinot B, Michel F-B. Nasal challenge with pollen grains, skin-prick tests and specific IgE in patients with grass pollen allergy. Clin Allergy 1987; 17:529–536.
27. Frostad AB, Grimmer O, Sandvik L, Aas K. Hyposensitization. Comparing a purified (refined) allergen preparation and a crude aqueous extract from timothy pollen. Allergy 1980; 35:81–95.
28. Moller C, Björksten B, Nilsson G, Dreborg S. The precision of the conjunctival provocation test. Allergy 1984; 39:37–41.
29. Moller C, Dreborg S, Lanner A, Björksten B. Oral immunotherapy of children with rhinoconjunctivitis due to birch pollen allergy. A double blind study. Allergy 1986; 41:271–279.
30. Creticos PS, Adkinson NF, Kagey-Sobotka A, et al. Nasal challenge with ragweed pollen in hay fever patients. Effect of immunotherapy. J Clin Invest 1985; 76:2247–2253.
31. Bousquet J, Becker WM, Hejjaoui A, Chanal I, Lebel B, Dhivert H, Michel F-B. Differences in clinical and immunologic reactivity of patients allergic to grass pollens and to multiple-pollen species. II. Efficacy of a double-blind, placebo-controlled, specific immunotherapy with standardized extracts. J Allergy Clin Immunol 1991; 88:43–53.
32. Furin MJ, Norman PS, Creticos PS, Proud D, Kagey-Sobotka A, Lichtenstein LM, Naclerio RM. Immunotherapy decreases antigen-induced eosinophil cell migration into the nasal cavity. J Allergy Clin Immunol 1991; 88:27–32.
33. Iliopoulos O, Proud D, Adkinson NFJ, Creticos PS, Norman PS, Kagey-Sobotka A, Lichtenstein LM, Naclerio RM. Effects of immunotherapy on the early, late, and rechallenge nasal reaction to provocation with allergen: changes in inflammatory media-

tors and cells. J Allergy Clin Immunol 1991; 87:855–866.
34. Otsuka H, Mezawa A, Ohnishi M, Okubo K, Seki H, Okuda M. Changes in nasal metachromatic cells during allergen immunotherapy. Clin Exp Allergy 21:115–119.
35. Hedlin G, Silber G, Naclerio R, Proud D, Lamas AM, Eggleston P, Adkinson NFJ. Comparison of the in-vivo and in-vitro response to ragweed immunotherapy in children and adults with ragweed-induced rhinitis. Clin Exp Allergy 1990; 20:491–500.
36. Durham S, Varney V, Gaga M, Jacobson M, Frew A, Kay A. Grass pollen immunotherapy decreases mast cell numbers in the skin. Proc Am Assoc Phys 1998. Submitted.
37. Rak S, Lowhagen O, Venge P. The effect of immunotherapy on bronchial hyperresponsiveness and eosinophil cationic protein in pollen-allergic patients. J Allergy Clin Immunol 1988; 82:470–480.
38. Jutel M, Muller UR, Fricker M, Rihs S, Pichler WJ, Dahinden C. Influence of bee venom immunotherapy on degranulation and leukotriene generation in human blood basophils. Clin Exp Allergy 1996; 26:1112–1118.
39. Hedlin G, Silber G, Schieken L, Naclerio R, Proud D, Eggleston P, Adkinson NFJ. Attenuation of allergen sensitivity early in the course of ragweed immunotherapy. J Allergy Clin Immunol 1989; 84:390–399.
40. Tsicopoulos A, Tonnel A-B, Wallaert B, Joseph M, Ramon P, Capron A. A circulating suppressive factor of platelet cytotoxic functions after rush immunotherapy in Hymenoptera venom hypersensitivity. J Immunol 1989; 142:2683–2686.
41. Rak S, Hallden G, Sorenson S, Margari V, Scheynius A. The effect of immunotherapy on T-cell subsets in peripheral blood and bronchoalveolar lavage fluid in pollen-allergic patients. Allergy 1993; 48:460–465.
42. Nagata M, Shibasaki M, Sakamoto Y, Fukuda T, Makino S, Yamamoto K, Dohi Y. Specific immunotherapy reduces the antigen-dependent production of eosinophil chemotactic activity from mononuclear cells in patients with atopic asthma. J Allergy Clin Immunol 1994; 94:160–166.
43. Rak S, Bjornson A, Hakanson L, Sorenson S, Venge P. The effect of immunotherapy on eosinophil accumulation and production of eosinophil chemotactic activity in the lung of subjects with asthma during natural pollen exposure. J Allergy Clin Immunol 1991; 88:878–888.
44. Rak S. Effects of immunotherapy on the inflammation in pollen asthma. Allergy 1993; 48:143–144.
45. Kuna P, Alam R, Kuzminska B, Rozniecki J. The effect of preseasonal immunotherapy on the production of histamine-releasing factor (HRF) by mononuclear cells from patients with seasonal asthma: results of a double-blind, placebo-controlled, randomized study. J Allergy Clin Immunol 1989; 83:816–824.
46. Des Roches A, Paradis L, Knani J, Hejjaoui A, Dhivert H, Chanez P, Bousquet J. Immunotherapy with a standardized *Dermatophagoides pteronyssinus* extract 5. Duration of the efficacy of immunotherapy after its cessation. Allergy 1996; 51:430–433.
47. Durham S, Varney V, Gaga M, Frew A, Jacobson M, Kay A. Grass pollen immunotherapy remains effective 3 years after discontinuation: a double-blind, placebo-controlled withdrawal study. Clin Exp Allergy 1998. In press.
48. Mosmann TR, Coffman RL. T_HI and T_H2 cells: different patterns of lymphokine secretion lead to different functional properties. Annu Rev Immunol 1989; 7:145–173.
49. Paliard X, Yssel H, Blanchard D, Waitz JA, DeVries JE, Spits H. Antigen specific and MHC nonrestricted cytotoxicity of T cell receptor alpha beta$^+$ and gamma delta$^+$ human T cell clones isolated in IL-4. J Immunol 1988; 143:452–457.
50. Maggi E, Del Prete G, Macchia D, Parronchi P, Tiri A, Chrétien I, Ricci M, Romagnani S. Profiles of lymphokine activities and helper function for IgE in human T cell clones. Eur J Immunol 1988; 18:1045–1050.
51. Parronchi P, Macchia D, Piccinni MP, Biswas P, Simonelli C, Maggi E, Ricci M, Ansari AA, Romagnani S. Allergen- and bacterial antigen-specific T-cell clones established from atopic donors show a different profile of cytokine production. Proc Natl Acad Sci USA 1991; 88:4538–4542.

52. Romagnani S. Lymphokine production by human T cells in disease states. Annu Rev Immunol 1994; 12:227–257.
53. Del Prete GF, De Carli M, Mastromauro C, Biagiotti R, Macchia D, Falagiani P, Ricci M, Romagnani S. Purified protein derivative of *Mycobacterium tuberculosis* and excretory–secretory antigen(s) of *Toxocara canis* expand in vitro human T cells with stable and opposite (type 1 T helper or type 2 T helper) profile of cytokine production. J Clin Invest 1991; 88:346–350.
54. Yssel H, Shanafelt MC, Soderberg C, Schneider PV, Anzola J, Peltz G. *Borrelia burgdorferi* activates a T helper type 1-like T cell subset in Lyme arthritis. J Exp Med 1991; 174:593–601.
55. Parronchi P, Manetti R, Simonelli C, Rugiu FS, Piccinni MP, Maggi E, Romagnani S. Cytokine production by allergen (Der p 1)-specific $CD4^+$ T cell clones derived from a patient with severe atopic disease. Int J Clin Lab Res 1991; 21:186–189.
56. Wierenga EA, Snoek M, De Groot C, Chrétien I, Bos JD, Jansen HM, Kapsenberg ML. Evidence for compartmentalization of functional subsets of $CD2^+$ T lymphocytes in atopic patients. J Immunol 1990; 144:4651–4656.
57. Yssel H, Johnson KE, Schneider PV, Wideman J, Terr A, Kastelein R, De Vries JE. T cell activation-inducing epitopes of the house dust mite allergen Der p 1. Proliferation and lymphokine production patterns by Der p 1-specific $CD4^+$ T cell clones. J Immunol 1992; 148:738–745.
58. Pène J, Rousset F, Brière F, Chrétien I, Bonnefoy JY, Spits H, Yokota T, Arai N, Arai K, Banchereau J, De Vries JE. IgE production by normal human lymphocytes is induced by interleukin 4 and suppressed by interferons gamma and alpha and prostaglandin E_2. Proc Natl Acad Sci USA 1988; 85:6880–6884.
59. Pène J, Rousset F, Brière F, Chrétien I, Paliard X, Banchereau J, Spits H, De Vries JE. IgE production by normal human B cells induced by alloreactive T cell clones is mediated by IL-4 and suppressed by IFN-gamma. J Immunol 1988; 141:1218–1224.
60. Del Prete G, Maggi E, Parronchi P, Chrétien I, Tiri A, Macchia D, Ricci M, Banchereau J, De Vries J, Romagnani S. IL-4 is an essential factor for the IgE synthesis induced in vitro by human T cell clones and their supernatants. J Immunol 1988; 140:4193–4198.
61. Vercelli D, Jabara HH, Arai K, Geha RS. Induction of human IgE synthesis requires interleukin 4 and T/B cell interactions involving the T cell receptor/CD3 complex and MHC class II antigens. J Exp Med 1989; 169:1295–1307.
62. Dolecek C, Steinberger P, Susani M, Kraft D, Valenta R, Boltznitulescu G. Effects of IL-4 and IL-13 on total and allergen specific IgE production by cultured PBMC from allergic patients determined with recombinant pollen allergens, Clin Exp Allergy 1995; 25:879–889.
63. Pawankar RU, Okuda M, Hasegawa S, Suzuki K, Yssel H, Okubo K, Okumura K, Ra CS. Interleukin-13 expression in the nasal mucosa of perennial allergic rhinitics. Am J Respir Crit Care Med 1995; 152:2059–2067.
64. De Vries JE, Zurawski G. Immunoregulatory properties of IL-13: its potential role in atopic disease. Int Arch Allergy Immunol 1995; 106:175–179.
65. Garraud O, Nkenfou C, Bradley JE, Nutman TB. Differential regulation of antigen-specific IgG4 and IgE antibodies in response to recombinant filarial proteins. Int Immunol 1996; 8:1841–1848.
66. Levy F, Kristofic C, Heusser C, Brinkmann V. Role of IL-13 in CD4 T cell-dependent IgE production in atopy. Int Arch Allergy Immunol 1997; 112:49–58.
67. Lundgren M, Persson U, Larsson P, Magnusson C, Smith CI, Hammarstrom L, Severinson E. Interleukin 4 induces synthesis of IgE and IgG4 in human B cells. Eur J Immunol 1989; 19:1311–1315.
68. Gascan H, Gauchat JF, Aversa G, Van Vlasselaer P, De Vries JE. Anti-CD40 monoclonal antibodies or $CD4^+$ T cell clones and IL-4 induce IgG4 and IgE switching in purified human B cells via different signaling pathways. J Immunol 1991; 147:8–13.
69. Gascan H, Gauchat JF, Roncarolo M-G, Yssel H, Spits H, De Vries JE. Human B cell

clones can be induced to proliferate and to switch to IgE and IgG4 synthesis by interleukin 4 and a signal provided by activated CD4+ T cell clones. J Exp Med 1991; 173:747–750.

70. Punnonen J, Aversa G, Cocks BG, McKenzie AN, Menon S, Zurawski G, De Waal-Malefyt R, De Vries JE. Interleukin 13 induces interleukin 4-independent IgG4 and IgE synthesis and CD23 expression by human B cells. Proc Natl Acad Sci USA 1993; 90:3730–3734.
71. Carballido JM, Schols D, Namikawa R, Zurawski S, Zurawski G, Roncarolo MG, De Vries JE. IL-4 induces human B cell maturation and IgE synthesis in SCID-hu mice—inhibition of ongoing IgE production by in vivo treatment with an IL-4/IL-13 receptor antagonist. J Immunol 1995; 155:4162–4170.
72. Marshall JD, Secrist H De Kruyff RH, Wolf SF, Umetsu DT. IL-12 inhibits the production of IL-4 and IL-10 in allergen-specific human CD4+ T lymphocytes. J Immunol 1995; 155:111–117.
73. De Kruyff RH, Fang Y, Wolf SF, Umetsu DT. IL-12 inhibits IL-4 synthesis in keyhole limpet hemocyanin-primed CD4+ T cells through an effect on antigen-presenting cells. J Immunol 1995; 154:2578–2587.
74. Bradley LM, Dalton DK, Croft M. A direct role for IFN-gamma in regulation of Th1 cell development. J Immunol 1996; 157:1350–1358.
75. Hilkens CMU, Snijders A, Vermeulen H, Van Der Meide PH, Wierenga EA, Kapsenberg ML. Accessory cell-derived IL-12 and prostaglandin E(2) determine the IFN-gamma level of activated human CD4(+) T cells. J Immunol 1996; 156:1722–1727.
76. Lopez AF, Sanderson CJ, Gamble JR, Campbell HD, Young IG, Vadas MA. Recombinant human interleukin 5 is a selective activator of human eosinophil function. J Exp Med 1988; 167:219–224.
77. Walker C, Virchow J Jr, Bruijnzeel PL, Blaser K. T cell subsets and their soluble products regulate eosinophilia in allergic and nonallergic asthma. J Immunol 1991; 146:1829–1835.
78. Bentley AM, Meng Q, Robinson DS, Hamid Q, Kay AB, Durham SR. Increases in activated T lymphocytes, eosinophils, and cytokine mRNA expression for interleukin-5 and granulocyte/macrophage colony-stimulating factor in bronchial biopsies after allergen inhalation challenge in atopic asthmatics. Am J Respir Cell Mol Biol 1993; 8:35–42.
79. Kelso A. Th1 and Th2 subsets: paradigms lost? Immunol Today 1995; 16:374–379.
80. Maggi E, Biswas P, Del-Prete G, Parronchi P, Macchia D, Simonelli C, Emmi L, De-Carli M, Tiri A, Ricci M, Romagnani S. Accumulation of Th-2-like helper T cells in the conjunctiva of patients with vernal conjunctivitis. J Immunol 1991; 146:1169–1174.
81. Kapsenberg ML, Wierenga EA, Bos JD, Jansen HM. Functional subsets of allergen-reactive human CD4+ T cells. Immunol Today 1991; 12:392–395.
82. Hamid Q, Azzawi M, Ying S, et al. Expression of mRNA for interleukin-5 in mucosal bronchial biopsies from asthma. J Clin Invest 1991; 87:1541–1546.
83. Robinson DS, Hamid Q, Ying S, Tsicopoulos A, Barkans J, Bentley AM, Corrigan C, Durham SR, Kay AB. Predominant TH2-like bronchoalveolar T-lymphocyte population in atopic asthma. N Engl J Med 1992; 326:298–304.
84. Durham SR, Ying S, Varney VA, Jacobson MR, Sudderick RM, Mackay IS, Kay AB, Hamid QA. Cytokine messenger RNA expression for IL-3, IL-4, IL-5, and granulocyte/macrophage-colony-stimulating factor in the nasal mucosa after local allergen provocation: relationship to tissue eosinophilia. J Immunol 1992; 148:2390–2394.
85. Robinson DS, Ying S, Bentley AM, Meng Q, North J, Durham SR, Kay AB, Hamid Q. Relationships among numbers of bronchoalveolar lavage cells expressing messenger ribonucleic acid for cytokines, asthma symptoms, and airway methacholine responsiveness in atopic asthma. J Allergy Clin Immunol 1993; 92:397–403.
86. Hamid Q, Naseer T, Minshall EW, Song YL, Boguniewicz M, Leung DYM. In vivo expression of IL-12 and IL-13 in atopic dermatitis. J Allergy Clin Immunol 1996; 98:225–231.
87. Wierenga EA, Snoek M, Bos JD, Jansen HM, Kapsenberg ML. Comparison of diversity

and function of house dust mite-specific T lymphocyte clones from atopic and non-atopic donors. Eur J Immunol 1990; 20:1519–1526.
88. Van Der Heijden FL, Wierenga EA, Bos JD, Kapsenberg ML. High frequency of IL-4-producing CD4+ allergen-specific T lymphocytes in atopic dermatitis lesional skin. J Invest Dermatol 1991; 97:389–394.
89. Rousset F, Robert J, Andary M, Bonnin JP, Souillet G, Chrétien I, Brière F, Pène J, De Vries JE. Shifts in interleukin-4 and interferon-gamma production by T cells of patients with elevated serum IgE levels and the modulatory effects of these lymphokines on spontaneous IgE synthesis. J Allergy Clin Immunol 1991; 87:58–69.
90. Gagnon R, Lian J, Boutin Y, Hebert J. Seasonal enhancement of IL-4 induced IgE synthesis by peripheral blood mononuclear cells of atopic patients. Clin Exp Allergy 1993; 23:498–503.
91. Gagnon R, Akoum A, Hebert J. Lol p 1-induced IL-4 and IFN-gamma production by peripheral blood mononuclear cells of atopic and nonatopic subjects during and out of the pollen season. J Allergy Clin Immunol 1993; 91:950–956.
92. Pène J, Rivier A, Lagier B, Becker WM, Michel F-B, Bousquet J. Differences in IL-4 release by PBMC are related with heterogeneity of atopy. Immunology 1994; 81:58–64.
93. Lagier B, Pons N, Rivier A, Chanal I, Chanez P, Bousquet J, Pène J. Seasonal variations of interleukin-4 and interferon-gamma release by peripheral blood mononuclear cells from atopic subjects stimulated by polyclonal activators. J Allergy Clin Immunol 1995; 96:932–940.
94. Fujishima H, Takeuchi T, Shinozaki N, Saito I, Tsubota K. Measurement of IL-4 in tears of patients with seasonal allergic conjunctivitis and vernal keratoconjunctivitis. Clin Exp Immunol 1995; 102:395–398.
95. André F, Pène J, André C. Interleukin-4 and interferon-gamma production by peripheral blood mononuclear cells from food-allergic patients. Allergy 1996; 51:350–355.
96. Esnault S, Benbernou N, Lavaud F, Shin HC, Potron G, Guenounou M. Differential spontaneous expression of mRNA for IL-4, IL-10, IL-13, IL-2 and interferon-gamma (IFN-gamma) in peripheral blood mononuclear cells (PBMC) from atopic patients. Clin Exp Immunol 1996; 103:111–118.
97. Garlepp MJ, Rose AH, Bowman RV, Mavaddat N, Dench J, Holt BJ, Baron-Hay M, Holt PG, Robinson BW. A clonal analysis of lung T cells derived by bronchoalveolar lavage of healthy individuals. Immunology 1992; 77:31–37.
98. Pène J, Lagier B, Rivier A, Chanez P, Vendrell JP, Bousquet J. Phenotype of T cell clones obtained from bronchial biopsies and peripheral blood from three asthmatics. Cell Biol Int 1993; 17:353–357.
99. Krug N, Madden J, Redington AE, Lackie P, Djukanovic R, Schauer U, Holgate ST, Frew AJ, Howarth PH. T-cell cytokine profile evaluated at the single cell level in BAL and blood in allergic asthma. Am J Respir Cell Mol Biol 1996; 14:319–326.
100. Durham SR, Varney V, Gaga M, Frew AJ, Jacobson M, Kay AB. Immunotherapy and allergic inflammation. Clin Exp Allergy 1991; 1:206–210.
101. Counsell CM, Greenstein JL, Garman RD, Ohman JL. Cat immunotherapy decreases T cell reactivity and skin test reactivity to Fel d 1, the major allergen of cat allergy (abstr). J Allergy Clin Immunol 1994; 93:231.
102. Varney VA, Hamid QA, Gaga M, Ying S, Jacobson M, Frew AJ, Kay AB, Durham SR. Influence of grass pollen immunotherapy on cellular infiltration and cytokine mRNA expression during allergen induced late phase cutaneous responses. J Clin Invest 1993; 92:644–651.
103. Durham SR, Ying S, Varney VA, Jacobson MR, Sudderick RW, McKay IS, Kay AB, Hamid OA. Grass pollen immunotherapy inhibits allergen-induced infiltration of CD4(+) T lymphocytes and eosinophils in the nasal mucosa and increases the number of cells expressing messenger RNA for interferon-gamma. J Allergy Clin Immunol 1996; 97:1356–1365.
104. Hamid QA, Schotman E, Jacobson MR, Walker SM, Durham SR. Increases in IL-12

messenger RNA⁺ cells accompany inhibition of allergen-induced late skin responses after successful grass pollen immunotherapy. J Allergy Clin Immunol 1997; 99:254–260.
105. Renz H, Lack G, Saloga J, Schwinzer R, Bradley K, Loader J, Kupfer A, Larsen GL, Gelfand EW. Inhibition of IgE production and normalization of airways responsiveness by sensitized CD8 T cells in a mouse model of allergen-induced sensitization. J Immunol 1994; 152:351–360.
106. Jutel M, Pichler WJ, Skrbic D, Urwyler A, Dahinden C, Muller UR. Bee venom immunotherapy results in decrease of IL-4 and IL-5 and increase of IFN-gamma secretion in specific allergen-stimulated T cell cultures. J Immuonl 1995; 154:4187–4194.
107. Secrist H, Chelen CJ, Wen Y, Marshall JD, Umetsu DT. Allergen immunotherapy decreases interleukin 4 production in $CD4^+$ T cells from allergic individuals. J Exp Med 1993; 178:2123–2130.
108. McHugh SM, Deighton J, Stewart AG, Lachmann PJ, Ewan PW. Bee venom immunotherapy induces a shift in cytokine responses from a T_H-2 to a T_H-1 dominant pattern: Comparison of rush and conventional immunotherapy. Clin Exp Allergy 1995; 25:828–838.
109. Ohashi Y, Nakai Y, Okamoto H, Ohno Y, Sakamoto H, Sugiura Y, Kakinoki Y, Tanaka A, Kishimoto K, Washio Y, Hayashi M. Serum level of interleukin-4 in patients with perennial allergic rhinitis during allergen-specific immunotherapy. Scand J Immunol 1996; 43:680–686.
110. Akoum H, Tsicopoulos A, Vorng H, Wallaert B, Dessaint J-P, Joseph M, Hamid Q, Tonnel A-B. Venom immunotherapy modulates interleukin-4 and interferon-gamma messenger RNA expression of peripheral T lymphocytes. Immunology 1996; 87:593–598.
111. Hoyne GF, Lamb JR. Peptide-mediated regulation of the allergic immune response. Immunol Cell Biol 1996; 74:180–186.
112. Racioppi L, Ronchese F, Matis LA, Germain RN. Peptide–major histocompatibility complex class II complexes with mixed agonist/antagonist properties provide evidence for ligand-related differences in T cell receptor-dependent intracellular signaling. J Exp Med 1993; 177:1047–1060.
113. Pfeiffer C, Stein J, Southwood S, Ketelaar H, Sette A, Bottomly K. Altered peptide ligands can control CD4 T lymphocyte differentiation in vivo. J Exp Med 1995; 1841:1569–1574.
114. HayGlass KT, Stefura BP. Anti interferon gamma treatment blocks the ability of glutaraldehyde polymerized allergens to inhibit specific IgE responses. J Exp Med 1991; 173:279–285.
115. De Kruyff RH, Fang Y, Umetsu DT. IL-4 synthesis by in vivo primed keyhole limpet hemocyanin specific $CD4^+$ T cells. I. Influence of antigen concentration and antigen presenting cell type. J Immunol 1992; 149:3468–3476.
116. Manetti R, Parronchi P, Giudizi MG, Piccinni M-P, Maggi E, Trinchieri G, Romagnani S. Natural killer cell stimulatory factor (interleukin 12 [IL-12]) induces T helper type 1 (Th1) specific immune responses and inhibits the development of IL-4 producing Th cells. J Exp Med 1993; 177:1199–1204.
117. Gajewski TF, Pinnas M, Wong T, Fitch FW. Murine Th1 and Th2 clones proliferate optimally in response to distinct antigen-presenting cell populations. J Immunol 1991; 146:1750–1758.
118. Schmitz J, Assenmacher M, Radbruch A. Regulation of T helper cell cytokine expression: functional dichotomy of antigen-presenting cells. Eur J Immunol 1993; 23:191–199.
119. Secrist H, De Kruyff RH, Umetsu DT. Interleukin 4 production by CD4(+) T cells from allergic individuals is modulated by antigen concentration and antigen-presenting cell type. J Exp Med 1995; 181:1081–1089.
120. Lamb JR, Skidmore BJ, Green N, Chiller JM, Feldmann M. Induction of tolerance in influenza virus-immune T lymphocyte clones with synthetic peptides of influenza hemagglutinin. J Exp Med 1983; 157:1434–1447.
121. Fasler S, Aversa G, Terr A, Thestrup-Pedersen K, De Vries JE, Yssel H. Peptide-induced anergy in allergen-specific human Th2 cells results in lack of cytokine production and B

cell help for IgE synthesis—reversal by IL-2, not by IL-4 or IL-13. J Immunol 1995; 155:4199–4206.

122. Hoyne GF, Kristensen NM, Yssel H, Lamb JR. Peptide modulation of allergen-specific immune responses. Curr Opin Immunol 1995; 7:757–761.

123. Yssel H, Fasler S, Lamb J, De Vries JE. Induction of non-responsiveness in human allergen-specific type 2 T helper cells. Curr Opin Immunol 1994; 6:847–852.

124. Hoyne GF, Askonas BA, Hetzel C, Thomas WR, Lamb JR. Regulation of house dust mite responses by intranasally administered peptide: transient activation of CD4(+) T cells precedes the development of tolerance in vivo. Int Immunol 1996; 8:335–342.

125. Hoyne GF, Bourne T, Krsitensen N, Hetzel C, Lamb J. From epitopes to peptides to immunotherapy. Clin Immunol Immunopathol 1996; 80:S23–S30.

126. De Vries JE, Yssel H. Modulation of the human IgE response. Eur Respir J 1996; 9:S58–S62.

127. Savelkoul HFJ, Vanommen R. Role of IL-4 in persistent IgE formation. Eur Respir J 1996; 9:S67–S71.

128. Higgins JA, Lamb JR, Marsh SG, Tonks S, Hayball JD, Rosen-Bronson S, Bodmer JG, O'Hehir RE. Peptide-induced nonresponsiveness of HLA-DP restricted human T cells reactive with *Dermatophagoides* spp. (house dust mite). J Allergy Clin Immunol 1992; 90:749.

129. Jarman ER, Hawrylowicz CM, Panagiotopolou E, O'Hehir RE, Lamb JR. Inhibition of human T cell responses to house dust mite allergens by a T cell receptor peptide. J Allergy Clin Immunol 1994; 94:844–852.

130. Lake RA, O'Hehir RE, Verhoef A, Lamb JR. CD28 mRNA rapidly decays when activated T cells are functionally anergized with specific peptide. Int Immunol 1993; 5:461–466.

131. Tsicopoulos A, Labalette M, Akoum H, Duez C, Wallaert B, Dessaint JP, Tonnel AB. CD28 expression is increased in venom allergic patients but is not modified by specific immunotherapy. Clin Exp Allergy 1996; 26:1119–1124.

132. Akdis CA, Akdis M, Blesken T, Wymann D, Alkan SS, Möller U, Blaser K. Epitope-specific T cell tolerance to phospholipase A_2 in bee venom immunotherapy and recovery by IL-2 and IL-15 in vitro. J Clin Invest 1996; 98:1676–1683.

133. Hoyne GF, O'Hehir RE, Wraith DC, Thomas WR, Lamb JR. Inhibition of T cell and antibody responses to house dust mite allergen by inhalation of the dominant T cell epitope in naive and sensitized mice. J Exp Med 1993; 178:1783–1788.

134. Hoyne GF, Callow MG, Kuo MC, Thomas WR. Inhibition of T cell responses by feeding peptides containing major and cryptic epitopes: studies with the Der p 1 allergen. Immunology 1994; 83:190–195.

135. Jenkins MD, Schwartz RH. Antigen presentation by chemically modified splenocyptes induces antigen-specific T cell unresponsiveness in vitro and in vivo. J Exp Med 1987; 165:302.

136. Briner TJ, Kuo MC, Keating KM, Rogers BL, Greenstein JL. Peripheral T-cell tolerance induced in naive and primed mice by subcutaneous injection of peptides from the major cat allergen Fel d 1. Proc Natl Acad Sci USA 1993; 90:7608–7612.

137. Rogers BL, Bond JF, Craig SJ, Nault AK, Segal DB, Morgenstern JP, Chen MS, Bizinkauskas CB, Counsell CM, Lussier AM, et al. Potential therapeutic recombinant proteins comprised of peptides containing recombined T cell epitopes. Mol Immunol 1994; 31:955–966.

138. Bauer L, Bohle B, Jahnschmid B, Widermann U, Daser A, Renz H, Kraft D, Ebner C. Modulation of the allergic immune response in BALB/c mice by subcutaneous injection of high doses of the dominant T cell epitope from the major birch pollen allergen Bet v 1. Clin Exp Immunol 1997; 107:536–541.

139. O'Hehir RE, Yssel H, Verma S, De Vries JE, Spits H, Lamb JR. Clonal analysis of differential lymphokine production in peptide and superantigen induced T cell anergy. Int Immunol 1991; 3:819–826.

140. O'Hehir RE, Aguilar BA, Schmidt TJ, Gollnick SO, Lamb JR. Functional inactivation of

Dermatophagoides spp. (house dust mite) reactive human T-cell clones. Clin Exp Allergy 1991; 21:209–215.

141. Faith A, Akdis A, Blaser K. Anergy induction in cloned phospholipase A_2-specific T cells of Th2 functional phenotype (abstr). J Allergy Clin Immunol 1996; 97:426.
142. Bond JF, Brauer AW, Segal DB, Nault AK, Rogers BL, Kuo MC. Native and recombinant Fel d 1 as probes into the relationship of allergen structure to human IgE immunoreactivity. Mol Immunol 1993; 30:1529–1541.
143. Norman PS, Ohman JL Jr, Long AA, Creticos P, Gefter MA, Shaked Z, Wood RA, Eggleston PA, Hafner KB, Rao P, Lichtenstein M, Jones NH, Nicodemus CF. Treatment of cat allergy with T-cell reactive peptides. Am J Respir Crit Care Med 1996; 154:1623–1628.
144. Simons FER, Imada M, Li Y, Watson WTA, HayGlass KT. Fel d 1 peptides: effect on skin tests and cytokine synthesis in cat-allergic human subjects. Int Immunol 1996; 8:1937–1945.
145. Müller U, Fricker M, Akdis J, Carballido J, Blaser K. Successful immunotherapy with T-cell epitopes of bee venom phospholipase A_2 (PLA) in patients with bee venom (BV) allergy (abstr). J Allergy Clin Immunol 1995; 97:426.

12

Objectives of Immunotherapy in Asthma

ANTHONY J. FREW

Southampton General Hospital
Southampton, England

I. Background

Asthma is a common chronic disease of young adults and children, with a considerable amount of morbidity. The economic effects of asthma are substantial, both because of lost working days and in terms of health care costs, with asthma now consuming 11% of the U.K. National Health Services' (NHS) drug bill. The prevalence of asthma appears to be rising in many Western countries including the United Kingdom (1); hospital admission rates for asthma have increased markedly over the last 30 years, particularly for children (2), and many adults with asthma lose time from work owing to asthma (3). Current forms of antiasthma treatment are aimed at suppressing the airways inflammation that is a characteristic feature of the disorder. None of these treatments is curative, and asthma recurs rapidly on ceasing treatment. Moreover, none of the current drug therapies is directed against agents that might cause asthma. Allergen avoidance has been proposed as a potentially useful maneuver in those with allergic asthma, but although extreme forms of allergen avoidance (e.g., admission to a hospital or sending children to holiday homes at higher altitudes), can improve the control of asthma (4,5), there is little evidence that such benefit can be achieved by the more modest forms of allergen avoidance that can be achieved in suburban homes (6,7), nor is the improvement seen at the higher altitudes sustained once the children return to sea level (5).

There is thus scope for improving asthma care and for identifying allergen-specific therapies. Specific-allergen immunotherapy (SIT) offers the possibility of deviating the immune response away from the allergic pattern toward a more-protective or less-damaging response. However, SIT remains controversial as a treatment for asthma because of limited trial data and various potential side effects. Another important, but separate possible use of SIT, is to treat patients at high risk of developing asthma in a manner to prevent or delay the onset of airways disease.

Allergen immunotherapy was introduced in the second decade of the 20th century by investigators at St. Mary's Hospital, London (8,9). This form of therapy became popular in North America and in Europe, but significant differences in practice have developed on either side of the Atlantic. There is no doubt that SIT is effective in the treatment of allergic rhinitis, and it remains the treatment of choice for severe wasp and bee venom hypersensitivity (10,11). The value of SIT as a primary treatment for asthma, however, has been more controversial. Immunotherapy was widely used to treat allergic asthma in the United Kingdom before 1986, but evidence of severe adverse reactions, including few fatalities, has led to SIT being abandoned for asthma treatment in the United Kingdom (12), although asthma remains a common indication for SIT in North America and continental Europe.

The efficacy of SIT in adult asthma has been assessed in many trials over the last 40 years. The results of these studies are often difficult to interpret, either because poor quality allergen extracts were used or because of poor study design. Many trials were not placebo-controlled; they were either open or single-blind, and usually, only small numbers of patients were treated.

II. Appropriate Subject Selection and Endpoints

The two main keys to success in designing any clinical trial are the application of appropriate criteria for subject recruitment and the selection of appropriate clinical endpoints (Table 1). When assessing improvement in asthma, it is important to remember that most patients with atopic asthma have relatively mild disease and are usually easy to control with standard doses of conventional antiasthma drugs. Cases of severe disease are relatively few, and the role of allergy in their disease is often less obvious than in mild cases. In mild cases, resting spirometry will often be close to predicted values, so there is little scope for improvement in simple spirometric measures, such as the 1-sec forced expiratory volume (FEV_1). Peak expiratory flow rates (PEFR) may show improvement, especially the early morning values, which are most likely to be reduced below the patient's best possible value. Objective measures of bronchial irritability are more useful markers; and a shift in the concentration of histamine or methacholine needed to induce a 20% fall in FEV_1 (PC_{20}) is commonly used. This measurement can be quite variable within individuals, so the minimum change that would be clinically significant is a change of at least one-doubling dilution in the PC_{20}. Other bronchial challenge tests, such as exercise challenge or adenosine inhalation, may provide additional insights into the ability of an

Table 1 Endpoints for Trials of Specific Immunotherapy in Asthma

Spirometry	Airflow obstruction	FEV_1, PEFR
	Bronchial irritability	Histamine/methacholine PC_{20}
Symptoms	Wheeze, nocturnal waking, cough, breathlessness, time off work or school (diary cards or visual analog scales)	
Drug use	Bronchodilator use as surrogate for symptoms	
Cost/benefit	Reduction in other drugs, lost work, compared with costs of SIT and time lost owing to SIT	
Safety		
Immunology	Allergen-specific IgG4 skin test responses	
	Nasal allergen challenge responses	
	Inhalation allergen challenge responses	

antiasthma treatment to prevent acute attacks. Both these parameters depend indirectly on the PC_{20}, so again, it is important to consider statistical and biological significance separately.

Although these challenge models are useful surrogates for evaluating antiasthma treatment, more credence is placed on improvements in the symptoms or progression of the disease than on protection against laboratory challenges. Two principal study designs are used for such field trials: (1) add-on studies that use the trial treatment in addition to existing therapy and assess efficacy in terms of improved lung function or improved symptom scores; (2) substitution studies in which the trial treatment is given and then an attempt is made to reduce concomitant medication while maintaining lung function and symptom scores at a constant level. Some studies try to combine these two approaches, but typically this results in unclear results or in poor statistical power. Lately, there has been a move to assess efficacy in terms of improvements in quality of life or as health gain per unit cost. These analyses are still relatively unsophisticated and require careful validation to ensure that the quality of life instrument is sensitive to the illness being studied and that the economic model is realistic.

Finally, many trials of SIT have used laboratory surrogate markers of efficacy, such as changes in IgG subclasses (13,14), in vivo challenges of the nose (15,16), or skin test responses (17). Although such measures undoubtedly do change, and may shed light on the mechanism of action of SIT, they cannot be used to provide direct evidence of clinical effectiveness until there is evidence that they discriminate between responders and nonresponders or correlate very tightly with changes in symptom or drug scores.

A. Measures of Efficacy in SIT Trials

Turning to look at trials of immunotherapy for asthma, three double-blind placebo-controlled (DBPC) studies have found that SIT has a beneficial effect in patients with grass pollen asthma; as assessed by a reduction in asthma symptom and treatment scores. In the first of these, a standardized grass pollen extract was given to nine patients aged 20–39 years with another nine patients receiving placebo. Efficacy was judged by a combined symptom and treatment score that was reduced by 47 points in the active group and by 17.8 points in the placebo group (18). In the other two studies, a formaldehyde-inactivated allergoid preparation was given to patients between 11 and 47 years of age. Just over half of these subjects had clinical asthma. A total of 36 received active treatment and 32 had placebo injections. The primary efficacy variable was symptom scores, which were four times higher in the placebo-treated groups than in the three active treatment groups (19,20). An important recent study has looked at SIT for ragweed allergy and found that patients who received active injections had an improvement in peak flow rates during the pollen season as well as reduced hay fever symptoms and reduced sensitivity to laboratory challenge with ragweed pollen extracts, as compared with the placebo group. In addition, the active group used less antiasthma medication. The economic analysis indicated that the cost-saving in asthma drugs was more than offset by the costs of SIT (21).

The use of SIT to treat allergy to domestic animals has been controversial, with many doctors believing that all the patient has to do is remove the animal from the home. In practice, it is actually quite difficult for patients to avoid cats and dogs, because these are present in 20–40 % of U.K. homes. People who live with domestic animals carry the allergens on their clothing, and cat allergens can be found in many public places, including schools, nurseries, taxis, aircraft, and others (22). For groups who make home visits, such as district nurses, priests, doctors, social workers, and such, domestic animals also present an occupational hazard. In asthmatic patients sensitive to cats, SIT with standardized aqueous extracts reduces the early asthmatic response to inhaled allergen (23,24) and attenuates responses to cat room exposure (23). Interestingly, this latter study showed a clear delay in onset of symptoms and an overall reduction in symptoms and peak flow recordings after exposure to cats in a "cat room," but there was no protection against allergen-induced increases in nonspecific bronchial hyperresponsiveness. The other major study of cat immunotherapy for asthma [25] used a depot preparation and found a reduction in both specific and nonspecific reactions (to cat extract and histamine, respectively). In contrast, SIT with a dog extract was unsuccessful [25].

Several DBPC studies have examined the effects of SIT in asthmatic patients sensitive to house dust mite. Most of these date from 1975 to 1985 and used tyrosine-adsorbed or depot preparations. In some respects, these studies have produced conflicting results. A total of 118 subjects received active treatment in six well-designed studies. Two of these were in asthmatic children aged 5–15 years (total 40 children). In this age band, substantial reductions in drug requirements were reported (26,27), but no such improvement in asthma control was found in the four adult studies (total 78 subjects aged 15–68 years) (28–31).

Specific immunotherapy with the mold *Cladosporium* reduced the drug score and early asthmatic response to inhaled allergen (37). However, there was a high incidence of systemic reactions in the treated group. In another small study of patients sensitive to the mold *Alternaria alernata*, the group receiving SIT ($n = 13$) showed reductions in nasal and respiratory symptoms compared with the placebo group ($n = 11$) (38). However, a formal diagnosis of asthma was made in less than 50% of each group (i.e., most of these patients had allergic rhinitis without asthma).

In laboratory-based evaluations, SIT has attenuated the late asthmatic reaction to allergen inhalation in children (26,34), but this has not been extensively studied in adults (20). In contrast, one study has suggested that SIT may actually increase nonspecific bronchial hyperreactivity in asthmatic children (35), although this has yet to be confirmed.

B. Comparison of SIT with Other Types of Treatment for Asthma

Most clinical trials of SIT have compared SIT either with historical controls or with a matched placebo-treated group. The effectiveness of specific SIT in asthma has not yet been compared with conventional management with avoidance measures and conventional inhaled or oral drugs. Such comparisons are needed before it will really be possible to assess the risk/benefit ratio of SIT compared with other treatments. In the present climate it is also important that any such trial should include an economic dimension because purchasers of health care are increasingly sophisticated in their demands for proof of efficacy and cost-effectiveness.

C. Safety

The main factor cited against the widespread adoption of SIT for asthma is the risk of serious adverse reactions. In the United Kingdom between 1957 and 1986, 26 fatal reactions to SIT were reported to the Committee on Safety of Medicines (12). In 17 of the fatal cases, the indication for SIT was documented: 16 of these 17 patients were receiving SIT to treat asthma (36). Similarly, in the American Academy of Allergy, Asthma, and Immunology's confidential inquiry into SIT-associated deaths, asthma appeared in virtually all the fatal cases. In those for which asthma was not cited as a contributory factor, documentation of asthma status was missing and certainly bronchospasm was a cardinal feature of the clinical course of the anaphylactic reactions (37–39). The incidence of systemic reactions in patients receiving SIT for asthma varies between series and has been reported to range from 5 to 35% (20). The central issue in using safety as an endpoint is to recognize that all treatments carry risks. Where differential risks exist between therapies, a more risky therapy can be justified only if that therapy offers substantial additional benefit over the safer therapy. The science of assessing risk/benefit ratios is still in its infancy, and it is undoubtedly true that different patients and agencies faced with the same facts can come to widely varying risk assessments.

D. Effects on Natural History of Allergic Disease

It has been suggested that SIT may modify the natural history of asthma in children who are known to be atopic, but have not yet developed asthma. It is undeniable that a proportion of patients with allergic rhinitis progress to asthma each year. This annual rate of progression has been estimated at 5% in college students (40), but this is, perhaps surprisingly, an area of considerable ignorance. Several long-term epidemiological studies are now in progress, under the auspices of the ISAAC program and should soon shed light on the rate of progression at different ages and the extent of regional and international variation. Only limited data is available to support the proposition that SIT may alter the natural rate of progression. One prolonged open study, using uncharacterized mixed allergen extracts, supports this view (41), but among other problems, this study failed to allow for the spontaneous improvement that often occurs in asthmatic patients. Thus, there is, as yet, no hard evidence that SIT modifies the natural history of allergic disease through childhood and into adult life. If such evidence were to become available, it would have a major bearing on the economic and clinical arguments surrounding SIT and asthma. There is also as yet no evidence to support claims that SIT is different from pharmacotherapy in terms of influencing the evolution of established asthma. Studies that have investigated withdrawal of therapy have found rapid recurrence of symptoms (20,27,42).

III. Conclusions

Specific immunotherapy is a controversial type of treatment for asthma. Although it seems entirely logical to try to treat allergic disorders by specifically suppressing the immune response to the triggering agents, the critical issue is whether SIT, in its present form, is the best option for managing patients with asthma. To assess this requires proper comparisons of best current SIT versus best current drug therapy, with robust endpoints including symptoms, objective measures of lung function, evaluation of cost/benefit ratios, safety, and quality of life. In vitro and in vivo measures such as skin test responses or allergen-specific IgG4 measurements are not sufficiently specific or sensitive to serve as surrogates for clinical efficacy. Thus far, there have been few well-controlled studies of SIT in asthma, but there is convincing evidence that benefit has been found in grass pollen asthma. The clinical efficacy of SIT in adult asthmatic patients sensitive to house dust mite, cats, or molds is less certain, and no comparative studies with conventional treatment have been performed. Further clinical trials are indicated, particularly in mild to moderate childhood asthma and also in patients with atopic disease who have not yet developed asthma, but are at high risk of progression to asthma.

References

1. Burney PGJ, Chinn S, Rona RJ. Has the prevalence of asthma increased in children? Br Med J 1990; 300:1306–1310.
2. Ninan TK, Russell G. Respiratory symptoms and atopy in Aberdeen schoolchildren: evidence from two surveys. Br Med J 1992; 304:873–875.

3. Sheffer AL. International consensus report on diagnosis and management of asthma. Eur Respir J 1992; 5:601–641.
4. Platts-Mills TAE, Tovey ER, Mitchell EB, Mozarro H. Long-term effects of living in a dust-free room on patients with allergic asthma—reversal of bronchial hyperreactivity. Monogr. Allergy 1983; 18:153–155.
5. Boner AL, Niero E, Antolini T, Valletta EA, Gaburro D. Pulmonary function and bronchial hypereactivity in asthmatic children with house dust mite allergy during prolonged stay in the Italian Alps (Misurina 1756 m). Ann Allergy 1985; 54:42–45.
6. Ehnert B, Lau-Schadendorf S, Weber A, Buettner P, Schou C, Wahn U. Reducing domestic exposure to dust mite allergen reduces bronchial hyperreactivity in sensitive children with asthma. J Allergy Clin Immunol 1992; 90:135–138.
7. Marks GB, Tovey ER, Green W, Shearer M, Salome CM, Woolcock AJ. House dust mite allergen avoidance: a randomised controlled trial of surface chemical treatment and encasement of bedding. Clin Exp Allergy 1994; 24:1078–1083.
8. Noon L. Prophylactic inoculation against hay fever. Lancet 1911; 1:1572.
9. Freeman J. Vaccination against hay fever: report of results during the first three years. Lancet 1914; 1:1178.
10. Malling HJ, Weeke B. Immunotherapy. European Academy of Allergology and Clinical Immunology position paper. Allergy 1993; 48(S14):7–35.
11. British Society for Allergy and Clinical Immunology. Injection immunotherapy. Clin Exp Allergy 1993; 23(S3):1–44.
12. Committee on the Safety of Medicines. CSM update: desensitizing vaccines. Br Med J 1986; 293:948.
13. Creticos P, van Metre TE, Mardingley MR, Rosenberg GL, Adkinson NF. Dose–response of IgE and IgG antibodies during ragweed immunotherapy. J Allergy Clin Immunol 1984; 73:94–104.
14. Djurup R, Malling HJ. High IgG4 antibody level is associated with failure of immunotherapy with inhalant allergens. Clin Allergy 1987; 17:459–468.
15. Iliopoulos O, Proud D, Adkinson NF, Creticos PS, Norman PS, Kagey-Sobotka A, Lichtenstein LM, Naclerio RM. Effects of immunotherapy on the early, late and rechallenge nasal reaction to provocation with allergen: changes in inflammatory mediators and cells. J Allergy Clin Immunol 1991; 87:855–866.
16. Furin MJ, Norman PS, Creticos PS, Proud D, Kagey-Sobotka A, Lichtenstein LM, Naclerio RM. Immunotherapy decreases antigen-induced eosinophil migration into the nasal cavity. J Allergy Clin Immunol 1991; 98:27–32.
17. Ohman JL. Allergen immunotherapy in asthma: evidence for efficacy. J Allergy Clin Immunol 1989; 84:133–139.
18. Reid MJ, Moss RB, Yao-Pi Hsa MS, Kwasnicki JC, Commerford TM, Nelson BL. Seasonal asthma in northern California. Allergic causes and efficacy of immunotherapy. J Allergy Clin Immunol 1986; 78:590–600.
19. Bousquet J, Maasch HJ, Hejjaoui A, Skassa-Brociek W, Wahl R, Dhivert H, Michel FB. Double blind placebo-controlled immunotherapy with mixed grass pollen allergoids. III. Efficacy and safety of unfractionated and high molecular weight preparations in rhinoconjunctivitis and asthma. J Allergy Clin Immunol 1989; 84:546–556.
20. Bousquet J, Hejjaoui A, Michel FB. Specific immunotherapy in asthma. J Allergy Clin Immunol 1990; 86:292–305.
21. Creticos PS, Reed CE, Norman PS, Khoury J, Adkinson NF, Buncher CR, Busse WW, Bush RK, Gadde J, Li JT, Richerson HB, Solomon WR, Steinberg P, Yunginger JW. Ragweed immunotherapy in adult asthma. N Engl J Med 1996; 334:501–506.
22. Bollinger ME, Eggleston PA, Flanagan E, Wood RA. Cat antigen in homes with and without cats may induce allergic symptoms. J Allergy Clin Immunol 1996; 97:907–914.
23. Ohman JL, Findlay SR, Leitermann KM. Immunotherapy in cat-induced asthma. Double-blind trial with evaluation of in vivo and in vitro responses. J Allergy Clin Immunol 1984; 74:230–239.

24. van Metre TE, Marsh DG, Adkinson NF, et al. Immunotherapy for cat asthma. J Allergy Clin Immunol 1988; 82:1053–1058.
25. Sundin B, Lilja G, Graff-Lonnevig V, Hedlin G, Heilborn H, Norrlind K, Peglow KO, Lowenstein H. Immunotherapy with partially purified and standardized animal dander extracts. 1. Clinical results from a double-blind study on patients with animal dander asthma. J Allergy Clin Immunol 1986; 77:478–487.
26. Warner JO, Price JF, Soothill JF, Hey EN. Controlled trial of hyposensitization to *Dermatophagoides pteronyssinus* in children with asthma. Lancet 1978; 2:912–915.
27. Price JF, Warner JO, Hey EN, Tuner MW, Soothill JF. A controlled trial of hyposensitization with tyrosine-adsorbed *Dermatophagoides pteronyssinus* antigen in childhood asthma. In vivo aspects. Clin Allergy 1984; 14:209–219.
28. Gaddie J, Skinner C, Palmer KNV. Hyposensitization with house dust mite vaccine in bronchial asthma. Br Med J 1976; 2:561–562.
29. British Thoracic Association. A trial of house dust mite extract in bronchial asthma. Br J Dis Chest 1979; 73:260–270.
30. Pauli G, Bessot JC, Bigot H, et al. Clinical and immunologic evaluation of hyposensitization with tyrosine-adsorbed *Dermatophagoides pteronyssinus* extract: a double-blind placebo-controlled trial. Clin Allergy 1984; 14:209–219.
31. Bousquet J, Calvayrac P, Guérin B, Hejjaoui A, Dhivert H, Hewitt B, Michel FB. Immunotherapy with standardized *Dermatophagoides pteronissinus* extract. I. In vivo and in vitro parameters after a short course of immunotherapy. J Allergy Clin Immunol 1985; 76:734–744.
32. Dreborg S, Agrell B, Foucard T, Kjellman NM, Koivikko A, Nilsson S. A double-blind, multicenter immunotherapy trial in children using a purified and standardized *Cladosporium herbarum* preparation. I. Clinical results. Allergy 1986; 41:131–140.
33. Horst M, Hejjaoui A, Horst V, et al. Double-blind, placebo-controlled rush immunotherapy with a standardized *Alternaria* extract. J Allergy Clin Immunol 1990; 85:460–472.
34. Van Bever HP, Bosmans J, De Clerk LS, Stevens WJ. Modification of the late asthmatic reaction by hyposensitiziation in asthmatic children allergic to house dust mite (*Dermatophagoides pteronyssinus*) or grass pollen. Allergy 1988; 43:378–385.
35. Murray AB, Ferguson AC, Morrison BJ. Non-allergic bronchial hyperreactivity in asthmatic children decreases with age and increases with mite immunotherapy. Ann Allergy 1985; 54:541–544.
36. Rawlins MD, Wood SM, Mann RD. Hazards with desensitizing vaccines. Arb Paul Ehrlich Inst 1988; 82:147–151.
37. Lockey RF, Benedict LM, Turkeltaub PC, Bukantz SC. Fatalities from immunotherapy and skin testing. J Allergy Clin Immunol 1987; 79:660–667.
38. Reid MJ, Lockey RF, Turkeltaub PC, Platts-Mills TAE. Fatalities from immunotherapy and skin testing (abstr). J Allergy Clin Immunol 1990; 85:180.
39. Reid MJ, Lockey RF, Turkeltaub P, Platts-Mills TAE, Lehrer SB. Fatalities from immunotherapy 1990–91. J Allergy Clin Immunol 1992; 89:abstr 823.
40. Horak F. Manifestation of allergic rhinitis in latent sensitised patients. A prospective study. Arch Otorhinolaryngol 1985; 242:242–249.
41. Johnstone DE, Dutton A. The value of hyposensitization therapy for bronchial asthma in children. A 14 year study. Pediatrics 1968; 42:793–802.
42. Mosbech H, Osterballe O. Does the effect of immunotherapy last after termination of treatment? Follow-up study in patients with grass pollen rhinitis. Allergy 1988; 43:523–529.

13

Allergen-Specific Immunotherapy for Asthma

Metanalysis of Randomized Controlled Trials

MICHAEL J. ABRAMSON and JOHN M. WEINER

Monash Medical School
Alfred Hospital
Prahran, Australia

ROBERT M. PUY

Alfred Hospital
Prahran, Australia

I. Introduction

Allergen-specific immunotherapy (hyposensitization or desensitization) has long been a controversial treatment for asthma. Although beneficial effects based on clinically relevant outcomes have been demonstrated in randomized controlled trials, there remains a risk of severe and sometimes fatal anaphylaxis. The recommendations of professional bodies have ranged from cautious acceptance (1) to outright dismissal (2).

We have previously conducted a metanalysis of 20 randomized controlled trials of allergen immunotherapy for asthma published between 1954 and 1990 (3). Overall, subjects randomized to immunotherapy were 3.2 times more likely to report fewer asthma symptoms, 4.2 times more likely to require less asthma medication, and 6.8 times more likely to demonstrate reduced bronchial hyperreactivity (BHR) than those randomized to placebo. The overall effect of immunotherapy on all continuous outcomes (including symptom and medication scores, lung function, and indices of BHR; such as PD_{20}) corresponded to a mean 7.1% predicted increase in 1-sec forced expiratory volume (FEV_1).

During the last 6 years, there has been increasing interest in new allergen preparations, such as allergen–antibody complexes, and new methods of delivery, including oral, sublingual, and inhaled immunotherapy. Recombinant peptides containing the relevant epitopes, but lacking the ability to cross-link IgE bound to mast cells are currently in preclinical trials, at least for hay fever. Finally, the advent of the Cochrane collaboration has led to major improvements in the statistical software for performing metanalysis. Thus, the time was opportune to update our systematic review of allergen-specific immunotherapy for asthma.

A. Objectives

1. To identify all published randomized controlled trials of allergen-specific immunotherapy (hyposensitization or desensitization) in allergic asthma.
2. To assess the methodological quality of these randomized controlled trials.
3. To estimate the overall efficacy of allergen-specific immunotherapy on asthmatic symptoms, medication requirements, lung function, nonspecific BHR, and allergen-specific BHR.

B. Selection Criteria

This review was restricted to randomized controlled trials (RCT), which provide the strongest evidence for the efficacy of any medical treatment. Only studies that focused on asthma were included. Studies of immunotherapy for hay fever were considered only if the results for subjects with asthma were separately identified. For the purposes of this review, allergen-specific immunotherapy included the administration of extracts of house dust mites, pollens, animal danders, or molds; chemically modified allergoids; or antigen–antibody complexes. Only the subcutaneous route of administration was considered. Oral, sublingual, intranasal, and inhaled immunotherapy will be the topics of future reviews.

Placebo-controlled trials are methodologically stronger, although studies that have administered house dust or other relatively antigenically inactive preparations to the control group were also considered. Double-blind trials were preferred, but single-blind and open studies were also reviewed for possible inclusion.

At least one of the following clinical outcomes had to be reported:
Asthmatic symptoms (including symptom scores)
Asthma medication requirements
Lung function (including FEV_1, peak expiratory flow, and thoracic gas volume)
Nonspecific bronchial hyperreactivity (to histamine or methacholine)
Allergen-specific bronchial hyperreactivity

Studies that reported only nonclinical outcomes, such as allergen-specific IgE (by radio allergo sorbent test [RAST] or skin-prick test) or other in vitro results were excluded.

Studies published in languages other than English were considered if the translated abstract indicated that the study was a randomized, controlled trial (RCT) of allergen immunotherapy for asthma and a translator was sought (see acknowledgments).

C. Search Strategy

MEDLINE searches were undertaken from 1966 to 1996 for studies of immunotherapy and asthma. Review articles identified in this process were surveyed for additional and earlier citations. Dissertation Abstracts and the WorldCat and ArticleFirst databases were also searched to identify more recently published and unpublished studies.

A search was performed of the Asthma database maintained by the Cochrane Airways Group at St. Georges Hospital Medical School, London. This database included all studies with the keywords "asthma" or "wheeze" from the MEDLINE, EMBASE, and CINAHL databases, together with other studies identified by handsearching. A total of 660 nonunique citations were identified with the keywords "immunotherap" or "hyposensiti" or "desensiti" and were examined for possible inclusion.

II. Methods

Inclusion of studies in the review was decided by a simple majority of all three reviewers, who independently read the methods sections of papers identified by the search strategy and applied the stated criteria. Quality assessment was performed by two reviewers (RMP and JMW), who independently assessed the concealment of allocation following the guidelines of the Cochrane Collaboration (4).

A. Statistical Considerations

The planned comparisons were:

1. Allergen immunotherapy versus placebo
2. Allergen immunotherapy versus antigenically inactive control
3. House dust versus placebo
4. Allergen immunotherapy versus untreated control

These comparisons were performed separately for each outcome; namely, asthma symptoms, medication, lung function, nonspecific BHR, and allergen-specific BHR, whenever the results were reported.

Outcome data were extracted and entered into RevMan 3.0 for statistical analysis (5). Categorical outcomes were analyzed as odds ratios (OR) and 95% confidence intervals (95% CI) calculated by Peto's method for individual studies. The odds ratio is simply the ratio between the immunotherapy and control groups for the odds of subjects being the same or worse to subjects being better after treatment. The convention of the Cochrane collaboration is to consider odds ratios greater than

1.0 as indicating clinically undesirable outcomes (in this review, worse symptoms, increased medication, deteriorating lung function, and increased nonspecific and allergen-specific BHR).

Continuous outcomes (symptom and medication scores, lung function parameters, and indices of nonspecific and allergen-specific BHR) were also extracted from tables of results. Where the results were presented only in graphs, these were digitized and then converted to numbers with Un-Scan-It v4.0 (Silk Scientific Corporation, 1996). Continuous outcomes were analyzed as standardized mean differences (SMD). The SMD is a statistic that expresses the difference in means between immunotherapy and control groups in units of the pooled standard deviation.

Fixed effects models were used to obtain summary statistics for the overall efficacy of allergen immunotherapy on both categorical and continuous outcomes and χ^2 tests were performed to assess heterogeneity between studies. In this context, a p value < 0.05 indicates significant differences between studies and raises questions of whether the results can be meaningfully combined.

B. Description of Studies

Fifty-one randomized controlled trials published in 57 papers (6–62) between 1954 and 1996 were identified that satisfied the inclusion criteria. The methods, participants, interventions, and outcomes of included studies are listed in Table 1. There were 21 studies reporting immunotherapy for mite allergy, generally *Dermatophagoides pteronyssinus* or *D. farinae*, although one study (10) used extracts of the storage mite *Lepidoglyphus destructor*. A further two studies (6,11) used extracts of house dust, which has generally been considered antigenically inactive. There were 14 studies of immunotherapy for pollen allergy, utilizing extracts of Bermuda, orchard, timothy, cocksfoot, velvet, sweet vernal, ryegrass, or ragweed pollen. Eight studies reported immunotherapy for animal dander allergy, particularly to cats and dogs. Two studies utilized extracts of the mold *Cladosporium* and 4 attempted simultaneous immunotherapy for multiple aeroallergens. Four studies from one group of investigators (34–37) used allergen–antibody complexes for immunotherapy.

A further 80 studies reported in 88 papers (63–151) were excluded from this review, and the reasons for their exclusion are listed in Table 2. The most common reasons were that the studies were not randomized (24), not controlled (14), did not report clinically relevant outcomes (9), or involved only subjects with rhinitis, rather than asthma (9). We identified several clinical trials of oral immunotherapy (12), inhaled or intranasal immunotherapy (6), and sublingual immunotherapy (4), which will be the subject of a subsequent review. Finally there were three abstracts, which contained insufficient information for further assessment.

C. Methodological Quality

The only criterion for assessing the quality of randomized controlled trials for which there is evidence of a relationship to the potential for bias in the results is concealment of allocation following randomization to active treatment or control. The following criteria have been suggested by the Cochrane collaboration (4) for judging concealment schemes to be *adequate*:

1. Some form of centralized randomization scheme, such as having to provide details of an enrolled participant to an office by phone to receive the treatment group allocation.
2. Some form of randomization scheme controlled by a pharmacy.
3. Numbered or coded containers, such as in a pharmaceutical trial in which capsules from identical-looking, numbered bottles are administered sequentially to enrolled participants.
4. An on-site computer system, given that the allocations are in a locked, unreadable file that can be accessed only after inputting the characteristics of an enrolled participant. If assignment envelopes were used, the report should at least specify that they were sequentially numbered, sealed, opaque, envelopes.
5. Other combinations of described elements of the process that provide assurance of adequate concealment. This may include statements that imply an approach similar to one of those just listed, along with reassuring comments that the person who generated the allocation scheme did not administer it. Some schemes may be innovative and not fit any of the foregoing approaches, but still seem to provide adequate concealment. This "other" category is necessary, but it is likely to include only a small percentage of all trials deemed to have used adequate allocation concealment.

Approaches to concealment of allocation that are considered clearly *inadequate* by the Cochrane collaboration (4) include the following:

1. Alternation
2. Reference to case record numbers, dates of birth, day of the week, or any other such approach
3. Any allocation procedure that is entirely transparent before assignment, such as an open list of random numbers or assignments

For this review, concealment of allocation was assessed as clearly adequate (category A) in only 11 studies (6,15,17,18,19,23,31,42,47,51,58). The adequacy or otherwise of 35 studies could not be determined from the details published in the papers (category B), and further information has been sought from the authors. Only three studies used a clearly inadequate method for concealment of allocation (category C). There was almost perfect agreement between reviewers.

Although not explicitly considered as part of the quality assessment, blinding of subjects or evaluators is another design feature that reduces bias in randomized controlled trials. Forty-two of the 51 studies were double-blind, 2 single-blind, 1 mixed, 2 open, and the remainder unclear. Forty-three studies were placebo-controlled trials of allergen-specific immunotherapy, 3 compared immunotherapy with

Table 1 Characteristics of Included Studies

Study	Methods	Participants	Interventions	Outcomes
Aas (6)	RCT, colored sugar phenol placebo, double-blind	80 asthmatic children, age 2–14 yr	Subcutaneous house dust immunotherapy	Clinical state (subjective parental impression) Specific bronchial hyperreactivity to house dust
Alvarez-Cuesta (7)	RCT, histamine placebo, double-blind	28 patients with rhinoconjunctivitis and asthma, age 15–28 yr	Subcutaneous *Fel d* I immunotherapy	Symptom medication scores Nonspecific and allergen-specific bronchial hyperreactivity
Amaral-Marques (8)	RCT, unstated placebo, double-blind	28 asthmatics, age 12–55 yr with positive skin tests to house dust mite	Tyrosine adsorbed *D. pteronyssinus* subcutaneous immunotherapy	Symptoms, medication
Armentia Medina (10)	RCT, double-blind	35 (25 asthmatic) patients sensitized to storage mite (*Lepidoglyphus destructor*)	Subcutaneous immunotherapy with *L. destructor* extract	Subjective clinical assessment based on symptoms and drug intake Nonspecific (methacholine) BHR
Armentia Medina (9)	RCT, placebo, double-blind	30 (21 asthmatic) patients with Bermuda grass pollen allergy	Subcutaneous Bermuda grass pollen immunotherapy	Nonspecific (methacholine) and allergen (Bermuda grass pollen) specific BHR
BTA (11)	RCT, carbol saline placebo, double-blind	96 asthmatic patients, mean age 24	House dust subcutaneous immunotherapy	Symptoms, medication, peak expiratory flow
BTA (12)	RCT, glycerated extract placebo, double-blind	70 asthmatic patients	House dust mite subcutaneous immunotherapy	Symptoms, medications, FEV_1
Baur (13)	RCT, crossover design, placebo-controlled, single-blind	39 asthmatics, age 18–45 yr	Pollen, house dust mite, and fungal subcutaneous immunotherapy	Allergen-specific BHR
Bertelsen (14)	RCT, untreated controls, open study	27 dog- or cat-allergic children	Dog and cat subcutaneous immunotherapy	Allergen-specific BHR
Bousquet (15)	RCT, unstated placebo, double-blind	30 patients with perennial asthma, age 18–42 yr	*D. pteronyssinus* subcutaneous immunotherapy	Allergen-specific BHR
Bousquet (16)	RCT, unstated placebo	48 (39 asthmatic) patients with grass pollen allergy, age 10–51 yr	Subcutaneous immunotherapy with *D. glomerata* extracts. Rush immunotherapy with standardized lyophilized extract was compared with classic immunotherapy with alum-precipitated pyridine-extracted material.	Symptom medication scores

Bousquet (17)	RCT, untreated controls, open study	215 patients with perennial asthma, age 3–72 yr	House dust mite subcutaneous immunotherapy	Symptoms, medication, FEV_1
Bousquet (18)	RCT, placebo phenol histamine in normal saline Mixed design: 3 groups double-blinded, 1 open	60 (38 asthmatic) patients with grass pollen allergy	Subcutaneous immunotherapy with high molecular weight formalinized allergoid, unfractionated allergoid and standardized orchard grass pollen extract	Symptoms, medication
Bousquet (19)	RCT, phenol saline placebo, double-blind	57 (30 asthmatic) patients with orchard grass pollen allergy, age 11–45 yr	Subcutaneous immunotherapy with high molecular weight formalinized allergoid in high- and low-dose schedules	Symptoms
Bruce (20)	RCT, colored histamine placebo, stratified allocation, blinding not specified	39 ragweed allergic seasonal asthmatics	Subcutaneous immunotherapy with aqueous ragweed extract	Symptoms Allergen-specific BHR
Buchanan (21)	RCT, saline placebo, double-blind	55 asthmatic patients	House dust mite subcutaneous immunotherapy	Symptoms (self-assessed), Medication and asthma attacks (physician-assessed)
Choovoravech (22)	RCT, house dust control, single-blind	57 adult asthmatics	*D. pteronyssinus* and *D. farinae* subcutaneous immunotherapy	Symptom scores Physician evaluation based on examination, PEF and, medication requirements
Creticos (23)	RCT, placebo, double-blind	77 adult asthmatics	Ragweed pollen subcutaneous immunotherapy	Symptom scores Medication scores Peak expiratory flow Allergen-specific BHR
D'Souza (24)	RCT, carbol saline placebo, double-blind	91 (83 asthmatic) patients with house dust mite allergy, age over 10 yr	House dust mite subcutaneous immunotherapy	Symptoms, medication
Dreborg (25)	RCT, histamine placebo, double-blind	30 children with *Cladosporium* allergy age 5–17 yr	*Cladosporium* subcutaneous immunotherapy	Symptoms, medication, peak expiratory flow (no SD reported) Allergen-specific BHR
Frankland (26)	RCT, phenol saline and ultrafiltrate controls, double-blind	200 (57 asthmatic) patients with pollen allergy, age over 10 yr	Subcutaneous immunotherapy with mixed timothy and cocksfoot grass pollen extract, purified pollen protein	Symptoms

(continued)

Table 1 Continued

Study	Methods	Participants	Interventions	Outcomes
Gaddie (27)	RCT, placebo-controlled, double-blind	55 patients with perennial asthma	Subcutaneous immunotherapy with tyrosine-adsorbed depot *D. pteronyssinus* preparation	Symptoms, medication, FEV_1 (no SD reported)
Haugaard (28)	RCT, histamine control with burnt glucose, double-blind	24 asthmatics allergic to cat and dog dander	Subcutaneous immunotherapy with cat epithelium and dog dander extracts	Symptoms Nonspecific (histamine) BHR Allergen-specific BHR
Hill (29)	RCT, 1 PNU ryegrass pollen, placebo, double-blind	20 asthmatic children, age 9–14 yr, with ryegrass pollen allergy	Subcutaneous immunotherapy with aqueous ryegrass pollen extract	Symptoms, medications (medians only reported, no SD)
Johnstone (30)	RCT, buffered saline control, double-blind	112 (72 asthmatic) children with pollinosis	Subcutaneous immunotherapy with ragweed pollen extract, administered by 3 regimens	Asthma symptoms reported by mother
Johnstone (31)	RCT, buffered saline control, double-blind, 4-yr follow-up	173 children with perennial asthma	Subcutaneous immunotherapy with relevant allergen extracts, administered by 3 regimens	Asthma symptoms reported by mother
Johnstone (32)	RCT, buffered saline control, double-blind	130 children with perennial asthma followed to age 16 yr	Subcutaneous immunotherapy with relevant allergens administered by 3 regimens	Asthma symptoms reported by mother
Kuna (33)	RCT, saline placebo, double-blind	24 patients with seasonal asthma	Subcutaneous immunotherapy with glutaraldehyde-modified tyrosine-adsorbed grass pollen extracts	Symptoms FEV_1 (only baseline results reported) Nonspecific (histamine) BHR
Machiels (34)	RCT, albumin buffer placebo-controlled, double-blind, 2 yr follow-up	39 asthmatic patients with *D. pteronyssinus* allergy, age 16–57 yr	Subcutaneous immunotherapy with *D. pteronyssinus* allergen–antibody complexes by 2 regimens	Symptoms, medication, peak expiratory flow Nonspecific (acetylcholine) BHR Allergen-specific BHR
Machiels (35)	RCT, albumin phenol buffer control, double-blind	30 (18 asthmatic) patients with grass pollen allergy, age 14–57 yr	Intradermal immunotherapy with grass pollen antibody complexes	Asthma symptoms Medication (vasconstrictors, antihistamines, oral steroids)
Machiels (36)	RCT, albumin phenol saline buffer placebo-controlled, double-blind	51 grass pollen hypersensitive patients, age 12–51 yr Including 12 previously treated patients	Subcutaneous immunotherapy with grass pollen allergen antibody complexes by 2 regimens	Symptoms, medications
Machiels (37)	RCT, albumin buffer placebo-controlled, double-blind, 4-yr follow-up	39 asthmatic patients with *D. pteronyssinus* allergy, age 16–57 yr	Subcutaneous immunotherapy with *D. pteronyssinus* allergen–antibody complexes by 2 regimens	Symptoms, medication, FEV_1, TLV, SGaw Nonspecific (acetylcholine) BHR Allergen-specific BHR

Malling (38–40)	RCT, caramellized histamine placebo-controlled, double-blind	22 adult asthmatics with *Cladosporium* allergy, age 16–60 yr	Subcutaneous immunotherapy with lyophilized partially purified *C. herbarum* extract	Symptoms, medication Allergen-specific BHR
Maunsell (41)	RCT, house dust control, double-blind	34 asthmatic patients with house dust allergy, age 16–56 yr	Subcutaneous immunotherapy with *D. farinae* extracts	Symptoms (clinical improvement)
Mosbech (42–44)	RCT, placebo-controlled, double-blind	46 house dust mite allergic asthmatics, age 18–56 yr	Subcutaneous immunotherapy with *D. pteronyssinus* and monomethoxypolyethylene glycol-modified extracts	Symptoms, medications, Peak expiratory flow Nonspecific BHR to histamine Allergen-specific BHR
Murray (45)	RCT, caramel carbol and glycerol saline placebo-controlled, double-blind	13 asthmatic children with *D. farinae* allergy	Subcutaneous immunotherapy with glycerinated *D. farinae* +/– relevant pollen extracts	Symptoms Nonspecific (histamine) BHR Allergen-specific BHR
Newton (46)	RCT, normal saline placebo-controlled, double-blind	14 patients with perennial asthma and house dust mite allergy, age 18–44 yr	Subcutaneous immunotherapy with alum-precipitated *D. farinae* extracts	Symptoms, medication Peak expiratory flow Allergen-specific BHR
Ohman (47)	RCT, histamine placebo-controlled, double-blind	17 asthmatic patients with cat allergy, age 22–48 yr	Subcutaneous immunotherapy with cat pelt extract	Symptoms and peak expiratory flow on cat exposure Nonspecific (methacholine) BHR Allergen-specific BHR
Ortolani (48)	RCT, riboflavin-colored Coca solution placebo-controlled, double-blind	15 grass pollen allergic asthmatic patients, age 15–45 yr	Cutaneous immunotherapy with aqueous velvet, sweet vernal, and timothy grass pollen extracts	Symptoms Allergen-specific BHR (medians only presented)
Pauli (49)	RCT, tyrosine phenol placebo-controlled, double-blind	18 patients with perennial asthma, age 19–40 yr	Subcutaneous immunotherapy with tyrosine-adsorbed *D. pteronyssinus* extract	Symptoms, medication Peak expiratory flow
Price (50)	RCT, saline placebo-controlled, double-blind Continuation of study by Warner et al. (1978) for second year with placebo group crossed over to active immunotherapy	25 children with perennial asthma, age 5–15 yr	Subcutaneous immunotherapy with *D. pteronyssinus* extracts	Symptoms, medication Lung function (TGV)
Reid (51)	RCT, nongrass extract placebo-controlled, double-blind	18 patients with seasonal asthma and grass pollen allergy	Subcutaneous immunotherapy with ryegrass pollen extract	Symptom medication scores

(*continued*)

Table 1 Continued

Study	Methods	Participants	Interventions	Outcomes
Sabbah (52)	RCT, placebo-controlled, double-blind	52 perennial asthmatics with house dust mite allergy, mean age 28.7 yr	Subcutaneous immunotherapy with alpha fraction slow-release *D. pteronyssinus* extract	Symptoms (patient self-evaluation) Medication (physician's opinion)
Smith (53)	RCT, human skin scale control, double-blind	22 asthmatic patients with house dust mite allergy, age 11–48 yr	Subcutaneous immunotherapy with *D. pteronyssinus*	Symptoms, medication Peak expiratory flow
Sundin (54)	RCT, histamine albumin aluminium hydroxide control, double-blind	39 asthmatic patients with cat or dog allergy, age 8–47 yr	Subcutaneous immunotherapy with cat or dog dander extracts	Symptoms (patient subjective assessment) Nonspecific (histamine) BHR Allergen-specific BHR
Taylor (55)	RCT, phenol saline placebo-controlled, double-blind	42 asthmatic children with house dust mite allergy, age 6–15 yr	Subcutaneous immunotherapy with mite-fortified house dust extract	Height and weight Lung function (PEF, $FEV_{.75}$, VC, Raw, FRC, TGV) Chest examination
Taylor (56)	RCT, placebo-controlled, double-blind	10 patients with cat-induced asthma	Subcutaneous immunotherapy with cat pelt extract	Nonspecific (histamine) BHR Allergen-specific BHR
Tuchinda (57)	CCT, low allergen dose control	15 asthmatic children, age 9–16 yr	Subcutaneous immunotherapy with aqueous extracts of multiple allergens	Medication Peak expiratory flow Allergen-specific BHR
Valovirta (58,59)	RCT, caramel histamine placebo-controlled, double-blind	27 asthmatic children allergic to dog dander, age 5–18 yr	Subcutaneous immunotherapy with aluminium hydroxide–bound dog dander extract	Symptoms Allergen-specific BHR
Van Bever (60)	RCT, histamine placebo, double-blind	18 asthmatic children, with late reaction to *D. pteronyssinus* bronchial challenge	Subcutaneous immunotherapy with standardized aqueous *D. pteronyssinus* extracts	Nonspecific (histamine) BHR Allergic-specific BHR
Van Metre (61)	RCT, histamine placebo-controlled, double-blind	22 asthmatic patients allergic to cats, age 21–52 yr	Subcutaneous immunotherapy with cat hair and dander extract	Nonspecific (methacholine) BHR Allergen-specific BHR
Warner (62)	RCT, tyrosine placebo-controlled, double-blind	51 asthmatic children, age 5–14 yr, with positive *D. pteronyssinus* challenge	Subcutaneous immunotherapy with tyrosine-adsorbed *D. pteronyssinus* extracts	Symptoms, medication Lung function (PEF, $FEV_{.75}$, TGV) Allergen-specific BHR

Table 2 Characteristics of Excluded Studies

Study identifier	Reason for exclusion
Adamek-Guzik (63)	Relevant outcomes not reported separately for patients with asthma
Almagro (64)	Sublingual immunotherapy
Bessot (65)	Abstract: insufficient detail reported
Botey (66)	Probably not randomized: inadequate reporting of outcomes
Bousquet (67)	No asthma outcomes reported
Bruun (68)	Not randomized controlled trial: alternate allocation
Choovoravech (69)	Uncontrolled study
Choovoravech (70)	Uncontrolled study
Chu (71)	Uncontrolled study
Cleveland (72)	Not randomized: untreated controls
Cooper (73)	Oral immunotherapy
Corbetta (74)	Not randomized controlled trial
Crimi (75)	Local immunotherapy
D'Amato (76)	Only 12/36 patients had asthma: results not presented separately
Engstrom (77)	Retrospective uncontrolled case series
Eriksson (78)	Subjects had hay fever, not asthma
Fanti (79)	All patients received allergen immunotherapy
Feliziani (80)	Sublingual immunotherapy
Ferreira (81)	Nonrandomized trial
Formgren (82)	Abstract only: insufficient results reported
Giovane (83)	Oral immunotherapy
Goldstein (84)	Uncontrolled study
Goor (85)	Not randomized; not all subjects asthmatic
Gordon (86)	Results for asthma symptoms not reported separately
Grammer (87)	Hay fever subjects only
Grammer (88)	Asthmatic subjects not clearly identified
Haahtela (89)	Subjects had only hay fever
Haugaard (90)	Nonrandom allocation
Hedlin (91)	Patients randomized to placebo in previous study [Sundin et al. (54)] subsequently treated with allergen immunotherapy in an open fashion
Henocq (92)	Nonrandomized trial
Hirsch (93)	Subjects had only hay fever
Horst (94)	Subjects had only hay fever
Jarisch (95)	Not a randomized controlled trial
Kalla (96)	Uncontrolled trial
Laetsch (97)	Oral immunotherapy
Leng (98)	Oral immunotherapy
Levin (99)	Not randomized controlled trial
Lichtenstein (100)	Hay fever subjects only

(*continued*)

Table 2 Continued

Study identifier	Reason for exclusion
Lilja (101)	Second year of study reported by Sundin et al. (54)—placebo-treated patients crossed over to active immunotherapy, thus uncontrolled study
Mallet (102)	Not randomized controlled trial, asthmatics not clearly identified
Martorell (103)	Not randomized controlled trial, comparison of 2 groups treated for different durations
Maruo (104)	Not randomized controlled trial
Matoga (105)	Not randomized controlled trial
McAllen (106)	Not randomized trial
Metzger (107)	Abstract only: insufficient results reported
Miguel Lozano (108)	Uncontrolled study
Mischler (109)	Rhinitis subjects only
Moller (110)	Oral immunotherapy for rhinoconjunctivitis
Mosbech (111)	All subjects desensitized with different extracts, not randomized
Moscato (112)	Comparison of inhaled with parenteral immunotherapy
Moshkevich (113)	Inhaled immunotherapy
Munoz-Lejarazu (114)	Not randomized
Munoz-Lopez (115)	Not randomized controlled trial
Munoz-Lopez (116)	Topical intranasal immunotherapy
Munro-Ashman (117)	Uncontrolled trial
Nagata (118)	Uncontrolled study
Nagata (119)	Not randomized
Norman (120)	Only hay fever subjects
Novembre (121)	Sublingual immunotherapy
Oppenheimer (122)	Oral immunotherapy
Osterballe (123)	Not randomized, comparison of immunotherapy regimens
Pence (124)	Asthma symptom score not reported separately
Petersen (125)	26/54 subjects had asthma, but only global symptoms reported, and results not reported separately
Rak (126)	No clinical outcomes reported
Rak (127)	Not randomized controlled trial: no relevant outcomes reported
Rebien (128)	Oral immunotherapy
Reinert (129)	Uncontrolled study
Reinert (130)	Oral immunotherapy
Rocha (131)	30 controls received immunotherapy, but not analyzed by intention to treat
Rohatgi (132)	Uncontrolled study
Sadan (133)	Hay fever subjects only
Sanchez (134)	Comparison of oral with parenteral immunotherapy
Sanders (135)	Matched pairs, but not clearly randomized; global symptoms score, asthmatics not clearly identified

Table 2 Continued

Study identifier	Reason for exclusion
Swineford (136)	Not a randomized controlled trial
Sychlowy (137)	Uncontrolled study
Tari (138)	Sublingual immunotherapy
Tari (139)	Inhaled immunotherapy
Taub (140)	Editorial with personal experience: not randomized controlled trial
Taudorf (141)	Oral immunotherapy
Taudorf (142)	Oral immunotherapy
Tuadorf (143)	Oral immunotherapy
Turner (144)	No clinical outcomes reported
Urbanek (145)	Oral immunotherapy
Van Bever (146)	Not randomized controlled trial
Van Bever (147)	Not randomized
Van Bever (148)	All patients received immunotherapy during first year
Wahn (149)	Not a randomized controlled trial
Weyer (150)	No clinical outcomes reported
Wuthrich (151)	Uncontrolled study

an antigenically inactive control (22,41,57), 2 compared house dust with placebo (6,11), 2 used untreated controls (14,17), and Murray et al. (45) had both a placebo and an untreated control group.

III. Results

An overview of the metanalysis for each outcome is presented in Figure 1. More detailed results for the individual placebo-controlled trials are presented in Figures 2–11. Symptom scores were reported by 13 studies, although neither Dreborg et al. (25), nor Hill et al. (29) published standard deviations (SD), thereby preventing the calculation of the standardized mean differences (SMD) for these studies. The combined SMD for symptom scores was –0.92 with a 95% confidence interval from –1.13 to –0.71, which excluded 0, thus indicating an overall significant improvement in asthma symptoms following immunotherapy (Fig. 2). However, there was significant heterogeneity between these results ($\chi^2 = 70.3$; $p < 0.0005$), with three studies (20,34,58) not reporting any reduction in symptoms.

Symptoms were simply reported as worse, the same, or improved in 6 studies of children and 17 studies of adults. The combined odds ratio (OR) was 0.28, with a 95% CI from 0.21 to 0.36, which excluded 1, again indicating that patients randomized to immunotherapy were significantly less likely to report a deterioration in asthma symptoms than those randomized to placebo (Fig. 3). Although the results of studies of children were relatively homogeneous, there was significant

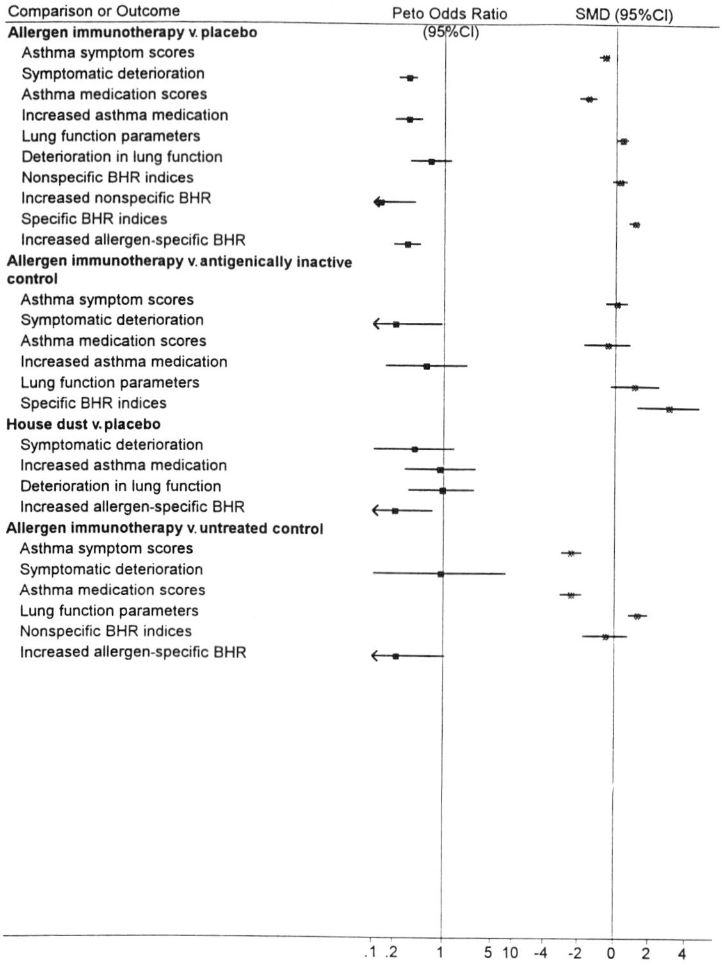

Figure 1 Metanalysis of allergen immunotherapy for asthma: summary odds ratios and standardized mean differences (with 95% confidence intervals) for each outcome within each comparison.

heterogeneity among the results of adult studies ($\chi^2 = 40.0$; $p < 0.001$). The BTA (12) and Buchanan et al. (21) actually found symptoms more likely in treated patients.

Asthma medication scores were reported by 5 studies, with Dreborg et al. (25) and Hill et al. (29) again failing to publish any SDs. The combined SMD was –1.8 (95% CI, –2.1 to –1.4), indicating a significant reduction in medication following immunotherapy (Fig. 4). Medication requirements were simply reported as increased, unchanged, or decreased in 15 studies. The combined OR was 0.28 (95% CI, 0.19–

Study	Weight %	SMD (95%CI Fixed)	Quality
Kuna(33)	2.0	-4.099 [-5.615,-2.583]	B
Alvarez-Cuesta(7)	3.5	-3.009 [-4.154,-1.864]	B
Ortolani(48)	2.1	-2.442 [-3.926,-0.957]	B
ArmentiaMedina(10)	5.7	-2.196 [-3.088,-1.303]	B
Bousquet(19)	9.7	-2.009 [-2.694,-1.324]	A
Reid(51)	3.9	-1.279 [-2.366,-0.192]	A
Bousquet(18)	11.6	-0.804 [-1.431,-0.178]	A
Machiels(34)	8.2	-0.486 [-1.231,0.259]	B
Creticos(23)	21.6	-0.485 [-0.945,-0.026]	A
Bousquet(16)	7.0	-0.485 [-1.291,0.321]	A
Machiels(35)	8.2	-0.346 [-1.093,0.400]	B
Valovirta(58,59)	7.3	-0.263 [-1.056,0.529]	A
xDreborg(25)	0.0	0.000 [0.000,0.000]	B
xHill(29)	0.0	0.000 [0.000,0.000]	B
Bruce(20)	9.1	0.084 [-0.623,0.791]	B
Total (95%CI)	**100.0**	**-0.920 [-1.134,-0.707]**	
Chi-square 70.33 (df=12) Z=8.44			

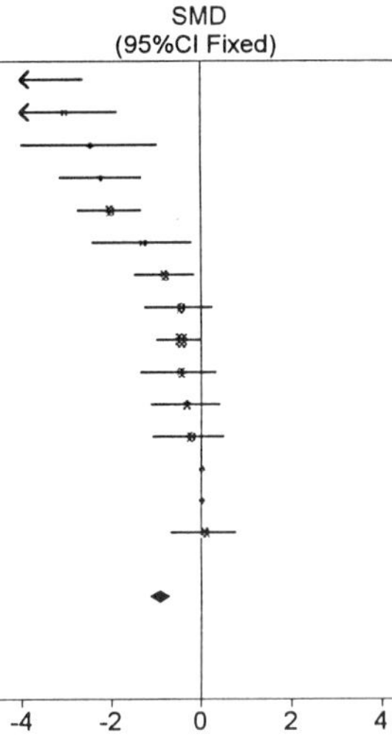

Figure 2 Metanalysis of asthma symptom scores from placebo-controlled trials: standardized mean differences (with 95% confidence intervals) for each study and all studies combined.

0.42), indicating that patients randomized to immunotherapy were significantly less likely to require more medication than those randomized to placebo (Fig. 5). Although there was significant heterogeneity among the studies reporting medication scores ($\chi^2 = 28.0$; $p < 0.0005$), there was substantial homogeneity among the results of these 14 studies.

Lung function results were reported by nine studies, with several studies failing to provide SDs. The SD of FEV_1 was estimated as 10% of the predicted value and the SD of thoracic gas volume in children as 18% predicted (152). There was no overall improvement in lung function parameters following immunotherapy (Fig. 6), and marked heterogeneity among studies ($\chi^2 = 134$; $p < 0.0001$). Lung function was simply reported as worse, the same, or improved in seven studies. Although there was homogeneity among these studies and an overall trend against a deterioration in lung function following immunotherapy, this did not achieve statistical significance (Fig. 7).

Indices of nonspecific bronchial hyperreactivity (such as $PC_{20}FEV_1$ to histamine challenge) were reported by ten studies. There was significant heterogeneity among the results of these studies ($\chi^2 = 61.1$; $p < 0.0005$) and no overall reduction in nonspecific BHR following immunotherapy (Fig. 8). Nonspecific BHR was simply reported as increased, unchanged, or reduced in four small studies. There was homogeneity among these studies and the combined OR of 0.13 (95% CI, 0.05–0.34), indicated that patients randomized to immunotherapy were significantly less

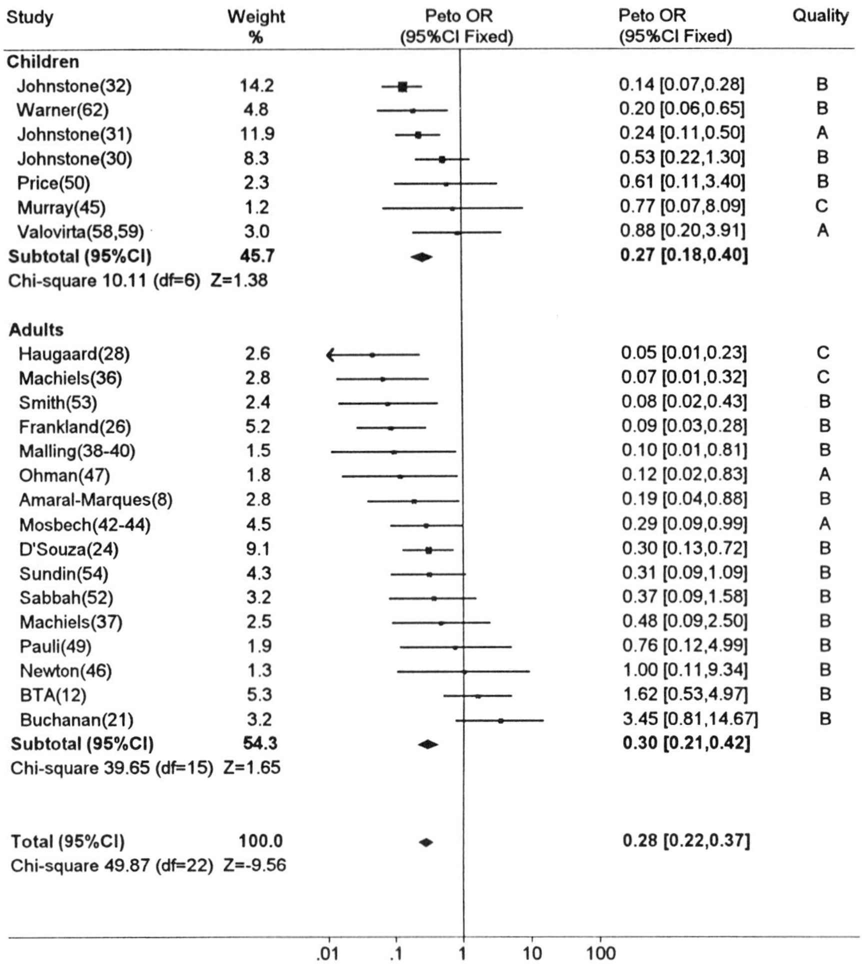

Figure 3 Metanalysis of symptomatic deterioration from placebo-controlled trials: odds ratios (with 95% confidence intervals) for each study, pediatric and adult studies and all studies combined.

likely to develop increased nonspecific BHR than those randomized to placebo (Fig. 9).

Indices of allergen-specific BHR (such as $PD_{20}FEV_1$ to allergen challenge) were reported by 13 studies. Although there was significant heterogeneity among studies ($\chi^2 = 46.5$; $p < 0.0005$), the overall SMD was 0.69 (95% CI, 0.44–0.93), indicating a significant reduction in allergen-specific BHR following immunotherapy (Fig. 10). Allergen-specific BHR was simply reported as increased, unchanged, or reduced by 17 studies. There was homogeneity among studies, and the combined

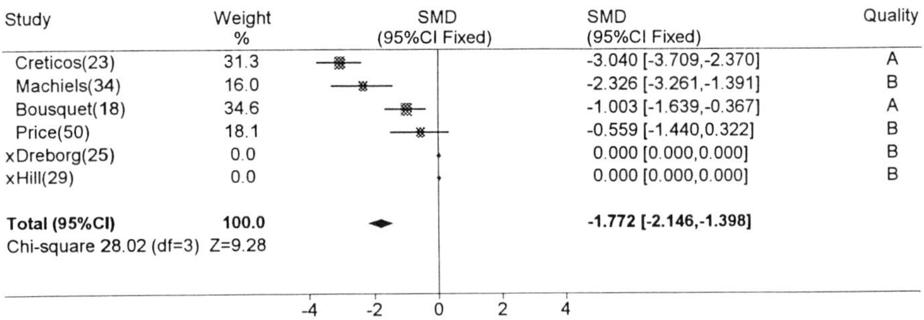

Figure 4 Metanalysis of asthma medication scores from placebo-controlled trials: standardized mean differences (with 95% confidence intervals) for each study and all studies combined.

OR of 0.28 (95% CI, 0.19–0.41) indicated that patients randomized to immunotherapy were significantly less likely to develop increased allergen-specific BHR (Fig. 11).

Because of the small number and disparate outcomes reported by the non–placebo-controlled randomized trials, only limited metanalysis could be performed. Choovoravech (22) did not find a significant reduction in asthma symptoms com-

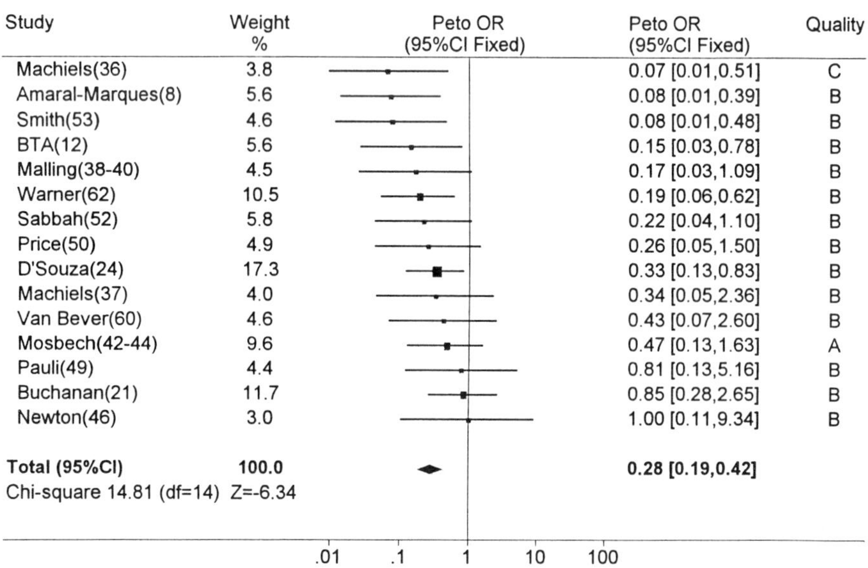

Figure 5 Metanalysis of increased asthma medication requirements from placebo-controlled trials: odds ratios (with 95% confidence intervals) for each study and all studies combined.

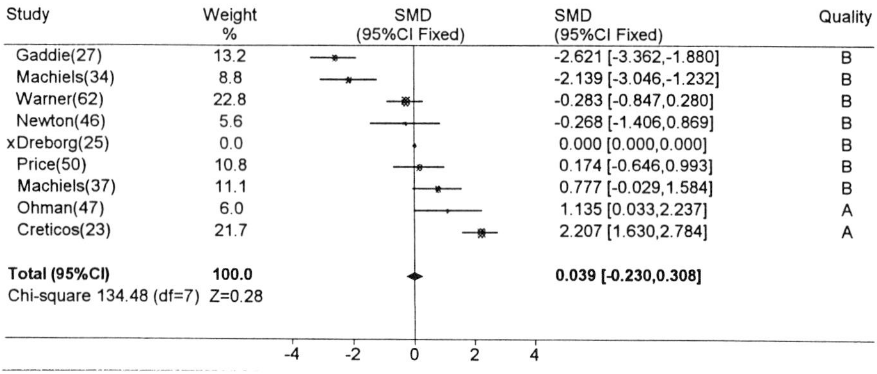

Figure 6 Metanalysis of lung function parameters from placebo-controlled trials: standardized mean differences (with 95% confidence intervals) for each study and all studies combined.

paring house dust mite (HDM) immunotherapy with house dust (SMD = –0.23; 95% CI, –0.77 to 0.30). However Maunsell et al. (41) did find that patients randomized to HDM were significantly less likely to report asthma symptoms than those randomized to house dust (OR = 0.2; 95% CI, 0.05–0.8). Neither Tuchinda and Chai (57) nor Choovoravech (22) found any significant reduction in asthma medications following immunotherapy (SMD = –0.73; 95% CI, –1.9 to 0.46 and OR = 0.5; 95% CI, 0.15–1.7, respectively). Tuchinda and Chai (57) found a trend to improved lung function, although this did not achieve statistical significance (SMD = 0.72; 95% CI, –0.47 to 1.9). Finally, Tuchinda and Chai (57) did find a significant reduction in allergen-specific BHR following immunotherapy (SMD = 2.4; 95% CI, 0.9–4.0).

The two studies (6,11) that compared house dust extracts with placebo found negative results for most outcomes. Subjects randomized to house dust were less

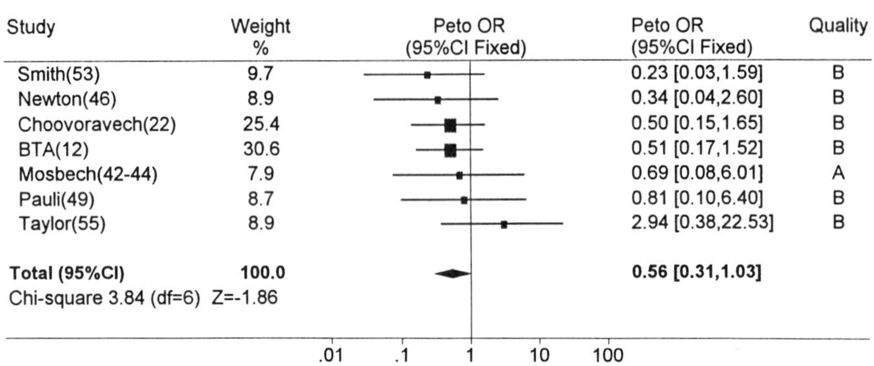

Figure 7 Metanalysis of deterioration in lung function from placebo-controlled trials: odds ratios (with 95% confidence intervals) for each study and all studies combined.

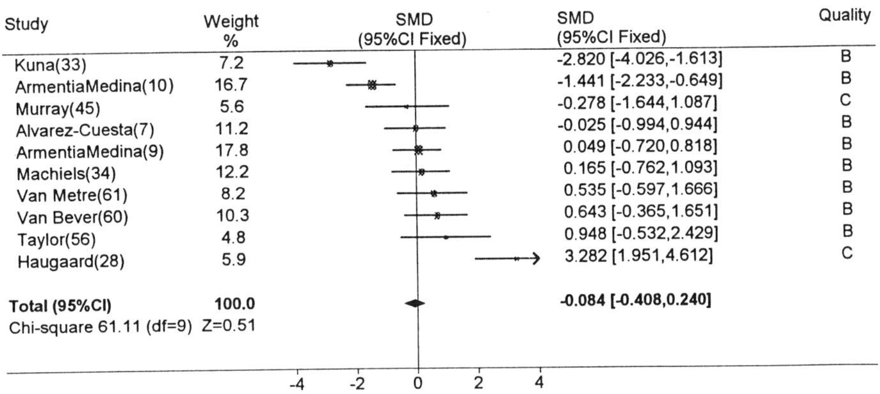

Figure 8 Metanalysis of indices of nonspecific bronchial hyperreactivity from placebo-controlled trials: standardized mean differences (with 95% confidence intervals) for each study and all studies combined.

likely to report worse asthma symptoms, but the combined effect of both studies did not achieve statistical significance (OR = 0.35; 95% CI, 0.11–1.1). In the BTA study (11), those randomized to house dust had minimal reduction in asthma medication (OR = 0.76; 95% CI, 0.27–2.2) and were marginally less likely to demonstrate deterioration in lung function (OR = 0.79; 95% CI, 0.3–2.1). However, Aas (6) found that asthmatic children randomized to house dust had significantly reduced allergen-specific BHR (OR = 0.19; 95% CI, 0.06–0.59).

On the other hand, studies with untreated controls reported several positive results of allergen immunotherapy. Bousquet et al. (17) found that patients randomized to immunotherapy demonstrated significant reductions in asthma symptoms (SMD = –2.5; 95% CI, –3.1 to –2.0) and medication (SMD = –2.6; 95% CI, –3.1 to 2.0) and a significant improvement in lung function (SMD = 0.91; 95% CI, 0.47–

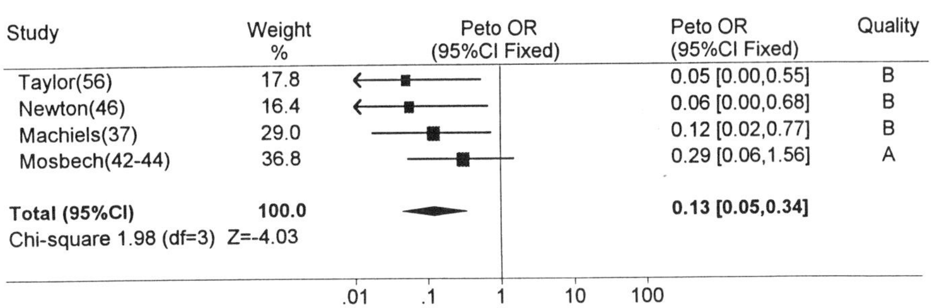

Figure 9 Metanalysis of increased nonspecific bronchial hyperreactivity from placebo-controlled trials: odds ratios (with 95% confidence intervals) for each study and all studies combined.

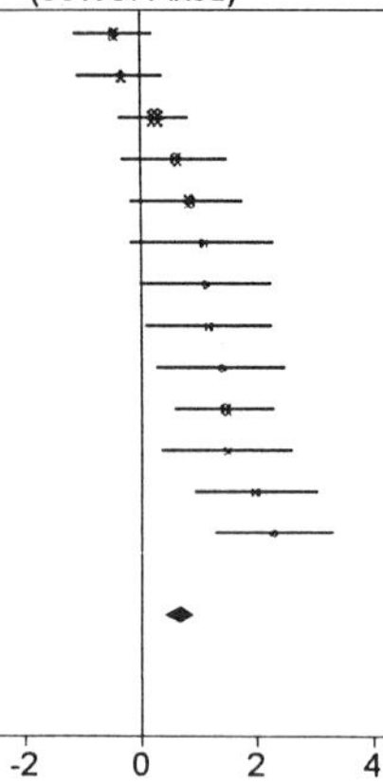

Study	Weight %	SMD (95%CI Fixed)	Quality
Baur(13)	13.6	-0.450 [-1.104,0.205]	B
Sundin(54)	12.3	-0.333 [-1.023,0.357]	B
Creticos(23)	18.0	0.256 [-0.313,0.825]	A
Malling(38-40)	7.3	0.587 [-0.310,1.484]	B
Van Metre(61)	6.6	0.803 [-0.136,1.743]	B
Newton(46)	3.9	1.079 [-0.145,2.303]	B
Ohman(47)	4.8	1.131 [0.029,2.232]	A
Alvarez-Cuesta(7)	5.1	1.177 [0.107,2.248]	B
Van Bever(60)	4.8	1.382 [0.278,2.486]	B
ArmentiaMedina(9)	7.8	1.445 [0.582,2.308]	B
Machiels(34)	4.8	1.495 [0.395,2.594]	B
Haugaard(28)	5.2	2.000 [0.939,3.061]	C
Bousquet(15)	5.8	2.298 [1.295,3.301]	A
Total (95%CI)	**100.0**	**0.685 [0.443,0.926]**	

Chi-square 46.46 (df=12) Z=5.56

Figure 10 Metanalysis of indices of allergen-specific bronchial hyperreactivity from placebo-controlled trials: standardized mean differences (with 95% confidence intervals) for each study and all studies combined.

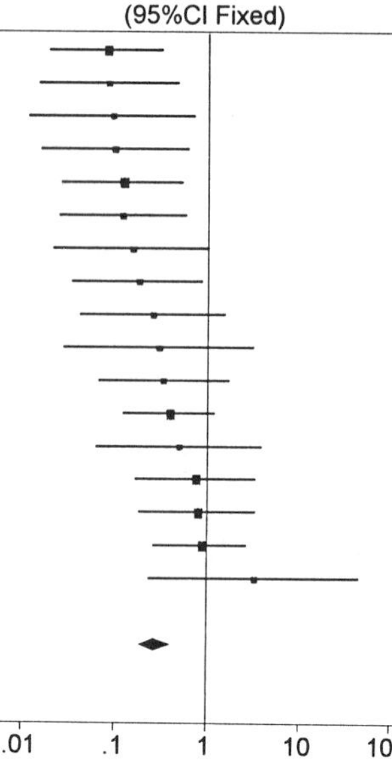

Study	Weight %	Peto OR (95%CI Fixed)	Quality
Sundin(54)	7.8	0.08 [0.02,0.32]	B
Van Metre(61)	5.1	0.09 [0.02,0.48]	B
Alvarez-Cuesta(7)	3.5	0.09 [0.01,0.72]	B
Machiels(37)	4.5	0.10 [0.02,0.62]	B
Dreborg(25)	6.8	0.12 [0.03,0.52]	B
Bousquet(15)	6.1	0.12 [0.03,0.59]	A
Van Bever(60)	4.1	0.15 [0.02,1.02]	B
Malling(38-40)	5.6	0.18 [0.03,0.90]	B
Machiels(34)	4.6	0.25 [0.04,1.53]	B
Murray(45)	2.7	0.31 [0.03,3.23]	C
Valovirta(58,59)	5.6	0.34 [0.07,1.74]	A
Creticos(23)	12.1	0.39 [0.13,1.19]	A
Ohman(47)	3.6	0.50 [0.07,3.80]	A
Mosbech(42-44)	7.0	0.75 [0.17,3.25]	A
Bruce(20)	7.4	0.79 [0.19,3.27]	B
Warner(62)	11.2	0.86 [0.27,2.73]	B
Taylor(56)	2.2	3.32 [0.24,46.04]	B
Total (95%CI)	**100.0**	**0.28 [0.19,0.41]**	

Chi-square 21.97 (df=16) Z=-6.50

Figure 11 Metanalysis of increased allergen-specific bronchial hyperreactivity from placebo-controlled trials: odds ratios (with 95% confidence intervals) for each study and all studies combined.

1.4). A small study by Murray et al. (45) found that children randomized to immunotherapy were marginally less likely to report asthma symptoms than were untreated controls (OR = 0.77; 95% CI, 0.11–5.5), but there was no significant effect of immunotherapy on nonspecific BHR (SMD = –0.75; 95% CI, –1.9 to 0.39). Finally, Bertelsen et al. (14) found that those randomized to immunotherapy were significantly less likely to develop increased allergen-specific BHR (OR = 0.2; 95% CI, 0.05–0.9).

IV. Discussion

This updated systematic review of allergen immunotherapy for asthma has identified an additional 31 randomized controlled trials, which were not covered by our previous review (3) of double-blind, placebo-controlled studies published in English up to 1990. Of the additional studies, 7 were published since 1990, 8 were not placebo-controlled, 9 were not double-blind, and 2 were published in languages other than English. Most of the non-English language publications on allergen immunotherapy were not randomized controlled trials. A total of 80 studies were excluded from the review, primarily because they were not randomized, not controlled, did not report clinically relevant outcomes, or involved only subjects with rhinitis.

Given the well-recognized bias favoring the publication of positive studies, it is quite possible that some additional negative studies have been conducted, but that their results have not been published in the medical literature. This problem could be avoided in the future by prospective registration of all clinical trials of allergen immunotherapy, as has been attempted in other clinical disciplines. Unfortunately, the methodological quality of most studies, particularly the concealment of allocation following randomization could not be clearly determined from the information presented in the papers. We would encourage authors of future papers to follow the CONSORT guidelines (153) and fully report such details.

This metanalysis has confirmed that allergen-specific immunotherapy can significantly reduce asthma symptoms and medication requirements. The heterogeneity of symptom and medication scores is likely to have arisen from the different scoring schemes used in different studies. Standardization of asthma symptom and medication scores is required for easier interpretation of future studies. However, we do not believe that the heterogeneity of the results means that the studies could not be meaningfully combined or that this invalidates the conclusions.

There is no consistent effect of immunotherapy on lung function. The marked heterogeneity probably arises from the attempt to combine such diverse measures of lung function as FEV_1 peak expiratory flow, and thoracic gas volume. These parameters presumably reflect different aspects of the pulmonary pathophysiology of asthma, such as reduced airway caliber, variable airflow limitation, and hyperinflation. A further problem is the need to infer some SDs from studies of normal subjects, who are likely to have more reproducible measurements than asthmatic patients. In contrast, our previous metanalysis (3) did find a modest improvement in lung function. However, in retrospect, this conclusion resulted substantially from the post hoc exclusion of one negative study (50) in response to a reviewer's concerns.

Whereas in our previous metanalysis, nonspecific and allergen-specific BHR were combined, they were analyzed separately in this review. Although patients randomized to immunotherapy were significantly less likely to develop increased nonspecific BHR, there was no consistent effect on indices of nonspecific BHR. The heterogeneity is likely to have arisen from the combination of such diverse indices of nonspecific BHR as $PC_{20}FEV_1$ to histamine, $PD_{20}FEV_1$ to methacholine, and $PC_{35}SGaw$ to acetylcholine. There is an additional statistical problem, in that such indices of BHR are normally considered to follow a log-normal distribution (i.e., the geometric mean is the most appropriate summary measure). However, RevMan required the arithmetic means and standard deviations to be entered to calculate the SMD.

Allergen immunotherapy significantly reduced allergen-specific BHR. The heterogeneity among studies is again likely to have resulted from combining such diverse indices of allergen-specific BHR as $PD_{15}PEF$, $PD_{25}PEF$, $PD_{20}FEV_1$, and $PD_{35}SGaw$. It would be desirable for future studies to use a standardized protocol for bronchial allergen challenges and to report the results in a consistent fashion. Not surprisingly, it would appear that allergen immunotherapy has a greater effect on allergen-specific BHR than on nonspecific BHR.

Less importance should be attached to the results of the relatively few non–placebo-controlled trials. There is some evidence that house dust mite extracts may reduce asthma symptoms and allergen-specific BHR compared with house dust extracts. One study even suggested that house dust extracts alone could reduce allergen-specific BHR, challenging the view that such extracts are antigenically inactive. However, taken together, these results are consistent with the greater efficacy of house dust mite extracts compared with placebo. Studies with untreated controls are particularly susceptible to bias and may overestimate the true benefit of treatment. The effects of immunotherapy on symptoms, medication, and lung function found in one such study are beyond the upper confidence limits for placebo-controlled studies.

The results of this systematic review are consistent with our previous metanalysis (3) and, importantly, the positive findings have not been overturned by the inclusion of 31 additional randomized controlled trials of allergen immunotherapy. In the previous metanalysis, we intuitively calculated the combined odds ratios for symptomatic improvement, reduction in medication, and BHR. These odds ratios can be converted to the Cochrane convention of clinically unfavorable outcomes being greater than 1 by taking their reciprocals. When the reciprocals are compared with the odds ratios from the present review, the results are strikingly similar and always lie within the 95% confidence intervals. Unfortunately, the overall effect of immunotherapy on continuous outcomes cannot be directly compared because quite different statistical methods have been used.

Although this evidence confirms the efficacy of immunotherapy, it gives no direct guidance concerning its clinical application. We have previously stated the well-accepted principles that we follow in using immunotherapy in asthma (3). We believe that immunotherapy should be considered when asthma is extrinsic and an unavoidable clinically relevant allergen can be identified. A specific effective extract must be available, and there should be flexibility in the dosage schedule. The question of side effects must be fully discussed with the patient. The patient must be observed long enough to deal with any major systemic reactions (in our practice 45 min) and adequate resuscitation measures must be available because of the well-known possibility of anaphylaxis. There must be access to expert advice at all times. These issues are discussed more fully in the recently published Australian and New Zealand guidelines (154) and also receive further attention elsewhere in this volume.

However, certain questions remain to be answered: What are the most important determinants of the clinical relevance of an allergen? Which patient is the ideal recipient of immunotherapy? Is the result better when there is a narrow range of positive skin tests, or is it just as effective in panreactors? Is monocomponent immunotherapy better than the use of a cocktail of allergens to which the patient reacted? What is the optimal length of treatment and the best duration of effect? The answers to some of these questions may be present in the studies currently available, but others will require new and better randomized controlled trials.

Acknowledgments

We wish to thank Daniel Czarny, Rosa Dias Santilhiano, Andrei Saramovich, Fiona Savio, and Georg Schäppi for their assistance in translating studies published in languages other than English. The German Assistant (Microtac software) was used to translate papers published in German. The Cochrane Airways Group database was searched by Steve Milan. David Badger and Vivienne Moore from the Australasian Cochrane Centre provided helpful advice on the use of RevMan.

References

1. Weeke B. The future for immunotherapy. Clin Exp Allergy 1991; 21(suppl 1):86–92.
2. Henry RL, Landau LI, Mellis C, et al. Childhood asthma: application of the international view of management in Australia and New Zealand. J Paediatr Child Health 1990; 26:72–74.
3. Abramson M, Puy R, Weiner J. Is allergen immunotherapy effective in asthma? A meta-analysis of randomised controlled trials. Am J Respir Crit Care Med 1995; 151:969–974.
4. Oxman A, ed. Section VI. Preparing and maintaining systemic reviews: assessment of methodological quality. In: Sackett D, ed. Cochrane Collaboration Handbook, 1994.

5. Duley L, Fischer M, Moustgaard R. Guide to using the Cochrane Review Manager (RevMan) version 3.0 for Windows. Cochrane Collaboration, 1996.
6. Aas K. Hyposensitization in hose dust allergy asthma. A double-blind controlled study with evaluation of the effect on bronchial sensitivity to house dust. Acta Paediatr Scand 1971; 60:264–268.
7. Alvarez Cuesta E, Cuesta Herranz J, PuyanaRuiz J, Cuesta Herranz C, Blanco Quiros A. Monoclonal antibody-standardized cat extract immunotherapy: risk–benefit effects from a double-blind placebo study J Allergy Clin Immunol 1994; 93:556–566.
8. Amaral Marques R, Avila R. Results of a clinical trial with a *Dermatophagoides pteronyssinus* tyrosine adsorbed vaccine. Allergol Immunopathol 1978; 6:231–235.
9. Armentia Medina A, Blanco Quiros A, Martin Santos JM, Alvarez Cuesta E, Moneo Goiri I, Carreira P, Losada Cosmes E. Rush immunotherapy with a standardized Bermuda grass pollen extract. Ann Allergy 1989; 63:127–135.
10. Armentia Medina A, Tapias JA, Martin JF, Ventas P, Fernandez A. Immunotherapy with the storage mite *Lepidoglyphus destructor*. Allergol Immunopathol 1995; 23:211–223.
11. British Tuberculosis Association. Treatment of house dust allergy. Br Med J 1968; 3:774–777.
12. British Thoracic Association. A trial of house dust mite extract in bronchial asthma. Br J Dis Chest 1979; 73:260–270.
13. Baur X. Hyposensitization in bronchial asthma—still a current therapeutic procedure? Med Klin 1989; 84:439–444.
14. Bertelsen A, Andersen JB, Christensen J, Ingermann L, Kristensen T, Ostergaard PA. Immunotherapy with dog and cat extracts in children. Allergy 1989; 44:330–335.
15. Bousquet J, Calvayrac P, Guerin B, et al. Immunotherapy with a standardised *Dermatophagoides pteronyssinus* extract I. In vivo and in vitro parameters after a short course of treatment. J Allergy Clin Immunol 1985; 76:734–744.
16. Bousquet J, Guerin B, Dotte A, et al. Comparison between rush immunotherapy with a standardised allergen and an alum adjuved pyridine extracted material in grass pollen allergy. Clin Allergy 1985; 15:179–193.
17. Bousquet J, Hejjaiou A, Clauzel AM, Guerin B, Dhivert H, Skassa-Brociek W, Michel FB. Immunotherapy with a standardised *Dermatophagoides pteronyssinus* extract II. Prediction of efficacy of immunotherapy. J Allergy Clin Immunol 1988; 82:971–977.
18. Bousquet J, Maasch HJ, Hejjaoui A, Skassa-Brociek W, Wahl R, Dhivert H, Michel FB. Double blind placebo controlled immunotherapy with mixed grass pollen allergoids. III. Efficacy and safety of unfractionated and high molecular weight preparations in rhinoconjunctivitis and asthma. J Allergy Clin Immunol 1989; 84:546–556.
19. Bousquet J, Hejjaoui A, Soussana M, Michel FB. Double-blind, placebo-controlled immunotherapy with mixed grass-pollen allergoids. IV. Comparison of the safety and efficacy of two dosages of a high-molecular-weight allergoid. J Allergy Clin Immunol 1990; 85:490–497.
20. Bruce CA, Norman PS, Rosenthal RR, Lichtenstein LM. The role of ragweed pollen in autumnal asthma. J Allergy Clin Immunol 1977; 59:449–459.
21. Buchanan DJ, Hillis A, Williams PN. A double blind controlled trial of Bencard house dust mite (Migen) hyposensitisation in Zambian asthmatics. Med J Zambia 1981; 15:14–16.
22. Choovoravech P. Effect of immunotherapy in bronchial asthma: treatment with extracts of house dust and mite. J Med Assoc Thai 1974; 57:445-449.
23. Creticos PS, Reed CS, Norman PS, et al. Ragweed immunotherapy in adult asthma. N Engl J Med 1996; 334:501–506.
24. D'Souza MF, Pepys J, Wells ID, Tai E, Palmer F, Overell BG, McGrath IT, Megson M. Hyposensitisation with *Dermatophagoides pteronyssinus* in house dust allergy: a controlled study of clinical and immunological effects. Clin Allergy 1973; 3:177–193.
25. Dreborg S, Agrell B, Foucard T, et al. A double blind multicentre immunotherapy trial in

children using a purified and standardised *Cladosporium herbarum* preparation. Allergy 1986; 41:131–140.
26. Frankland AW, Augustin R. Prophylaxis of summer hayfever and asthma. Lancet 1954; 1:1055–1057.
27. Gaddie J, Skinner C, Palmer KNV. Hyposensitisation with house dust mite vaccine in bronchial asthma. Br Med J 1976; 2:561–562.
28. Haugaard L, Dahl R. Immunotherapy in patients allergic to cat and dog dander. I. Clinical results. Allergy 1992; 47:249–254.
29. Hill DJ, Hosking CS, Shelton MJ, Turner MW. Failure of hyposensitisation in treatment of children with grass-pollen asthma. Br Med J 1982; 284:306–309.
30. Johnstone DE. Study of the role of antigen dosage in the treatment of pollenosis and pollen asthma. Am J Dis Child 1957; 94:1–5.
31. Johnstone DE, Crump L. Value of hyposensitisation therapy for bronchial asthma in children. Pediatrics 1961; 27:39–44.
32. Johnstone DE, Dutton A. The value of hyposensitisation therapy for bronchial asthma in children—a 14 year study. Pediatrics 1968; 42:793–802.
33. Kuna P, Alam R, Kuzminska B, Rozniecki J. The effect of preseasonal immunotherapy on the production of histamine-releasing factor (HRF) by mononuclear cells from patients with seasonal asthma: results of a double-blind, placebo-controlled, randomized study. J Allergy Clin Immunol 1989; 83:816–824.
34. Machiels JJ, Somville MA, Lebrun PM, Lebecque SJ, Jacquemin MG, Saint Remy JMR. Allergic bronchial asthma due to *Dermatophagoides pteronyssinus* hypersensitivity can be efficiently treated by inoculation of allergen–antibody complexes. J Clin Invest 1990; 85:1024–1035.
35. Machiels JJ, Buche M, Somville MA, Jacquemin MG, Saint-Remy JM. Complexes of grass pollen allergens and specific antibodies reduce allergic symptoms and inhibit the seasonal increase of IgE antibody. Clin Exp Allergy 1990; 20:653–660.
36. Machiels JJ, Somville MA, Jacquemin MG, Saint-Remy JMR. Allergen–antibody complexes can efficiently prevent seasonal rhinitis and asthma in grass pollen hypersensitive patients. Allergen–antibody complex immunotherapy. Allergy 1991; 46:335–348.
37. Machiels JJ, Lebrun PM, Jacquemin MG, Saint-Remy JM. Significant reduction of nonspecific bronchial reactivity in patients with *Dermatophagoides pteronyssinus*-sensitive allergic asthma under therapy with allergen–antibody complexes. Am Rev Respir Dis 1993; 147:1407–1412.
38. Malling HJ. Diagnosis and immunotherapy of mould allergy. With special reference to *Cladosporium herbarum*. Dan Med Bull 1990; 37:12–22.
39. Malling HJ, Dreborg S, Weeke B. Diagnosis and immunotherapy of mould allergy. V. Clinical efficacy and side effects of immunotherapy with *Cladosporium herbarum*. Allergy 1986; 41:507–519.
40. Malling HJ, Dreborg S, Weeke B. Diagnosis and immunotherapy of mould allergy. VI. IgE-mediated parameters during a one-year placebo-controlled study of immunotherapy with *Cladosporium*. Allergy 1987; 42:305–314.
41. Maunsell K, Wraith DG, Hughes AM. Hyposensitisation in mite asthma. Lancet 1971; 1:967–968.
42. Mosbech H, Dreborg S, Frolund L, Ljungstedt Pahlman I, Svendsen UG, Soborg M, Taudorf E, Weeke B. Hyposensitisation in asthmatics with mPEG modified and unmodified house dust mite extract. I. Clinical effect evaluated by diary cards and a retrospective assessment. Allergy 1989; 44:487–498.
43. Mosbech H, Dreborg S, Frolund L, Ljungstedt-Pahlman I, Svendsen UG, Soborg M, Taudorf E, Weeke B. Hyposensitisation in asthmatics with mPEG modified and unmodified house dust mite extract II. Effect evaluated by challenges with allergen and histamine. Allergy 1989; 44:499–509.
44. Mosbech H, Dirkson A, Dreborg S, Frolund L, Heinig JH, Svendsen UG, Soborg M,

Taudorf E, Weeke B. Hyposensitization in asthmatics with mPEG-modified and unmodified house dust mite extract. IV. Occurrence and prediction of side effects. Allergy 1990; 45:142–150.

45. Murray AB, Ferguson AC, Morrison BJ. Non allergic bronchial hyperreactivity in asthmatic children decreases with age and increases with mite immunotherapy. Ann Allergy 1985; 54:541–544.
46. Newton DAG, Maberly DJ, Wilson R. House dust mite hyposensitisation. Br J Dis Chest 1978; 72:21–28.
47. Ohman JL, Findlay SR, Leitermann KM. Immunotherapy in cat induced asthma. Double blind trial with evaluation of in vivo and in vitro responses. J Allergy Clin Immunol 1984; 74:230–239.
48. Ortolani C, Pastorello E, Moss RB, Hsu YP, Restuccia M, Joppolo G, Miadonna A, Cornelli U, Halpern G, Zanussi C. Grass pollen immunotherapy: a single year double blind placebo controlled study in patients with grass pollen induced asthma and rhinitis. J Allergy Clin Immunol. 1984; 73:283–290.
49. Pauli G, Bessot JC, Bigot H, Delaume G, Hordle DA, Hirth C, Thierry R. Clinical and immunologic evaluation of tyrosine adsorbed *Dermatophagoides pteronyssinus* extract: a double blind placebo controlled trial. J Allergy Clin Immunol 1984; 74:524–535.
50. Price JF, Warner JO, Hey EN, Turner MW, Soothill JF. A controlled trial of hyposensitisation with adsorbed tyrosine *Dermatophagoides pteronyssinus* antigen in childhood asthma: in vivo aspects. Clin Allergy 1984; 14:209–219.
51. Reid MJ, Moss RB, Hsu YP, Kwasnicki JM, Commerford TM, Nelson BL. Seasonal asthma in northern California: allergic causes and efficacy of immunotherapy. J Allergy Clin Immunol 1986; 78:590–600.
52. Sabbah A, Bonnaud F, Sonneville A, Bonneau JC, Pinon H. Specific immunotherapy with delayed release *D. pteronyssinus* alpha fraction. A double blind study in asthma. Allergie Immunol 1991; 23:58–60.
53. Smith AP. Hyposensitisation with *Dermatophagoides pteronyssinus* antigen: trial in asthma induced by house dust. Br Med J 1971; 4:204–206.
54. Sundin B, Lilja G, Graff-Lonnevig V, Hedlin G, Heilborn H, Norrlind K, Pegelow KO, Lowenstein H. Immunotherapy with partially purified and standardised animal dander extracts. I. Clinical results from a double blind study on patients with animal dander asthma. J Allergy Clin Immunol 1986; 77:478–487.
55. Taylor B, Sanders SS, Norman AP. A double blind controlled trial of house mite fortified house dust vaccine in childhood asthma. Clin Allergy 1974; 4:35–40.
56. Taylor WW, Ohman JL, Lowell FC. Immunotherapy in cat induced asthma. Double blind trial with evaluation of bronchial responses to cat allergen and histamine. J Allergy Clin Immunol 1978; 61:283–287.
57. Tuchinda M, Chai H. Effect of immunotherapy in chronic asthmatic children. J Allergy Clin Immunol 1973; 51:131–138.
58. Valovirta E, Koivikko A, Vanto T, Viander M, Ingeman L. Immunotherapy in allergy to dog: a double blind clinical study. Ann Allergy 1984; 53:85–88.
59. Valovirta E, Viander M, Koivikko A, Vanto T, Ingeman L. Immunotherapy in allergy to dog. Immunologic and clinical findings of a double-blind study. Ann Allergy 1986; 57:173–179.
60. Van Bever HP, Stevens WJ. Effect of hyposensitisation upon the immediate and late asthmatic reaction and upon histamine reactivity in patients allergic to house dust mite (*Dermatophagoides pteronyssinus*). Eur Respir J 1992; 5:318–322.
61. van Metre TE, Marsh DG, Adkinson NF, Kagey-Sobotka A, Khattignavong A, Norman PS, Rosenberg GL. Immunotherapy for cat asthma. J Allergy Clin Immunol 1988; 82:1055–1068.
62. Warner JO, Price JF, Soothil JF, Hey EN. Controlled trial of hyposensitisation to *Dermatophagoides pteronyssinus* in children with asthma. Lancet 1978; 2:912–915.
63. Adamek-Guzik T, Szczeklik A, Woloszynski J. Multicentre controlled trial of de-

sensitisation treatment of pollen induced hay fever and asthma with Pollinex vaccine. Pol Tyg Lek 1979; 34:1111–1113.

64. Almagro E, Asensio O, Bartolome JM, et al. Multicentric study of pharmacovigilance of sublingual immunotherapy in allergic patients. Allergol Immunopathol 1995; 23:153–159.
65. Bessot JC, Delaume G, Meyer PD, Pauli G. Hyposensitization with *Dermatophagoides pteronyssinus* tyrosine absorbate in bronchial asthma Allergol Immunopathol 1980; 8:351–352.
66. Botey J, Eseverri JL, Marin A, et al. Double blind trial of hyposensitization to *Dermatophagoides farinae* and *D. pteronyssinus* in asthmatic children. Allergie Immunol 1981; 13:16–19.
67. Bousquet J, Becker WM, Hejjaiou A, Chanal I, Lebel B, Dhivert H, Michel FB. Differences in clinical and immunologic reactivity of patients allergic to grass pollens and to multiple pollen species. II. Efficacy of a double blind placebo controlled specific immunotherapy with standardized extracts. J Allergy Clin Immunol 1991; 88:43–53.
68. Bruun E. Control examination of the specificity of specific desensitisation in asthma. Acta Allergol 1949; 2:122–128.
69. Choovoravech P. Effect of immunotherapy: treatment with mite and other aeroallergens in Thai allergic patients. J Med Assoc Thai 1980; 63:506–511.
70. Choovoravech P, Yongpanich Y, Choovoravech N. Effect of immunotherapy in bronchial asthma: treatment with mite extract adsorbed on tyrosine. Curr Med Res Opin 1976; 4:330–339.
71. Chu JC, Wun TH, Chen XJ. Treatment of asthmatic patients sensitive to mites (*Dermatophagoides farinae*); a four year study of immunotherapy with an extract of *Dermatophagoides farinae*. Ann Allergy 1981; 47:107–109.
72. Cleveland CH, Metzger WJ. Immunotherapy with pollens and fungi. Immunol Allergy Clin North Am 1992; 12:39–52.
73. Cooper PJ, Darbyshire J, Nunn AJ, Warner JO. A controlled trial of oral hyposensitization in pollen asthma and rhinitis in children. Clin Allergy 1984; 14:541–550.
74. Corbetta L, Pesiri P, Ferro G, Mander A. Improvement of fog and exercise-induced bronchoconstriction after local and subcutaneous immunotherapy in mite asthma. Allergol Immunopathol 1992; 20:61–66.
75. Crimi E, Voltolini S, Troise C, Gianiorio P, Crimi P, Brusasco V, Negrini AC. Local immunotherapy with *Dermatophagoides* extract in asthma. J Allergy Clin Immunol 1991; 87:721–728.
76. D'Amato G, Kordash TR, Liccardi G, et al. Immunotherapy with Alpare in patients with respiratory allergy to *Parietaria* pollen: a two year double blind placebo controlled study. Clin Exp Allergy 1995; 25:149–158.
77. Engstrom I, Kraepelien S. Specific desensitisation in bronchial asthma in childhood. Acta Paediatr 1957; 46:81–89.
78. Eriksson NE, Ahlstedt S, Lovhagen O. Immunotherapy in spring-time hay fever. A clinical and immunological study comparing two different treatment extract compositions. Allergy 1979; 34:233–247.
79. Fanti A, Coccoli M, Pompili T, Angeloni M, DellOrco G, Cafaggi R, DiMolfetta M. Randomized double-blind trial of a combination of cromoglycate disodium administration and specific desensitization treatment in adults with perennial extrinsic asthma and nonspecific bronchial hyperreactivity. Lotta Contro Tuber Mal Polm Soc 1988; 58:658–663.
80. Feliziani V, Lattuada G, Parmiani S, DallAglio PP. Safety and efficacy of sublingual rush immunotherapy with grass allergen extracts. A double blind study. Allergol Immunopathol 1995; 23:224–230.
81. Ferreira N, Trindade JC. Specific immunotherapy 3 years follow-up in asthmatic children. Allergol Immunopathol 1993; 21:185–192.
82. Formgren H, Lanner A, Lindholm N, Lowhagen O, Dreborg S. Effects of immunotherapy on specific and nonspecific sensitivity of the airways. J Allergy Clin Immunol 1984; 73:140.

83. Giovane AL, Bardare M, Passalacqua G, Ruffoni S, Scordamaglia A, Ghezzi E, Canonica GW. A three-year double-blind placebo-controlled study with specific oral immunotherapy to *Dermatophagoides*: evidence of safety and efficacy in paediatric patients. Clin Exp Allergy 1994; 24:53–59.
84. Goldstein GL, Chai H. Efficacy of rush immunotherapy in decreasing bronchial sensitivity to inhaled antigens in perennial childhood asthma. Ann Allergy 1981; 47:333–337.
85. Goor W, Wuthrich B. Specific therapy of pollinosis. Results of desensitization with two different semi-depot allergen extracts (Allpyral and Suspal). Schweiz Med Wochenschr 1971; 101:1217–1221.
86. Gordon VH, Caplinger KJ, Meade JH Jr, Thompson C. Correlation of type specific fluorescent antibodies to ragweed with symptomatology: double-blind study. Ann Allergy 1972; 30:507–517.
87. Grammer LC, Zeiss CR, Suszko IM, et al. A double-blind, placebo-controlled trial of polymerized whole ragweed for immunotherapy of ragweed allergy. J Allergy Clin Immunol 1982; 69:494–499.
88. Grammer LC, Shaughnessy MA, Suszko IM, et al. A double-blind histamine placebo-controlled trial of polymerized whole grass for immunotherapy of grass allergy. J Allergy Clin Immunol 1983; 72:448–453.
89. Haahtela T, Wihl JA, Munch E, et al. Hyposensitization in hay fever with grass pollen extracts: a three-year study comparing a dialysed alum adsorbed extract with Allpyral. Ann Allergy 1984; 52:355–362.
90. Haugaard L, Dahl R, Jacobsen L. A controlled dose–response study of immunotherapy with standardized, partially purified extract of house dust mite: clinical efficacy and side effects. Allergy Clin Immunol 1993; 91:709–722.
91. Hedlin G, Heilborn H, Lilja G, et al. Long term follow-up of patients treated with a three year course of cat or dog immunotherapy. J Allergy Clin Immunol 1995; 96:879–885.
92. Henocq E, Garcelon M, Berrens L. Photo-inactivated allergens II. Clinical experience with house dust allergen in pulmonary function tests and in immunotherapy. Clin Allergy 1973; 3:461–469.
93. Hirsch SR, Kalbfleisch JH, Cohen SH. Comparison of Rinkel injection therapy with standard immunotherapy. J Allergy Clin Immunol 1982; 70:183–190.
94. Horst M, Hejjaiou A, Horst V, Michel FB, Bousquet J. Double blind placebo controlled rush immunotherapy with a standardised *Alternaria* extract. J Allergy Clin Immunol 1990; 85:460–472.
95. Jarisch R, Sandor I, Gotz M, Krummer F. Immunotherapy of allergic disease: studies on 460 patients. Hautarzt 1979; 30:365–370.
96. Kalla M, Rozniecki J, Polanska Z, Swatko A. Evaluation of the effectiveness of desensitisation in bronchial asthma caused by house mites or grass pollen in the light of clinical results and the histamine and polymyxin inhalation test. Pol Tyg Lek 1979; 34:865–868.
97. Laetsch C, Wuthrich B. Towards the oral desensitization of inhalational allergies in childhood: treatment-results. Schweiz Med Wochenschr 1973; 103:342–347.
98. Leng X, Fu YX, Ye ST, Duan SQ. A double-blind trial of oral immunotherapy for *Artemisia* pollen asthma with evaluation of bronchial response to the pollen allergen and serum-specific IgE antibody. Ann Allergy 1990; 64:27–31.
99. Levin SJ. Hyposensitising (immunising) injections in hay fever and asthma. Pediatr Clin North Am 1959; 6:698–708.
100. Lichtenstein LM, Norman PS, Winkenwerder WL. A single year of immunotherapy for ragweed hay fever: immunologic and clinical studies. Ann Intern Med 1971; 75:663.
101. Lilja G, Sundin B, Graff-Lonnevig V, Hedlin G, Heilborn H, Norrlind K, Pegelow KO, Lowenstein H. Immunotherapy with cat- and dog-dander extracts. IV. Effects of 2 years of treatment. J Allergy Clin Immunol 1989; 83:37–44.
102. Mallet A, Lluch M, Valero AL, Casanovas M. Clinical and immunological effects of

immunotherapy with glutaraldehyde modified house dust mite extract. Allergol Immunopathol 1994; 22:226–232.

103. Martorell Aragones A, Vila Martinez R, Colomer Sala J. Bronchial asthma. Clinical evolution with hyposensitization Anal Espan Pediatr 1980; 13:87–100.

104. Maruo H, Hashimoto K, Shimoda K, Shimanuki K, Nakayama T, Yamaguchi H, Shiigai N, Uchimura K, Mitsubayashi T, Ajkasaka T. Long-term follow up studies of bronchial asthma in children. II. Prognosis and complications, treatment and allergic evaluations. Arerugi 1990; 39:662–669.

105. Matoga S, Scislicki A, Haluszka J, Kurzwa R. Results of immunotherapy with HDM (Bencard) in children with bronchial asthma. Pediatr Pol 1989; 64:167–172.

106. McAllen MK, Heaf PJD, McInroy P. Depot grass pollen injections in asthma: effect of repeated treatment on clinical response and measured bronchial sensitivity. Br Med J 1967; 1:22–25.

107. Metzger WJ, Donnelly A, Richerson HB. Modification of late asthmatic responses during immunotherapy for *Alternaria* induced asthma. J Allergy Clin Immunol 1983; 71:119.

108. Miguel Lozano R, Guerra Pasadas F, Arenas Vacas A, Daza Munoz JC, Torres Murillo P, Sanchez Guijo P. Monitoring of various types of immunotherapy with gramineal pollens. I. Variation of clinical and biochemical parameters. Allergol Immunopathol 1992; 20:230–234.

109. Mischler TW, OBrien WM, Rugloski RJ, et al. A multiclinic trial with glutaraldehyde-modified tyrosine-adsorbed ragweed pollen immunotherapy (Pollinex). Curr Ther Res 1981; 29:745–756.

110. Moller C, Dreborg S, Lanner A, Bjorksten B. Oral immunotherapy of children with rhinoconjunctivitis due to birch pollen allergy. A double blind study. Allergy 1986; 41:271–279.

111. Mosbech H. Who will benefit from hyposensitisation? Allergy 1990; 45:209–212.

112. Moscata G, Rossi G, Dellabianca A, Pisati A, Vinci G, Biale C. Local immunotherapy by inhalation of a powder extract in asthma due to house dust mite *Dermatophagoides pteronyssinus*: a double-blind comparison with parenteral immunotherapy. J Invest Allergol Clin Immunol 1991; 1:383–394.

113. Moshkevich VS. Local immunotherapy for chronic respiratory allergic pathology with allergen aerosols. II. Treatment of bronchial asthma. Allergol Immunopathol 9815; 13:317–321.

114. Munoz Lejarazu D, Bernaola G, Fernandez E, Audicana M, Ventas P, Martin S, Fernandez De Corres L. Seasonal versus perennial immunotherapy: evaluation after three years of treatment. J Invest Allergol Clin Immunol 1993; 3:210–216.

115. Munoz-Lopez F. Immunotherapy—methods of treatment and results in children. Allergol Immunopathol 1981; (suppl 9):171–173.

116. Munoz-Lopez F, Martin Mateos A, Moreira A, Martinez Marin F. Topical nasal immunotherapy with *Dermatophagoides pteronyssinus* extract. Allergol Immunopathol 1994; 22:132–134.

117. Munro-Ashman D, Frankland AW. Treatment of allergy to house dust with pyridine-extracted alum-precipitated extracts of the house dust mite. Ann Allergy 1976; 36:95–98.

118. Nagata M, Tabe K, Yamamoto H, Maruo H, Kiuch H, Sakamoto Y, Yamamoto K, Dohi Y. The analysis of factors contributing to the safety and efficacy of rush immunotherapy in bronchial asthma. Arerugi 1993; 42:628–634.

119. Nagata M, Yamamoto H, Tabe K, Kimura I, Houya I, Kuramitsu K, Kiuchi H, Yangihara Y, Sakamoto Y, Yamamoto K, Dohi Y. Effect of rush immunotherapy in house-dust-mite (HDM)-sensitive adult bronchial asthma: changes in in vivo and in vitro responses to HDM. Intern Med 1993; 32:702–709.

120. Norman PS, Lichtenstein LM. The clinical and immunologic specificity of immunotherapy. J Allergy Clin Immunol 1978; 61:370–377.

121. Novembre E, Marano E, Bernardini R, Caria M, Dini L, Vierucci A. Sublingual immu-

notherapy in the treatment of allergic asthma in children: a controlled study. Riv Ital Pediatr 1991; 17:75–78.
122. Oppenheimer J, Areson JG, Nelson HS. Safety and efficacy of oral immunotherapy with standardized cat extract. J Allergy Clin Immunol 1994; 93:61–67.
123. Osterballe O. Immunotherapy with grass pollen major allergens. Allergy 1982; 37:379–388.
124. Pence HL, Mitchell DQ, Greely RL, Updegraff BR, Selfridge HA. Immunotherapy for mountain cedar pollinosis: a double blind controlled study. J Allergy Clin Immunol 1976; 58:39–50.
125. Petersen BN, Janniche H, Munch EP, Wihl JA, Bowadt H, Opsen H. Lowenstein H. Immunotherapy with partially purified and standardized tree pollen extracts. I. Clinical results from a three-year double-blind study of patients treated with pollen extracts either of birch or combinations of alder, birch and hazel. Allergy 1988; 43:353–362.
126. Rak S, Ahlstedt S, Bjorksten B, Fabbri L, Dahl R. Effects of immunotherapy on the inflammation in pollen asthma. Allergy Suppl 1993; 48:125–128.
127. Rak S, Hallden G, Sorenson S, Margari V, Scheynius A. The effect of immunotherapy on T-cell subsets in peripheral blood and bronchoalveolar lavage fluid in pollen-allergic patients. Allergy 1993; 48:460–465.
128. Rebien W, Wahn U, Puttonen E, Maasch HJ. Comparative study on the immunological and clinical efficacy of oral and subcutaneous hyposensitization. Allergologie 1980; 3:101–106.
129. Reinert M, Biro G. Hyposensitization with tyrosine-allergoids. Prax Klin Pneumol 1981; 35:71–75.
130. Reinert M, Reinert U. Oral hyposensitization with pollen solutions and placebos. Prax Klin Pneumol 1983; 37:228–231.
131. Rocha EM. Effect of 2 therapeutic protocols in minor forms of respiratory allergy. Allergie Immunol 1986; 18:29–41.
132. Rohatgi N, Dunn K, Chai H. Cat or dog induced immediate and late asthmatic responses before and after immunotherapy. J Allergy Clin Immunol 1988; 82:389.
133. Sadan N, Rhyne MB, Mellits ED, et al. Immunotherapy of pollinosis in children: investigation of the immunologic basis of clinical improvement. N Engl J Med 1969; 280:623–627.
134. Sanchez Palacios A, Schamann Medina F, Lamas Rua-Figueroa A, Bosch Millares C, Ramos Santos S, Garcia Marrero JA. Comparative clinical–immunológical study of oral and subcutaneous immunotherapy in children with extrinsic bronchial asthma. Allergol Immunopathol 1989; 17:323–329.
135. Sanders S. The treatment of seasonal hay fever and asthma in children. A controlled trial of pre-seasonal depot pollen therapy. Practitioner 1966; 196:811–815.
136. Swineford O, Cumbia JW, Berger KW, Lucas DC. Treatment of pollen hay fever and asthma with aerosols of pollen extracts. J Allergy 1955; 26:305–319.
137. Sychlowy A, Lukas A, Nowak W, Maruszewski W. Treatment of asthma caused by house dust mites with a combination of Intal and vaccine adsorbed on tyrosine. Pediatr Pol 1979; 54:1295–1298.
138. Tari MG, Mancino M, Monti G. Efficacy of sublingual immunotherapy in patients with rhinitis and asthma due to house dust mite. A double-blind study. Allergol Immunopathol 1990; 18:277–284.
139. Tari MG, Mancino M, Monti G. Immunotherapy by inhalation of allergen in powder in house dust allergic asthma—a double-blind study. J Invest Allergol Clin Immunol 1992; 2:59–67.
140. Taub SJ. Ragweed hayfever and asthma. Ill Med J 1969; 135:706–707.
141. Taudorf E, Weeke B. Orally administered grass pollen. Allergy 1983; 38:561–564.
142. Taudorf E, Laursen LC, Djurup R, et al. Oral administration of grass pollen to hay fever patients. An efficacy study in oral hyposensitization. Allergy 1985; 40:321–335.

143. Taudorf E, Laursen LC, Lanner A, et al. Oral immunotherapy in birch pollen hay fever. J. Allergy Clin Immunol 1987; 80:153–161.
144. Turner MW, Yalcin I, Soothill JF, Price JF, Warner JO, Hey EN, Chapman MD, Platts-Mills TA. In vitro investigations in asthmatic children undergoing hyposensitization with tyrosine-adsorbed *Dermatophagoides pteronyssinus* antigen. Clin Allergy 1984; 14:221–231.
145. Urbanek R, Gehl R. Efficacy of oral hyposensitization treatment in house dust mite allergy. Monatsschr Kinderheilk 1982; 130:150–152.
146. Van Bever JP, Bosmans J, De Clerck LS, Stevens WJ. Modification of the late asthmatic reaction by hyposensitisation in asthmatic children allergic to house dust mite (*Dermatophagoides pteronyssinus*) or grass pollen. Allergy 1988; 43:378–385.
147. Van Bever HP, Stevens WJ. Suppression of the late asthmatic reaction by hyposensitization in asthmatic children allergic to house dust mite (*Dermatophagoides pteronyssinus*). Clin Exp Allergy 1989; 19:399–404.
148. Van Bever HP, Stevens WJ. Evolution of the late asthmatic reaction during immunotherapy and after stopping immunotherapy. J Allergy Clin Immunol 1990; 86:141–146.
149. Wahn U, Siraganian RP. Efficacy and specificity of immunotherapy with laboratory animal allergen extracts. J Allergy Clin Immunol 1980; 65:413–421.
150. Weyer A, Donat N, L'Heritier C, et al. Grass pollen hyposensitization versus placebo therapy. Allergy 1981; 36:309.
151. Wuthrich B, Hafner G. Pollinosis II. Specific hyposensitisation: indications and results of treatment. A study with the allergen preparation Stallergenes-Depot in the pollen season of 1976, 1977 and 1978. Schweiz Med Wochenschr 1980; 110:281–290.
152. Cotes J. Lung Function—Assessment and Application in Medicine, 4th ed. Oxford: Blackwell Scientific, 1979.
153. CONSORT Group. Improving the quality of reporting of randomised controlled trials: the CONSORT statement. JAMA 1996; 276:637–639.
154. Specific allergen immunotherapy for asthma—a position statement of the Thoracic Society of Australia and New Zealand and the Australasian Society of Clinical Immunology and Allergy. Med J Aust 1997; 167:540–544.

14

Noninjective Immunotherapy
Present Knowledge and Experimental Evidence

GIOVANNI PASSALACQUA and GIORGIO WALTER CANONICA

University of Genoa
Genoa, Italy

GIAN ENRICO SENNA

Verona General Hospital
Verona, Italy

I. General Aspects

A. Historical Background

Although the mechanisms underlying the allergic reactions were almost unknown, the possibility of obtaining a desensitization against the offending allergens by administering increasing doses of the allergen itself, has been envisaged since the first years of the century. The original aim of such a treatment was to achieve an *immunization*, similar to that obtained with other vaccinations, thus evoking a protective response to the antigen. The early pioneering attempts in humans provided encouraging results (1,2); therefore, the kind of prophylaxis, in the following years, assumed more and more clinical relevance, and the term allergen-specific *immunotherapy* (IT) became of common use. Subsequently, the *subcutaneous* IT (SIT) was clinically used and prescribed on a mere empirical basis. Since the 1970s, many controlled studies demonstrated the clinical effectiveness of SIT in asthma and rhinitis treatment (3–20) and some problems, previously unexpected, emerged. These problems particularly concerned (1) characterization, standardization, and purification of the extracts; (2) risks and safety of the treatment; (3) dosage and schedules for SIT administration; (4) comparison with pharmacological treatments; (5) duration of SIT effects after suspension; and (6) mechanisms of action. Both clinical and basic immunology studies performed during the last 15 years solved many of the foregoing problems. In particular, aims and clinical indications of SIT and its prophylactic rationale (21–23) were satisfactorily defined. Nevertheless, the problem of the possible severe adverse events persisted and made the use of SIT questionable (24). Actually, prospective studies showed that technical errors or incorrect prescription or executions of SIT were often responsible for the severe adverse events observed (25), and a strenuous and continuous educational effort (26–29) was made to improve its safety. In addition, several routes for IT administration began to be developed and investigated with the primary aim of avoiding the occurrence of severe adverse events.

B. Noninjective Immunotherapy

The term noninjective (or local) immunotherapy (NIIT) indicates the nonparenteral routes for IT administration (i.e., oral [OIT], sublingual [more properly *sublingual–oral*, SLIT], local nasal [LNIT], and local bronchial [LBIT]). The term *alternative routes*, presently used, should be abandoned because it may generate confusion with other treatments (30). Attempts to achieve systemic or local hyposensitization through oral, nasal, or bronchial routes were made in the first decades of the century (31–33), but a renewed interest in NIIT arose in Europe in the 1970s and increased after the reports of fatalities caused by subcutaneous IT (24–25). In fact, the overall aim of noninjective routes of IT is to reduce the risk of severe untoward effects and to provide a well-tolerated and accepted treatment for the patients (26). The literature now provides several well-controlled clinical studies, and allows us to define the possible role of NIIT in the management of respiratory allergic disease.

C. NIITs in Respiratory Allergy: Evaluation of Efficacy

An objective, rigorous, and quantitative assessment of the efficacy of IT is obviously needed to support its routine clinical use and, also, a careful risk/benefit ratio has to be established. Consequently, we will herein consider only those trials published in English in peer-reviewed journals, conducted in a double-blind, placebo-controlled fashion, performed with a correct experimental design and adequate statistical treatment.

As a matter of fact, the only possible and reasonable assessment of the efficacy of IT can be made by evaluation of clinical aspects: symptoms and drugs intake. Thus, in the available clinical trials, the main parameters considered were (1) presence and grade of clinical symptoms, usually performed under *natural allergenic exposure* through a diary card kept by the patient, or on the basis of clinical visits. *Standardized exposure devices* (Vienna Challenge Chamber, apartment exposure), can also be employed for the clinical evaluation. (2) *Rescue medication intake* or symptomatic drug consumption, recorded by diary cards.

Additional (*paraclinical*) parameters of efficacy also can be considered: (1) *target organ* (nose, conjunctiva, or bronchi) *reactivity*; threshold allergen provocative dose; nonspecific bronchial hyperresponsiveness; indexes of nasal obstruction; or skin reactivity; (2) *systemic immunological parameters* (total IgE, specific IgE, specific IgG, and specific IgG1 and IgG4). These parameters are of interest from a pathophysiological perspective, but they should be considered as adjuncts to clinical evaluation, which still remains the main objective measurement of IT efficacy.

II. Experimental Evidence

To establish objectively the effectiveness of NIIT, only the double-blind, placebo-controlled (DBPC) studies, published in English, in peer-reviewed journals and performed with adequate design and statistical analysis will be considered.

A. Oral Route

The oral route (OIT) was studied in the treatment of both asthma and rhinoconjunctivitis. Thirteen DBPC studies aimed at assessing the efficacy of OIT have now been performed (34–46). Nevertheless, six (34–39) of them did not provide complete information or showed a poor study design (incorrect statistical analysis, low doses of extract, or small numbers of patients); thus, these studies will not be considered herein to be conclusive from a clinical perspective. Of the remaining seven studies (40–46), only three (40,42,43) evaluated the effects of OIT on asthma symptoms. In the study by Moller et al. (40), most of the patients had hay fever, nevertheless a protective effect of OIT on the development of asthma was observed. In the study by Giovane et al. (42) a significant improvement of asthma symptoms and drug intake was observed during the second year of treatment. The study by Mosbech et al. (43) failed to demonstrated a significant effect of OIT on grass-induced asthma. Nevertheless, it is noteworthy that systemic immunological responses were observed, in some studies (36,37,42,47), resembling those induced by subcutaneous IT, and that a nasal–conjunctival-specific reactivity reduction was also described in some trials (36,40,42). The duration of the treatment appeared to be crucial, because a clear-cut clinical improvement was observed after only 12 months of treatment (42). Nevertheless, it is difficult to reach a balanced conclusion because different allergen preparations (i.e., drops, tablets, and enteric-coated capsules) were employed in the clinical trials.

B. Sublingual Route

Ten eligible studies are now available (48–57), but six of them evidenced methodological or sample size problems (48–53), and their results, although encouraging (49,50,52), cannot be assumed as objectively demonstrating the effectiveness of the treatment. Four studies (54–57) clearly demonstrated the clinical efficacy of SLIT (administered as sublingual–oral), as summarized in Table 1.

Table 1 SLIT Controlled Studies

Author (Ref.)	Allergen	Duration (mo)	Patients[a] (A/P)	Age (yr)	Disease[b]	Efficacy	Adverse events
Tari (54)	Mite	18	30/28	5–12	R/A	Yes	3 urticaria 3 asthma
Sabbah (56)	Grass	1.5	29/29	13–51	R	Yes	No severe
Troise (57)	*Parietaria*	10	15/16	17–60	R	Yes	No severe
Feliziani (55)	Grass	3.5	18/16	14–18	R/A	Yes	No severe

[a]Patients: A, active; P, placebo.
[b]Disease: R, rhinitis; A, asthma.

The SLIT significantly reduced both asthma symptoms and drug intake in patients suffering from respiratory allergy caused by dust mite (54), and grass (56) or *Parietaria* (57) pollen. In addition, SLIT appeared clinically effective when administered as preseasonal "rush" in grass pollen allergy (55).

Also, for SLIT, systemic immunological effects (i.e., IgG1 or IgG4 increase, and skin reactivity reduction) were observed (51,52,54,58), and a target organ sensitivity reduction was described. (54,57). Finally, two favorable double-blind, placebo-controlled studies of SLIT with birch and grass extracts (58–59) are available as abstracts. The one performed with grass extract (59) demonstrated a significant steroid-sparing effect of SLIT in a large population of rhinitic patients.

C. Local Nasal Route

Numerous clinical trials of LNIT are now available (60–79). Seven of these studies (60–66) cannot be assumed to prove with certainty the effectiveness of LNIT because of methodological limits. Twelve of the 13 remaining papers demonstrate a significant improvement of nasal symptoms both in perennial and seasonal rhinitis (Table 2). Furthermore, a reduction of the nasal reactivity and local allergic inflammation was also evidenced, whereas systemic immunological changes were undetectable or were equivocal. This may suggest that the effectiveness of LNIT is restricted to only the target organ. In general, the effectiveness of LNIT seems to be dose-related and, at least for pollen allergy, a preseasonal course should be repeated every year (Passalacqua G, et al., submitted). Aqueous and powdered extracts appeared more effective than the modified ones.

D. Local Bronchial Route

The local bronchial IT (LBIT) is supported by much experimental evidence from clinical and basic immunology, and several clinical attempts using this route have been made (80–81). Two controlled clinical trials of LBIT to mite antigens are available (82–83): their results are controversial. After a 4-week course of LBIT, a reduction of only early specific bronchial reactivity was demonstrated, with no significant clinical improvement by diary card scores (82). In another study, the symptomatological improvement was significant after an 18-month treatment, and an increase in bronchial challenge threshold dose was also observed (83). The small number of patients observed, and the equivocal results, currently discourage the clinical use of LBIT. On the other hand, it represents a speculative, interesting model of local desensitization for further investigation.

E. Safety

For OIT, relevant adverse reactions clearly related to the treatment were observed only in the study employing very high doses of extract (45), whereas in other studies, asthma or rhinitis were also observed in the placebo groups (43,46). Indeed,

Table 2 LNIT Controlled Studies

Author (Ref.)	Allergen	Extract[a]	Duration (wk)	Patients[a] (A/P)	Efficacy	Adverse events
Johansson (67)	Grass	Aq	14	12/11	Yes	12 rhinitis
Nickelsen (68)	Ragweed	Aq (mod)	12	38 (35)/34	Yes	72 rhinitis
Welsh (69)	Ragweed	Aq	20	18/15	Yes	No
Schumacher	Grass	Pwd	10	8/7	No	No
Georgitis (71,72)	Grass	Pwd (mod)	10	16 (15)/13	Yes	No
Georgitis (62,63)	Ragweed	Aq (mod)	10	15 (14)/16	Yes (no)	Rhinitis
Andri (73)	*Parietaria*	Pwd (mod)	18	8 (8)/8	Yes	No
Andri (74)	Mite	Pwd	52	11/10	Yes	No
Passalacqua (76)	*Parietaria*	Pwd	20	9/9	Yes	No
D'Amato (75)	*Parietaria*	Pwd	32	10/10	Yes	3 asthma
Andri (77)	Birch	Pwd	22	14/14	Yes	No
Andri (78)	Grass	Pwd	26	13/15	Yes	No
Cirla (79)	Birch/alder	Pwd	16	11/11	Yes	No

[a]Extract: Aq, aqueous; mod, modified; Pwd, powdered.
[b]Patients: A, active; P, placebo.

some gastrointestinal side effects were observed in several studies, but none of these patients required discontinuation of the treatment.

The most frequently reported side effect with SLIT was the onset of oral–sublingual itching; this phenomenon was always described as mild and self-resolving. Headache, rhinorrhea, constipation, or urticaria were described only sporadically, and no severe adverse event was reported in the quoted studies. A study of pharmcovigilance for SLIT (84) has been recently published. The incidence of side effects was indeed low: oropharyingeal itching represented about 50% of the untoward effects, followed by rhinorrhea and constipation. Urticaria and asthma were very rare. Ninety percent of the effects were mild to moderate and systemic anaphylaxis was never described.

For LNIT, the earliest aqueous extract, although effective, appeared beset by troublesome local side effects (rhinitis); this made the usefulness of LNIT somewhere questionable (85). Conversely, the modified extracts showed reduced side effects, but also appeared less effective. The recently introduced dried powder extracts showed more efficacy than the aqueous ones, and they appear devoid of local side effects. The hypothesized risk of asthma attack induction is not substantiated by evidence, and such an occurrence has been described only anecdotally in a single study (75). Finally, in the studies of LBIT, asthma attacks (even if mild) that required bronchodilators were reported as frequent. Thus, the risk/benefit ratio does not support LBIT for clinical use.

F. Combination and Comparison with Subcutaneous Immunotherapy

The use of OIT as an extension and follow-up of a course of subcutaneous IT was investigated in two clinical trials (86,87). These studies provided controversial results with grass extracts. Therefore, on the basis of the literature, no conclusive statement can be provided, and the use of NIIT as an extension of a build-up course of injection treatment is not presently justified.

Several clinical trials (88–94) attempted to compare the clinical effectiveness of NIITs and subcutaneous IT, with controversial results. Two studies (88,89) reported NIIT to be less effective than subcutaneous IT. Three studies conducted with LBIT (91) and SLIT (93,94), respectively, showed NIITs to be more effective and better tolerated than the injective route. Finally, one study (92) showed that injective IT induces systemic immunological effects that are more pronounced than NIITs.

The only study performed in a double-blind, double-dummy fashion (94), demonstrated that SLIT has a clinical efficacy equivalent to SIT, with no side effects.

G. Mechanisms of Action: Immunological Evidence

The mechanisms of action of subcutaneous IT has only recently begun to be clarified (95–97). Similar evidence is still lacking for NIIT, but an imposing number of basic immunology studies provide interesting information and hypotheses. The "tolerogenicity" of the oral route has been demonstrated in animal models (98–100); it appears to involve the Th1–Th2 differentiation (101) and the regulation of IgE production (100). In addition, dendritic cells of the oral mucosa are able to act as efficient antigen-presenting cells (102,103) and to produce interleukin (IL)-12, which affects the Th1–Th2 balance (104). In humans, a significant enhancement of mucosal IgA production following OIT has also been described (105)

Also, similar mechanisms appear to operate in the lung (106,107). In the so-called high IgE responder mice, a certain tolerance (decreased IgE production) is achieved after inhalation allergen administration (108,109), although in some cases, the systemic and local immunity appears to be dissociated (110). In humans, the mucosal antibody response and the systemic changes appear unrelated to the clinical efficacy; thus, they remain of uncertain importance and cannot be considered as the main mechanism of action. Finally, LNIT has been able to reduce nasal allergic inflammation (76) after specific allergen challenge (decrease of inflammatory cell infiltration and ICAM-1 expression on nasal epithelium).

Only sparse data on the kinetics (absorption and fate) of the allergenic extracts are yet available for NIIT (111–114). Preliminary kinetic data in healthy humans demonstrate that the gastroenteric absorption is quantitatively the most relevant absorption route for both SLIT and LNIT, although a significant involvement of local immunity is also likely to occur (115).

III. Clinical Indications

The NIITs share with SIT the same rationale: they should be used with the aim of modifying the clinical history of the disease and of preventing its evolution, possibly reducing the drug intake. Accordingly, NIIT should not be used in the late course of the disease, when nonreversible damages are present and the progression cannot be modified.

The clinical effectiveness of OIT (tablets, capsules, or drops) is not sufficiently supported by experimental data. SLIT (administered as sublingual–oral), has been effective in asthma treatment. It is indicated in patients with allergic rhinoconjunctivitis or asthma, when the offending allergen cannot be avoided by environmental care. The sublingual–oral route is particularly suitable for pediatric patients because it is well accepted and tolerated, although further specific studies are needed. For now, LBIT must be considered an experimental attempt, and its use in clinical practice is not recommended. LNIT is strictly indicated in rhinitis: because of its peculiar administration technique, careful training of the patients (preferably adult) is required.

Finally, in general, NIITs are suggested in patients showing low compliance with SIT, or in those with previous severe adverse reactions. Importantly, NIIT should not to be considered a substitute for subcutaneous IT, but rather, as a complementary or additional therapeutic tool. NIIT and SIT might also be used in various combinations, to optimize both the compliance of the patient and the therapeutic effect.

IV. Practical Aspects of NIIT

A. Prescription

Because NIIT is self-administered, we strongly suggest that the prescription is made only by a specialist. Furthermore, similarly to SIT, a proper etiologic diagnosis (involving skin testing, RAST, and specific nasal–conjunctival challenge) is required (26–28,116). Patients must be instructed to carefully follow the manufacturer's schedule of administration and to have a clinical visit every 3 months, at least in the early phase of the treatment.

B. Administration Technique

The administration schedules vary from manufacturer to manufacturer, but usually an NIIT course involves a buildup phase, during which the extract is administered at increasing doses; and a maintenance phase, during which the maximal dose is administered two or three times a week. Furthermore, NIIT can be administered either preseasonally or continuously, depending on the allergen; rush schedules for preseasonal IT are also available.

Oral Route

The allergenic extract is consumed as drops or tablets in the morning, after the patient has fasted, and swallowed with water or juice.

Sublingual Route

Two administration techniques exist: the extract can be kept sublingually for 1 or 2 min and then swallowed (properly called *sublingual–oral*), or it can be kept sublingually and then spit out (*sublingual–spit*). The preliminary kinetic study, suggests that the sublingual–oral route is preferable to take advantage of both local immunity and enteric absorption.

Intranasal Route

The allergenic extract (aqueous or powdered) has to be sprayed into a nostril while vocalizing. Some manufacturers suggest a premedication with nasal cromolyn.

C. Extracts

The problem of an unequivocal standardization of the allergenic extracts (and of their preparation) still remains of primary interest, and it is also a matter of debate (117–118) for NIIT extracts.

Extracts of a wide variety of allergens have been used in the reviewed NIIT clinical trials (e.g., grass, *Parietaria*, birch, ragweed, dust mite, and animal dander). Each producer applies an in-house method for standardization (RAST-inhibition, biological assays) and provides arbitrary units (allergenic units, biological units, or other); therefore, a comparison of potency of the different extracts is impossible. For the pharmacological preparation, allergenic extracts are usually produced as aqueous solutions for SLIT. The problem is more complex for OIT, which can be dispensed either as drops, enteric-coated capsules, or tablets. LNIT and LBIT can be dispensed either as aqueous solution or in powder form; this latter preparation appeared to be more safe and effective.

D. Precautions

Some of the rules suggested (26–28) for subcutaneous IT should also be observed with NIIT: (1) age: although several studies in pediatric patients provide favorable results, for children younger than 5 years, NIIT prescription should be made by a specialist. (2) Pregnancy: it is not a reason for discontinuing an ongoing NIIT course; nevertheless, as a prudential rule, NIIT should be not instituted in pregnant women. (3) Contraindications: these include severe immunological disorders or deficiencies, malignancies, severe or uncontrolled asthma, or oral allergic syndrome.

The routine clinical use and the controlled trials of NIIT are a matter of the last 15 years. Therefore, no empirically supported rule can be given about modification or adjustment of the doses in the event of adverse events. On the other hand, relevant adverse events have been very rarely reported. Thus, because the severity of adverse reactions seem to be dose-related, as with subcutaneous IT, a dose reduction (or no dose increase) is suggested for adverse events.

V. Conclusions

In general, IT has been effective in reducing asthma symptoms (119), in preventing the progression of allergic disease, and is capable of modifying the natural history of the disorder. Indeed, most of the controversies over the use of IT in asthma originate from an incorrect prescription. In fact, during the last 15 years, IT was prescribed as a last-choice treatment, with the expectation of a dramatic clinical outcome when pharmacological treatment failed to control symptoms. This is not actually true; we now know that respiratory allergy is a complex inflammatory disorder involving inherited characters, allergen exposure, immune inflammation, and bronchial hyperreactivity. We also are well aware that the available drug treatments (i.e., β_2-adrenergic agonists, corticosteroids, xanthines) act only nonspecifically on the epiphenomena of the disorder (i.e., bronchospasm, cell migration, and recruitment) and do not affect the allergen-driven immune response. On the contrary, IT appears able to specifically modify the characteristics of the immunological response

Table 3 Immunotherapy Costs per Year (Approximate Data from Italian Market)

	OIT/SLIT LNIT ($)	SIT ($)	
Patient's costs	400 4 refills	200 2 refills	Treatment
	—	200	12 injections per year
	300 3 visits	200 2 visits	Allergist's controls
Social cost	—	480	Loss of working time per 12 injections
Total	700	1080	

to the offending allergen. Thus, IT must be considered a prophylactic treatment (or biological response modifier) for allergic asthma, to be used in association with drugs and environmental care. The prophylactic effect of IT would also suggest its use in children and in the earliest phases of the disease (120,121).

Actually, some aspects of NIITs have to be further investigated and developed: (1) allergen standardization, (2) schedule definition and treatment duration, (3) kinetics of the extracts, and (4) the effectiveness of other allergens and further comparison with subcutaneous IT. Nevertheless, the data now available indicate a significant clinical efficacy and safety of LNIT and SLIT (sublingual–oral); hence, their clinical use can be suggested in everyday clinical practice, also considering the likely improved compliance of patients.

Most importantly, NIIT must not be considered to be a substitute for subcutaneous IT, but rather, as a complementary or additional therapeutic tool. Consequently, as a hypothesis, NIIT and subcutaneous IT might also be used in various combinations for different allergens to optimize both the compliance of the patient and the therapeutic effect, although this has to be proved. Finally, NIITs may allow a not negligible socioeconomic saving, for they have a reduced social cost (Table 3); an important feature of a prophylactic treatment (122).

Note Added in Proof

Since the time of submission of the present chapter, three further papers (among them Ref. 123) on sublingual immunotherapy have been published in international journals. A panel of experts of the World Health Organization, in a position paper (124), have officially recognized the nasal and sublingual immunotherapy as suitable alternatives to injection immunotherapy.

References

1. Noon L. Prophylactic inoculation against hayfever. Lancet 1911; 1:1572.
2. Freeman J. Vaccination against hay fever: report of results during the first 3 years. Lancet 1914; 1:1178.
3. Reid MJ, Moss RB, Yao Pi Sha MS, Kwasnicki JC, Commerford TL, Nelson BL. Seasonal asthma in northern California. Allergic causes and efficacy of immunotherapy. J Allergy Clin Immunol 1986; 78:590–600.
4. Bousquet J, Maasch HJ, Heijaoui A, Skassa-Brociek W, Wahl R, Dhivert H, Michel FB. Double blind placebo controlled immunotherapy with grass pollen allergoids. III. Efficacy and safety of unfractionated and high molecular weight preparations in rhinoconjunctivitis and asthma. J Allergy Clin Immunol 1989; 84:546–556.
5. Bousquet J, Heijaoui J, Michel FB. Specific immunotherapy in asthma. J Allergy Clin Immunol 1990; 86:292–305.
6. Ohman JL, Findlay SR, Leitermann KM. Immunotherapy in cat-induced asthma. Double blind trial with evaluation of in vitro and in vivo response. J Allergy Clin Immunol 1984; 74:230–239.
7. Sundin B, Lilja G, Graff-Lonnevig V, Hedlin G, Heilborn H, Norrlind K Peglow KO, Lowenstein H. Immunotherapy with partially purified and standardized animal dander extracts. I. Clinical results from a double blind study on patients with animal dander asthma. J Allergy Clin Immunol 1986; 77:478–487.
8. van Metre TE, Marsh DG, Adkinson NF. Immunotherapy for cat asthma. J Allergy Clin Immunol 1988; 82:1053–1058.
9. Dreborg S, Agrell B, Foucard T, Kjellmann NM, Koiikko A, Nilsson S. A double blind multicenter immunotherapy trial in children using a purified and standardized *Cladosporium herbarum* preparation. I. Clinical results. Allergy 1986; 41:131–140.
10. Horst M, Heijaoui A, Horst V. Double blind placebo controlled rush immunotherapy with a standardized *Alternaria* extract. J Allergy Clin Immunol 1990: 85:460–462.
11. Price JF, Warner JO, Hey EN, Turner MW, Soothill JF. A controlled trial of hyposensitization with tyrosine adsorbed *Dermatophagoides pteronyssinus* antigen in childhood asthma. In vivo aspects. Clin Allergy 1984; 14:209–219.
12. Warner JO, Price JF, Soothill JF, Hey EN. Controlled trial of hyposensitization to *Dermatophagoides pteronyssinus* in children with asthma. Lancet 1978; 2:912–915.
13. Bousquet J, Calvayrac P, Guerin B, Heijaoui A, Dhivert H, Hewitt B, Michel FB. Immunotherapy with standardized *Dermatophagoides pteronyssinus* extract. I. In vivo and in vitro parameters after a short course of immunotherapy. J Allergy Clin Immunol 1985; 76:734–744.
14. Pauli G, Bessot JC, Bigot H, et al. Clinical and immunological evaluation of hyposensitization with tyrosine adsorbed *Dermatophagoides pteronyssinus* extract: a double blind placebo controlled trial. Clin Allergy 1984; 14:209–219.
15. Creticos PS, Reed CE, Norman PS. Ragweed immunotherapy in adult asthma. N Engl J Med 1996; 334:501–506.
16. Corrado OJ, Pastorello E, Ollier S, Cresswell L, Zanussi C, Ortolani C, Incorvaia A, Fugazza A, Lovely J, Harris RI, Watson KH, Avies RJ. A double blind study of hyposensitization with an alginate conjugated extract of *Dermatophagoides pteronyssinus* in patients with perennial rhinitis. Allergy 1989; 44:108–115.
17. Lichtenstein LM, Norman PS, Winkenwerder WL. A single year of immunotherapy for ragweed hayfever: immunological and clinical studies. Ann Int Med 1971; 75:663–671.
18. Brunet CV, Bedard PM, Lavoise A, Jobin M, Herbert J. Allergic rhinitis to ragweed pollen. Reassessment of the effects of immunotherapy on cellular and humoral responses. J Allergy Clin Immunol 1992; 89:76–86.
19. Ewan PW, Alexander MM, Shape C, Ind PW, Agrell B. Effective hyposensitization in allergic rhinitis using a potent partially purified extract of house dust mite. Clin Allergy 1988; 18:501–508.

20. Mc Hugh SM, Lavelle B, Kemeney DM, Patel S, Ewan PW. A placebo controlled trial of immunotherapy with two extracts of *D. pteronyssinus* in allergic rhinitis comparing clinical outcome with changes in antigen specific IgE and IgG subclasses. J Allergy Clin Immunol 1990; 86:521–532.
21. Johnstone D. A study of the natural history of bronchial asthma in children. Am J Dis Child 1968; 115:213–221.
22. Johnstone D, Dutton A. The value of hyposensitization therapy for bronchial asthma in children: a 14 years study. Pediatrics 1968; 42:793–799.
23. Rachemann FN, Edwards MC. Asthma in children. A follow up study on 688 patients after an interval of 20 years. N Engl J Med 1952; 246:915–918.
24. Committee on the Safety of Medicines. CSM update. Desensitizing vaccines. Br Med J 1986; 293:948.
25. Lockey RF, Benedict LM, Turkeltaub PC, Bukantz SC. Fatalities from immunotherapy and skin testing. J Allergy Clin Immunol 1987; 79:660–677.
26. Malling HJ, Weeke B, eds. EAACI Immunotherapy position paper. Allergy 1993; 48:1–81.
27. SIAIC. Memorandum sull'immunoterapia specifica. G It Allergol Immunol Clin 1991; 1:99.
28. BSACI. Position paper on allergen specific immunotherapy. Clin Exp Allergy 1993; 23(3).
29. Anderson JA, Chai H, Claman HJ, et al. Personnel and equipment to treat systemic reactions caused by immunotherapy with allergenic extracts. Position statement. J Allergy Clin Immunol 1991; 77:271–275.
30. Watkins AD. The role of alternative therapies in the treatment of allergic diseases. Clin Exp Allergy 1994; 24:813–825.
31. Black JH. The oral administration of pollen. J Lab Clin Med 1927; 12:1156.
32. Dunbar WP. The present state of knowledge of hayfever. J Hyg 1913; 13:105.
33. Black JH. The oral administration of ragweed pollen. Allergy 1939; 10:156.
34. Urbanek R, Gehl R. Wirksamkeit Oral Huposensibilisierung bei Hausstabmilbenallergie. Montasschr Kinderheilkd 1982; 130:150–152.
35. Taudorf E, Weeke B. Orally administered grass pollen. Allergy 1983; 38:561–564.
36. Bjorksten B, Moller C, Broberger U, Ahlsted S, Dreborg S, Johansson SGO, Juto P, Lanner A. Clinical and immunological effects of oral immunotherapy with standardized birch pollen extract. Allergy 1986; 41:290–295.
37. Leng X, Fu YX, Ye ST, Duan SQ. A double blind trial of oral immunotherapy for *Artemisia* pollen asthma with evaluation of bronchial response to pollen allergen and serum specific IgE antibody. Ann Allergy 1990; 64: 27–31.
38. Creticos PS, Naclerio RM, Adkinson F, Norman PS. Efficacy, safety and kinetics of oral ragweed immunotherapy in the treatment of seasonal allergic rhinitis. J Allergy Clin Immunol 1990; 85:165–170.
39. Bordignon V, DiBerardino L. Efficacia di una nuova immunoterapia ad assorbimento orale per Graminacee. Studio in doppio cieco eseguito per tre anni. G It Allergol Immunol Clin 1994; 4:153–159.
40. Moller C, Dreborg S, Lanner A, Bjorksten B. Oral immunotherapy of children with rhinoconjunctivitis due to birch pollen allergy. Allergy 1986; 41:271–279.
41. Taudorf E, Laursen CL, Lanner A, Bjorksten B, Dreborg S, Seborg M, Weeke B. Oral immunotherapy to birch pollen hay fever. J Allergy Clin Immunol 1987; 80:153–161.
42. Giovane A, Bardare M, Passalacqua G, Ruffoni S, Scordamaglia A, Ghezzi E, Canonica GW. A three year double blind placebo-controlled study with specific oral immunotherapy to *Dermatophagoides*: evidence of safety and efficacy in pediatric patients. Clin Exp Allergy 1994; 24:53–59.
43. Cooper PJ, Darbyshire J, Nunn AJ, Warner JO. A controlled trial of oral hyposensitization in pollen asthma and rhinitis in children. Clin Allergy 1984; 14:541–550.
44. Taudorf E, Laursen LC, Djurup R, Kappelgaard E, Pederson CT, Soborg M, Wilkinson P, Weeke B. Oral administration of grass pollen to hay fever patients. An efficacy study in oral hyposensitization. Allergy 1985; 40:321–335.

45. Mosbech H, Dreborg S, Madsenn F, Ohlsson H, Stahl Skov P, Taudorf E, Weeke B. High dose grass pollen tablets used for hyposensitization in hay fever patients. A one year double blind placebo controlled study. Allergy 1987; 42:451–455.
46. Oppenheimer J, Areson JG, Nelson HS. Safety and efficacy of oral immunotherapy with standardized cat extract. J Allergy Clin Immunol 1994; 93:61–67.
47. Taudorf E, Lanner A, Laursen L, Bjorksten B, Dreborg S, Weeke B. Specific IgG IgE and IgA antibody response to oral immunotherapy in birch pollenosis. J Allergy Clin Immunol 1989; 83:589–594.
48. Scadding K, Brostoff J. Low dose sublingual therapy in patients with allergic rhinitis due to dust mite. Clin Allergy 1986; 16:483–491.
49. Van Niekerk CH, De Wet JI. Efficacy of grass–maize pollen oral immunotherapy in patients with seasonal hay fever: a double blind study. Clin Allergy 1987; 17:507–513.
50. Feliziani V, Marfisi RM, Parmiani S. Rush immunotherapy with sublingual administration of grass allergen extract. Allergol Immunopathol 1993; 21:173–178.
51. Nelson HS, Oppenheimer J, Vatsia GA, Bucheimer A. A double blind placebo controlled evaluation of sublingual immunotherapy with standardized cat extract. J Allergy Clin Immunol 1993; 92:229–236.
52. Casanovas M, Guerra F, Moreno C, Miguel R, Maranon F, Daza JC. Double blind placebo controlled clinical trial of preseasonal treatment with allergenic extracts of *Olea europaea* pollen administered sublingually. J Invest Allergol Clin Immunol 1994; 4:305–314.
53. Reilly D, Taylor MA, Beattle NGM, Campbell JH, McSharry C, Aitchson TC, Carter R. Is evidence for homeopathy reproducible? Lancet 1994; 344:1601–1606.
54. Tari MG, Mancino M, Monti G. Efficacy of sublingual immunotherapy in patients with rhinitis and asthma due to house dust mite. A double blind study. Allergol Immunopathol 1990; 18:277–284.
55. Feliziani V, Lattuada G, Parmiani S, Dall'Aglio PP. Safety and efficacy of sublingual rush immunotherapy with grass allergen extracts. A double blind study. Allergol Immunoathol 1995; 23:173–178.
56. Sabbah A, Hassoun S, Le Sellin J, Andre C, Sicard H. A double blind placebo controlled trial by the sublingual route of immunotherapy with a standardized grass pollen extract. Allergy 1994; 49:309–313.
57. Troise C, Voltolini S, Canessa A, Pecora S, Negrini AC. Sublingual immunotherapy in *Parietaria* pollen induced rhinitis: a double blind study. J Invest Allergol Clin Immunol 1995; 5:25–30.
58. Horak F, Jager S, Erger U, Marks B, Temmel A, Toth J. Sublingual birch pollen extract for IT. Allergy 1995; 50:279.
59. Clanel R, Couturier P, Basset D, et al. Reduction of corticosteroid therapy by sublingual immunotherapy. Double blind study against placebo of a standardized grass pollen extract in rhinitis. Allergy 1995; 50:279.
60. Metha SB, Smith JM. Nasal hyposensitization and hay fever. Clin Allergy 1975; 5:279–284.
61. Welsh PW, Butterfield JH, Yunginger W, Agarwal MK, Gleich GJ. Allergen controlled study of intranasal immunotherapy for ragweed hay fever. Allergy Clin Immunol 1983; 71:454–460.
62. Georgitis JW, Nickelsen JA, Wypych JI, Kane JH, Reisman RE. Local nasal immunotherapy. Efficacy of low-dose aqueous ragweed extract. J Allergy Clin Immunol 1985; 75:496–500.
63. Georgitis JW, Nickelsen JA, Wypych JI, Barde SH, Clayton WF, Reisman RE. Local internasal immunotherapy with high-dose polymerized ragweed extract. Int Archs Allergy Appl Immun. 1986; 76:170–173.
64. Filiaci, Zambetti G, LoVecchio A. Specific local immunotherapy with macronized dust in the treatment of seasonal allergic rhinopathy due to Graminacee. Persp ENT Immunol 1989; 3:170–176.

65. Gasparini A, Di Franco G, Malavenda A. Preliminary evaluation of the nasal local specific immunotherapy in mites-sensitive respiratory patients. Persp ENT Immunol 1991; 5:29–33.
66. Ariano R, Panzani RC, Chiapella M, Augeri G, Falagiani P. Local immunotherapy of seasonal allergic rhinitis in children due to *Parietaria* pollen: a preliminary report. Pediatr Asthma Allergy Immunol 1993; 7:227–237.
67. Johansson SGO, Deuschl H, Zetterstrom O. Use of glutaraldehyde-modified timothy grass pollen extract in nasal hyposensitization of hay fever. Int Arch Allergy Appl Immunol 1979; 60:447–460.
68. Nickelsen JA, Goldstein S, Mueller U, Wypych J, Reisman RE, Arbesman CE. Local intranasal immunotherapy for ragweed allergic rhinitis: clinical response. J Allergy Clin Immunol 1981; 68:33–40.
69. Welsh PW, Zimmermann EM, Yunginger JW, Kern EB, Gleich GJ. Preseasonal intranasal immunotherapy with nebulized short ragweed extract. J Allergy Clin Immunol 1981; 67:237–242.
70. Schumacher MJ, Pain MCF. Intranasal immunotherapy with polymerized grass pollen allergens. Allergy 1981; 37:241–245.
71. Georgitis JW, Reisman RE, Clayton WF, Muller U, Wypych J, Arbesman CE. Local nasal immunotherapy for grass allergic rhinitis. J Allergy Clin Immunol 1983; 71:71–76.
72. Georgitis JW, Clayton WF, Wypich JI, Barde SH, Rasman RE. Further evaluation of local nasal immunotherapy with aqueous and allergoid grass extract. J Allergy Clin Immunol 1984; 74:694–700.
73. Andri L, Senna GE, Betteli C, Givanni S, Andri G, Falagiani P. Local nasal immunotherapy for *Dermatophagoides*-induced rhinitis: efficacy of a powder extract. J Allergy Clin Immunol 1993; 91:587–596.
74. Andri L, Senna GE, Betteli C, Givanni S, Andri G, Falagiani P, Lugo G. Local nasal immunotherapy in allergic rhinitis to *Parietaria*. Allergy 1992; 47:318–323.
75. D'Amato G, Lobefalo G, Liccardi G, Cazzola M. A double blind placebo controlled trial of local nasal immunotherapy in allergic rhinitis to *Parietaria* pollen. Clin Exp Allergy 1995; 25:141–148.
76. Passalacqua G, Albano M, Ruffoni S, Pronzato C, Riccio A, DiBerardino L, Scordamaglia A, Canonica GW. Local nasal immunotherapy to *Parietaria*: evidence of reduction of allergic inflammation. Am J Respir Crit Care Med 1995; 152:461–466.
77. Andri L, Senna GE, Andri G, Dama A, Givanni S, Betteli C, Dimitri G, Falagiani P, Mezzelani P. Local nasal immunotherapy for birch allergic rhinitis with extract in powder form. Clin Exp Allergy 1995; 25:1092–1099.
78. Andri L, Senna GE, Betteli C, Givanni S, Andri G, Dimitri G, Falagiani P, Mezzelani P. Local nasal immunotherapy with extract in powder form is effective and safe in grass pollen rhinitis. A double blind study on 32 patients. J Allergy Clin Immunol 1996; 97:37–41.
79. Cirla AM, Sforza N, Roffi GP, Alessandrini A, Stanizzi R, Dorigo R, Sala E, Della Toree F. Preseasonal intranasal immunotherapy in birch-alder rhinitis. A double blind study. Allergy 1996; 51:299–305.
80. Herxheimer H, Prior EN. Further observations in induced asthma and bronchial hyposensitization. Int Archs Allergy Appl Immunol 1952; 3:159–161.
81. Moshkevic VS, Esanzanovo GM. Local specific treatment of dust bronchial asthma. Ther Arch 1982; 4:72–74.
82. Crimi E, Voltolini S, Troise C, Gianiorio P, Crimi P, Brusasco V, Negrini AC. Local immunotherapy with *Dermatophagoides* extract in asthma. J Allergy Clin Immunol 1991; 87:721–728.
83. Tari MG, Mancino M, Monti G. Immunotherapy by inhalation of allergen in powder in house dust allergic asthma. J Invest Allergy Clin Immunol 1992; 2:59–67.
84. Almangro E, Assensio O, Bartolome' JM, Bousque M, De la Hoz B, Dolz I, Elorza J, Ferreiro M, Garcia JM, Losada E, Luna I, Mandrazo JL, Malek T, Marco T, Mariscal J,

Meseguer J, Nieto A, Oliveto A, Perez-Frances C, Sanchez-Cano M, Sastre A, Tejedor MA, De la Torre F. Estudio multicentrico de farmacovigilancia de imunoterapia sublingual en pacientes alergicos. Allergol Immunopathol 1995; 23:153.

85. Bjorksten B. Local immunotherapy is not documented for clinical use. Allergy 1994; 49:299–301.
86. Horak F, Wheeler AW. Oral hyposensitization with enteric coated allergens as extension therapy following a basic subcutaneous course of injections. Int Arch Allergy Appl Immunol 1987; 84:74–78.
87. Trede NS, Urbanek R. Combination of parenteral and oral immunotherapy in grass pollen allergic children. Allergy 1989; 44:272–280.
88. Rebien W, Puttonen E, Maasch HJ, Stix E, Wahn U. Clinical and immunological response to oral and subcutaneous immunotherapy with grass pollen extracts. Eur J Pediatr 1982; 138:341–344.
89. Palacios AS, Medina FS, Rua-Figueroa AL, Millares CB, Santos SR, Marrero JAG. Comparative clinical immunological study of oral and subcutaneous immunotherapy in children with extrinsic bronchial asthma. Allergol Immunopathol 1989; 17:323–329.
90. Moscato G, Rossi G, Dellabianca A, Pisati A, Vinci G, Viale C. Local immunotherapy by inhalation of a powder extract in asthma due to house dust mite: a double blind comparison with parenteral immunotherapy. J Invest Allergol Clin Immunol 1991; 1:383–394.
91. Corbetta L, Pesiri P, Ferro G, Mander A. Improvement of fog and exercise induced asthma after local and subcutaneous immunotherapy in mite asthma. Allergol Immunopathol 1992; 20:60–66.
92. Piazza I, Bizzarro N. Humoral response to subcutaneous oral and nasal immunotherapy for allergic rhinitis due to *Dermatophagoides pteronyssinus*. Ann Allergy 1993; 71:461–469.
93. Bernardis P, Agnoletto M, Puccinelli P, Parmiani S, Pozzan M. Injective vs sublingual immunotherapy in *Alternaria tenuis* allergic patients. J Invest Allergol Clin Immunol 1996; 6:55–62.
94. Quirino T, Iemoli E, Siciliani E, Parmiani S. Sublingual vs injective immunotherapy iin grass pollen allergic patients: a double blind double dummy study. Clin Exp Allergy 1996; 26:42–48.
95. Rak S, Hakanson L, Venge P. Immunotherapy abrogates the generation of eosinophil and neutrophil chemotactic activity. J Allergy Clin Immunol 1990; 86:706–711.
96. Varney VA, Hamid QA, Gaga M. Influence of grass pollen immunotherapy on cellular infiltration and cytokine mRNA expression during late phase cutaneous response. Clin Invest 1993; 92:644–450.
97. Nagata M, Shibasaki M, Sakamoto Y, Fukuda T, Makino S, Yamamoto K, Dohi Y. Specific immunotherapy reduces the antigen-dependent production of eosinophil chemotactic activity from mononuclear cells in patients with atopic asthma. J Allergy Clin Immunol 1994; 94:160–166.
98. Chen Y, Kuchroo VK, Inobe J, Hafler DA, Weiner HL. Regulatory T cell clones induced by oral tolerance: suppression of autoimmune encephalomyelitis. Science 1994; 265:1237–1240.
99. Mowart AM. The regulation of immune response to dietary proteins. Immunol Today 1987; 8:93–96.
100. Holt PG, Vines J, Britten D. Sublingual allergen administration. I. Selective suppression of IgE production in rats with high allergen doses. Clin Allergy 1988; 18:229–234.
101. Miller A, Lider O, Roberts AB, Sporn MB. Suppressor T cells generated by oral tolerization to myelin basic protein suppress both in vitro and in vivo immune response by the release of TGF-beta following antigen specific triggering. Proc Natl Acad Sci USA 1992; 89:421–425.
102. Van Wilsem EJ, Van Hoogstraten IM, Breve J, Scheper RJ, Kraal G. Dendritic cells of the oral mucosa and the induction of oral tolerance. A local affair. Immunology 1994; 93:128–132.

103. Hasseus B, Dahlgren W, Bergenholtz G, Jontell M. Antigen presenting capacity of Langerhans cells from rat oral epithelium. J Oral Pathol Med 1995; 24:56–60.
104. Macatinia SE, Hosken NA. Dendritic cells produce IL-12 and direct the development of T_H1 cells from naive $CD4^+$ T cells. J Immunol. 1995; 154:5071–5079.
105. Taudorf E, Moller C, Russel MW. Secretory IgA response in oral immunotherapy. Investigation in birch pollinosis. Allergy 1984; 49:760–765.
106. Holt PG, Sedgwick JD. Suppression of IgE response following antigen inhalation: a natural homeostatic mechanism which limits sensitizations to aeroallergens. Immunol Today 1987; 8:14–15.
107. Holt PG, McMenamin C. Defense against allergic sensitization in healthy lung: the role of inhalation tolerance. Clin Exp Allergy 1989; 19:55–62.
108. Holt PG, Britten D, Sedgewick JD. Suppression of IgE responses by antigen inhalation: studies on the role of genetic and environmental factors. Immunology 1987; 60:97–102.
109. Holt PG, Batty JE, Turner KJ. Inhibition of specific IgE responses in mice by pre exposure to inhaled antigen. Immunology 1981; 42:409–417.
110. Holt PG, Reid M, Britten D, Sedgwick J, Bazin H. Suppression of IgE responses by passive antigen inhalation: dissociation of local and systemic immunity. Cell Immunol 1987; 104:434–439.
111. Swarbrick ET, Stokes CR, Soothill JF. Absorption of antigens after oral immunisation and the simultaneous induction of specific tolerance. Gut 1979; 20:121–123.
112. Einarsson R, Renck B, Taudorf E. In vitro studies of degradation of birch and timothy pollen allergen preparations by human duodenal juice. Allergy 1988; 43:469–475.
113. Mistrello G, Roncarolo D, Gentili M, Zanoni D, Falagiani P. Modified Par j 1 allergen from *P. judaica* pollen and its rate of absorption in rats. Immunol Lett 1993; 40:31–36.
114. Mistrello G, Rapisarda G, Falagiani P. Detection of IgE-binding activity in serum after intranasal treatment of normal rabbits with *P. judaica* extracts. Allergy 1991; 46:52–55.
115. Canonica GW, Bagnasco M, Passalacqua G, Motta C, Bartolomei M, Mariani G. Kinetics of radiolabelled allergen administered by sublingual and oral route. J Allergy Clin Immunol 1996; 97:191.
116. Malling HJ. Principles of successful immunotherapy. Clin Exp Allergy 1991; 21:216–220.
117. Turkeltaub PC. Biological standardization of allergenic extracts. Allergol Immunopathol 1989; 17:53–65.
118. Dreborg S, Frew A. Allergen standardization and skin tests. Allergy 1993; 48:49–82.
119. Abramson MJ, Puy RM, Weiner JM. Is allergen immunotherapy effective in asthma? A meta-analysis of randomized controlled trials. Am J Respir Crit Care Med 1995; 151:969–974.
120. Holt PG. A potential vaccine strategy for asthma and allied atopic disease during childhood. Lancet 1994; 344:456–458.
121. Holt PG. Immunoprophylaxis of atopy. Light at the end of tunnel? Immunol Today 1994; 15:484–489.
122. Passalacqua G, Canonica GW. Alternative routes for allergen specific immunotherapy. J Invest Allergol Clin Immunol 1996; 6:81–87.
123. Passalacqua G, et al. Randomised controlled trial on local allergoid immunotherapy on allergic inflammation in mite-induced rhinoconjunctivitis. Lancet 1998; 351:629–632.
124. World Health Organization position paper. Specific immunotherapy: therapeutical vaccines for allergic diseases. Allergy 1998; 53(supp).

15

Pediatric Issues in Immunotherapy

ERKKA VALOVIRTA

Turku Allergy Center
Turku, Finland

I. Introduction

The efficacy of allergen subcutaneous immunotherapy in allergic rhinitis and asthma has been demonstrated in several double-blind, placebo-controlled studies in adults and also in children, at least with the following extracts: mite, *Cladosporium*, cat, and dog (1–8). Local immunotherapy (nasal, bronchial, oral, and sublingual) has been carefully evaluated by the working group in local immunotherapy formed by the Immunotherapy Subcommittee of EAACI (European Academy of Allergology and Clinical Immunology) and the Immunotherapy Committee of ESPACI (European Society of Pediatric Allergology and Clinical Immunology). Bronchial and oral immunotherapy are not recommended for clinical practice, except as part of controlled studies. Nasal and sublingual–swallow immunotherapy are not indicated for normal clinical use in children. More studies are needed until these forms of local immunotherapy can be recommended for general use in children as an alternative to subcutaneous immunotherapy (5).

The use of allergen immunotherapy in children requires a specialist assessment because there are several special problems and questions concerning specific allergen immunotherapy in this age group: At what age to start? With which allergens? With what dose regimens? What is the optimal dose? For how long a time?

What are the measurements of efficacy? The mechanisms of allergen injection immunotherapy have been evaluated only in studies with adult patients. There are no studies in children relative to the compliance of injection immunotherapy with different disease entities (i.e., allergic rhinoconjunctivitis and asthma bronchiale).

Immunotherapy started in the early phase of the allergic disorder should modify the spontaneous long-term progress of the allergic inflammation and disease (10,11). Some pediatricians recommend treatment in children at 1–2 years of age, but it is important to evaluate in controlled studies the benefits of immunotherapy in patients younger than 5 years. It is still unknown whether immunotherapy should be administered to very young children. When immunotherapy is indicated in children, it is mandatory that the physician has full experience in the treatment of possible systemic reactions and has mastered the establishment of an intravenous line (10). Continual education in the field of immunotherapy is imperative for medical personnel and doctors treating allergic children, thereby ensuring their patients the optimal allergy treatment. As a consequence, the natural history of the allergic disorders in children may be positively influenced.

Specific allergy diagnosis forms the basis of the selection of patients and allergens and allergen extracts for immunotherapy. The clinical diagnosis of allergy is always based on the combination of clinical evaluation (clinical history, monitoring of symptoms, and use of medication) and the results of the diagnostic tests. The diagnosis of allergic rhinoconjunctivitis and allergic asthma in very young children is difficult and demands special assessment (11).

Motivation for allergen injection immunotherapy is crucially needed both from the child, depending on the age, and from the parents, to produce good compliance for the treatment and to avoid discontinuation of immunotherapy. Good compliance is achieved with proper allergy diagnosis and with adequate information and injection protocol, including the information on the adverse reactions during the treatment period. During allergen immunotherapy, the regular visits to the clinic and to the doctor responsible for the treatment offer the child and the parents a unique opportunity to have close control of the multifactorial allergic disease.

II. Advantages of Immunotherapy in Children

It has been suggested that immunotherapy should be introduced to the patients in the early phase of the allergic disease (10) to modify the natural course of the allergic disorder (12) before further sensitizations take place.

Theoretically, specific immunotherapy should be used early in the course of the allergic disease to prevent the destruction and remodeling observed in asthma with long-standing disease. Therefore, specific immunotherapy has been considered to be more effective in children than in adults. Long-lasting, severe nonreversible disease does not respond to immunotherapy. Specific immunotherapy may give relief soon after the onset of the allergic disease so that children do not need to have symptoms for many years before they are introduced to adequate treatment (i.e., specific allergen immunotherapy).

It has been proposed that specific immunotherapy, when introduced to children with only allergic rhinoconjunctivitis, may stop the development of asthma (13). Johnstone and Dutton (13) used several different nonstandardized allergens for immunotherapy in children. Twenty-eight percent of those who received immunotherapy developed asthma, compared with 78% in placebo-treated children.

To answer the question "Does specific allergen immunotherapy stop the development of asthma?", the Preventive Allergy Treatment (PAT) study (14,15) has been started as a multicenter study in Europe for birch or timothy pollen allergic children, from 5 to 13 years old; who are suffering from allergic rhinoconjunctivitis, with no symptoms of clinical asthma and with no clinically important perennial allergies. The PAT study is a prospective, randomized controlled trial using high-quality allergen extracts with the aim of investigating the possible preventive effect on the development of asthma. The results (15) of this study show that immunotherapy has a preventive effect for the development of asthma in children suffering from allergic rhinitis caused by birch or timothy pollen. The preventive use of immunotherapy opens a new era for doctors dealing with children suffering from allergic rhinitis. In the study by Adkinson et al. (16) on immunotherapy for asthma in allergic children, the only subgroups in which there was a trend toward a benefit from immunotherapy were the children with milder disease and the younger children, which could reflect a shorter duration of disease. Future investigations should focus on the potential prophylactic use of immunotherapy in children with allergic rhinitis who are at high risk for asthma, or in highly allergic children with the recent onset of mild asthma.

In polysensitized children, immunotherapy has not prevented the development of clinical sensitization against new allergens, as has been shown in children sensitive to only house dust mite (12). This prospective case–controlled study has been performed in 44 asthmatic children, 2–6 years of age, who were monosensitized to house dust mite. During the treatment and the follow-up of 3 years, all 22 children in the control group developed new sensitizations, measured by skin prick testing and allergen-specific IgE in serum, compared with 12/22 children with new sensitivities in the immunotherapy group. The conclusion of this study suggests that immunotherapy in children sensitized to only house dust mite may alter the natural course of allergy by preventing the development of new sensitizations.

Adverse reactions of allergen immunotherapy in infants and children are less common than in adults. This was shown in a 3-year prospective study performed in children 4–16 years of age (17). For systemic reactions, epinephrine is better tolerated by children than by adults.

During infancy and early childhood, severe allergic reactions to Hymenoptera venoms are extremely rare, and fatalities are still more rare. Only in the heavily exposed cases, such as children of beekeepers, with severe reactions is venom immunotherapy started before the age of 5 years, and it should always be given by a pediatric allergist who is well trained in establishing a venous access in small children (18).

III. Points to Be Considered When Using Immunotherapy in Children

1. It is unknown how the immune system of very young children is influenced by specific-allergen immunotherapy.
2. The use of local immunotherapy is not recommended for children. Further, placebo-controlled studies are urgently needed.
3. The optimal dose of allergen injected for small children is unknown.
4. Aluminum hydroxide is used as an adjuvant to allergen extracts. There are no data on possible side effects in children. In adults, no patient has had any clinical evidence of aluminum toxicity (19).
5. In Hymenoptera venom allergy, immunotherapy may be started in very well-selected children only by a pediatric allergist.

IV. Indications for Immunotherapy in Children

1. IgE-mediated allergic rhinoconjunctivitis and asthma.
2. Severe systemic anaphylactic reactions to Hymenoptera venoms.
3. A specific allergy diagnosis assessed by a trained pediatrician or an allergist with special experience in the field of pediatric allergology.
4. Avoidance and elimination procedures performed as far as practically possible.
5. Standardized allergen extract available.
6. Adequate treatment schedule with proper administration of allergen extract.
7. Trained personnel, following the guidelines recommended by EAACI (10,18,20).
8. The child and the family are motivated for specific-allergen immunotherapy (i.e., there is good compliance).
9. There are no contraindications for immunotherapy.

V. Contraindications for Immunotherapy in Children

A. Absolute Contraindications

1. Noncompliance
2. Immunological disease and malignancies
3. Severe heart or lung diseases
4. Continuous systemic corticosteroid treatment

B. Relative Contraindications

1. Treatment with β-adrenergic blockers
2. Children younger than the age of 5 years

VI. Summary

Allergen-specific injection immunotherapy for children is demanding treatment for the whole family and for all those persons who are in contact with the child. Cooperation with the family is most important for good compliance in all age groups. Preschool children have problems different from those of school-age and adolescents, but all demand the special knowledge of a pediatrician. A child younger than the age of 15 years always needs an adult with them when coming to the clinic for injection(s). The restrictions in sports after the immunotherapy injection during the same day must be understood not only by the child, but also by parents, teachers, relatives, and the child's friends.

Specific allergen immunotherapy in children should be recommended as follows:

1. Children with allergic rhinitis should be treated with immunotherapy because symptoms are reduced for many years after the treatment period of 3 years. Usually symptoms are reduced in a dose-dependent manner. The asthmatic symptoms are reduced early in the course of immunotherapy in patients with pollen allergy, but not in chronic asthmatics.
2. Immunotherapy reduces the allergic component of rhinitis and asthma, acting as an anti-inflammatory treatment.
3. Immunotherapy should be given in the early phase of asthma, before permanent tissue damage occurs in the bronchi. Immunotherapy should be recommended only for children affected by stable asthma. Patients affected by severe, unstable asthma have a high risk of adverse reactions during immunotherapy.

References

1. Aas K. Hyposensitization in house dust allergy asthma. A double blind controlled study with evaluation of the effect on bronchial sensitivity to house dust. Acta Paediatr Scand 1971; 60:264.
2. Bertelsen A, Andersen JB, et al. Immunotherapy with dog and cat extracts in children. Allergy 1989; 44:330.
3. Dreborg S, Agrell B, et al. A double-blind multi-centre immunotherapy trial in children, using a purified and standardized *Cladosporium herbarum* preparation. I. Clinical results. Allergy 1986; 41:131.
4. Sundin B, Lilja G, et al. Immunotherapy with partially purified and standardized animal dander extracts. I. Clinical results from a double-blind study on patients with animal dander asthma. J Allergy Clin Immunol 1986; 77:478.
5. Hedlin G, Heilborn H, et al. Long-term follow-up of patients treated with a three-year course of cat or dog immunotherapy. J Allergy Clin Immunol 1995; 96:87.
6. Valovirta E, Koivikko A, et al. Immunotherapy in allergy to dog: a double-blind clinical study. Ann Allergy 1986; 53:85.
7. Wahn U, Schweter C, et al. Prospective study on immunologic changes induced by two different *Dermatophagoides pteronyssinus* extracts prepared from whole mite culture and mite bodies. J Allergy Clin Immunol 1988; 82:360.

8. Warner JO, Price JF, et al. Controlled trial of hyposensitization to *Dermatophagoides pteronyssinus* in children with asthma. Lancet 1978; 2:912.
9. Local immunotherapy. In: Malling H-J, Bousquet J, eds. Position paper by the working group on local immunotherapy of EAACI Immunotherapy Subcommittee and the ESPACI Immunotherapy Committee. Allergy 1998. In press.
10. Malling H, Weeke B. Immunotherapy. Position paper of the European Academy of Allergology and Clinical Immunology. Allergy 1993; 48:suppl 14.
11. Ownby DR, Adinoff AD. The appropriate use of skin testing and allergen immunotherapy in young children. J Allergy Clin Immunol 1994; 94:662.
12. Des-Roches A, Paradis L, et al. Immunotherapy with a standardized *Dermatophagoides pteronyssinus* extract. VI. Specific immunotherapy prevents the onset of new sensitizations in children. J Allergy Clin Immunol 1997; 99:450.
13. Johnstone D, Dutton A. The value of hyposensitization therapy for bronchial asthma in children: a fourteen-year study. Pediatrics 1968; 42:793.
14. Jacobsen L. The benefit of specific allergy treatment. In: Basomba A, Sastre J, eds. Proceedings of the XVI European Congress of Allergology and Clinical Immunology. Bologna, Italy: Monduzzi Editore, 1995:745.
15. Valovirta E. Capacity of specific immunotherapy in prevention of allergic asthma in children: the preventive allergy treatment study (PAT). J Invest Allergol Clin Immunol Sept–Oct 1997; 7(5):369.
16. Adkinson NF Jr, Eggleston PA, et al. A controlled trial of immunotherapy for asthma in allergic children. N Engl J Med 1997; 336:324.
17. Businco L, Zannino L, et al. Systemic reactions to specific immunotherapy in children with respiratory allergy: a prospective study. Pediatr Allergy Immunol 1995; 6:44.
18. Muller U, Mosbech H. Immunotherapy with Hymenoptera venoms. Position Paper of the European Academy of Allergology and Clinical Immunology. Allergy 1993; 48(suppl 14).
19. Glinert RJ, Burnatowska-Hledin M. Serum and urinary aluminium levels in patients receiving alum-precipitated allergenic extracts. Ann Allergy 1988; 461:433.
20. Bousquet J, Lockey RF, Malling H-J. WHO position paper. Allergen immunotherapy: therapeutic vaccines for allergic diseases. Allergy 1998; 53(suppl 44).

16

International Recommendations

HANS-JØRGEN MALLING

National University Hospital
Copenhagen, Denmark

I. Introduction

Injection immunotherapy in asthma is considered controversial by many physicians (1,2). One editorial concludes that "drug therapy, combined when possible with the avoidance of allergens, is the recommended approach to the management of asthma" (3). This statement is primarily based on the results of a single ragweed immunotherapy study (4) that reinvestigated the effects of immunotherapy in patients who were selected with the suspicious diagnosis of a primary ragweed-induced asthma. Rather than using the outcome of this study as an argument against immunotherapy, the reasons for not showing convincing efficacy should be discovered. The Creticos study (4) is a repetition of an unsuccessful study from 1977 (5), which documented that autumnal asthma is caused primarily by mold allergens and not by ragweed. Consequently, as the authors have used an inappropriate indication, the outcome will inevitably be a failure. Therefore, this should not be used as an argument for immunotherapy being ineffective as a treatment principle. Although the magnitude of clinical efficacy might be debated, the recently published metanalysis of the clinical efficacy of immunotherapy in asthma clearly documents its applicability (6). The British Society of Allergy takes the position of recommending the use immunotherapy for asthmatic patients only as part of a controlled study (2).

The use of immunotherapy in the treatment of asthma has decreased in connection with the introduction of potent inhaled corticosteroids and long-acting β_2-adrenergic agonists (7,8). In the ongoing debate about the use of immunotherapy in asthma, pros and cons of several aspects should be considered (9). The optimal treatment of asthma should focus on patient compliance, long-term preventive aspects, efficacy and side effects, patient awareness of factors inducing symptoms and exacerbations, cost and duration of treatment, and identification of patients most likely to respond to distinctive treatments. For many physicians, the treatment of asthma does not represent many options, because asthma, in their opinion, should be treated exclusively with drugs. However, a debate could be raised about whether having the possibility of "playing on different strings" may improve the treatment of asthma. To improve asthma treatment (i.e., to reduce morbidity and mortality) intervention in the pathophysiological mechanisms by different routes may both improve patient compliance and efficacy, and reduce the risk of treatment-related side effects. It is of paramount importance to follow the guidelines for the indication of immunotherapy, contraindications, and the monitoring of immunotherapy, as well as some practical rules for prevention and treatment of immunotherapy-induced side effects, and some guidelines relative to top dose and dose modifications. International recommendations on immunotherapy have been provided by several recent position statements, status articles, and review articles (2,9–17). The present recommendations apply only to injection (subcutaneous) immunotherapy. Treatment by other routes (i.e., local immunotherapy is dealt with in Chapter 14).

II. Indications for Immunotherapy

The arguments for including immunotherapy in the general treatment strategy of asthma are based on the aims to (1) reduce morbidity and mortality; (2) prevent progressive decline in lung function; and (3) improve quality of life (14). Specific immunotherapy appears to be the only treatment that might modify the course of the disease, either by preventing the development of new sensitizations or by altering the natural history of asthma (12). The most important aspect in making immunotherapy successful is to identify the patients most likely to respond positively. When trying to define the indications for immunotherapy in allergic asthma, several aspects have to be taken into consideration. These include both the general and the more specific aspects that are related to the individual patient.

A. General Guidelines

The general guidelines apply to all patients. For asthma, immunotherapy should be seriously considered in patients with disease caused by allergens for which clinical efficacy and safety have been documented by placebo-controlled, double-blind studies, and for which sufficient disease control could not be obtained by allergen avoidance or allergen reduction (14). Allergen avoidance or reduction is, by nature, the most logical way of preventing the initiation of the damaging allergic inflammatory cascade that is caused by the allergen–IgE interaction in the mucous membranes of atopic individuals. Although allergen reduction is possible for only a few allergens (primarily animal dander and house dust mites), it should always constitute the basic line of intervention. With animal dander, the indirect exposure to allergens may clinically represent the most importance source of disease-inducing factors, which are practically impossible to avoid (14). Immunotherapy should be considered in patients with allergic asthma when allergen reduction is impossible, or when the disease responds insufficiently to allergen reduction, even when symptomatic relief can be achieved with pharmacological therapy (18). Because of the controversial nature of immunotherapy in asthma, it is recommended in daily clinical practice, to initiate immunotherapy only with allergens for which the clinical efficacy has been documented in appropriately designed, placebo-controlled, double-blind studies giving adequate information on indication, randomization, allergen extracts, and statistics, and using a duration of treatment sufficient to ensure the validity of conclusions. Furthermore, the safety (i.e., the frequency of severe systemic side effects) should document a beneficial, or at least not damaging efficacy–side effect profiles (14).

According to previous recommendations, the indications for immunotherapy were restricted to include only patients not responding adequately to drug treatment, or presenting with side effects (17). A shift toward a more liberal indication has emerged, based on the concept of trying to interfere in the natural progression of the asthma disease in the early course, before damage has occurred and while still having the capacity to modulate (i.e., to prevent, rather than reduce, the chronic inflammation and to prevent the further development of severe disease; 14). The consequence of this approach is to recommend immunotherapy relatively early in life.

As inhalant allergens play only a minor role in the overall disease severity of patients younger than the age of 5, immunotherapy is only rarely indicated in infants (14). Furthermore, more side effects have been associated with immunotherapy in patients younger than 5 years of age (19). When immunotherapy is indicated in infants, it is mandatory that the physician manages all aspects of coping with the treatment of systemic reactions in this age group (14). When discussing immunotherapy in children, the natural history of asthma should be considered. Although some children outgrow their asthma, many asthmatic children will continue having symptoms in adulthood (20–22). The preventive capacity of immunotherapy is insufficiently investigated and primarily based on dated uncontrolled evidence. Rackemann and Edwards (23) reported that in a 20-year follow-up study of 688 children, 3 out of 4 treated by immunotherapy became asthma-free in adulthood. Likewise, a 14-year follow-up study showed that 2 out of 3 actively treated patients became free of asthma, in contrast with 1 in 4 in the placebo group (24). These studies are uncontrolled and include a number of extracts that, from a modern point of view, have no documented efficacy. However, the spontaneous outcome in asthmatic children treated with modern drugs does not indicate that inhaled corticosteroids have the capacity to prevent childhood asthma from progressing into adulthood asthma. The clinical documentation of the value of inhaled corticosteroids in asthma is almost exclusively based on short-term studies (25), and the explanation of this schism is probably impossible, as long-term placebo-controlled inhaled corticosteroid studies would be considered unethical. From a theoretical point of view, the fundamental anti-inflammatory capacity of immunotherapy (26) might have the potential for changing the natural history of asthma. This is in contrast with drug treatment, which only seems to have anti-inflammatory effects when administered (27). The immunotherapy-induced transformation of cells orchestrating inflammation to a more "normal-like" (i.e., a nonatopic phenotype) cellular response is of interest (28).

B. Individual Guidelines

Individual guidelines relate to the individual patients and their special situations. When considering immunotherapy, a very careful evaluation of individual factors has to be performed. This implies a careful diagnosis of the allergic component in exacerbations and the overall severity of the disease. In the individual patient, several nonspecific factors, such as irritants, exercise, viral infections, psychological stress, occupational factors, and air pollution, may play a more important role than allergens in inducing symptoms (16). Immunotherapy should be considered only in patients who (based on a careful monitoring of the factors that are responsible for the severity of the disease) have a primarily allergen-induced disease (14). Furthermore, the number of allergens used for injection should be restricted to a minimum (i.e., only those that are responsible for most of the symptoms). In multiallergic patients, it is problematic to conclusively define the allergens that are of importance for the combination of symptoms. Furthermore, the clinical effect of immunotherapy in polysensitized patients may be inferior to that of monosensitized patients (29). To obtain a successful outcome of immunotherapy, the availability of a potent, standardized allergen extract, the administration of a sufficiently high dose (to ensure an immunological response), and treatment for a proper time period are crucial. Other considerations that should be included in the indications for immunotherapy in asthma are (1) the patient's attitude to the relief of symptoms with drugs, versus trying to interfere with the pathophysiological mechanisms of the disease (specific treatment); (2) the severity and duration of symptoms; (3) the requirement for and the effect of drugs; (4) the risk incurred by the treatment and by the disease; and (5) psychological factors.

1. Given the growing insight of patient awareness of the risks of using synthetic drugs, physicians are often faced with a patient request for a treatment that intervenes with the natural course of the disease (immunotherapy), in contrast to continuing to take drugs that only diminish their symptoms.

2. The indication for immunotherapy in allergic asthma is related to both the severity of the disease and to the duration of symptoms. Mild symptoms that respond adequately to prn β_2-adrenergic agonists are no argument for instituting immunotherapy. Symptoms requiring repeated courses of inhaled corticosteroids (regardless of the duration of the allergen season), or perennial symptoms (even if these symptoms are rather mild and respond adequately to pharmacological treatment), may be arguments in favor of initiating immunotherapy (14). It seems that young children respond better to treatment than adults do (30). This may be related to the actual age of the patient, but is more likely related to the duration of the disease, implying that attempts to interfere with the natural course of the disease should be introduced at a time when the patient has the capacity to respond positively (i.e., before the disease deteriorates to a chronic, irreversible airway obstruction; 10,14). Patient with severe asthma (i.e., requiring constant or regular course systemic corticosteroids) and patients with persistent lung functions below 70% of the predicted despite optimal drug treatment do not seem to benefit from immunotherapy (12).
3. The requirement for intensive drug treatment, especially patients with a need for several daily intakes of prophylactic drugs (inhaled corticosteroids) strengthens the rationale for adding immunotherapy to the treatment strategy (to reduce the amount of corticosteroids needed and the requirement for prn β_2-agonists). Optimal results of immunotherapy are obtained in patients with mild disease (i.e., requiring a rather modest pharmacological treatment). To restrict immunotherapy to patients who do not respond adequately to drug treatment or present with side effects from drug treatment is a common fallacy (14).
4. Risk/benefit assessments of possible treatments and possible deteriorations of the disease constitute important aspects in the indication for immunotherapy. Generally, allergic asthma is, when in the mild form, a bothersome disease, and in more severe cases a disease implying a risk of life-threatening asthmatic attacks and even a risk of developing chronic respiratory failure (31,32). The disabling natures of allergic asthma in relation to diminishing performance capacity in school work, job, and social contacts are of great importance for the quality of life. The risk of immunotherapy is strictly related to the risk of inducing anaphylactic reactions. The rate of severe systemic reactions in asthmatics treated with high-potency extracts is approximately 5% of the injections (33), primarily in the dose-escalation phase (14). However, systemic reactions represent a general limitation in the use of immunotherapy; therefore, the indication for and possibly also the practical treatment of the patient, must be ascertained and performed by a specialist, who is aware of the risks of immunotherapy, and who is capable of dealing with these systemic reactions (12,14).

5. Psychological factors have an influence on compliance in the intake of medicine and the patients' fixation on the disease character. In studies of drug compliance in asthmatic patients, only approximately half the prescribed drugs are actually taken (34,35). Compliance may be higher in seasonal asthma, owing to the shorter duration of symptoms in seasonal allergies, but patients often tend to tolerate some symptoms (in a considerable number of patients, rather severe symptoms) without substituting the prn-based use of β_2-agonists by the more effective inhaled corticosteroids (25). An important issue in treating allergic diseases is to be aware of the patient's individual perception of disease severity and the psychological motivation and the scientific understanding of the rationale for treating the allergic inflammation, in contrast with only diminishing the inconvenience of symptoms. In spite of a massive amount of information on the safety of inhaled corticosteroids, "steroid phobia" and inadequate steroid treatment still represent a problem excluding patients from an effective drug treatment.

In the discussion about the treatment of allergic asthma, several aspects have to be taken into consideration: Generally speaking, no definite rules for the indication of immunotherapy in asthma can be laid down. The indications are based on a careful balancing of the advantages and disadvantages, taking into consideration the patient's attitude to both symptoms and possible treatments. In this way immunotherapy does not take the position of being an ultimate treatment, but represents a supplement to both allergen avoidance and drug treatment when used in the early phase of the disease (14). Immunotherapy is recommended in highly selected patients (Table 1). Immunotherapy may, in carefully selected patients (using allergen extracts and induction regimens that have a documented efficacy and safety profile), represent a profitable supplement to drugs to improve patient compliance, obtain long-term preventive aspects, increase efficacy and reduce side effects, improve patient awareness of factors inducing symptoms and exacerbations, and reduce costs and duration of treatment. Immunotherapy in no way represents an alternative to drug therapy in asthma—but should be considered a complementary treatment (36). Identifying patients most likely to respond to immunotherapy is of crucial importance for the success of the treatment. Only patients with sensitization to a few allergens, symptoms primarily induced by these allergens, and with fully reversible disease, should be considered candidates for immunotherapy. In contrast to drugs, which could be used in all asthmatics, immunotherapy is probably applicable to only about 10–20% of the asthmatic population. Still, immunotherapy may be a valuable option in the treatment strategy of asthma.

The best documentation of efficacy (based on the number of studies and the degree of symptom and medication reduction) is obtained in pollen asthma (37–40). A few studies have documented the beneficial effects of immunotherapy in house dust mite allergies (41,42), in patient allergic to cats (43–45) and to molds belong-

Table 1 Considerations for the Indications of Immunotherapy

- The nature of the disease
  - Immunotherapy is indicated only in unequivocal allergic asthma.
- The severity and duration of symptoms
  - Mild and sporadic symptoms responding well to drugs are not indications for immunotherapy.
  - Severe chronic symptoms have a reduced likelihood of responding positively to immunotherapy.
- The importance of allergens in exacerbations and symptoms
  - The offending allergen(s) should be the primary cause of symptoms and the overall severity of the disease.
  - Nonspecific hyperreactivity should play only a minor role in exacerbations and symptoms.
- The offending allergens
  - Only high-quality, standardized allergens with a documented clinical efficacy and safety profile should be applied.
- The practicability of allergen avoidance
  - If allergen avoidance can eliminate symptoms, it is the treatment of choice.
- The response to treatment
  - Optimal pharmacotherapy (e.g., systemic corticosteroids) should have the capacity to eradicate symptoms and normalize lung function.
- Cost, efficacy, and side effects of possible treatments
  - The indication for immunotherapy is based on a careful balance of cost, efficacy, and side effects connected with allergen avoidance, pharmacotherapy, and immunotherapy in the individual patient.
- Patient handling of disease and treatment
  - The psychological attitude toward the intensity of treatment versus the tolerance to suffer some symptoms is critical in ensuring optimal patient compliance.

ing to the *Cladosporium* and *Alternaria* species (46,47). Consequently, pollen-induced asthma is a suitable indication for immunotherapy, especially in pollen rhinitic patients who experience asthma during the height of the pollen season. In house dust mites allergic asthma, allergen reduction represents the first line of intervention, and only if this is insufficient in controlling the symptoms necessitating that the patient use regular prophylactic inhaled drugs, immunotherapy may be considered. This is mainly in children and young adults who are primarily allergic to mites and who have a documented exposure to mites, and in whom an irreversible decrease in lung function has been excluded by appropriate drug treatment. In cat asthma, allergen avoidance is the treatment of choice, and only in patients who are unable to avoid the indirect exposure to cat allergens and who present with inconvenient symptoms, immunotherapy may be indicated. In mold allergies, the diagnosis may be problematic, and the quality of allergen extracts is of crucial importance when considering immunotherapy.

III. Contraindications

Absolute contraindications are the presence of concurrent immunological diseases, other severe disease, and malignancies. Likewise, conditions interfering with the treatment of anaphylaxis (β-blockers) or contraindicating the administration of epinephrine (severe coronary heart disease and severe hypertension), and a lack of patient compliance are considered absolute contraindications for the initiation of immunotherapy (14). Most allergists do not advise the use of immunotherapy in children younger than age 5 years (symptoms rarely caused by inhalation allergens), in pregnancy (relates mainly to induction phase, whereas a well-tolerated immunotherapy might be continued), and in severe allergic disease (increased risk of inducing anaphylactic reactions and low-grade efficacy).

IV. Discontinuation of Immunotherapy

Immunotherapy is usually intended as a treatment administered for a defined period of years. Efficacy is normally manifest after 1 year of treatment, and if no improvement in the clinical state is observed after 2 years of treatment, the chance of obtaining efficacy is low, and immunotherapy should be terminated (14). Short-term treatment has no protracted effect after the treatment is discontinued. Traditionally, immunotherapy (in responding patients) has been performed for 3 years. Given the relatively slow onset of action, and the recent knowledge of the likely mechanisms, a tendency toward extending the treatment period to 5 years has emerged (e.g., venom allergy) (48,49). This is not based on scientific data in case of inhalant allergies, but is rather an attempt to reduce the risk of relapses. However, in patients who respond to treatment, the discontinuation of immunotherapy after less than 3 years results in a high frequency of relapses (10,50,51). In patients who show an effect during allergen administration, and deterioration after terminating immunotherapy, treatment could be prolonged. In nonresponders (i.e., patients showing marginal or no efficacy after 1 year of treatment) the indication for immunotherapy should be carefully reassessed and the possibility of the development of concurrent sensitizations being responsible for the symptoms should be investigated (14). Patients responding insufficiently to immunotherapy should be withdrawn after no more than 2 years of treatment. Likewise, in patients presenting with severe anaphylactic reactions, alternative treatments should be chosen, which is also true for patients who do not comply (52).

V. Monitoring

A. Safety Monitoring

The primary target for the monitoring of immunotherapy is related to safety monitoring (14). Safety monitoring is undertaken with the aim of reducing the risk of immunotherapy-induced systemic reactions, and includes evaluation of the patient before, after, and between injections (9,14,53–55). Safety monitoring should include verbal and written information and instructions involving the patients in the monitoring of immunotherapy, with the aim of making patients more responsible for their own safety. Monitoring should be supervised by the staff administering the injections. Registering the actual state of the patient, amount of the allergen injected, lung function, and possible side effects in special record forms is recommended, as well as a uniform registration of reason for dose reductions and grading of side effects.

Special attention should be focused on reactions to previous injections, deterioration of allergic disease, and intercurrent infections. In patients with bronchial asthma, including those having allergic rhinitis with bronchial asthma, it is essential that all regular antiasthmatic drugs are continued, especially on the day of injection (14). It is recommended that peak flow be measured before and 30 min after the injection. In patients with peak flows below 80% of normal value, injections should be postponed, and likewise, it is not advisable to give injections when there are signs of an ongoing or recent viral infection, recent allergen exposure, or when the patient has forgotten to use the routine prescribed drugs.

It is mandatory that the patient waits in the physician's clinic for at least 30 min after the injection. The patient should be instructed to report immediately any symptoms appearing during the observation period. The injection site has to be inspected before the patient leaves the clinic. The patient should be informed to consult the physician or emergency room in case of a more severe delayed reaction. The patient should be carrying short-acting β_2-agonists for rescue treatment. It is recommended to separate vaccinations against infectious diseases from immunotherapy injections with at least 1 week.

B. Efficacy Monitoring

An important aspect in the quality validation of immunotherapy is to monitor the clinical efficacy. This is to ensure that the desired result is achieved (i.e., that the treatment results in a reduction in clinical symptoms, a reduction in the need for drugs, and an improvement in the quality of life). Negligence of efficacy monitoring implies the risk of continuing an ineffective treatment, resulting only in inconvenience and a risk of inducing life-threatening side effects.

Efficacy monitoring should be performed by methods reflecting the severity of the disease. No in vivo or in vitro parameters are useful here. In daily clinical practice, the parameter mirroring disease severity is the use of drugs. In patients pharmacologically optimally treated (monitored by lung function, need for rescue β_2-agonists, daily performance, exacerbations, and emergency visits), the capability to reduce pharmacotherapy during immunotherapy implies a clinical efficacy of allergen administration (7). In controlled studies, a more meticulous monitoring of symptom and medication scores is advisable, including a scoring system ensuring a high patient compliance and strict rules for intensifying pharmacotherapy (14).

Simple subjective patient estimation of efficacy, and especially efficacy that is based on the doctor's own opinion implies a risk of continuing an ineffective treatment.

VI. Practicals

A. Safety of Immunotherapy

In the elucidation of immunotherapy-induced side effects, a differentiation of severity is important. Large local reactions are almost inevitable (i.e., diffuse swellings persisting for a day or more). These local reactions are annoying, but are in no way dangerous, and do not predict systemic reactions. Systemic reactions may be subdivided into nonspecific, mild, moderate, and life-threatening. Nonspecific symptoms (grade 1) include malaise, lethargy, headaches, and such (probably not IgE-mediated). Mild reactions (grade 2) include rhinitis and mild asthma responding promptly to minimal drug treatment. Moderate reactions (grade 3) include urticaria, angioedema, and severe asthma, requiring more intensive treatment. The life-threatening side effects (grade 4) constitute anaphylactic shock and other anaphylactic reactions. The severe life-threatening systemic reactions and rare fatalities represent the major problem in a more widespread use of immunotherapy.

The frequency of systemic side effects in some high-dose immunotherapy studies applying accelerated dose-escalation regimens is high, but this risk does not apply to standard immunotherapy. The noncritical systemic reactions (mild asthma and rhinitis) are noted more frequently, and in some studies in which aggressive dosing is used, noncritical systemic reactions are reported following 20% of injections in the majority of patients (46). A study of rush immunotherapy in children, showed 100% systemic reactions following doses of 10,000–100,000 SQ-U/mL (56). The frequency of systemic side effects in placebo-controlled, double-blind asthma studies is often in the range of 20–30% of patients having reactions. Asthmatic attacks seem to be the most prevalent form of reaction. Anaphylaxis is reported in only a few of the newer studies, with a frequency below 10% of patients (39,46,57–61).

The frequency of systemic side effects is related to the dosage regimen (the rush schedule being the most dangerous), and to high-dosage regimens in highly sensitive subjects (62). In routine immunotherapy following the guidelines of the EAACI Immunotherapy Position Paper (14), systemic reactions were observed in 5% of the patients (in 9500 injections no anaphylactic shock or life-threatening reactions were registered; 2). Even in pregnancy immunotherapy for allergic disease is safe (63). Immune complexes have been associated with immunotherapy, but long-term adverse reactions are rarely documented (64).

The prevalence of immunotherapy-induced fatalities has been analyzed in both the United Kingdom (65) and the United States (66,67). The U.K. survey indicates 26 fatalities during a 31-year period, with a tendency to increase during the last 10 years. The first U.S. retrospective study (66) reviewed 24 fatalities from immunotherapy in the period 1959–1984. Not included in these figures are 16 additional fatalities from skin testing and immunotherapy, with information not sufficiently detailed to permit further analysis. However, the risk of a fatal reaction to immunotherapy is low, as seven to ten million allergen injections are administered annually in the United States (66). The second U.S. survey (67) reports 17 fatalities for the years 1985–1989. The most important factors associated with death were asthma (76%), high sensitivity (71%), and dose-increase phase (56%). Other factors were changing to a new vial, dosing error or inappropriate dose adjustment, allergen seasons, symptoms before injection, not waiting after injection, and home injection.

Although fatal reactions to immunotherapy are rare, exposing asthmatic patients to the risk of anaphylaxis and even death must be carefully balanced with the probability of obtaining a significant clinical improvement. To reduce the risk to a minimum, the availability of emergency resuscitative equipment and trained personnel, as well as meticulous observation of the patient after injection and strict guidelines for dosage adjustment, are essential (14,53).

B. Prevention and Treatment of Side Effects

The risk of inducing systemic side effects depends on various factors, and identifying these might exclude high-risk patients from starting immunotherapy (68). Asthma itself seems to be a risk factor in relation to experiencing systemic reactions, compared with patients who suffer only hay fever. In a prospective study (following the guidelines of EAACI Immunotherapy Subcommittee; 14) of immunotherapy in 419 patients, 84% of systemic side effects were observed in asthmatic patients, although asthmatics constituted only 57% of the study population (33). In immunotherapy fatalities, asthma has likewise been identified as a risk factor (67), and the risk is further increased when the asthmatic patient is steroid-dependent, has experienced recent hospitalizations or visits to the accident and emergency department, has unstable asthma, or has complicating cardiovascular disease (14). The severity of asthma is a key factor. Bousquet et al. (58) showed that a lung function persistently below 70% of predicted value in patients receiving an optimal drug therapy was highly associated with side effects and, furthermore, indicates a poor clinical efficacy. The age of the patient is also of importance in relation to the frequency of systemic reactions. Children younger than the age of 5 years experience more side effects (19). Some studies have identified a slightly increased risk in females, but in practice, gender is of minimal importance as a risk factor (67). High sensitivity, as identified by skin test or radioallergosorbent technique (RAST) score is a risk factor for anaphylaxis (66,69). Treatment during allergen season has been identified as a risk factor for anaphylaxis (67), and based on that, dose escalation should not be performed during the season (14). Treatment with β-blockers is, by some authors, considered a risk factor. However, the risk is not related to an increased probability of inducing systemic reactions (70), but rather, to more severe systemic reactions or to interfering with and reducing the effect of adrenergic drugs used in the treatment of systemic reactions (71). Patients with other diseases or conditions that complicate the treatment of anaphylaxis, such as symptomatic coronary heart diseases and severe hypertension, also have an increased risk of developing systemic reactions that may end fatally (14). During ongoing immunotherapy, recent heavy intakes of alcohol might, owing to interaction with diamine oxidase, lower the threshold of allergen tolerance and, thereby, increase the risk of inducing systemic reactions in patients with ongoing uncomplicated immunotherapy (72). The magnitude of the delayed local reaction is widely used as an indicator to reduce allergen dosages (73,74). Controlled studies of the predictive value of local reactions do not, however, substantiate that the size of the local reactions is of use to predict systemic side effects (46,69).

Large and inconvenient local swellings may be treated successfully with ice bags or topical corticosteroids. Mild adverse reactions including mild urticaria or rhinitis can be treated with oral or parenteral antihistamines. These patients should be observed carefully, as these symptoms may be an early warning of an impending more serious reaction (14). In an immediate, mild or moderately severe bronchial obstruction, especially when occurring in patients treated with depot allergen extracts, it is advisable not only to use a β_2-agonist, but also to add oral corticosteroids to prevent delayed reactions. Severe bronchial obstruction (FEV_1 below 50% of the predicted value) might be treated with inhaled and parenteral β_2-agonist, although some prefer to use epinephrine given by inhalation. Patients with generalized urticaria might be treated with parenteral antihistamine, but most patients require epinephrine.

Anaphylactic reactions may progress rapidly, terminating in death within a few minutes (66,67). The early signs and symptoms of anaphylaxis include pruritus of the palms and scalp, intense erythema of the skin, conjunctival injection, and cough. Angioedema, laryngeal edema, severe asthma, hypotension, and shock may follow rapidly. Epinephrine is the only curative drug, and it should be administered promptly in sufficient doses (injected subcutaneous or intramuscular; 75). The patient should be placed in the Trendelenburg position, and an intravenous line should be set up, whereby intravenous fluids are administered rapidly. Steroids and antihistamines represent supplements in the treatment of anaphylaxis as well as antiasthmatic drugs and oxygen. In some patients, local infiltration of epinephrine at the site of the allergen injection, combined with a tourniquet, may be helpful to delay the absorption of allergens. In severe cases of anaphylactic reactions, further doses of epinephrine may be required. In patients with inadequate peripheral circulation and no response to subcutaneous or intramuscular epinephrine, intravenous or even intracardiac injections of the diluted drug may be needed (76). Patients should be hospitalized for intensive observation for approximately 24 h owing to the risk of delayed anaphylactic reactions. In some centers prophylactic antihistamines are used before injections to reduce the number and severity of side effects. A study of pretreatment with terfenadine in honeybee venom allergic patients showed a reduction in cutaneous symptoms, but no reduction in the more severe respiratory and cardiovascular symptoms (77). In a placebo-controlled, double-blind study of inhalant immunotherapy (78), pretreatment with loratidine showed a reduction in the number of patients experiencing systemic side effects of more than 50% and also a significant reduction in the severity of systemic reactions. A further advantage of antihistamine pretreatment was a diminished frequency of dose reductions and, thereby, a reduction in the number of injections to reach the maintenance dose. The advantages of antihistamine pretreatment in routine immunotherapy needs further evaluation before it can be recommended for general use.

C. Dosage Regimens and Dose Modifications

Several studies document that low-dose immunotherapy is inadequate in ensuring a pronounced clinical efficacy (79). On the other hand, high-dose immunotherapy implies an increased risk of eliciting life-threatening side effects. Ideally, the maintenance dose achieved should be the highest tolerated dose not eliciting side effects (i.e., the optimum dose) 14,61,62). From several controlled studies, allergen doses required to ensure efficacy are in the range of 5–20 μg major allergen (55). Allergen doses in the lower range appear to be the most appropriate as a guideline for an effective, but still safe dose. Studies designed to administer the maximal-tolerated dose result in a high frequency of side effects (55).

The maintenance dose may be less than the one recommended by the manufacturer, but it may also be higher. The dosage schedules supplied by the manufacturers serve as only a guide in uncomplicated immunotherapy (14). In sensitive patients, dose escalation must be modified, implying the administration of reduced doses, repetition of doses, or reduced increments. Highly sensitive patients may require smaller initial and top doses. No gold standard dosage schedule exists, for tolerance to injections depends on nonstandardized patients presenting with a variety of interfering factors, such as severity of disease, subclinical exposure to allergens, and nonspecific hyperreactivity.

The scheduled dose should be modified to administering either a reduced dose, repetition of the previous dose (i.e., no increment), or omitting the dose in the event of adverse reactions. Some guidelines relative to dose modifications may be suggested (14). These general guidelines are useful, but should not be followed religiously. Allergen doses should be adjusted in relation to the individual, and the obligatory evaluation of the patient's sensitivity and allergic state before each injection. The safety of the patient is the most important aspect, and it is advisable to reduce the dose if uncertain (14). The magnitude of the dose reduction depends on the individual situation. Guidelines that have been presented in international position papers stipulate the magnitude of allergen dose reduction relative to immediate and late local reactions, systemic reactions, and exceeding the time intervals between injections (14,55).

References

1. Grant IWB. Does immunotherapy have a role in the treatment of asthma? Clin Allergy 1986; 16:7–16.

2. BSACI Position Paper on Immunotherapy. Clin Exp Allergy 1993; 23:1–44.
3. Barnes PJ. Is immunotherapy for asthma worthwhile? N Engl J Med 1996; 334:351–352.
4. Creticos PS, Reed CE, Norman PS, et al. Ragweed immunotherapy in adult asthma. N Engl J Med 1996; 334:501–506.
5. Bruce CA, Norman PS, Rosenthal RR, Lichtenstein LM. The role of ragweed pollen in autumnal asthma. J Allergy Clin Immunol 1977; 59:449–459.
6. Abramson MJ, Puy RM, Weiner JM. Is allergen immunotherapy effective in asthma? A meta-analysis of randomized controlled trials. Am J Respir Crit Care Med 1995; 151:969–974.
7. International Consensus Report on Diagnosis and Management of Asthma. National Institutes of Health. Publication No. 92-3091, 1992.
8. Bousquet J, Dhivert H, Michel F-B. Current trends in the management of allergic diseases. Allergy 1994; 49:31–36.
9. Malling H-J. Immunotherapy in Europe. Clin Exp Allergy 1994; 24:515–521.
10. Bousquet J, Hejjaoui A, Michel F-B. Specific immunotherapy in asthma. J Allergy Clin Immunol 1990; 86:292–305.
11. Bousquet J, Michel F-B. Advances in specific immunotherapy. Clin Exp Allergy 1992; 22:889–896.
12. Bousquet J, Michel F-B. Specific immunotherapy in asthma: is it effective? J Allergy Clin Immunol 1994; 94:1–11.
13. Frew AJ. Conventional and alternative allergen immunotherapy: do they work? are they safe? Clin Exp Allergy 1994; 24:416–422.
14. Malling H-J, Weeke B. EAACI Immunotherapy Position Paper, Allergy 1993; 48:9–35.
15. Norman PS, Lichtenstein LM. The great debate: immunotherapy and asthma. Clin Allergy 1986; 16:269–271.
16. Ohman JL. Allergen immunotherapy in asthma: evidence for efficacy. J Allergy Clin Immunol 1989; 84:133–140.
17. Thompson RA. The current status of allergen immunotherapy (hyposensitisation). Report of WHO/IUIS working group. Allergy 1989; 44:369–379.
18. van Metre TE, Adkinson NF. Immunotherapy for aeroallergen disease. In: Middleton E, Reed CE, Ellis EF, Adkinson NF, Yunginger JW, eds. Allergy: Principles and Practice, 3rd ed. St Louis, MO: CV Mosby, 1988;1327–1343.
19. Hejjaoui A, Dhivert H, Michel FB, Bousquet J. Immunotherapy with standardized *Dermatophagoides pteronyssinus* extract. IV. Systemic reactions according to the immunotherapy schedule. J Allergy Clin Immunol 1990; 85:473–479.
20. Johnstone DE. Some aspects of the natural history of asthma. Ann Allergy 1982; 49:257–264.
21. Jenkins MA, Hopper SL, Bowes G, Carlin SB, Flander LB, Giles GG. Factors in childhood as predictors of asthma in adult life. Br Med J 1994; 309:90–93.
22. Roorda RS, Gerritsen J, Van Aalderen WM, Schouten JP, Veltman JC, Weiss ST, Knol K. Risk factors for the persistence of respiratory symptoms in childhood asthma. Am Rev Respir Dis 1993; 148:1490–1495.
23. Rackemann FM, Edwards MC. Asthma in children. A follow-up study of 688 patients after an interval of twenty years. N Engl J Med 1952; 246:815–863.
24. Johnstone DE, Dutton A. The value of hyposensitization therapy for bronchial asthma in children—a 14-year study. Pediatrics 1968; 42:793–802.
25. Barnes PJ, Pedersen S. Efficacy and safety of inhaled corticosteroids in asthma. Am Rev Respir Dis 1993; 148:1–26.
26. Malling H-J. Current status of allergen-specific immunotherapy. In: Kurth R, Haustein D, eds. Regulatory Control and Standardization of Allergenic Extracts. Arbeit Paul-Ehrlich-Instit 1994; 87:169–177.
27. Robinson D, Hamid Q, Ying S, Bentley A, Assoufi B, Durham S, Kay AB. Prednisolone treatment in asthma is associated with modulation of bronchoalveolar lavage cell interleukin-4, interleukin-5, and interferon-gamma cytokine gene expression. Am Rev Respir Dis 1993; 148:401–406.

28. Kelso A. Th1 and Th2 subsets: paradigms lost? Immunol Today 1995; 16:374–379.
29. Bousquet J, Becker WM, Hejjaoui A, Chanal I, Lebel B, Chivert H, Michel FB. Differences in clinical and immunologic reactivity of patients allergic to grass pollens and to multiple-pollen species. II. Efficacy of a double-blind, placebo-controlled, specific immunotherapy with standardized extracts. J Allergy Clin Immunol 1991; 88:43–53.
30. Bousquet J, Hejjaoui A, Clauzel AM, Guérin B, Dhivert H, Skassa-Brociek W, Michel F-B. Specific immunotherapy with a standardized *Dermatophagoides pteronyssinus* extract. II. Prediction of efficacy of immunotherapy. J Allergy Clin Immunol 1988; 82:971–977.
31. Peat JK, Woolcock AJ, Cullen K. Rate of decline of lung function in subjects with asthma. Eur J Respir Dis 1987; 70:171–179.
32. Bousquet J, Chanez P, Lacoste JY, et al. Asthma: a disease remodeling the airways. Allergy 1992; 47:3–11.
33. Tabar AI, Garcia BE, Rodriguez A, Olaguibel JM, Muro MD, Quirce S. A prospective safety-monitoring study of immunotherapy with biologically standardized extracts. Allergy 1993; 48:450–453.
34. Allessandro F, Vincenzo ZG, Marco S, Marcello G, Enrica R. Compliance with pharmacologic prophylaxis and therapy in bronchial asthma. Ann Allergy 1994; 73:135–140.
35. Yeung M, O'Connor SA, Parry DT, Cochrane GM. Compliance with prescribed drug therapy in asthma. Respir Med 1994; 88:31–35.
36. Czarny D. Asthma and allergy. What is the connection? Aust Fam Physician 1993; 22:1967–1970.
37. Reid MJ, Moss RB, Hsu Y-P, Kwasnicki JM, Commerford TM, Nelson BL. Seasonal asthma in northern California: allergic causes and efficacy of immunotherapy. J Allergy Clin Immunol 1986; 78:590–600.
38. Bousquet J, Maasch H, Hejjaoui A, Skassa-Brociek W, Wahl R, Dhivert H, Michel F-B. Double blind, placebo-controlled immunotherapy with mixed grass-pollen allergoids. III. Efficacy and safety of unfractionated and high-molecular-weight preparations in rhinoconjunctivitis and asthma. J Allergy Clin Immunol 1989; 84:546–556.
39. Bousquet J, Hejjaoui A, Soussana M, Michel F-B. Double-blind, placebo-controlled immunotherapy with mixed grass-pollen altergoids. IV. Comparison of the safety and efficacy of two dosages of a high-molecular-weight allergoid. J Allergy Clin Immunol 1990; 98:490–497.
40. Machiels JJ, Somville MA, Jacquemin MG, Saint-Remy JMR. Allergen-antibody complexes can efficiently prevent seasonal rhinitis and asthma in grass pollen hypersensitive patients. Allergy 1991; 46:335–348.
41. Bousquet J, Calvayrac P, Guérin B, Hejjaoui A, Dhivert H, Hewitt B, Michel F-B. Immunotherapy with a standardized *Dermatophagoides pteronyssinus* extract. I. In vivo and in vitro parameters after a short course of treatment. J Allergy Clin Immunol 1985; 76;734–744.
42. Machiels JJ, Somville MA, Lebrun PM, Lebecque SJ, Jacquemin MG, Saint-Remy J-MR. Allergic bronchial asthma due to *Dermatophagoides pteronyssinus* hypersensitivity can be efficiently treated by inoculation of allergen–antibody complexes. J Clin Invest 1990; 85:1024–1035.
43. Ohman JL, Findlay SR, Leitermann KM. Immunotherapy in cat-induced asthma. Double-blind trial with evaluation of in vivo and in vitro responses. J Allergy Clin Immunol 1984; 74:230–239.
44. Hedlin G, Graff-Lonnevig V, Heilborn H, Lilja G, Norrlind K, Pegelow K, Sundin B, Löwenstein H. Immunotherapy with cat- and dog-dander extracts. V. Effects of 3 years of treatment. J Allergy Clin Immunol 1991; 87:955–964.
45. Alvarez-Cuesta E, Cuesta-Herranz J, Puyana-Ruiz J, Cuesta-Herranz C, Blanco-Quirós A. Monoclonal antibody-standardized cat extract immunotherapy: risk–benefit effects from a double-blind placebo study. J Allergy Clin Immunol 1994; 93:556–566.
46. Malling H-J, Dreborg S, Weeke B. Diagnosis and immunotherapy of mould allergy. V. Clinical efficacy and side effects of immunotherapy with *Cladosporium herbarum*. Allergy 1986; 41:507–519.

47. Horst M. Hejjaoui A, Horst V, Michel F-B. Double blind, placebo-controlled rush immunotherapy with a standardized *Alternaria* extract. J Allergy Clin Immunol 1990; 85:460–472.
48. Keating MU, Kagey-Sobotka A. Hamilton RG, Yunginger JW. Clinical and immunologic follow-up of patients who stop venom immunotherapy. J Allergy Clin Immunol 1991; 88:339–348.
49. Golden DB, Kwiterovich KA, Kagey-Sobotka A, Valentine MD, Lichtenstein LM. Discontinuing venom immunotherapy: outcome after five years. J Allergy Clin Immunol 1996; 97:579–587.
50. Des Roches A, Paradis L, Knani J, Hejjaoui A, Dhivert H, Chanez P, Bousquet J. Immunotherapy with a standardized *Dermatophagoides pteronyssinus* extract. V. Duration of efficacy of immunotherapy after its cessation. Allergy 1996; 51:430–433.
51. Hedlin G, Heilborn H, Lilja G, Norrlind K, Pegelow K-O, Schou C, Løwenstein H. Long-term follow-up of patients treated with a three-year course of cat or dog immunotherapy. J Allergy Clin Immunol 1995; 96:879–885.
52. Cohn RJ, Pizzi A. Determinants of patient compliance with allergen immunotherapy. J Allergy Clin Immunol 1993; 91:734–737.
53. AAAI Board of Directors. Guidelines to minimize the risk from systemic reactions caused by immunotherapy with allergenic extracts. J Allergy Clin Immunol 1994; 93:811–812.
54. Norman PS. Safety of allergen immunotherapy. J Allergy Clin Immunol 1989; 84:438–439.
55. Norman PS, van Metre TE. The safety of allergenic immunotherapy. J Allergy Clin Immunol 1990; 85:522–525.
56. Sundin B, Lilja G, Graff-Lonnevig V, Hedlin G, Heilborn H, Norrlind K, Pegelow KO, Løwenstein L. Immunotherapy with partially purified and standardized animal dander extracts. I. Clinical results from a double-blind study on patients with animal dander asthma. J Allergy Clin Immunol 1986; 77:478–487.
57. Ortolani C, Pastorello E, Moss RB, Hsu Y-P, Restuccia M, Joppolo G, Miadonna A, Cornelli U, Halpern G, Zanussi C. Grass pollen immunotherapy: a single year double-blind, placebo-controlled study in patients with grass pollen induced asthma and rhinitis. J Allergy Clin Immunol 1984; 73:283–290.
58. Bousquet J, Hejjaoui A, Dhivert H, Clauzel AM, Michel FB. Specific immunotherapy with a standardized *Dermatophagoides pteronyssinus* extract. III. Systemic reactions during the rush protocol in patients suffering from asthma. J Allergy Clin Immunol 1989; 83:797–802.
59. Armentia-Medina A, Blanco-Quiros A, Martin-Santos JM, Alvarez-Cuesta E, Moneo-Goiri I, Carreira P, Losada-Cosmes E. Rush immunotherapy with a standardized Bermuda grass pollen extract. Ann Allergy 1989; 63:127–135.
60. Haugaard L, Dahl R, Jacobsen L. A controlled dose–response study of immunotherapy with standardized, partially purified extract of house dust mite: clinical efficacy and side effects. J Allergy Clin Immunol 1993; 91:709–722.
61. Hejjaoui A, Ferrando R, Dhivert H, Michel FB, Bousquet J. Systemic reactions occurring during immunotherapy with standardized pollen extracts. J Allergy Clin Immunol 1992; 89:925–933.
62. Stewart GE II, Lockey RF. Systemic reactions from allergen immunotherapy. J Allergy Clin Immunol 1992; 90:567–578.
63. Shaikh WA. A retrospective study of the safety of immunotherapy in pregnancy. Clin Exp Allergy 1993; 23:857–860.
64. Taylor RJ, Hypersensitivity vasculitis occurring in a patient receiving immunotherapy. J Allergy Clin Immunol 1991; 88:889–890.
65. Committee on the Safety of Medicine. CMS update: desensitizing vaccines. Br Med J 1986; 293:948.
66. Lockey RF, Benedict LM, Turkeltaub PC, Bukantz SC. Fatalities from immunotherapy (IT) and skin testing (ST). J Allergy Clin Immunol 1987; 79:660–667.
67. Reid MJ, Lockey RF, Turkeltaub PC, Platts-Mills TAE. Survey of fatalities from skin testing and immunotherapy 1985–1989. J Allergy Clin Immunol 1993; 92:6–15.

68. Tinkelmann DG, Cole WQ, Tunno J. Immunotherapy: a one-year prospective study to evaluate risk factors of systemic reactions. J Allergy Clin Immunol 1995; 95:8–14.
69. Mosbech H, Dirksen A, Dreborg S, Frølund L, Heinig JH, Svendsen UG, Søborg M, Taudorf E, Weeke B. Hyposensitization in asthmatics with mPEG-modified and unmodified house dust mite extract. IV. Occurrence and prediction of side effects. Allergy 1990; 45:142–150.
70. Hepner MJ, Ownby DR, Anderson JA, Rose MS, Sears-Ewald D, Brown EB. Risk of systemic reactions in patients taking beta-blocker drugs receiving allergen immunotherapy injections. J Allergy Clin Immunol 1990; 86:407–411.
71. Toogood JH. Risk of anaphylaxis in patients receiving beta-blocker drugs. J Allergy Clin Immunol 1988; 81:1–5.
72. Wantke F, Demmer CM, Götz M, Jarisch R. Inhibition of diamine oxidase is a risk in specific immunotherapy. Allergy 1993; 48:552.
73. Löfkvist T, Agrell B, Dreborg S, Svensson G. Effects of immunotherapy with a purified standardized allergen preparation of *Dermatophagoides farinae* in adults with perennial allergic rhinoconjunctivitis. Allergy 1994; 49:100–107.
74. Varney VA, Gaga M, Frew AJ, Aber VR, Kay AB, Durham SR. Usefulness of immunotherapy in patients with severe summer hay fever uncontrolled by antiallergic drugs. Br Med J 1991; 302:265–269.
75. Anderson JA, Chai H, Claman HN, Ellis EF, Fink JN, Kaplan AP, Lieberman PL, Pierson WE, Salvaggio JE, Sheffer AL, Slavin RG. Personnel and equipment to treat systemic reactions caused by immunotherapy with allergenic extracts. J Allergy Clin Immunol 1986; 77:271–273.
76. Perkin RM, Anas NG. Mechanisms and management of anaphylactic shock not responding to traditional therapy. Ann Allergy 1985; 54:202–208.
77. Berchtold E, Maibach R, Müller U. Reduction of side effects from rush immunotherapy with honeybee venom by pretreatment with terfenadine. Clin Exp Allergy 1992; 22:59–65.
78. Nielson L, Johnsen CR, Mosbech H, Poulsen LK, Malling H-J. Antihistamine premedication in specific cluster immunotherapy: a double-blind, placebo-controlled study. J Allergy Clin Immunol 1996; 97:1207–1213.
79. Creticos PS. Immunotherapy with allergens. JAMA 1992; 268:2834–2839.

NEW FORMS OF SPECIFIC IMMUNOTHERAPY

17

Peptide-Mediated Immunomodulation as Therapy for Allergic Disorders

NANNA S. KRISTENSEN

Institute for Medical Microbiology
and Immunology
University of Copenhagen
Copenhagen, Denmark

HANS YSSEL

INSERM U454
Hôpital Arnaud de Villeneuve
Montpellier, France

JONATHAN R. LAMB

Respiratory Medicine Unit
University of Edinburgh Medical School
Edinburgh, Scotland

I. Introduction

Atopic disorders, including asthma, atopic dermatitis, and allergic rhinitis are caused by an inappropriate immune response to common environmental antigens (allergens) in genetically susceptible individuals. It is estimated that between 10 and 20% of the population in developed countries suffer from atopic disorders, and the prevalence is increasing. The allergic immunopathology is characterized by an overproduction of allergen-specific IgE and infiltration of the disease site with lymphocytes, mast cells, and basophils. IgE molecules are able to bind to high-affinity Fcε receptors (FcεRI) on the surface of mast cells and basophils. Reexposure to the allergen will induce FcεRI cross-linking and trigger the release of inflammatory and vasoactive mediators, chemotactic factors, and cytokines, responsible for the allergic cascade. In addition to mast cells and basophils, eosinophils also appear to be involved in the allergic reaction, because these cells accumulate at the site of inflammation and, furthermore, are capable of inducing tissue damage by release of toxic products.

Desensitization immunotherapy with intact native allergen has proved effective in some allergic disorders, such as bee venom allergy (1), hay fever (2,3), and cat asthma (4), but has been less successful for others. Because administration of native allergen, containing B-cell epitopes that might be recognized by IgE, confers a potential risk of anaphylactic shock, attention has been focused on developing immunotherapies based on allergen derivatives (5–8). In this chapter, we will discuss peptide-mediated immunotherapy that targets CD4⁺ T cells involved in the allergic reaction, with emphasis on the immunological basis underlying the mechanisms leading to induction of nonresponsiveness, or anergy.

II. Involvement and Activation of $CD4^+$ T-Cell Subsets in Allergy

Our understanding of the immunological basis of allergic disorders has advanced in recent years. Although the effector elements are allergen-specific IgE, mast cells, basophils, and eosinophils, their differentiation and expansion is regulated in part by $CD4^+$ T cells through the production of certain cytokines and chemokines. IgE production by B cells is induced by interleukin-4 (IL-4) and is inhibited by interferon gamma (IFN-γ), IFN-γ, and prostaglandin-E_2 (PGE_2) (9). IL-4 also costimulates CD40-induced B-cell activation, clonal expansion, and induces isotope switching for the production of IgE and IgG4 (see Refs. 9,10). IL-13 is another cytokine that is capable of inducing IgE and IgG4 synthesis independently from IL-4 (11), and IL-5 is an important eosinophil differentiation and chemotactic factor (12,13), which has also been implicated in induction of B-cell differentiation (14). In addition, $CD4^+$ T cells produce chemokines, such as RANTES, a chemoattractant for monocytes, as well as memory $CD4^+$ T cells, and production of eotaxin, which is an important activator and attractor of eosinophils, is regulated in vivo by T cells (15). Thus, activation of allergen-specific $CD4^+$ T cells is a key step in the initiation of allergic sensitization.

It has been proposed that at least two signals are required for optimal activation of T cells: the first signal is provided by transient ligation of the T-cell receptor (TCR) by an antigen-derived peptide bound to the peptide-binding groove of a major histocompatibility complex (MHC) class II molecule on the surface of an antigen-presenting cell (APC). Engagement of several TCR molecules will trigger TCR dimerization (16) and result in signal transduction into the nucleus by a phosphokinase cascade (reviewed in Ref. 17). The second, costimulatory, signal is provided by triggering of cell surface molecules on the APC, such as the B7 (CD80 and CD86) family, which are ligands for the CD28 or CTLA-4 molecules on the T cell. In addition, adhesion molecules strengthen the interaction between T cells and APC, whereas cytokines and other soluble factors deliver costimulatory signals as well.

Murine $CD4^+$ helper T cells can be divided into, at least two subsets defined by the cytokines they produce (reviewed in Ref. 18): T cells of the type 1 subset (Th1) secrete IL-2, IFN-γ, and tumor necrosis factor-β (TNF-β). Th1 cells are involved in inflammatory reactions and their activation leads to cell-mediated immunity. By inducing macrophage activation and providing help for cytotoxic cells, they play an important role in combating intracellular microbes. Mouse $CD4^+$ T-cell clones of the type 2 subset (Th2), on the other hand, produce IL-4, IL-5, IL-6, IL-10, and IL-13. These cytokines are important for humoral immune responses and, in addition, IL-4, IL-10, and IL-13 have strong anti-inflammatory effects. Although this dichotomy in cytokine production has also been reported for human T-cell clones (reviewed in Ref. 1), a major proportion of in vitro-derived human T-cell clones display intermediate (Th0) cytokine profiles (see Refs. 20,21). Th0 cells may be precursor cells with the potential of differentiating into either Th1 or Th2 cells or, alternatively, Th0 cells may have effector functions in their own right.

Studies in the mouse have demonstrated that various factors can influence whether a naive T cell will differentiate into a Th1 or a Th2 cell on activation. High ligand (i.e., peptide–MHC class II complex) density on the surface of the APC and a strong interaction with the TCR selects for a Th1 response, whereas commitment to the Th2 phenotype is favored by a lower ligand density and a weaker interaction of the ligand with the TCR (22,23). The type of APC delivering the activating signals will also influence the outcome of activation: macrophages tend to favor the induction of Th1 cells, whereas B cells prime for Th2 responses (24,25). Recently, it has been suggested that the B7 family of costimulatory molecules, notably CD80 (B7-1) and CD86 (B7-2), deliver different signals to naive T cells. Ligation of CD28 on naïve murine T cells by CD86, but not by CD80, reportedly induced IL-4 production by these cells (26). Similar results were obtained from in vivo antibody-inhibition studies, which suggested that ligation via CD80 or CD86 induces Th1 or Th2 differentiation, respectively (27). However, in vitro studies using human peripheral lymphocytes did not reveal any intrinsic differences between CD80 and CD86 in the ability to induce cytokine secretion (28). Soluble factors, such as cytokines and prostaglandins, which are present in the microenvironment in which cell–cell interactions take place, also play an important role in determining whether a T cell is committed to a Th1- or a Th2-dominant phenotype on activation. Studies in TCR transgenic mice have indicated that T cells expressing identical TCRs can differentiate into either Th1- or Th2-like effector cells, depending on the priming conditions. IL-4, in particular, has been implicated in the selection for a Th2-dominant phenotype, which is inhibited by the action of IFN-γ, secreted by Th1 cells (29–30).

It has been argued that normal in vivo immune responses will involve Th0 cells or a mixed population of effector cells, each capable of producing and secreting only one cytokine (31), and that differentiation into either the Th1 or the Th2 subset is an extreme situation that requires repeated stimulation with antigen and appropriate priming conditions. However, in certain pathological conditions, such as autoimmune lesions (32), helminth infestation, and exposure to environmental allergens (19), chronic antigen stimulation is present and, therefore, can lead to differentiation into the Th1 or Th2 subset, respectively. Evidence from both in in vivo and in vitro studies (33,34) lends strong support to the notion that a key feature of allergic disorders is a polarization of allergen-specific T cells toward an IL-4–producing Th2-dominant phenotype. T cells with a Th2-like phenotype, producing

IL-4 and IL-5, accumulate in the diseased tissues and in allergen-induced, cutaneous late-phase reactions in atopic individuals (33–37). Furthermore, allergen-specific T-cell clones, isolated from atopic individuals, secrete high amounts of IL-4 and IL-5 and to give help to B cells for the synthesis of IgE. However, most of these cells are capable of secreting low levels of IFN-γ and, therefore, do display an Th0/Th2 phenotype (21,38). In vitro analysis of the kinetics of cytokine secretion by allergen-specific Th0 clones has revealed that IL-4 production, after activation, precedes that of IFN-γ by several hours, thereby emphasizing their Th2 function (Yssel H, Verhoef A, Lamb J, unpublished data). The Th2-dominant phenotype is not inherent for individuals with atopic disorders, for they are capable of mounting a Th0/Th1 response after stimulation with nonallergens, such as tetanus toxoid and mycobacterial antigens (21). In addition, the ability to respond to allergens is not unique to patients with atopic disorders; however, T-cell responses to allergens in nonatopic individuals are predominantly of a Th1 type, and these T cells fail to support IgE synthesis (38,39). Thus, the current hypothesis is that, in individuals predisposed to atopic disorders, chronic or seasonal repeated exposure to allergen will lead to a preferential differentiation of naive $CD4^+$ T cells into a Th2- or Th0-dominant, IL-4–producing phenotype, by mechanisms that still remain to be elucidated. The latter cells, in turn, are responsible for allergic disease, by supporting production of allergen-specific IgE as well as accumulation of eosinophils in the affected tissue.

In broad terms, the goal of immunotherapy is to ameliorate the clinical severity of allergic disorders through a decrease in the ratio of allergen-induced Th2 to Th1 cytokines. This can, in theory, be accomplished in two different ways: by downregulating the functional activity of allergen-specific Th2-type cells, or alternatively, by inducing, or upregulating, a population of allergen-specific T cells with a Th1-dominant phenotype. Downregulation of a Th2 response may be achieved by inducing tolerance or clonal anergy, which can result in modulation of the cytokine secretion pattern of the T cells, as will be discussed later. It has been previously reported that murine Th2 cells seem less susceptible in vivo to tolerogenic signals mediated by nominal antigens than are Th1 cells (40,41). Recent studies, however, have demonstrated that tolerance can be induced in vitro in mouse Th2 cells by high doses of peptide, or as a result of partial activation (42–44). A preferential induction of allergen-specific Th1 cells has been achieved in vitro as well as in vivo by using cytokines, such as IFNγ, IFN-α, and IL-12 (29,45–47). Alternatively, Th1 cells may be upregulated by using adjuvants or vehicles that select for a Th1 phenotype, such as allergen expressed in recombinant mycobacteria or by plasmid DNA. Strategies that aim at upregulating allergen-specific Th1-dominant cells have potential advantages over those that aim only at downregulating Th2 responses: First, some of the Th1 effector responses, such as IgG production and macrophage activation, will actively aid in clearing allergen from the system. Second, a Th1 response is likely to inhibit the function of already established allergen-specific Th2 cells, because the Th1 cytokine IFN-γ strongly inhibits IgE production (9).

III. Traditional Immunotherapy

Studies into the immunological mechanisms underlying traditional allergen-mediated immunotherapy, in which increasing doses of purified allergen are administered subcutaneously under defined clinical conditions, have yielded promising data. It appears that the decrease in severity of clinical allergy following immunotherapy is partly due to a shift in allergen-induced CD4$^+$ T-cell cytokine patterns. Following successful immunotherapy in patients with allergic rhinitis to inhalant allergens, the quantity of IL-4 produced by CD4$^+$ allergen-specific memory T cells was reduced to levels produced by T cells from nonatopic individuals. The production of IFN-γ and IL-2 as well as the serum levels of total IgE were, however, not significantly influenced by the treatment (48). When the influence of immunotherapy on cytokine mRNA expression in skin from patients with grass pollen allergy was examined during allergen-induced late-phase cutaneous responses, no effect on Th2 cytokines was seen, whereas the expression of Th1-type cytokines was enhanced (49).

Immunotherapy has also been reported to induce peripheral T-cell tolerance in allergen-specific T cells (50). Subcutaneous administration of bee venom resulted in suppression of allergen-induced proliferation, Th2 cytokine secretion (IL-4, IL-5, and IL-13), as well as Th1 cytokine secretion (IFN-γ) in vitro. In an earlier study, proliferation and Th2 cytokine production was reduced, whereas IFN-γ secretion was increased, following immunotherapy with bee venom (51). However, the cytokine production was measured following stimulation of polyclonal T cells by anti-CD3 monoclonal antibody (MAb), instead of allergen-specific stimulation, which may account for the reported differences between these two studies. In addition, it was concluded from the results of this study that serum levels of allergen-specific IgE initially increased (after 2 months of therapy) and decreased (after 9 months), whereas IgG levels continued to increase throughout the treatment (51). The more recent report partly supports this finding: serum levels of specific IgE, as well as IgG4, increased during 2 months of therapy; however, the IgE/IgG4 ratio declined owing to a greater increase of serum IgG4 (50). Although these observations initially appear slightly discrepant, one should remember that the allergen-specific T cells used in these studies were obtained from different disease sites, and that patients with different types of allergies were studied (systemic versus mucosal exposure to allergen). Taken together, these studies support the notion that immunotherapy ameliorates the immunopathology of allergic disorders by altering the cytokine patterns induced in CD4$^+$ T cells after allergen exposure. This may be achieved either by inducing allergen-specific peripheral tolerance, by down-regulating subpopulations. However, because of the possible presence of B-cell epitopes that may be recognized by IgE, the use of whole-allergen extracts for immunotherapy confers a risk of anaphylactic shock, and even fatalities; accordingly, it is desirable to develop immunotherapies that target T cells only. Therefore, the rest of this chapter will be devoted to the discussion of peptide-mediated modulation of allergen-specific T-cell responses, based on the use of allergen derivatives and their potential importance for immunotherapy of allergic disorders.

IV. Peptide-Mediated Immunomodulation In Vitro

The ability of peptides to modulate the effector functions of T cells was initially observed for human Th0-type T-cell clones specific for influenza virus hemagglutinin. Exposure of the T cells to supraoptimal amounts of specific peptide, in the absence of APC, induced a state of unresponsiveness (anergy) after antigenic rechallenge, which could be reversed by the addition of IL-2 (52,53). This observation has been expanded to include human Th2-like cells specific for the house dust mite allergen *Dermatophagoides pteronissynus* 1 (Der p 1; 54,55), as well as Th2/Th0 T-cell clones, specific for the bee venom allergen phospholipase A_2 (PLA; 56). Although anergized T cells express the B-cell costimulatory molecule CD40 ligand, they fail to support IgE production by B cells, even in the presence of exogenous IL-4 or IL-13 (44). It is thus possible to modulate antibody responses by specifically targeting T cells in vitro. Murine T-cell clones, unlike their human counterparts, do not express MHC class II. However, peptide-mediated anergy can be induced in murine T cells by presenting specific peptide on chemically fixed APC (44,57). The induction phase following the stimulation of T-cell clones with relevant peptides is accompanied by a downregulation of the TCR–CD3 receptor complex and upregulation of CD2 and CD25 (55,58). Restoration of TCR expression without recovery of function does, however, suggest that it is not TCR downregulation that accounts for the anergic state (44). Furthermore, anergic murine T cells display altered inositol phosphate, calcium, and tyrosine kinase signaling (59). In addition, CD28-mediated costimulation has been reported to prevent the induction of anergy (60). Analysis of anergic Th1 and Th2 cells has revealed that a defect in IL-2 production, a result of posttranscriptional regulation, precedes the induction of unresponsiveness (57,60,61). The transcription of other cytokines has been reported to be upregulated by anergy induction in a human Th0 clone, although the increase in mRNA levels was not accompanied by an increase in cytokine secretion (62). In contrast, murine Th2 clones, rendered anergic following partial activation, retained the ability to secrete cytokines (particularly IL-4), albeit at reduced levels (43,56).

Modulation of specific T-cell responses has also been reported using analogues of immunogenic peptides, presented by live, unmodified APC. In the original study, Evavold and Allen introduced conservative amino acid substitutions, at positions in an immunogenic peptide that supposedly do not contribute to MHC-binding, and tested the ability of these altered peptide ligands (APLs) to induce cytokine secretion in a murine Th clone. One APL was identified that, although unable to stimulate proliferation, could induce IL-4 secretion and support cognate B-cell help in a specific Th2 clone. Addition of IL-1, which costimulates activation of Th2 cells, restored the proliferative response to normal levels (63). Partial activation by APL has also been demonstrated using murine Th1 clones (64). Interestingly, stimulation of both Th1 (64) and Th2 (43) clones with APL, presented by live APC, induced a long-lasting state of anergy.

This form of anergy seems to be different from the model described by Jenkins and Schwartz in which it was demonstrated that murine T cells could be anergized by stimulation with immunogenic peptides presented by chemically modified APC, which eliminates the costimulatory signal, during TRC triggering of the TCR (60). These anergized cells no longer respond to stimulation by the TCR, although they still retained the ability to proliferate following incubation in IL-2. Furthermore, this costimulatory signal can block the induction of anergy in T-cell clones (59). In contrast, the state of anergy induced by APL cannot be prevented by simply providing a costimulatory signal, indicating that different pathways are being affected in these two experimental models of anergy induction. It is clear from the observed biological responses using APL that these peptides, which in most instances have only a single amino acid residue substitution, as compared with the wild-type agonistic peptide, directly affect TCR-mediated signaling events. Indeed, a unique pattern of phosphorylation of the TCRζ-chain and a failure to activate the TCR-associated ZAP-70 kinase was detected following stimulation of a murine T-cell clone with an APL that induces partial activation (65). From these observations, it has been proposed that partial activation of T cells, using APL result in a major decrease in the pathway, which involves signaling by TCRζ-chain, ZAP-70, and nuclear factor of transcription (NFAT), whereas the Ras pathways and the costimulation pathway by CD28 appear to be activated, and the integration of these signals leads to the particular phenotype of partial T-cell activation (reviewed in Ref. 66) Importantly, according to this model, any stimulation of T cells through a limited subset of signaling pathways, would lead to a similar phenotype, which is indeed so during the induction of anergy in the absence of costimulatory signals (67).

Allergen-specific human T-cell clones, of the Th0 as well as the Th2 phenotype, are also susceptible to modulation by APL. Recently, two studies have shown that different analogues were able to induce various peptide analogues of effector functions in T-cell clones. Interestingly, several analogues, derived from Japanese cedar pollen allergen (Cry j 1) (68), as well as Der p 2 (69), were identified that were capable of altering the IFN-γ/IL-4 ration of allergen-specific T-cell clones, by selectively enhancing IFN-γ production, and additional APL have been found that are capable of selectively increasing, by more than tenfold, IFN-γ secretion by allergen-specific TH0 clones without affecting the production of IL-4. In addition, one of these Der p 2–derived APL, significantly enhances tolerogenic activity, as compared with the native peptide, when incubated with T-cell clones in the absence of APC (Verhoef A, Lamb J, unpublished observations).

Thus, by modifying the stimulus delivered by the TCR–CD3 complex, it is possible, at least in vitro, to prevent clonal expansion of effector cells, downregulate B-cell help, and occasionally, also modify cytokine secretion patterns. These observations have encouraged studies into peptide-mediated modulation of T-cell responses in vivo, especially those causing allergic as well as autoimmune, disorders.

V. Peptide-Mediated Modulation of In Vivo Immune Responses

The clinical application of peptides for specific immunotherapy of allergic diseases has only recently begun to be evaluated. However, reports from murine models on the ability of peptides to alter responses of autoantigen or allergen-specific T cells in vivo have proved promising and will be discussed later, together with the limited data available on peptide-mediated immunotherapy of atopic disorders.

Two independent studies on experimental autoimmune encephalomyelitis (EAE) have shown that APLs can deviate pathogenic immune responses in vivo. EAE is a demyelinating disease resulting in paralysis, in which autoreactive Th1 cells are believed to be the pathogenic mediators (70), whereas regulatory T cells that suppress the development of the disease display a Th2-like phenotype (71). In one model, immunization of mice with a myelin proteolipid protein (PLP)-derived peptide generates PLP-specific Th1 cells and induces EAE. In addition, the disease can be induced in naive animals by adoptively transferring these T cells, following in vitro activation (72). Altering the primary TCR-contact point in the PLP peptide, generated an APL that induced T cells that, in addition to Th1 cytokines, also produced IL-4 and IL-10. Mice that were preimmunized with this APL did not, or only partially develop EAE following subsequent injection of disease-inducing PLP-specific Th1 cells. Furthermore, adoptive transfer of T-cell lines, induced by the APL and activated in vitro by either the same APL or the native peptide, respectively, conferred protection against EAE induced by immunization with the native peptide (73). In another murine EAE model, the disease can be induced by adoptive transfer of a T-cell clone specific for a myelin basic protein (MBP)-derived peptide. By treating mice in vivo with an APL, either directly after transfer or after paralysis was established, it was possible to prevent induction of EAE and reverse paralysis. In this model, the APL appears to confer protection by altering the cytokine profile of the disease-including T-cell clone, which produces high levels of tumor necrosis factor (TNF)-α and low amounts of IL-4, after stimulation with the native peptide, whereas stimulation with the APL substantially downregulated the TNF-α production.

Experimental animal models have also been studied to evaluate the effects of the route of administration of allergen derivatives on immune responses. One system examined the modulation of murine T-cell responses to a major cat allergenic protein, *Felis domesticus* 1 (Fel d 1), following subcutaneous administration of allergen-derived peptides. Fel d 1 consist of two disulfide-linked polypeptide chains, which both contain epitopes recognized by T cells (74,75). However, most human T-cell responses to Fel d 1 are directed against epitopes contained within amino acid residues 7–55 on chain 1 (76). T-cell response in B6×CBAF_1 mice, immunized with Fel d 1, are also directed primarily at this region. Subcutaneous administration of two 27-amino acid peptides (designated IPC-1 and IPC-2) comprising this region, has been reported to induce peripheral T-cell tolerance in B6×CBAF_1 mice after subsequent peptide challenge, measured as suppression of peptide-induced secretion of the cytokines IL-2, IL-4, and IFN-γ in vitro. In mice primed with Fel d 1, a situation that may better reflect the clinical condition of allergic disorders, subcutaneous peptide administration resulted in the abrogation of ongoing T-cell responses to chain 1. Importantly, this treatment also downregulated the in vivo production of specific IgE (76). In another study from the same group, subcutaneous administration of a recombinant fusion protein, containing three linked T-cell epitopes from chain 1 of Fel d 1, was also reported to induce peripheral T-cell tolerance in mice (77).

Mucosal administration of soluble antigen has proved an effective way of modulating both $CD4^+$ and $CD8^+$ T-cell response, and oral and nasal administration of whole antigen or peptides has been proposed as a possible way of regulating inappropriate immune responses in allergic as well as autoimmune disorders (78–81). The intranasal administration to $H\text{-}2^b$ mice of a single peptide, amino acid residues 111–139 of Der p 1—which contains an immunodominant T-cell epitope—before priming with Der p 1 inhibits peptide-induced T-cell, as well as antibody, responses in vitro. More importantly, administration of the dominant peptide also induced tolerance to other minor T-cell epitopes within Der p 1, as well as to the whole allergen. Furthermore, as in the Fel d 1 model, the peptide treatment was effective, whether administered before or after sensitization with the allergen, indicating the possibility to module ongoing T-cell response (82). Similar results were obtained by feeding recombinant fusion proteins, containing the dominant peptide (83).

Although the immunological mechanisms underlying the induction of unresponsiveness remain to be elucidated, the results from these experimental models are promising and suggest that it is possible to modulate ongoing immune responses to whole allergens by mucosal or subcutaneous administration of allergen derivatives. Thus, successful immunotherapy in patients suffering from allergic disorders may, in theory, be achieved using a restricted number of immunodominant peptides. Initial results from studies on human atopic patients who received synthetic Fel d 1–derived peptides, indicated that a dose-related reduction of allergic symptoms, such as decreased bronchial reactivity and decreased skin responses was observed, following peptide treatment (6–8,83,84). Successful immunotherapy using a mixture of three T-cell epitopes, derived from bee venom PLA has also been reported (5). In the latter study, three patients exhibited a decrease in specific IgE and IgG4, and tolerated provocation with native PLA as well as a bee sting challenge after three weekly doses of 100 μg of peptide. However, conflicting data on the efficacy of peptide-mediated immunotherapy has recently been published in a study during which the Fel d 1-derived peptides IPC-1 and IPC-2 where administrated by subcutaneous injection to cat-allergic individuals. Subjects receiving immunotherapy did not tolerate significantly more allergen, measured as immediate and late-phase skin test reactivity, than did subjects who received placebo. Furthermore, no changes in allergen-induced cytokine expression (IL-4, IL-10, and IFN-γ) by peripheral lymphocytes was evident following immunotherapy. However, the study did not report whether or not the clinical condition of the patients improved (85).

VI. Concluding Remarks

The mechanisms whereby allergen-specific Th2 cells, producing IL-4 and IL-13, are selected in atopic patients remains to be determined, and a better understanding of these selection processes will result in the improved ways to therapeutically intervene in atopic diseases. Immunotherapy using intact native allergen with the aim to desensitize atopic patients has proved highly effective in certain allergic disorders, and it has been demonstrated in these cases that the success of immunotherapy was accompanied by a shift in the balance of cytokine production by $CD4^+$ T cells, by reducing the production of IL-4, or increasing the production of IFN-γ. There is now a body of evidence to suggest that in vitro stimulation of $CD4^+$ T cells with short, immunogenic peptides or with peptides in which certain amino acid residues have been substituted will lead to qualitative changes in their responses to specific antigen. In this respect, the use of modified allergen-derived peptides has been found to result in a decrease of the ratio of Th2 to Th1 cytokine production, and this information will be applied to generate peptide analogues that modulate the function and cytokine production of allergen-specific T cells in vivo.

Extensive diversity of antigen and MHC class II restriction specificity of allergen recognition has been observed in the T-cell repertoires of different patients. To avoid the problem of MHC restriction, mixtures of overlapping or modified peptides representing the major T-cell activation-inducing epitopes on the corresponding native allergen could be administered. The advantage of this approach is that it does not require precise MHC class II typing of the patients. In addition, it has been demonstrated in vivo that an immunodominant peptide of Der p 1 may downregulate an established response to the intact molecule, suggesting that mapping of all T-cell activation epitopes is not required. Because the short, allergen-derived peptides do not react with IgE and, therefore, are not able to induce anaphylactic reactions, they seem to be well suited to induced altered T-cell responses in vivo. However, in spite of the promising results to modulate T-cell responses in vitro, the success of specific immunotherapy using allergen-derived peptides will depend on the results of clinical trials.

References

1. Creticos P. Immunotherapy with allergens. JAMA 1992; 286:2834–2839.
2. Varney V, Gaga M, Frew A, Aber V, Kay A, Durham S. Usefulness of immunotherapy in patients with severe summer hay fever uncontrolled by antiallergic drugs. Br Med J 1991; 302:265–269.
3. Bousquet J, Becker W, Hejjaoui A, Chanal I, Lebel B. Dhivert H, Michel F. Differences in clinical and immunological reactivity of patients allergic to grass pollens and to multiple pollen species. II. Efficacy of a double-blind, placebo controlled, specific immunotherapy with standardized extracts. J Allergy Clin Immunol 1991; 88:43–53.
4. van Metre TJ, Marsh D, Adkinson NJ, Kagey-Sobotka A, Khattignavong A, Norman PJ, Rosenberg G. Immunotherapy for cat asthma. J Allergy Clin Immunol 1988; 82:1055–1068.

5. Müller U, Fricker M, Akdis A, Carballido J, Blaser K. Successful immunotherapy with T-cell epitopes of bee venom phospholipase A_2 (PLA) in patients with bee venom (BV) allergy (abstr). J Allergy Clin Immunol 1995; 97:426.
6. Creticos P, Spector S, Busse W, Israel E, Nicodemus C, Jones N, Olson T, Gefter M, Lichtenstein L, Norman P. Evaluation of T cell epitope defined peptides from cat allergen by bronchial challenge (abstr). Allergy Clin Immunol 1995; 95:390.
7. Norman P, Ohman J, Long A, Creticos P, Shaked Z, Wood R, Eggleston P, Jones N, Nicodemus C. Early clinical experience with T cell reactive peptides from cat allergen *Fel d* 1 (abstr). Allergy Clin Immunol 93:231.
8. Norman P, Ohman J, Long A, Creticos P, Gefter M, Shaked Z, Wood R, Eggleston P, Lichtenstein L, Jones N, Nicodemus C. Follow on study of the first clinical trial with T cell defined peptides from cat allergen Fel d 1 (abstr). Allergy Clin Immunol 95:259.
9. Pene J, Rousset F, Brière F, Chrétien I, Bonnefoy J-Y, Spits H, Yokota T, Arai N, Arai K-I, Banchereau J. IgE production by normal human lymphocytes is induced by interleukin 4 and suppressed by interferons γ and α and prostaglandin E_2. Proc Natl Acad Sci USA 1988; 85:6880–6884.
10. Carballido J, Schols D, Namikawa R, Zurawski S, Zurawski G, Roncarolo M, de Vries J. IL-4 induces human B cell maturation and IgE synthesis in SCID-hu mice. Inhibition of ongoing IgE production by in vivo treatment with an IL-4/IL-13 receptor antagonist. J Immunol 1995; 155:4162–4170.
11. Punnonen J, Aversa A, Cocks B, McKenzie A, Menon S, Zurawski G, De Waal Malefyt R, De Vries J. Interleukin 13 induces interleukin 4 independent IgG4 and IgE synthesis and CD23 expression by human B cells. Proc Natl Acad Sci USA 1993; 90:3730–3734.
12. Walker C, Virchow CJ, Bruijnzeel P, Blaser K. T cell subsets and their soluble products regulate eosinophilia in allergic and nonallergic asthma. J Immunol 1991; 146:1829–1835.
13. Stern M, Meagher L, Savill J, Haslett C. Apoptosis of human eosinophils: programmed cell death in the eosinophil leads to phagocytosis by macrophages and is modulated by IL-5. J Immunol 1992; 148:3543–3549.
14. Swain S. Role of BCGFII in the differentiation to antibody secretion of normal and tumor B cells. J Immunol 1985; 134:3934–3943.
15. MacLean J, Ownby R, Luster A. T cell-dependent regulation of eotaxin in antigen-induced pulmonary eosinophilia. J Exp Med 1996; 184:1461–1469.
16. Valitutti S, Müller S, Cella M, Padovan E, Lanzavecchia A. Serial triggering of many T-cell receptors by a few peptide-MHC complexes. Nature 1995; 375:148–151.
17. Weiss A. The role of proteins tyrosine kinases in and protein tyrosine phosphatases in T cell antigen receptor signal transduction. Ann Rev Immunol 1994; 12:555–592.
18. Mosmann T, Coffman R. TH1 and TH2 cells: different patterns of lymphokine secretion lead to different functional properties. Annu Rev Immunol 1989; 7:145–173.
19. Romagnani S. Lymphokine production by human T cells in disease states. Annu Rev Immunol 1994; 12:227–257.
20. Palliard X, De Waal Malefijt R, Yssel H, Blanchard D, Chretien I, Abrams J, De Vries J, Spits H. Simultaneous production of IL-2, IL-4 and IFN-γ by human $CD4^+$ and $CD8^+$ T cell clones. J Immunol 1988; 141:849–855.
21. Parronchi P, Macchia D, Piccinni M, Biswas P, Simonelli C, Maggi E, Ricci M, Ansari A, Romagnani S. Allergen- and bacterial antigen-specific T cell clones established from atopic donors show a different profile of cytokine production. Proc Natl Acad Sci USA 1991; 88:4538–4542.
22. Racioppi L, Ronchese F, Matis L, Germain R. Peptide-major histocompatibility complex class II complexes with mixed agonist/antagonist properties provide evidence for ligand-related differences in T cell receptor dependent signalling. J Exp Med 1993; 177:1047–1060.
23. Pfeiffer C, Stein J, Southwood S, Ketelaar H, Sette A, Bottomly K. Altered peptide ligands can control CD4 T lymphocyte differentiation in vivo. J Exp Med 1995; 181:1569–1574.
24. Gajewski T, Pinnas M, Wong T, Fitch F. Murine Th1 and Th2 clones proliferate optimally in response to distinct antigen presenting cell populations. J Immunol 1991; 24:1750–1758.

25. Schmitz J, Assenmacher M, Radbruch A. Regulation of T helper cell cytokine expression: functional dichotomy of antigen-presenting cells. Eur J Immunol 1993; 23:191–199.
26. Freeman G, Boussiotis V, Anumanthan A, Bernstein G, Ke X, Rennert P, Gray G, Gribben J, Nadler L. B7-1 and B7-2 do not deliver identical costimulatory signals, since B7-2 but not B7-1 preferentially costimulates the initial production of IL-4. Immunity 1995; 2:523–532.
27. Kuchroo V, Das M, Brown J, Ranger A, Zamvil S, Sobel R, Weiner H, Nabavi N, Glimcher L. B7-1 and B7-2 costimulatory molecules activate differentially the Thl/Th2 developmental pathways: application to autoimmune disease therapy. Cell 1995; 80:707–718.
28. Levine B, Ueda Y, Craighead N, Huang M, June C. CD28 ligands CD80 (B7-2) and CD86 (B7-1) induce long-term autocrine growth of $CD4^+$ T cells and induce similar patterns of cytokine secretion in vitro. Int Immunol 1995; 7:891–904.
29. Hsieh C, Heimberger A, Gold J, O'Garra A, Murphy K. Differential regulation of T helper phenotype development by interleukins 4 and 10 in an $\alpha\beta$ T cell–receptor transgenic system. Proc Natl Acad Sci USA 1992; 89:6065–6069.
30. Seder R, Paul W, Davis M, Fazekas-de-St-Groth B. The presence of interkeukin 4 during in vitro priming determines the lymphokine producing potential by $CD4^+$ cells. J Exp Med 1992; 176:1091–1098.
31. Kelso A. Thl and Th2 subsets: paradigms lost? Immunol Today 1995; 16:374–379.
32. Del Prete G, Tiri A, Mariotti S, Parronchi P, Pinchera A, Romagnani S, Ricci M. Thyroiditis as a model of organ specific autoimmune disease. Clin Exp Rheumatol 1989; 7:41–45.
33. Maggi E, Biswas P, Del Prete G, Parronchi P, Macchia D, Simonelli C, Emmi L, De Carli M, Tiri A, Ricci M, Romagnani S. Accumulation of Th2 like helper T cells in the conjuctiva of patients with vernal conjunctivitis. J Immunol 1991; 146:1169–1174.
34. Van der Heijden F, Wierenga E, Bos J, Kapsenberg M. High frequency of IL-4 producing $CD4^+$ allergen specific T lymphocytes in atopic dermatitis lesional skin. J Invest Dermatol 1991; 97:389–394.
35. Hamid Q, Azzawi M, Ying S, Moqbel R, Wardlaw A, Corrigan C, Bradley B, Durham S, Collins J, Jeffery P, Quint D, Kay A. Expression of mRNA for interleukin-5 in mucosal bronchial biopsies from asthma. J Clin Invest 1991; 87:1541–1546.
36. Robinson D, Hamid Q, Ying S, Tsicopoulos A, Barkans J, Bentley A, Corrigan C, Durham S, Kay A. Predominant Th2-like bronchoalveolar T-lymphocyte population in atopic asthma. N Engl J Med 1992; 326:295–304.
37. Kay A, Ying S, Varney V, Gaga M, Durham S, Moqbel R, Wardlaw A, Hamid Q. Messenger RNA expression of the cytokine gene cluster, interleukin-3 (IL-3, IL-4, IL-5 and granolocyte/macrophage colony-stimulating factor) in allergen-induced late-phase cutaneous reactions in atopic subjects. J Exp Med 1991; 173:775–778.
38. Wierenga E, Snoek M, Bos J, Jansen H, Kapsenberg M. Comparison of diversity and function of house dust mite specific T lymphocyte clones from atopic and non-atopic donors. Eur J Immunol 1990; 20:1519–1526.
39. O'Hehir R, Garman R, Greenstein J, Lamb J. The specificity and regulation of T-cell responses to allergens. Annu Rev Immunol 1991; 9:67–95.
40. Gilbert K, Hoang K, Wiegle W. Thl and Th2 clones differ in their response to a tolerogenic signal. J Immunol 1990; 144:2063–2071.
41. Williams M, Shea C, Lichtman A, Abbas A. Antigen receptor-mediated anergy in resting T lymphocytes and T cell clones: correlation with lymphokine secretion patterns. J Immunol 1992; 149:1221–1226.
42. Garside P, Steel M, Worthey E, Satoskar A, Alexander J, Bluethman H, Liew F. Mowat A. T helper 2 cells are subject to high dose oral tolerance and are not essential for its induction. J Immunol 1995; 154:5649–5655.
43. Sloan-Lancaster J, Evavold B, Allen P. Th2 cell clonal anergy as a consequence of partial activation. J Exp Med 1994; 180:1195–1205.
44. Yssel H, Fasler S, Lamb J, de Vries J. Induction of non-responsiveness in human allergen-specific type 2 helper T cells. Curr Opin Immunol 1994; 6:847–852.

45. Manetti R, Parronchi P, Giudizi M-G, Piccinni M-P, Maggi E, Trinchier G, Romagnani S. Natural killer cell stimulatory factor (IL-12) induces T helper type 1 (Th1)-specific immune responses and inhibits the development of IL-4 producing T cells. J Exp Med 1993; 177:1199–1204.
46. Lack G, Renz H, Saloga J, Bradley K, Loader J, Leung D, Larsen G, Gelfald E. Nebulized but not paranteral IFN-γ decreases IgE production and normalizes airway function in a murine model of allergen sensitization. J Immunol 1994; 152:2546–2554.
47. Maggi E, Paronchi P, Manetti R, Simonelli C, Piccinni M-P, Santoni Rugiu F, de Carli M, Ricci M, Romagnini S. Reciprocal effects of IFN-γ and IL-4 on the in vitro development of human Th 1 and Th 2 clones. J Immunol 1992; 148:2142–2147.
48. Secrist H, Chelen C, Wen Y, Marshall J, Umetsu D. Allergen immunotherapy decreases interleukin 4 production in $CD4^+$ T cells from allergic individuals. J Exp Med 1993; 177:2123–2130.
49. Varney V, Hamid Q, Gaga M, Ying S, Jacobsen M, Frew A, Kay A, Durham S. Influence of grass pollen immunotherapy on cellular infiltration and cytokine mRNA expression during allergen induced late phase cutaneous responses. J Clin Invest 1993; 92:644–651.
50. Akdis CA, Akdis M, Blesken T, Wymann D, Alkan SS, Müller U, Blaser K. Epitope-specific T cell tolerance to phospholipase A_2 in bee venom immunotherapy and recovery by IL-2 and IL-15 in vitro. J Clin Invest 1996; 98:1676–1683.
51. Jutel M, Pichler W, Skrbic D, Urwyler A, Dahinden C, Muller U. Bee venom immunotherapy results in decrease of IL-4 and IL-5 and an increase in IFN-gamma secretion in specific allergen stimulated cultures. J Immunol 1995; 154:4187–4194.
52. Lamb J, Skidmore B, Green N, Chiller J, Feldman M. Induction of tolerance in influenza virus immune T lymphocyte clones with synthetic peptides of influenza haemagglutinin. J Exp Med 1983; 157:1434–1447.
53. Essery G, Feldmann M, Lamb J. Interleukin-2 can prevent and reverse antigen-induced unresponsiveness in cloned T lymphocytes. Immunology 1988; 64:413–417.
54. O'Hehir R, Yssel H, Verma S, De Vries J, Spits H, Lamb J. Clonal analysis of differential lymphokine secretion in peptide and superantigen induced anergy. Int Immunol 1991; 3:819–826.
55. O'Hehir R, Aguilar B, Schmidt T, Gollnick S, Lamb J. Functional inactivation of *Dermatophagoides* spp. (house dust mite) reactive human T cell clones. Clin Exp Allergy 1991; 21:209–215.
56. Faith A, Akdis A, Blaser K. Anergy induction in cloned phospholipase A_2-specific T cells of Th2 functional phenotype (abstr). J Allergy Clin Immunol 1996; 97:426.
57. Jenkins MK, Schwartz RH. Antigen presentation by chemically modified splenocytes induces antigen-specific T cell unresponsiveness in vitro and in vivo. J Exp Med 1987; 165:302–319.
58. O'Hehir R, Lamb J. Induction of specific clonal anergy in human T lymphocytes by *Staphylococcus aureus* enterotoxin. Proc Natl Acad Sci USA 1990; 87:8884–8888.
59. Gajewski T, Qian D, Fields P, Fitch F. Anergic T lymphocytes have altered inositol phosphate, calcium, and tyrosine kinase signalling pathways. Proc Natl Acad Sci USA 1994; 91:38–42.
60. Harding FA, McArthur JG, Gross JA, Raulet DH, Allison JP. CD28-mediated signalling co-stimulates murine T cells and prevents induction of anergy in T cell clones. Nature 1992; 356:607–609.
61. Kang SM, Beverly B, Tran AC, Brorson K, Schwartz RH, Lenardo MJ. Transactivation by AP-1 is a molecular target of T cell clonal anergy. Science 1992; 257:1134–1138.
62. Schall T, O'Hehir R, Goeddel D, Lamb J. Uncoupling of cytokine mRNA expression and protein secretion during the induction phase T cell anergy. J Immunol 1992; 146:381–387.
63. Evavold B, Allen P. Separation of IL-4 production from Th cell proliferation by an altered T cell receptor ligand. Science 1991; 252:1308–1310.
64. Sloan-Lancaster J, Evavold B, Allen P. Induction of T cell anergy by altered T cell receptor ligand on live antigen presenting cells. Nature 1993; 363:156–159.

65. Sloan-Lancaster J, Shaw AS, Rothbard JB, Allen PM. Partial T cell signaling: altered phospho-ζ and lack of zap70 recruitment in APL-induced T cell anergy. Cell 1994; 79:913–922.
66. Kersh GJ, Allen PM. Essential flexibility in the T cell recognition of antigen. Nature 1996; 380:495–498.
67. Schwartz RH. A cell culture model for T lymphocyte clonal anergy. Science 1990; 2481:1349–1356.
68. Ikagawa S, Matsushita S, Chen Y, Ishikawa T, Nishimura Y. Single amino acid substitutions on a Japanese cedar pollen allergen (Cry j 1)-derived peptide induced alterations in human T cell responses and T cell receptor antagonism. J Allergy Clin Immunol 1996; 97:53–64.
69. Tsitoura D, Verhoef A, Gelder C, O'Hehir R, Lamb J. Altered T cell ligands derived from a major house dust mite allergen enhance IFN-γ but not IL-4 production by human $CD4^+$ T cells. J Immunol 1996; 157:2160–2165.
70. Miller S, Karpus W. The immunopathogenesis and regulation of T cell-mediated demyelinating diseases. Immunol Today 1994; 15:356–361.
71. Chen Y, Kuchroo V, Inobe J, Hafler D, Weiner H. Regulatory T cell clones induced by oral tolerance: suppression of autoimmune encephalomyelitis. Science 1994; 265:1237–1240.
72. Sobel RA, Greer JA, Kuchroo VK. Autoimmune responses to myelin proteolipid protein. Neurochem Res 1994; 19:915–920.
73. Nicholson L, Greer J, Sobel R, Lees M, Kuchroo V. An altered peptide ligand mediates immune deviation and prevents autoimmune encephalomyelitis. Immunity 1995; 3:397–405.
74. Duffort O, Carreira J, Nitti G, Polo F, Lombardero M. Studies on the biochemical structure of the major cat allergen *Felis deomsticus* I. Mol Immunol 1991; 28:301–309.
75. Morgenstern J, Griffith I, Brauer A, Rogers B, Bond J, Chapman M, Kuo M. Amino acid sequence of Fel d 1, the major allergen of the domestic cat: protein sequence analysis and cDNA cloning. Proc Natl Acad Sci USA 1991; 88:9690–9694.
76. Briner T, Kuo M, Keating K, Rogers B, Greenstein J. Peripheral T cell tolerance induced in naive and primed mice by subcutaneous injection of peptides from the major cat allergen Fel d 1. Proc Natl Acad Sci USA 1993; 90:7608–7612.
77. Rogers B, Bond J, Craig S, Nault A, Segal D, Morgenstern J, Chen M-S, Bizinkauskas C, Counsell C, Lussier A, Luby T, Kuo M-C, Briner T, Garman R. Potential therapeutic recombinant proteins comprised of peptides containing recombined T cell epitopes. Mol Immunol 1994; 31:955–966.
78. Mowat A. The regulation of immune responses to dietary antigens. Immunol Today 1987; 8:93–98.
79. Holt P, McMenamin C. Defense against allergic sensitisation in the healthy lung: the role of inhalation tolerance. Clin Exp Allergy 1989; 19:255–262.
80. Weiner H, Friedman A, Miller A, Khoury S, Al-Sabbagh A, Santos L, Sayegh M, Nussenblatt R, Trentham D, Hafler D. Oral tolerance: immunologic mechanisms and treatment of animal and human organ-specific autoimmune diseases by oral administration of autoantigens. Annu Rev Immunol 1994; 12:809–837.
81. Hoyne G, Callow M, Kuo M-C, Thomas W. Inhibition of T cell responses by feeding peptides containing major and cryptic epitopes. Studies with the Der p 1 allergen. Immunology 1994; 83:190–195.
82. Hoyne G, O'Hehir R, Wraith D, Thomas W, Lamb J. Inhibition of T cell and antibody responses to the major house dust mite allergen in naive and sensitised mice. J Exp Med 1993; 178:1783–1788.
83. Counsell C, Greenstein J, Garman R, Ohman J. Cat immunotherapy decreases T cell reactivity and skin test reactivity to Fel d 1, the major allergen of cat allergy (abstr). J Allergy Clin Immunol 1994; 93:231.

84. Norman P, Pasatiempo A, Creticos P, Nicodemus C, Jones N, Lichtenstein L, Gefter M. Intravenous administration of a potential T cell tolerogenic peptide to cat sensitive patients (abstr). J Allergy Clin Immunol 1996; 97:386.
85. Simons F, Imada M, Li Y, Watson W, HayGlass K. Fel d 1 peptides: effect on skin tests and cytokine synthesis in cat-allergic human subject. Int Immunol 1996; 8:1937–1945.

18

Potential of Recombinant Allergens as Immunotherapeutic Agents for Allergy and Asthma

SHYAM S. MOHAPATRA

University of South Florida College of Medicine
and VA Hospital
Tampa, Florida

I. Why Immunotherapy?

About one-quarter of the population suffers from an allergic disorder, including allergic rhinitis and asthma. The prevalence of allergies and asthma has increased throughout the world, including the United States, over the past two decades (1,2). Rates of death from asthma have increased from 0.8:100,000 in 1977–1978 to 2.0:100,000 in 1991, and these rates have increased in almost all age groups in the United States (3). Asthma is the most common cause of admission of children to the hospital and the most common chronic illness causing absence from school and work in North America. The total costs of illness related to asthma in 1990 were 6.2 billion dollars, a 53% increase in direct medical expenditures and a 23% increase in indirect costs since 1985 (4). The total estimated costs for the year 1995 for the treatment of allergic diseases, such as allergic rhinitis, asthma, chronic sinusitis, otitis media, and nasal polyps is about 10 billion dollars (5). Epidemiological studies have shown that there has been a global increase in the incidence of asthma; however, the reason for this is unclear. It has been suggested that this increase may be due to increasing air pollution. Besides allergen exposure, the main environmental factors investigated include tobacco smoke and increasing pollution from the release of NO, SO_2, ozone, and occupational exposure to certain chemicals (6,7). In a study of asthma patterns in an urban environment, asthma-related mortality in the Philadelphia area went from 0.68:100,000 persons in 1968 to 2.41:100,000 in 1991, despite an apparent decrease in the concentrations of major air pollutants during that time (8,9).

The rise in the prevalence of asthma may be attributed to several factors: (1) genetic predisposition (i.e., allergy and asthma are hereditary diseases, thus, about a quarter of the population remain genetically susceptible to develop allergy and asthma; 10); (2) life styles of the population that include living with pets and housing with high levels of allergens, and most importantly, (3) the therapeutic approaches against allergy and asthma, which have continually shifted in favor of pharmacotherapy, with a concomitant decrease in the use of allergen injection immunotherapy (IT; 11). Since the mid-1970s, inhaled β-adrenergic bronchodilator prescriptions have been issued at a markedly increasing rate. Corticosteroids are used in 15–20% of visits, but only recently has the inhaled route of administration become prominent. The overuse of anti-inflammatory therapy, including steroids, may be attributed to the increase in asthma prevalence, as well. A recent report indicated that glucocorticoids induce and support the proliferation of T-helper type-2 (Th2) cells (12), which have been implicated in the pathogenesis of asthma. The use of IT for allergy and asthma, as currently practiced using allergen extracts, has been controversial.

However, recently, progress has been made in the characterization of allergens by the application of genetic-engineering tools. This has led to the emergence of various novel immunotherapeutic approaches for allergy and asthma. This chapter will review the recent developments in the field of recombinant allergens, IT, and the potential of recombinant allergen-based therapeutic approaches.

II. Recombinant Allergens: The Nuts and Bolts

As reviewed previously, a diverse arsenal of rDNA and allied chemical synthesis technologies have been used for the molecular–immunological characterization of several allergens (13–15). With the advances in the field of molecular biology in general, new techniques are used for the isolation of clones of allergens, the characterization of isoallergens, and the identification of epitopes (13,14). The recent progress in different areas is summarized in the following.

A. Molecular Cloning, Sequencing, and Synthesis of Recombinant Allergens

The molecular cloning of allergens has led to the determination of the primary structure of numerous allergens. To date, most of the allergens have been cloned in the phage expression vectors. A list of allergens that have been molecularly cloned and sequenced using this strategy has recently been published (16). Thus, about 70 allergens have been characterized from diverse sources, such as mites, animals, molds, pollens (grasses, weeds, and trees), insects, and foods (for the list, see review). About five to ten new allergenic proteins are being added to this list every year. In addition to the cloned allergens, new allergens continue to be reported and presumably the cloning of these allergens is currently in progress. Most of these allergens have been cloned in plasmid vectors for high-level expression in *Escherichia coli*, which allows the synthesis of the allergenic protein, either (1) as a fusion protein (i.e., linked to β-galactosidase or glutathione *S*-transferase, or (2) as a recombinant allergen by itself. Recently, both yeast and baculovirus expression systems have been employed for the synthesis of certain recombinant allergens. A major application of molecular biology technologies for allergen characterization has been the expression cloning of allergens to enable production of the recombinant proteins in virtually unlimited amounts for use in basic as well as clinical studies (17).

B. Delineation of B- and T-Cell Epitopes and Cross-Reactivity

Knowledge of the B- and T-cell epitopes is mandatory for the formulation of any therapeutic modality based on epitopes. Therefore, the determination of the complete repertoire of epitopes of diverse environmental aeroallergens remains one of the most arduous and formidable tasks. As reviewed elsewhere (13–15), the availability of structural information has prompted studies on the delineation of the B-cell and T-cell epitopes of several major allergens of mites, cats; and tree pollens, ragweed, and grasses, using both human and model animal systems. The rapid characterization of epitopes has been possible through the following techniques: First, by methods that allowed the production of overlapping peptides; these include the expression cloning of overlapping cDNAs, the synthesis of the corresponding peptides in *E. coli*, and site-directed mutagenesis in conjunction with the polymerase chain reaction (PCR), which allowed the synthesis of allergens and peptides with the desired amino acid substitution. Additionally, overlapping peptides can be chemically synthesized by automated methods or by manual methods such as using polypropylene pins. These methods have aided in the identification of the B- and T-cell epitopes of several allergens. Second, the availability of allergens and peptides facilitated the analysis of B-cell epitopes, including human IgE-binding epitopes. The T-cell epitopes of many allergens were also examined by T-cell proliferation assays using peripheral blood mononuclear cells (PBMC) or T-cell lines and clones. Studies now suggest that (1) the major allergens have several epitopes, (2) the B- and T-cell epitopes appear to overlap, and (3) the epitopes recognized by individuals differ. Furthermore, the knowledge of their primary structures, and of the epitopes, led to the elucidation of cross-reactivities among different allergens, because of obvious implications in therapy and diagnosis. Cross-reactivities have been studied both at the B- and T-cell level, not only among allergens belonging to the same aeroallergen source, but also among different aeroallergens. In principle, the same methods as outlined previously for the identification of B- and T-cell reactivities have been used for the delineation of cross-reactivities among allergens and epitopes. The conservation of immunodominant residues among various allergens and their epitopes appears to be a principal reason for the extensive cross-reactivities observed among the allergens.

The availability of cDNA-encoding allergens, recombinant allergens, and synthetic allergenic peptides makes it possible to devise new immunotherapeutic approaches based on these reagents. The potential use of these allergens is provided in the following section.

III. Rationale for Allergen Immunotherapy for Asthma

Until recently, asthma has been defined purely as a clinical disease, with a focus on physiological change. This is reflected in a recent definition of asthma by the National Asthma Education Program expert panel report from the National Institutes of Health which states that: "Asthma is a lung disease with the following characteristics: (i) airway obstruction that is reversible (but not completely so in some subjects) either spontaneously or with treatment; (ii) airway inflammation; (iii) airway hyperresponsiveness (AHR) to a variety of stimuli" (18). The focus on airway inflammation has been expanded and the panel developing the International Guidelines defined asthma as follows: "Asthma is a chronic inflammatory disorder of the airway in which many cells play a role, including mast cells and eosinophils. In susceptible individuals this inflammation causes symptoms which are usually associated with widespread but variable airflow obstruction that is often reversible either spontaneously or with treatment, and causes an associated increase in airway responsiveness to a variety of stimuli" (19).

It is commonly recognized that most children with asthma (60–80%) have associated allergies. It is less well recognized that many adults with asthma also have allergies. If an *allergy* is defined as a positive skin test to an inhaled allergen, then 80% of 6- to 34-year olds, 70% of 35- to 54-year olds, and 40% of those older than 55, are allergic (20). There is a strong relationship between asthma and the presence of IgE. Furthermore, there appears to be a direct relation between serum IgE and AHR(21). The presence of allergen-specific IgE to inhalant allergens represents a risk factor for acute asthma and for death from asthma (22). Moreover, a positive association between allergen exposure, and emergency room visits and hospitalization for asthma was demonstrated (23). Although asthma can develop in certain individuals in the absence of elevated allergen-induced IgE, the latter constitutes a major risk factor for asthma in children and in adults. For the purpose of this chapter, I shall confine my comments to asthma with an etiology in an allergic condition.

A. Immunoglobulin E and T Helper Cell Type-2 Responses in Asthma

A persistently elevated IgE response is the hallmark of an allergic disease. Both immunologically specific and nonspecific mechanisms appear to control the inflammatory responses in allergic disorders. Initial sensitization involves the recognition of an allergen by the T cells and the synthesis of IgE to the specific allergen(s), such as pollens, molds, or mites, which constitutes the hallmark of human allergic diseases (24). As shown in Figure 1, the pathogenesis of an allergic condition may be divided into three sequential steps: First, antigen-presenting cells (APCs), such as dendritic cells or B cells, ingest and breakdown the incoming allergen into its constituent peptidic fragments and then present these to T cells. The latter recognize the peptide by its receptor, T-cell receptor, (TCR). The TCR interacts with a peptide histocompatibility complex (MHC) type II (binary complex) on the APC. The formation of this trimolecular interaction is essential and provides the foundation for a specific immune response (25). Furthermore, the interaction of the B7-family of molecules on APC and of CD28 on T cells, generates a second antigen–nonspecific signal, which is required for the full activation of T cells. Second, the activation of T cells leads to the production of effector cytokines (26). Data from both humans and animal systems suggest a polarization of T helper (Th) cell responses in allergic diseases toward the Th2 type (26,27). Th2 cells produce cytokines such as interleukin (IL)-4, IL-5, and IL-10, as opposed to the Th1 type of cells that produce IL-2 and interferon (IFN)-γ. The ratio of the major IgE-switch factor IL-4, and its counterregulator IFN-γ, determines the level of IgE synthesis. Moreover, IL-4 and IFN-γ also mediate the differentiation of Th2 and Th1 subsets, respectively

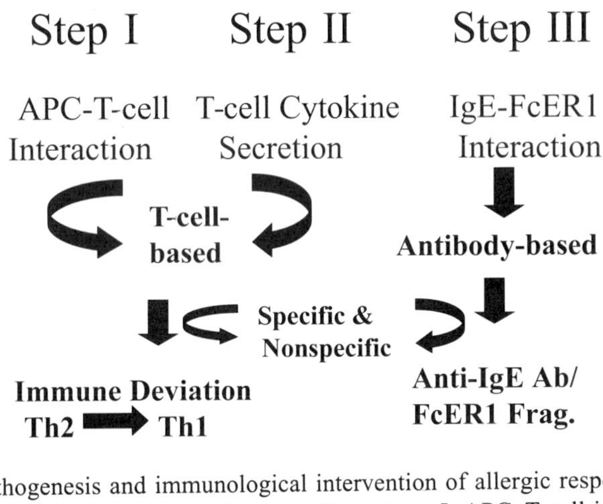

Figure 1 Pathogenesis and immunological intervention of allergic response. The initiation of an allergic immune response involves three steps: I. APC–T-cell interaction, II. T-cell activation and Th2-like cytokine (Il-4 and IL-13) secretion, and III. IgE antibody class switch and IgE receptor cross-bridging leading to mast cell degranulation. The experimental therapeutic approaches have been either at the T cell or at the antibody level. At the T-cell level efforts are focused on immune deviation, i.e., shifting T-cell response from a Th2-like to a Th1-like cytokine secretion. At the antibody level, the current efforts focus on developing therapies using humanized anti-IgE antibodies or fragments of the IgE receptor. The immune modulation may either be antigen-specific or nonspecific.

(26,28). In addition to IgE synthesis, airway inflammation and AHR are also controlled by activated $CD4^{+}T$ lymphocytes. Specifically, the Th2 cytokines IL-4 and IL-5 play pivotal roles in the pathogenesis of asthma and eosinophilia. Third, cytokines released by Th2 cells (e.g., IL-4 and IL-13) are involved in the class switch of antibodies and the production of IgE (26,27). IgE induces the stimulation of FcεR expression on mast cells and basophils. Additionally, IgE binds to the Fc receptors on the mast cells and basophils. Subsequent exposure of these cells to multivalent allergens results in the bridging of the cell-bound IgE and leads to the release of inflammatory mediators, including histamines (24). In allergic asthma, AHR may contribute to the exacerbation of asthma as a result of exposure to aeroallergens. Although IgE is produced by most individuals, it is the sustained production of allergen-specific IgE above a certain threshold level in conjunction with other inflammatory factors that is responsible for the clinical symptoms.

IV. Effectiveness of Immunotherapy

Immunotherapy has been a time-honored approach to the effective management of allergic rhinitis for years. The effectiveness of IT in treating asthma has been debated (30,34). However, a survey of the literature indicates that IT has been successfully used in selective asthmatic patients allergic to pollen, dust mites, or certain mold allergens, including *Alternaria*. IT appears to be of most use in those patients who are allergic to one, rather than many, allergens and whose asthma is not associated with other significant precipitating factors, such as chronic rhinosinusitis or aspirin sensitivity (30). In 1995, Abrahamson and associates conducted a metanalysis using a computerized bibliographic search, which revealed a total of 20 randomized, placebo-controlled, double-blind trials of allergen immunotherapy for asthma (33). This analysis indicated a combined odds of systematic improvements from immunotherapy with any allergen, including mite allergens. Another double-blind, placebo-controlled, multicenter trial using a purified extract of ragweed pollen in patients with asthma who were symptomatic during ragweed pollination, showed a small but significant increase in peak respiratory flow and a reduction in the use of asthma medications in the immunotherapy group (34).

V. Molecular and Cellular Mechanisms of Immunotherapy

Recent studies have recognized allergic inflammation as a major cause of asthma. The molecular and cellular mechanisms of IT and their effects on downregulating allergic inflammation are currently an area of intense investigation. Although some evidence supports the notion that IT leads to immune deviation from a Th2-like to a Th1-like response, other evidence favors the induction of total nonresponsiveness following IT (35–37). Given that multifarious changes occur as a result of IT, it is possible that more than one mechanism may be operational. In addition, specific

IT also plays a role in modulating immunological responses, including inflammatory mediator production (38–43). Specifically, several studies have reported the safety and effectiveness of IT on treatment of bronchial hyperreactivity (BHR) in both children (38,39) and adults (40,41). Such therapy not only induced a nonresponsive state in lymphocytes, but also reduced allergen-dependent production of eosinophil chemotactic factors in the mononuclear cells of asthmatics (42). Moreover, specific IT also reversed the secretion of endothelin-1, an endothelium-derived peptide, which is one of the most potent vasoconstrictors and bronchoconstrictors (43). These mechanistic studies support a role for IT in the future treatment of asthma.

Research endeavors, directed at suppressing allergic inflammation, continue on several fronts. Advances have been made in several areas; two are notable among these—the cytokine-based approach and approaches based on the blocking of IgE–FcεRI interaction—which may be combined with allergen–IT in the future for treating asthma.

VI. Allergen Immunotherapy for Asthma

A. At the Crossroads

Despite its proven effectiveness in selected patients with specific allergies, the use of IT for asthma continues to be debated. There are several drawbacks inherent with present IT. During its 85-year history, IT has been used essentially as described by Noon and other early investigators, which is cumbersome, expensive, and associated with the risk of fatal side effects (44). Most of the woes of IT stem from heterogeneous and often nonstandardized allergen extracts. In the early 1990s, IT came under severe criticism in several countries worldwide (45–47). In the light of the advances in various treatment modalities available for asthma, the question remains whether IT will continue to have a place in the treatment of allergy and asthma, and whether the existing IT can be and should be salvaged to make it more specific and more effective.

In view of the inconsistent and cumbersome nature of present allergen IT, and the recent proliferation of management strategies using anti-inflammatory drugs, the question arises of whether IT will continue to have a place in the treatment of allergy and asthma. It appears, however, that a significant proportion of allergic individuals may benefit from IT. A Swedish study of 7099 adult patients with asthma or rhinitis revealed that 44% of these were atopic (type I hypersensitivity). Interestingly, however, of these, 35% had remained monosensitized, whereas 24% had allergies against two aeroallergens (48). Furthermore, IT in individuals allergic to a limited number of allergens blocks sensitization to other related allergens and changes the natural course of the disease (49). These studies suggest that those individuals, who are sensitized to one or two major aeroallergens, may benefit from allergen-specific therapy. Preliminary preventive treatments with grass allergens resulted in the attenuation of BHR and lung function after 1 year of treatment (50).

Further progress has been made in the knowledge of the genetic predisposition factors of allergy and asthma, which may allow for the early prediction of susceptibility to these diseases. Together, these advances support the notion that immunologically specific therapeutic approaches for the prevention and management of allergic disorders are extremely important.

It has also been debated whether IT should be continued using allergen extracts or should be replaced, when feasible, with allergen-specific IT. The main drawback that limits the efficacy and use of current IT has been the lack of sufficient amounts of pure and standardized allergen extracts. To circumvent these limitations, several laboratories have recently employed rDNA techniques for the molecular characterization of the major allergens (13–15). Indeed, the last 5 years have seen spectacular advances in the field of allergen characterization, leading to the synthesis of several recombinant allergens in virtually unlimited quantities. Despite these advances, however, available recombinant allergens have yet to be used for IT, for the obvious reason that these recombinant allergens have to undergo rigorous testing by the Food and Drug Administration (FDA) before their approval for such studies. The compelling arguments in favor of purified allergens or recombinant allergens include (1) the assumption that the major goal of IT is to reduce the threshold of allergen-specific IgE levels in plasma and that a reduction of IgE of up to 80% should be sufficient, which can be achieved using major allergens; (2) demonstrations in the 1970s that, although the allergen extracts comprised of multiple allergenic constituents, often only a few, ranging from one up to about three allergens, contribute to a major portion (up to 80–90%) of the antibodies against the corresponding extract, possibly because of the extensive cross-reactivity among allergens of taxonomically related organisms; (3) two studies from Johns Hopkins University showed that the crude ragweed and purified extract preparations were equally efficacious for IT (51,52); and (4) the immunodominance of certain antigens and epitopes has already been reported for immune responses against certain aeroallergens (53). The availability of recombinant allergens makes it reasonably valid to examine the use of these allergens to improve existing IT with allergen extracts.

VII. Immunotherapy Using Recombinant Allergens

The advent of recombinant allergens makes it possible to identify the unique protein(s) to which the individual is sensitized; hence, it may be visualized that future allergen-specific IT will be based on the use of selective allergens. The other advantages of recombinant allergens, instead of crude extracts, for IT include the use of tailored extracts based on the determination of the major allergens to which the patient is sensitized, the administration of allergens in adequate amounts, better and more effective dosage control, and the possibility to modify IgE-binding structures, thereby increasing the safety of IT. However, in humans, because of the purity of recombinant allergen preparations, their anaphylactogenic index may be extremely high, and even at very low doses, extreme care may be required when they are administered by allergy specialists. Moreover, enteric-coated (54) or liposome-packed (55) recombinant allergens may also be useful for IT. Furthermore, approaches involving allergoids produced by formaldehyde polymerization (56) using recombinant allergens, "r-allergoids," may be useful for IT. The problem with presently available polymerized extracts (56) is that they are based on crude extracts and are indefinable in terms of their molecular properties. Because several allergens are present in varying concentrations in the extracts, it is difficult to ascertain whether all molecules have been polymerized to the same degree. Often batch-to-batch variation is excessive, and an analysis of each individual allergen is impossible. It is envisaged that a major improvement in allergen-specific IT may be achieved by the use of chemically modified recombinant allergens, which should render these regimens essentially nonallergenic, while retaining their antigenicity. Also, the conjugation with *N*-formyl-methionyl-leucyl-phenylalanine may be useful (57). On the basis of these methods, it is reasonable to predict that, in contrast with conventional IT, the use of relatively fewer injections of these modified recombinant allergens would lead to a safer and more efficacious therapy. The potential approaches are schematically illustrated in Figure 2.

A recently suggested modification to IT approaches involved the use of the allergen peptide–IT approach, which involves the parenteral injection of the defined

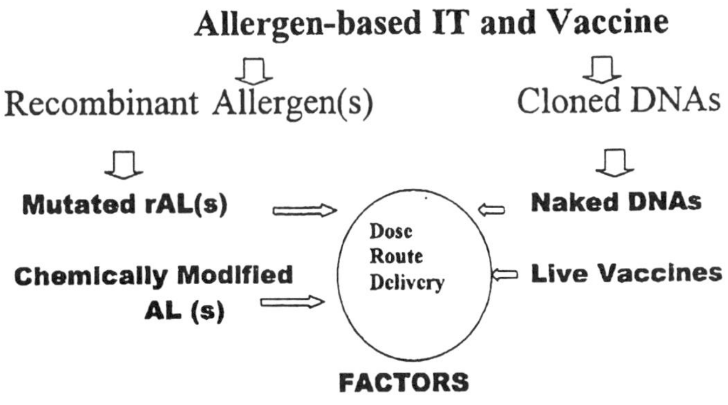

Figure 2 Scheme for allergen-based immunotherapy and vaccination in the future. It is anticipated that both recombinant allergen- and DNA-based strategies may be used. Further, recombinant allergen-based therapies may use allergens (ALs) mutated for IgE-binding epitopes, or recombinant allergens chemically modified with formaldehyde, or recombinant allergen(s) with a cytokine or another Th1-inducing adjuvant. The allergen DNAs may be used in the form of a cocktail of plasmids encoding requisite allergens, or in the form of live vaccines in appropriate host organisms. Both of these strategies have to be optimized for the dosage, route, and the delivery of the therapeutic regimen.

T-cell peptide(s) of allergens to the allergic patient instead of a crude extract. Studies in an animal model (58) and preliminary clinical studies in humans (59) are promising. However, theoretically, the T-cell peptide therapy appears to have several limitations (14,15): (1) major allergens appear to possess multiple T-cell epitopes; (2) allergic patients differ in their recognition of the peptide epitopes of diverse allergens; (3) sometimes B- and T-cell epitopes reside on the same peptide, this in conjunction with the multiplicity of epitopes raises the possibility that some of the therapeutic peptides may induce adverse systemic reactions as was seen with *Fel d* I peptides; and (4) a specific T-cell epitope may also provide help for Th2 cells, possibly by a costimulatory signal generated by unrelated events, such as a virus infection, and may actually boost the IgE production.

VIII. Immunotherapy with Recombinant Allergens and Cytokines

Demonstrations that Th2 cells play a critical role in the pathogenicity of allergic disorders, and that IFN-γ and IL-4, respectively, promote the polarization to Th1 and Th2 cell responses, have led to possibilities for developing methods for shifting allergen-specific responses from a Th2-type to a Th1-type for the suppression of allergic responses (60). Conceivably, allergen-induced changes in cytokine profiles could be a potential strategy in the treatment of allergic diseases. One approach has emerged from our in vitro studies, in collaboration with S. Romagnani's laboratory, using human peripheral blood lymphocytes. The culture of T-cell lines from atopic individuals with a recombinant allergen of the *Poa p* IX family of allergens and IFN-γ led to the development of "protective" (i.e., Th1 cells) instead of the "pathogenic" (i.e., Th2 cells) (61). Thus, the administration of recombinant allergens in conjunction with IFNs may aid in diverting allergen-specific immune responses from default Th2 to the Th1 type. This study suggested that a recombinant allergen(s), either singly, or in the form of a cocktail, can be used in conjunction with appropriate Th1-inducing adjuvants. For tailored IT, individuals allergic to certain antigens will be treated against the same allergens, the peripheral blood mononuclear cells of these patients may be cultured in vitro with the corresponding antigen and IFN and may be injected back into the same individual to boost a Th1-like response to these antigens, followed by an allergen booster. Alternatively, IT may be carried out with liposomes containing mixtures of recombinant allergens and a selected adjuvant.

IX. Development of Vaccines Against Allergies and Asthma

The concept of developing preventive vaccines against allergies is relatively new (60,62,63), although preseasonal IT against allergies has been practiced since the inception of IT. In view of the recent finding that the immune systems of neonates and adult mice are similar in terms of their ability to develop immune deviation, and the advances in genetics of atopy and asthma that may enable the prediction of susceptibility to these disorders, the preventive approach to IT using recombinant allergens holds great promise and needs to be further investigated.

The immune deviation hypothesis is based on the recent observations that: (1) most sensitization to allergens occurs between 6 months and 2 years of age (64); (2) long-lasting memory can be induced by initially deviating this response to a Th1-like response in genetically predisposed individuals, as has been shown for autoimmune disorders (65–67); (3) respiratory virus infections have no effect on established T-cell memory (68); and (4) early IT in children with sensitization to a few allergens at the initial phase decreases further progression to the chronic phase. These observations suggest that allergen exposure in childhood is an extremely important trigger for chronic allergies and asthma later in life; therefore, prophylactic vaccination aimed at inducing immune deviation can be an effective method of preventing or curing asthma (60,69). The foregoing studies suggest that an immunoprophylactic vaccine may be based on recombinant allergens with or without adjuvants, or on allergen–DNA molecules encoding allergens.

A. Vaccines Using Recombinant Allergen

We examined the possibility of redirecting specific antibody repertoires de novo in mice by immunization with a recombinant allergen–antigen chimeric (RAAC) protein and the Freund's Complete Adjuvant. These results indicated that the RAAC protein, when immunized with Freund's Complete Adjuvant (killed mycobacteria), promoted IgG2a production and suppressed antigen-specific IgE production; typical of a Th1-like response (70). On the other hand, dextran sulfate, similar to that of alum, induced elevated IgE production and a Th2-like response. This study, together with the demonstration that the T-cell profile of allergic individuals could be changed from a Th2 to a Th1 type in vitro after incubation with a recombinant allergen and IFN-α, suggest the potential to induce immune deviation in vivo with recombinant allergen(s) in conjunction with adjuvant factors (e.g., those inducing IFN-α) is very high.

The immune deviation potential of a recombinant allergen in the absence of adjuvants, as used in conventional IT in humans, was also examined (71). Thus, subcutaneous or intravenous treatment of mice with a recombinant allergen before their immunization with the recombinant allergen in alum, led to the induction of about 90% suppression of antibody responses to the recombinant allergen. This induction of IgE-specific tolerance was persistent insofar that IgE titers remained undetectable or low up to 81 days, despite three booster injections with the allergen (72). To establish the mechanism underlying this IgE suppression, we analyzed the cytokine patterns in mice undergoing vaccination with a recombinant allergen. The results indicated reductions in IL-2 and IL-4, and an in increase in IFN-γ production in mice vaccinated with the soluble recombinant allergen, compared with untreated controls, suggesting a preferential expansion of the Th1-like response. Moreover, treatment with the recombinant allergen followed by immunization with a Kentucky bluegrass (KBG) extract led to an increase in KBG-specific IgG1 and IgG2a titers and in IFN-γ production. Similarly, the treatment of mice already sensitized with recombinant allergen led to significant increases in IgG2a titers and in IFN-γ production. These results are similar to the cytokine changes reported in humans undergoing IT. The demonstration that a vaccination with a single major recombinant allergen of KBG pollen can modulate KBG-specific antibodies and cytokine production, resulting in immune deviation, suggests that vaccines comprising of a cocktail of recombinant allergens can be at least equally potent or even more potent than those using crude extracts.

B. Allergen–DNA Vaccines

The availability of cDNAs encoding allergens has prompted investigations to address the possibility of using the allergen genes and cDNAs for the suppression of allergen-specific IgE responses. The development of live vaccines, using allergen genes expressed in appropriate hosts, was suggested previously (73). In a recent study, immunization (by the oral route) of *Salmonella typhimurium*, expressing an allergen–cDNA also led to the development of IgG2a responses instead of default IgE responses (74); however, in only 10% of the immunized mice could an IgG2a response specific for Bet v 1 be detected. Two recent developments are noteworthy in this context. Recently, it was reported that immunization (i.d.) with an allergen–cDNA cloned in a plasmid vehicle resulted in the development of allergen-specific IgG2a and Th1-like responses and no detectable IgE response in mice (75,76) and in rats. Furthermore, the Th1 responses induced by gene immunization dominated an ongoing protein-induced Th2 response in an antigen-specific manner. This suggests that immunization by DNA encoding for an allergen may provide a novel type of vaccine for allergic diseases, including asthma. Although these are early studies, such approaches hold promise in terms of generating new techniques for the future development of vaccines.

X. Concluding Remarks

There has been tremendous progress in the molecular characterization of allergens; however, the application of this knowledge in clinical arenas is in its infancy. The synthesis of certain major recombinant allergens by fermentation and allied technologies is anticipated to expedite the use of these allergens for therapeutic studies. Cloned cDNAs and allergens may be used to modify existing IT or to develop new immunotherapeutic procedures based on rational immunological principles. When we take into account the complexity of allergic asthma, it is naive to expect that one form of allergen-specific IT would be effective in the treatment of all asthma. Clearly, for certain forms of allergenic asthma (e.g., grass), the protocol may involve a battery of recombinant allergens or allergen cDNAs. Furthermore, the knowledge of epitopes of allergens has advanced to a point at which allergen peptides of ragweeds and cats are in clinical trials. It is anticipated that these new forms of therapy may cure allergic asthma, or at least be effective enough that they will reduce the usage of the anti-inflammatory drugs, which appear to effectively control the symptoms, but may be harmful in the long term. As we continue to learn in greater detail the mechanisms involved in the establishment of allergic conditions, we may be able to devise additional and more effective protocols for management. Furthermore, as the genes for asthma are identified, it may be possible to accurately predict by genetic fingerprinting who is at risk to develop asthma and then, vaccinate these children with appropriate allergen vaccines based on their allergen exposure profiles.

References

1. Manfreda J, Becker AB, Wang PZ, Roos LL, Anthonisen NR. Trends in physician-diagnosed asthma prevalence in Manitoba between 1980 and 1990. 1993; Chest 103:151–157.
2. Reijula K, et al. Asthma prevalence and mortality in Finland. Chest 1996; 110:58.
3. Sly RM. Changing asthma mortality. Ann Allergy 1994; 73:259–268.
4. Weiss KB, Gergen PJ, Hodgson TA. An economic evaluation of asthma in the United States. N Engl J Med 1992; 326:862–866.
5. Baraniuk JN, Meltzer EO, Spector SL. Impact of allergic rhinitis and related airway disorders. J Respir Dis 1996; 17:S11.
6. Bascom R, Bromberg PA, Costa DA, et al. Health effects of outdoor air pollution. Am J Respir Crit Care Med 1996; 153:3.
7. Bascom R, Bromberg PA, Costa DA, et al. Health effects of outdoor air pollution. Am J Respir Crit Care Med 1996; 153:477.
8. Lang DM, Polansky M. Patterns of asthma mortality in Philadelphia from 1969 to 1991. N Engl J Med 1994; 331:1542.
9. Buist AS, Vollmer WM. Preventing deaths from asthma. N Engl J Med 1994; 331:1584.
10. Sandford A, Weir T, Pare P. The genetics of asthma. Am J Respir Crit Care Med 1996; 153:1749.
11. Terr AI, Bloch DA. Trends in asthma therapy in the United States: 1965–1992. Ann Allergy Asthma Immunol 1996; 76:273.
12. Ramirez F, Fowell DJ, Puklavec M, Simmonds S, Mason D. Glucocorticoids promote a Th2 cytokine response by CD4 T cells in vitro. J Immunol 1996; 156:2406–2412.
13. Mohapatra SS, Cao Y, Ni H, Salo D. In pursuit of the "holy grail": Recombinant allergens as catalysts for the allergen specific immunotherapy. Allergy 1995; 50(25 suppl):37–44.
14. Mohapatra SS, Mohapatra S. Application of molecular biology to diagnosis and treatment of allergic disease. Immunol Allergy Clin North Am 19–; 16:591–611.
15. Valenta R, Kraft D. Recombinant allergens for diagnosis and therapy of allergic disorders. Curr Opin Immunol 1995; 7:751–756.
16. Mohapatra SS. Modulation of allergen-specific antibody responses by T cell based peptide vaccines: principles and potential. Clin Rev Allergy 1994; 12:3.
17. Larson JN, Casals AB, From AB, et al. Characterization of recombinant *Bet v*1, the major allergen of *Betula verrucosa* (white birch) produced by fed batched fermentation. Int Arch Allergol Immunol 1993; 102:249.
18. Guidelines for the Diagnosis and Management of Asthma. National Asthma Education Program Expert Panel Report. US Department of Health and Human Services, NIH publication. 1991; 91–3042.
19. International Consensus Report on Diagnosis and Management of Asthma. US Department of Health and Human Services, NIH publication. 1992; 92–3091.

20. Burrows B, Martinez FD, Halonen M, et al. Association of asthma with serum IgE levels and skin test reactivity to allergens. N Engl J Med 1989; 320:271–277.
21. Sears MR, Burrows B, Flannery EM, et al. Relationship between airway hyperresponsiveness and serum IgE in children with asthma and in apparently normal children. N Engl J Med 1991; 325:1067–1071.
22. O'Hollaren MP, Yuninger JW, Offord KP, Somers MJ, O'Connell EJ, Ballard DJ, Sachs MI. Exposure to an aeroallergen as a possible precipitating factor in respiratory arrest in young patients with asthma. N Engl J Med 1991; 324:359.
23. Nelson RP, DiNicolo R, Fernandez-Caldas E, et al. Allergen specific IgE levels and mite allergen exposure in children with acute asthma first seen in an emergency department and in nonasthmatic control subjects. J Allergy Clin Immunol 1996; 98:258.
24. Bochner BS, Undem BJ, Lichtenstein LM. Immunological aspects of allergic asthma. Annu Rev Immunol 1994; 12:295.
25. Buss S, Sette A, Colon S, Miles C, Grey HM. The reaction between major histocompatibility complex (MHC) restriction and the capacity of Ia to bind immunogenic peptides. Science 1987; 235:1353-1358.
26. Finkleman FD, Holmes J, Katona IM, Urban JF Jr, Beckmann MP, Park LS, Schooley KA, Coffman RL, Mossmann TR, Paul WE. Lympokine control of in vivo immunoglobulin isotype selection. Annu Rev Immunol 1990; 8:303.
27. Romagnani S. Lymphokine production by human T cells in disease states. Annu Rev Immunol 1994; 12:227–257.
28. Van Oosterhout AJM, Nijkamp M. Lymphocytes and bronchial hyperresponsiveness. Life Sci 1990; 46:1255–1264.
29. Corrigan CJ, Kay AB. CD4 T lymphocyte activation in acute severe asthma. Relationship to disease severity and atopic status. Am Rev Respir Dis 1990; 141:970–977.
30. Bousquet J, Michel FB. Specific immunotherapy in asthma. Allergy Proc 1994; 15:329–333.
31. Norman PS, Barnes PJ. Is there a role for immunotherapy in the treatment of asthma? Am J Respir Crit Care Med 1996; 154:1225.
32. Adkinson NF, et al. A controlled trial of immunotherapy for asthma in allergic children. N Engl J Med 1997; 336:324.
33. Abrahamson MJ, Puy RM, Weiner JM. Is allergen immunotherapy effective in asthma? A meta-analysis of randomized controlled trials. Am J Respir Crit Care Med 1995; 151:969.
34. Creticos PS, Reed CE, Norman PS, et al. Ragweed therapy in adult asthma. N Engl J Med 1996; 334:501.
35. Secrist H, Chelen CJ, Wen Y, Marshall JD, Umetsu DT. Allergen immunotherapy decreases interleukin 4 production in $CD4^+$ T cells from allergic individuals. J Exp Med 1993; 178:2123–2130.
36. Jutel M, Pichler WJ, Skrbic D, et al. Bee venom immunotherapy results in decrease of Il-4 and IL-5 and increase of IFN-γ secretion in specific allergen-stimulated T cell cultures. J Immunol 1995; 154:4187–4194.
37. Varney VA, Hamid QA, Gaga M, Ying S, Jacobson M, Frew AJ, Kay AB, Durham S. Influence of grass pollen immunotherapy on cellular infiltration and cytokine mRNA expression during allergen-induced late-phase cutaneous responses. J Clin Invest 1993; 92:644–651.
38. Chen WY, Yu J, Wang YU. The effect of immunotherapy on bronchial hyperresponsiveness in asthmatic children. Asian Pac J Allergy Immunol 1994; 12:15–20.
39. Ferreira N, Trinidade JC. Specific immunotherapy 3 years follow-up in asthmatic children. Allergol Immunopathol 1993; 21:185–192.
40. Garcia-Ortega P, Merelo A, Marrugat J, Richart C. Decrease of skin and bronchial sensitization following short intensive scheduled immunotherapy in mite allergic asthma. Chest 1993; 103:183–187.
41. Armentia A, Martin-Santos JM, Quintero A, Fernandez, A, Barber D, Alonson E, Gil I. Baker's asthma: prevalence and evaluation of immunotherapy with a wheat flour extract. Ann Allergy 1990; 65:265–272.

42. Nagata M, Shibasaki M, Sakamoto Y, Fukuda T, Makino S, Yamamoto K, Dohi Y. Specific immunotherapy reduces the antigen-dependent production of eosinophil chemotactic activity from mononuclear cells in patients with atopic asthma. J Allergy Clin Immunol 1994; 94:160–166.
43. Chen WY, Yu J, Wang JY. Decreased production of endothlin-1 in asthmatic children after immunotherapy. J Asthma 1994; 32:29–35.
44. Lockey RF, Benedict LM, Turkeltaub PC, et al. Fatality from immunotherapy (IT) and skin testing (ST). J Allergy Clin Immunol 1987; 79:660.
45. Kay AB. Allergen injection immunotherapy (hyposensitization) on trial. Clin Exp Allergy 1989; 19:591.
46. Position paper on Allergen Immunotherapy Clin Exp Allergy 1993; 23:1–44.
47. CMS update: Desensitizing vaccines Br Med J 1986; 293:948.
48. Eriksson NE, Holmen A. In: Abstracts 5th International Congress on Aerobiology, Bangalore, 1994.
49. Des Roches A, Paradis L, Knanin J, Hejjaoui A, Dhibert H, Michel FB, Bousquet J. Specific immunotherapy prevents the onset of new sensitizations in monosensitized children. J Allergy Clin Immunol 1995; 95:309.
50. Jacobson L, Dreborg S, Moller C, et al. Immunotherapy as preventive allergy treatment (PAT). J Allergy Clin Immunol 1996; 97:232.
51. Norman PS, Winkenwerder WL, Lichtenstein LM. Immunotherapy of hay fever with ragweed antigen E: comparisons with whole pollen extract and placebos. J Allergy 1968; 42:93–108.
52. Lichtenstein LM, Norman PS, Winkenwerder WL. A single year of immunotherapy for ragweed hay fever: immunologic and clinical studies. Ann Intern Med 1971; 75:663–671.
53. Michael JG, Litwin A, Haserat V, et al. Modulation of the immune response to ragweed allergens by peptidic fragments. Clin Exp Allergy 1996; 20:669.
54. Wheeler AW, Henderson DC, Youlten LJ, et al. Immunogenecity in guinea pigs and tolerance in grass pollen-sensitive volunteers of enteric coated grass pollen allergens. Int Arch Allergy Appl Immunol 1987; 84:69.
55. Arora N, Fangal SV. Efficacy of liposome entrapped allergen in downregulation of IgE response in mice. Clin Exp Allergy 1992; 22:35.
56. Maasch HJ, Marsh DG. Standardized extracts of modified allergens—allergoids. Clin Rev Allergy 1987; 5:89.
57. Wheeler AW, Whittall N, Cook RM, et al. T cell reactivity of conjugates of *N*-formyl-methyl-leucyl-phenylalanine and rye grass pollen allergens. Int Arch Allergy Appl Immunol 1987; 84:69.
58. Briner TJ, Kuo M-C, Keating KM, Rogers BL, Greenstein JL. Peripheral T cell tolerance induced in naive and primed mice by subcutaneous injection of peptides from the major cat allergen, *Fel d* 1. Proc Natl Acad Sci USA 1993; 90:7608.
59. Norman PS. Therapeutic potential of peptides in allergic disease. Ann Allergy 1993; 71:330–333.
60. Mohapatra SS. An integrated approach to immune deviation and the prevention of allergies and asthma. Allergy Clin Immunol Int 1996; 8:164–168.
61. Parronchi P, Mohapatra S, Sampognaro S, et al. Effects of interferon on cytokine profile, T cell receptor repertoire and peptide reactivity of human allergen specific T cells. Eur J Immunol 1996; 26:697–703.
62. Holt P. Is immunization against allergic sensitization a realistic prospect for the future? Allergy Clin Immunol Int 1996; 8:169–171.
63. Holt PG. Immunoprophylaxis of atopy: light at the end of the tunnel? Immunol Today 1994; 15:484–489.
64. Borres MP, Einarsson R, Bjorksten B. Serum levels of interleukin-4, soluble CD23 and IFN gamma in relation to the developoment of allergic disease during the first 18 months of life. Clin Exp Allergy 1995; 25:543–548.
65. Golding B, Zaitseva M, Golding H. The potential for recruiting immune responses toward type 1 or type 2 T cell help. Am J Trop Med Hyg 1994; 50(supp):33–40.

66. Racke MK, Bonomo A, Scott DE, Cannella B, Levine A, Raine CS, Shevach EM, Rocken M. Cytokine-induced immune deviation as a therapy for inflammatory autoimmune disease. J Exp Med 1994; 180:1961–1966.
67. Finkelman FD. Relationships among antigen presentation, cytokines, immune deviation and autoimmune disease. J Exp Med 1995; 182:279–282.
68. Tripp RA, Hou S, McMickle A, Houston J, Doherty PC. Recruitment and proliferation of $CD8^+$ T cells in respiratory virus infections. J Immunol 1995; 154:6013–6021.
69. Holt PG. A potential vaccine strategy for asthma and allied atopic diseases. Lancet 1994; 344:956.
70. Zhang L, Mohapatra SS. Antigen- and isotype-specific immune responses to a recombinant antigen–allergen chimeric (RAAC) protein. J Immunol 1993; 151:791.
71. Cao Y, Luo Z, Yang M, Mohapatra SS. Vaccination with a multi-epitopic recombinant allergen (MERA) vaccine induces specific immune deviation via T cell anergy. Immunology 1997; 90:46.
72. Cao Y. Dissertation, University of Manitoba, 1996.
73. Mohapatra SS. Diagnosis and therapy of IgE mediated allergies with recombinant allergens. *Poa p* IX as a model. In: Debelic M, ed. Advances in Treatment of Allergic Diseases, Uppsala: Pharmacia Allergy Research Foundation, 1992: 4–15.
74. Vrtala S, Grote M, Ferreira F, et al. Humoral immune responses to recombinant tree pollen allergens (*Bet* 1 and *Bet* 2) in mice: construction of a live oral allergy vaccine. Int Arch Allergy Immunol 1995; 107:290.
75. Raz E, Tighe H, Sato Y, Swine S, Spiegelberg H, Caron D. Preferential induction of a Th1 immune response and inhibition of specific IgE antibody formation by plasmid DNA immunization. Proc Natl Acad Sci USA 1996; 93:5141.
76. Hsu C-H, Chua K-Y, Tao M-H, Lai Y-L, Wu H-D, Huang S-K, Hsieh K-H. Immunoprophylaxis of allergen-induced immunoglobulin E synthesis and airway hyperresponsiveness in vivo by genetic immunization. Nature Med 1996; 2:540.
77. Chen WY, Yu J, Wang JY. The effect of immunotherapy on bronchial hyperresponsiveness in asthmatic children. Asian Pac J Allergy Immunol 1994; 12:15–20.

19

Molecular Characterization of Allergens, Their B-Cell Epitopes and Allergen-Specific Antibodies for Allergy Prevention and Treatment

RUDOLF VALENTA, SUSANNE VRTALA, TANJA BALL, SYLVIA LAFFER, PETRA EIBENSTEINER, PETER STEINBERGER, SABINE FLICKER, SABINE FISCHER, IRENE MITTERMANN, SUSANNE SPITZAUER, and DIETRICH KRAFT

University of Vienna
Vienna General Hospital
Vienna, Austria

I. Introduction

Type I allergic diseases represent a health threat of increasing importance in industrialized countries (1). After cross-linking with effector cell-bound IgE antibodies, innocuous environmental allergens can immediately induce a cascade of allergic reactions comprising allergic rhinitis, conjunctivitis, dermatitis, asthma, and even anaphylactic shock (2). Although our knowledge of the genetics of atopy and the regulation of IgE synthesis has tremendously increased, scientific efforts focused on a general downregulation of IgE synthesis have not been successful, and in view of an eventual protective role of IgE (e.g., cancer or defense against parasitic infections) are questionable (3,4).

Since the introduction of molecular biological techniques into the field of allergen characterization, the knowledge on the nature of allergens has tremendously increased in the recent past (5). Unexpectedly, it turned out that because of their sequence and the immunological and structural similarities of relevant allergens, a possibly limited panel of allergens can be defined for diagnosis and possibly treatment of type I allergies (Table 1; 6). Recombinant allergens were produced in heterologous host systems, and the immunological equivalence of many recombinant allergens with their corresponding natural allergens as well as the homologous al-

Table 1 Steps on the Way to Defining Relevant Allergens for Specific Therapy of Type I Allergy

Molecular and structural characterization of the relevant allergens
Production and in vitro evaluation of relevant recombinant allergens for diagnosis of type I allergy
Establishment of suitable animal models for type I allergy
Mapping of the IgE- and IgG-binding sites of relevant allergens using recombinant DNA technology and competing antibodies
Production of allergen-specific antibodies and recombinant antibody fragments using the combinatorial library approach
In vivo evaluation of the biological activity of recombinant allergens, allergen derivatives, and antibodies
Development of concepts for specific active and passive therapy of type I allergy

lergens present in other species could be demonstrated (7–13). For plant allergies a few recombinant allergens have permitted successful in vitro and in vivo diagnosis of type I allergy (14–19) and allowed establishment of specific animal models for type I allergy (20,21). Now that a defined panel of model allergens can be defined for tree, grass pollen, and weed allergies, as well as for mite, cat, dog, and fungal allergies, studies on the interaction of these proteins with the human immune system has become possible (5,22). The molecular and structural analysis of the allergen–antibody interactions, as well as those of the allergen–cell interaction, should now permit us to elaborate preventive and therapeutic strategies for type I allergy that are focused on the interaction of the immune system with defined allergens.

II. Requirements for Specific Therapy of Type I Allergy Using Recombinant Allergens and Epitopes

Recent advances in the field of allergen characterization have indicated that, because of the structural similarities of the relevant allergens, only a limited panel of allergens can be produced for allergen-specific diagnosis and treatment of type I allergies. To pursue this concept, it is necessary to define those recombinant allergens that harbor relevant B-cell epitopes as well as T-cell epitopes for improved and component-based diagnosis and therapy. A rich panel of recombinant tree, grass, and weed allergens is already available that permits a precise and component-based in vitro and in vivo diagnosis of allergy against plant products (22). The IgE- and IgG-binding sites of the relevant allergens are currently being studied and attempts are planned to superimpose them on the three-dimensional structures of the corresponding allergens. The knowledge of IgE-binding sites should enable us to engineer recombinant allergen fragments (IgE-binding haptens) that can bind IgE of one specificity, but cannot cross-link effector cells. The nonanaphylactic IgE-binding haptens should be useful tools for passive therapy of type I allergy, by saturating effector cell-bound IgE molecules in the effector organs without inducing degranulation, or for active immunotherapy to induce blocking IgG against IgE epitopes. The nonanaphylactic potential of the IgE-binding haptens can be evaluated by histamine release assays and by skin-prick testing. For certain allergens for which no continuous IgE-binding sites can be defined (e.g., the major birch pollen allergen, Bet v 1 disruption of the allergens tertiary structure may lead to nonanaphylactic fragments containing the relevant T-cell epitopes.

By using the combinatorial library approach, it will be possible to generate a panel of human and mouse monoclonal antibodies (MAbs), against the most relevant plant allergens, which can be produced as recombinant Fab fragments in *Escherichia coli*, or as complete antibodies in transfected hybridoma cells. The recombinant allergen-specific antibodies and antibody fragments (Fabs) can be used to measure the allergen content in the environment as well as in plant-derived food to allow prevention of allergen exposure of high-risk persons (i.e., those from atopic risk families). This might be achieved by systematic monitoring of allergen content in plant-derived food as well as by selecting hypoallergenic cultivars for breeding. Recombinant antibodies and Fabs that block IgE binding to the corresponding allergens will be evaluated for their therapeutic potential using histamine release assays and skin-prick testing.

III. Model: Allergen-Specific and Patient-Tailored Therapy

As indicated in Figure 1 (22), we would suggest the selection of allergens according to the individual patient's IgE-binding pattern (i.e., allergen profile) for specific therapy of type I allergy. According to our own experimental experience, the qualitative pattern of IgE recognition in allergic patients seems to be subject to little variation, although the titers against certain components may vary, depending on natural exposure and booster mechanisms. Therefore, it is our strong contention that a component-based therapy, designed according to the patient's needs (i.e., including only those components against which significant levels of IgE are produced), may be superior to treatment with crude allergen mixtures that, in addition to the allergens, contain proteins, carbohydrates, nucleic acids, and other substances against which a patient is not sensitive. In fact, we have experimental evidence indicating that it is possible that patients treated with raw extracts can become sensitized against components for which they were not originally sensitized. Cross-reactivity studies indicate that, at least in the field of plant allergies, a few marker allergens that carry most of the IgE epitopes of related allergens from other species can be defined for specific therapy (22,23–25). Future strategies for specific therapy for allergy that are based on the analyses of allergen–IgE interactions are outlined in the following.

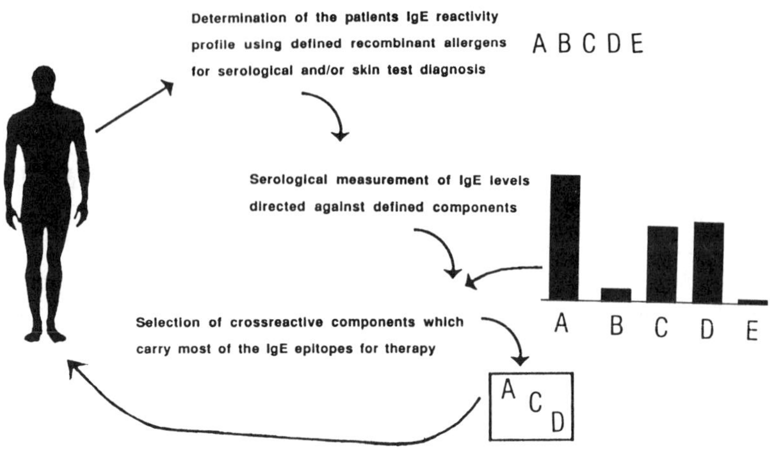

Figure 1 Component-based diagnosis and patient-tailored therapy based on recombinant allergens. The use of recombinant allergens will permit establishment of the patient's IgE-reactivity profile (allergogram). Those components against which high levels of specific IgEs are produced will be selected for specific immunotherapy.

IV. Immunoglobulin E–Binding Haptens for Passive Therapy: Saturation of Effector Cell–Bound IgE

The cross-linking of effector cell (i.e., mast cells or basophils)–bound IgE with specificity for at least two different epitopes is required to trigger release of biological mediators (histamine and leukotriens). The precise knowledge about IgE-binding sites, therefore, is crucial to dissect the allergic effector response. In a recent study we have identified an immunodominant IgE hapten of the major timothy grass pollen allergen, Phl p 1, which binds IgE, but does not induce effector cell activation (26). Therefore, it appears feasible to determine the IgE- and IgG-binding sites of relevant major allergens by gene fragmentation and superimposition on the three-dimensional structures of the allergens, as described for birch pollen profilin in a recent study (27). The dissection of allergens into IgE-binding haptens will provide reagents that are unable to trigger effector cell activation because they lack binding sites for additional IgE. As potential therapeutic application, the local saturation of effector cells is envisaged, such that subsequent exposure with complete allergens will fail to induce release of mediators and inflammation (Fig. 2).

V. Immunoglobulin E–Binding Haptens for the Induction of Blocking Antibodies by Active Immunotherapy

In addition to passive-blocking therapy, nonanaphylactic IgE-binding haptens should be considered for active immunotherapy to induce blocking IgG against the IgE-

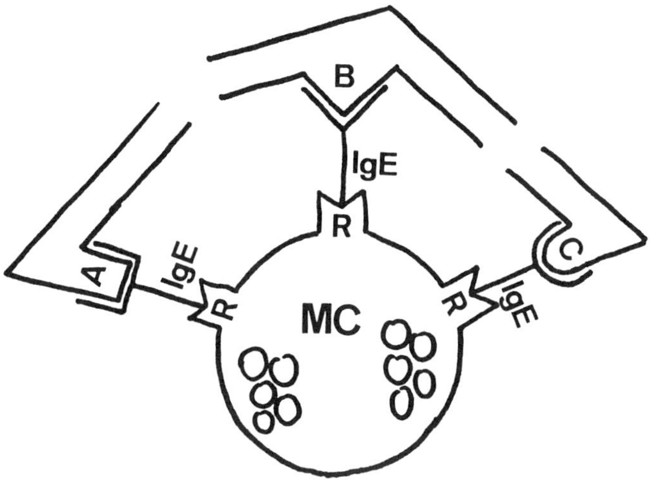

Figure 2 The allergen-induced release of biological mediators as possible target for specific therapy. IgE-binding haptens for saturation of surface-bound IgE without cell activation. Allergic effector cells (e.g., mast cells: MC) bind through high-affinity Fcε receptors (R), immunoglobulin E (IgE), with specificity for different allergen epitopes (A, B, C). IgE-binding haptens of allergens that contain only single epitopes (A, B, C) will bind to effector cells without induction of mediator release.

binding sites. The advantage of using IgE-binding haptens would be that higher doses of the fragments can be injected, thereby stimulating preferentially IgG synthesis. On the other hand, appropriate presentation as cyclic peptides, map peptides, or conjugates must be considered to maintain the immunogenicity of the fragments.

VI. Nonanaphylactic Modifications and Derivatives of Major Allergens Produced by Recombinant DNA Technology for Active Immunotherapy

In contrast with most plant allergens studied so far, no relevant continuous IgE epitopes could be identified on Bet v 1, the major birch pollen allergen. Therefore, we studied the interaction of patients IgE and Bet v 1 by using human and mouse monoclonal IgG (28–30). To produce fragments of Bet v 1 that contain the relevant T-cell epitopes, but are not recognized by IgE, we took advantage of the fact that Bet v 1 harbors conformational epitopes, and disrupted the allergen's three-dimensional structure by expressing two T-cell epitope-containing fragments in *E. coli* (31). Figure 3 shows the purified recombinant Bet v 1 halves, which indeed lost their tertiary structure, as analyzed by circular dichroism (31). In contrast with the complete recombinant Bet v 1, which presented a high content of both β-sheet and α-helical structure, the Bet v 1 fragments displayed random-coil structure, were un-

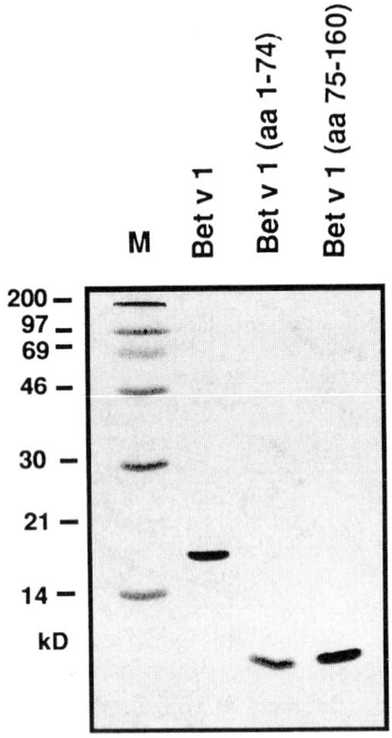

Figure 3 Purification of recombinant Bet v 1 fragments: 2 μg each of purified recombinant Bet v 1 and the two Bet v 1 fragments (amino acids 1–74 and 75–160) were analyzed by sodium dodecyl sulfate–polyacrylamide gel electophoresis (SDS–PAGE) and Coomassie Blue staining. A molecular weight marker was loaded in lane M.

able to bind IgE, and also failed to induce immediate-type skin reactions (Fig. 4). Therefore, both fragments may represent nonanaphylactic candidates for the active immunotherapy of Bet v 1-related allergies.

VII. Allergen-Specific Antibodies and Antibody Fragments for Passive Therapy in the Allergic Effector Organs

The occurrence of allergen-specific antibodies that do not belong to the "reaginic" class has been reported previously (32). Certain allergen-specific IgG molecules were able to inhibit anaphylactic reactions (33–35). Moreover, it was speculated that blocking antibodies, in particular those belonging to the IgG_4 subclass, might be induced by specific immunotherapy (36). Several studies failed, however, to correlate the presence or increase of allergen-specific IgG and IgG subclass levels with successful immunotherapy (37). Recently, it was proposed that specific immunotherapy might rather act by T-cell–mediated mechanisms that switch the cytokine patterns of allergen-specific T-cell clones toward a Th1 pattern (38). Although previous studies that investigated the role of allergen-specific IgG responses were hampered by the lack of well-defined allergen preparations, now, purified recombinant

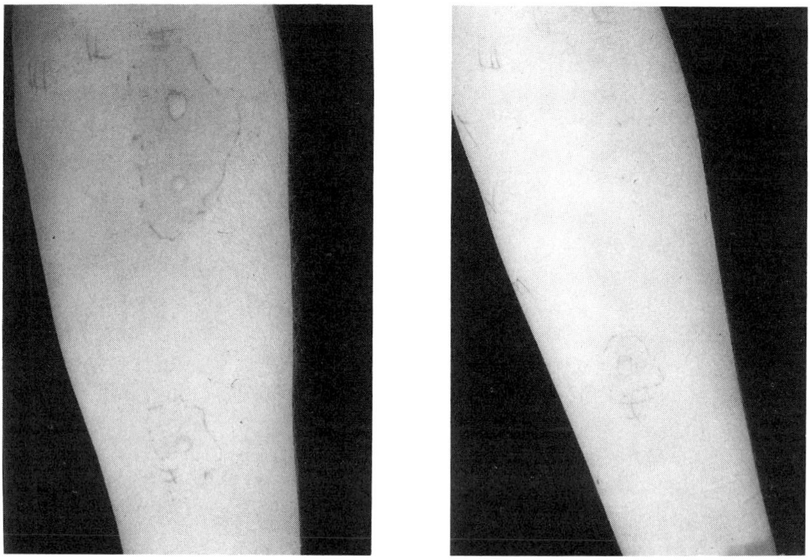

Figure 4 Comparison of the skin-prick activity of recombinant Bet v 1 and Bet v 1 fragments. Recombinant Bet v 1 amino acids (aa) 1–160 (A), and recombinant Bet v 1 fragments aa 1–74 (E) as well as Bet v 1 aa 75–160 (F) were tested in increasing concentrations (from bottom to top: 3:1 μg/mL, 2:10 μg/mL, 1:100 μg/mL) by skin-prick testing. H represents the histamine-positive control. The wheal area is surrounded by a closed line and the erythema by a broken line. The left photograph shows the forearm of a birch pollen allergic patient and the right photo shows the forearm of a nonallergic individual.

allergens have become available for measurements with defined components. Studies performed with recombinant Bet v 1 (17,18), the major birch pollen allergen, with recombinant timothy grass pollen allergens (Phl p 1, Phl p 2, Phl p 5) (16) and recombinant Der f 2 (39,40) showed that (1) sera from allergic and nonallergic persons contained allergen-specific IgG belonging to different subclasses; (2) levels of allergen-specific IgE are not correlated with certain IgG subclass responses; and (3) although certain allergic persons produce high levels of allergen-specific IgG, IgE responses against the same allergen can be measured, and skin sensitivity can be shown. On the other hand, evidence was provided that skin reactivity is reduced in individuals who possess high levels of allergen-specific IgG (41).

With epitopes prepared from major allergens by recombinant DNA technology it could be shown that IgE and IgG of allergic patients bind to the same and also different epitopes (40). This indicates that IgE and IgG responses in allergic persons may evolve preferentially in a nonsequential way and that IgE and IgG may possess different affinities or fine specificities for certain epitopes. Taken together it appears that the allergen-specific IgE and IgG response in allergic individuals is poorly synchronized for epitope recognition and, perhaps, affinity. These differences in epitope recognition of IgE and IgG were recently demonstrated for monoclonal human IgG specific for Bet v 1 (28). However, the demonstration that certain Bet v 1-specific IgGs were able to block IgE binding to Bet v 1 and to inhibit the Bet v 1-induced histamine release in several donors, clearly indicated that blocking IgG molecules are effective in reducing anaphylactic effects. Human and mouse monoclonal IgG specific for Bet v 1 strongly inhibited Bet v 1-induced histamine release (28,30; Fig. 5).

For the production of well-defined antibodies and antibody fragments, three approaches may be pursued. Animals can be immunized with allergens and monoclonal antibodies can be established using routine tissue culture techniques. Allergen-specific monoclonal antibodies can then be tested for whether they bind to the same epitopes as human IgE, or to different ones. Monoclonal antibodies that com-

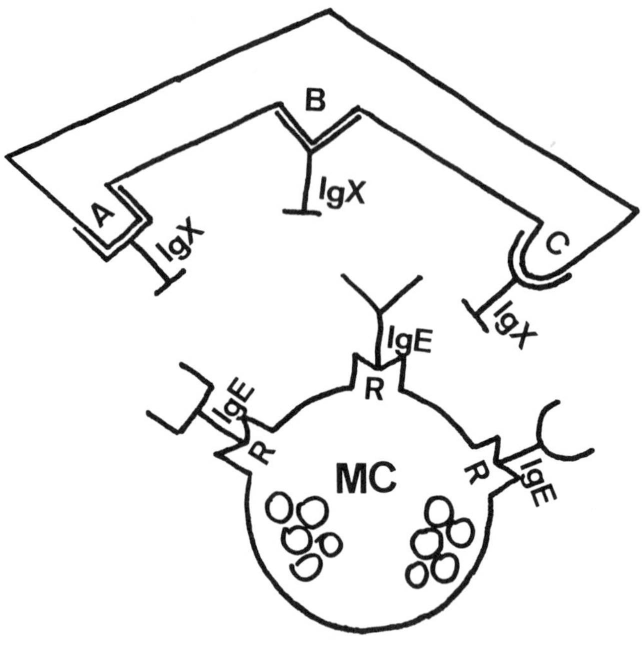

Figure 5 The allergen-induced release of biological mediators as possible target for specific therapy: Blocking antibodies (IgX: isotype different from IgE) bind to IgE epitopes (A, B, C) of the allergen before effector cell–bound IgEs are cross-linked. Allergic effector cells (e.g., mast cells: MC) that contain Fcε-receptor (R)-bound IgE will then not be activated. Blocking antibodies (IgX) may either be applied before allergen exposure to allergic effector organs (eyes, nose, or lung; passive therapy), or can be induced by active immunization using allergens or their B-cell epitopes.

pete with the IgE-binding may then be considered as potential tools for therapy of allergy (30). However, it may be necessary to modify such antibodies by humanization or to produce them as Fabs to reduce their immunogenicity.

Another method to obtain allergen-specific monoclonal antibodies would be to immortalize human B cells using the CD40 system or Epstein–Barr virus (EBV) transformation (28). With this approach IgGs, with specificity for Bet v 1, were obtained that blocked the patients' IgE binding to Bet v 1 and the Bet v 1-induced histamine release. Tissue culture methods are rather labor-intensive, require extensive culture work, and do not allow one to study the complete diversity of antibody responses. Therefore, it may be advantageous to use recombinant DNA technology for the production of recombinant allergen-specific antibody fragments. By using peripheral blood mononuclear cells (PBMCs) from allergic individuals, it is possible to generate cDNAs coding for heavy-chain fragments and light chains by reverse transcription and the polymerase chain reaction (PCR). Heavy-chain and light-chain cDNAs can then be combined and coexpressed in bacterial expression systems to represent the complete humoral diversity of the donor (42). Clones producing allergen-specific Fabs can then be selected using defined allergens by direct immunoscreening (42) or panning (43,44). In the last decade, considerable advances have been achieved in the expression of functional antibody fragments in *E. coli*. Basically, two systems allow the presentation of heavy- and light-chain variable regions on the surface of filamentous phage. The pCANTAB system (Pharmacia, Uppsala, Sweden) is designed to express single-chain variable fragments (sc-Fvs) of heavy and light chains that are artificially joined with a neutral linker (45). In contrast, the pCOMB system coexpresses heavy-chain fragments, including a portion of their constant region, together with the light chain (44). Both systems allow the efficient isolation of antigen-specific scFvs or Fabs by panning of the phage to a given antigen. The advantage of both systems over conventional cell culture techniques lies in the fact that both Fabs or scFvs can be produced in *E. coli*. The recombinant antibody fragments are small; hence, they are less immunogenic and can be subjected to in vitro manipulation (in vitro affinity maturation by mutagenesis or shuffling of heavy and light chains or the corresponding variable regions) (46). Because recombinant antibody fragments lack the major part or the complete constant region, they will not elicit effector reactions that are mediated by Fc receptors. With appropriate oligonucleotide primers, recombinant antibody fragments can be produced starting from cell lines, hybridomas of human or animal origin, or by constructing combinatorial libraries directly from a patient's B lymphocytes.

Recombinant human IgE Fabs with specificity for certain allergens might represent one of the ideal tools for studying the interaction of IgE with allergens, as well as for standardization and perhaps even therapy of type I allergy. Because of the extremely low levels of serum IgE, in particular of IgE with a given specificity, the low frequency of cells that secrete specific IgE, and the difficulties in immortalizing such cells, we have chosen the combinatorial library approach to obtain allergen-specific human IgE Fabs. A combinatorial IgE library was constructed from PBMCs obtained from a grass pollen allergic patient during the grass pollen season. By using the recombinant major timothy grass pollen allergens Phl p 1 and Phl p 5 for panning, phage-expressing specific IgE Fabs could be isolated (47). Recombinant human IgE Fabs cross-reacted with homologous allergens from other grass species, showed binding comparable with human IgE and, moreover, could be used to block IgE binding to the allergens. The recombinant IgE Fabs lack most parts of the constant region and, in particular, the Fcε receptor-binding site and, therefore, represent nonanaphylactic IgE fragments. Such IgE Fabs might be considered for local therapeutic application in allergic effector organs (nose, conjunctiva, and lung) to compete with the allergen–IgE interaction and to prevent allergen-induced allergic symptoms.

We suggest the use of recombinant allergen-specific Fabs for the investigation of allergen–IgE interactions, for standardization of allergen extracts, for environmental measurements of allergen concentrations, and for passive (blocking) therapy of type I allergy. In contrast with conventional monoclonal antibodies, which are used for standardization of allergen measurements, recombinant Fabs can be easily produced in bacterial expression systems and, thus, allow one to bypass tissue culture. Bacterially expressed Fabs can be modified by standard molecular biological techniques and engineered according to the desired application. To reduce the immunogenicity of an antibody fragment that is intended for passive therapy, it is possible to reduce the size of the molecule as well as to cut out immunogenic parts. Alternatively, mouse monoclonal antibodies can be humanized to reduce their immunogenicity. By in vitro maturation, using mutagenesis or CDR rearrangements, it is possible to improve the affinity of a recombinant Fab for its antigen. Such a manipulation might even increase the blocking activity of allergen-specific Fabs.

VIII. Summary

Almost 20% of the population in industrialized countries suffers from type I allergic symptoms (allergic rhinitis, conjunctivitis, dermatitis, asthma, and anaphylactic shock). These symptoms are due to cross-linking of effector cell-bound IgE by airborne, low molecular weight proteins from pollen, mites, or fungi, leading to release of anaphylactic mediators. Although the initial scientific efforts were mainly dedicated to investigating the regulation of IgE production, the recent advances in molecular allergen characterization indicate that, because of structural and immunological similarities among allergens, the number of proteins needed for diagnosis and specific therapy of type I allergy is less complex than anticipated. We have discussed the concept of producing relevant recombinant allergens, allergen epitopes, and derivatives with reduced anaphylactic potential, as well as allergen-specific antibodies for improved diagnosis and treatment of allergic diseases.

Acknowledgments

This study was supported by grant Y78GEN of the Austrian Science Foundation, by a grant of the Austrian Ministry of Research and Transports, and by Pharmacia–Upjohn AB, Uppsala, Sweden.

References

1. Miyamoto T. Increased prevalence of of pollen allergy in Japan. In: Godard P, Bousquet J, Michel FB, eds. Advances in Allergology and Clinical Immunology. Carnforth, UK: The Parthenon Publishing Group, 1992:343.
2. Segal DM, Taurog JD, Metzger H. Dimeric immunoglobulin E serves as a unit signal for mast cell degranulation. Proc Natl Acad Sci USA 1977; 41:457–461.
3. Steinberger P, Bohle B, di Padova F, Wrann M, Liehl E, Scheiner O, Kraft D, Valenta R. Allergen-specific IgE production of committed B cells from allergic patients in vitro. J Allergy Clin Immunol 1995; 96:209–218.
4. Dolecek C, Steinberger P, Susani M, Kraft D, Valenta R, Boltz-Nitulescu G. Effects of IL-4 and IL-13 on total and allergen specific IgE production by cultured PBMC from allergic patients determined with recombinant pollen allergens. Clin Exp Allergy 1995; 25:879–889.
5. Scheiner O, Kraft D. Basic and practical aspects of recombinant allergens. Allergy 1995; 50:384–391.
6. Valenta R, Kraft D. Recombinant allergens for diagnosis and therapy of allergic diseases. Curr Opin Immunol 1995; 7:751–756.
7. Breiteneder H, Pettenburger K, Bito A, Valenta R, Kraft D, Rumpold H, Scheiner O, Breitenbach M. The gene coding for the major birch pollen allergen, Bet v 1, is highly homologous to a pea diseases resistance response gene. EMBO J 1989; 8:1935–1938.
8. Valenta R, Duchêne M, Pettenburger K, Breitenbach M, Rumpold H, Kraft D, Scheiner O. Identification of profilin as a novel pollen allergen; IgE autoreactivity in sensitized individuals. Science 1991; 253:557–560.
9. Valenta R, Duchêne M, Ebner C, Valent P, Sillaber C, Deviller P, Feirrera F, Tejkl M, Edelmann H, Kraft D, Scheiner O. Profilins constitute a novel family of functional plant pan-allergens. J Exp Med 1992; 175:377–385.
10. Ebner C, Feirrera F, Szephalusi Z, Jilek A, Valenta R, Parronchi P, Maggi E, Romagnani S, Scheiner O, Kraft D. Identification of multiple T-cell epitopes on Bet v 1, the major birch pollen allergen using specific T cell clones and overlapping peptides. J Immunol 1993; 150:1047–1054.
11. Vrtala S, Sperr WR, Reimitzer I, vanRee R, Laffer S, Müller WD, Valent P, Lechner K, Rumpold H, Kraft D, Scheiner O, Valenta R. cDNA cloning of the major allergen from timothy grass (*Phleum pratense*) pollen: characterization of the recombinant Phl p 5 allergen. J Immunol 1993; 151:4773–4781.
12. Dolecek C, Vrtala S, Laffer S, Steinberger P, Kraft D, Scheiner O, Valenta R. Molecular characterization of Phl p 2, a major timothy grass (*Phleum pratense*) pollen allergen. FEBS Lett 1993; 335:299–304.
13. Laffer S, Valenta R, Vrtala S, Susani M, vanRee R, Kraft D, Scheiner O, Duchêne M. cDNA cloning of the major allergen Phl p 1 from timothy grass (*Phleum pratense*); recombinant Phl p 1 inhibits IgE binding to group I allergens from eight different grass species. J Allergy Clin Immunol 1994; 94:689–698.
14. Valenta R, Duchêne M, Vrtala S, Birkner T, Ebner C, Hirschwehr R, Breitenbach M, Rumpold H, Scheiner O, Kraft D. Recombinant allergens for immunoblot diagnosis of tree-pollen allergy. J Allergy Clin Immunol 1991; 88:889–894.
15. Valenta R, Vrtala S, Ebner C, Kraft D, Scheiner O. Diagnosis of grass pollen allergy with

recombinant timothy grass (*Phleum pratense*) pollen allergens. Int Arch Allergy Immunol 1992; 97:287–294.

16. Vrtala S, Susani M, Sperr WR, Valent P, Laffer S, Dolecek C, Kraft D, Valenta R. Immunologic characterization of purified recombinant timothy grass pollen (*Phleum pratense*) allergens (Phl p 1, Phl p 2, Phl p 5). J Allergy Clin Immunol 1996; 97:781–787.
17. Menz G, Dolecek C, Schönheit-Kenn U, Ferreira F, Moser M, Schneider T, Suter M, Boltz-Nitulescu G, Ebner C, Kraft D, Valenta R. Serological and skin-test diagnosis of birch pollen allergy with recombinant Bet v 1, the major birch pollen allergen. Clin Exp Allergy 1996; 26:50–60.
18. Pauli G, Oster P, Deviller P, Heiss S, Bessot J, Susani M, Ferreira F, Kraft D, Valenta R. Skin testing with recombinant allergens rBet v 1 and rBet v 2. Diagnostic value for birch pollen and associated allergies. J Allergy Clin Immunol 1996; 97:1100–1109.
19. Laffer S, Spitzauer S, Susani M, Pairleitner H, Schweiger C, Grönlund H, Menz G, Pauli G, Ishii T, Nolte H, Ebner C, Sehon AH, Kraft D, Eichler HG, Valenta R. Comparison of recombinant timothy grass pollen allergens with natural extract for diagnosis of grass pollen allergy in different populations. J Allergy Clin Immunol 1996; 98:652–658.
20. Ferreira FD, Mayer P, Sperr WR, Valent P, Seiberler S, Ebner C, Liehl E, Scheiner O, Kraft D, Valenta R. Induction of IgE antibodies with predefined specificity in rhesus monkeys with recombinant birch pollen allergens, Bet v 1 and Bet v 2. J Allergy Clin Immunol 1996; 97:95–103.
21. Vrtala S, Mayer P, Ferreira F, Susani M, Sehon AH, Kraft D, Valenta R. Induction of IgE antibodies in mice and rhesus monkeys with recombinant birch pollen allergens; different allergenicity of Bet v 1 and Bet v 2. J Allergy Clin Immunol 1996; 98:913–921.
22. Valenta R, Steinberger P, Duchêne M, Kraft D. Immunological and structural similarities among allergens: prerequisite for a specific and component-based therapy of allergy. Immunol Cell Biol 1996; 74:187–194.
23. Valenta R, Duchêne M, Vrtala S, Ball T, Ferreira F, Laffer S, Hirschwehr R, Ebner C, Sperr W, Valent P, Kraft D, Scheiner O. Recombinant allergens as candidates for immunotherapy of type I allergic diseases. In: Vaccines 93. Cold Spring Harbor, NY: Cold Spring Harbor Laboratory Press, 1993:37–42.
24. Valenta R, Kraft D. Type I allergic reactions to plant-derived food: a consequence of primary sensitization to pollen allergens. J Allergy Clin Immunol 1996; 97:893–895.
25. Laffer S, Duchêne M, Reimitzer I, Susani M, Mannhalter C, Kraft D, Valenta R. Common IgE-epitopes of a recombinant major timothy grass pollen allergen, Phl p 1, and natural group 1 grass pollen isoallergens. Mol Immunol 1996; 33:417–426.
26. Ball T, Vrtala S, Sperr WR, Valent P, Susani M, Kraft D, Valenta R. Isolation of an immunodominant IgE-hapten from an epitope expression cDNA library; dissection of the allergic effector reaction. J Biol Chem 1994; 269:28323–28328.
27. Fedorov AA, Ball T, Mahoney N, Valenta R, Almo S. Crystal structure and IgE-epitope mapping of birch pollen profilin: molecular basis for allergen cross-reactivity. Structure 1997; 5:33–45.
28. Visco V, Dolecek C, Denepoux S, Le Mao J, Guret C, Rousset F, Guinnepain MT, Kraft D, Valenta R, Weyer A, Banchereau J, Lebecque S. Human IgG monoclonal antibodies that modulate the binding of specific IgE to birch pollen Bet v 1. J Immunol 1996; 157:956–962.
29. Laffer S, Vangelista L, Steinberger P, Kraft D, Pastore A, Valenta R. Molecular characterization of Bip 1, a monoclonal antibody that modulates IgE binding to birch pollen allergen, Bet v 1. J Immunol 1996; 157:4953–4962.
30. Lebecque S, Dolecek C, Laffer S, Visco V, Denepoux S, Pin JJ, Guret C, Boltz-Nitulescu G, Weyer A, Valenta R. Immunologic characterization of monoclonal antibodies which modulate human immunoglobulin E binding to the major birch pollen allergen Bet v 1. J Allergy Clin Immunol 1997; 99:374–384.
31. Vrtala S, Hirtenlehner K, Vangelista L, Pastore A, Eichler HG, Sperr WR, Valent P, Ebner C, Kraft D, Valenta R. Conversion of the major birch pollen allergen, Bet v 1, into two

nonanaphylactic T-cell epitope-containing fragments; candidates for a novel form of specific immunotherapy. J Clin Invest 1997; 99:1673–1681.
32. Cooke RA, Bernhard JH, Hebald S, Stull A. Serological evidence of immunity with coexisting sensitization in hay fever type of human allergy. J Exp Med 1935; 62:733–750.
33. Lichtenstein LM, Holtzman NA, Burnett LS. A quantitative in vitro study of the chromatographic distribution and immunoglobulin characteristics of human blocking antibody. J Immunol 1968; 101:317–324.
34. Loveless MH. Immunological studies of pollinosis: I. The presence of 2 antibodies related to the same pollen-antigen in the serum of treated hay fever patients. J Immunol 1940; 38:25–50.
35. Maunsell K. Direct test for blocking antibody in treated hay-fever. Lancet 1946; 1:199–201.
36. Aalberse RC, Gaag R, Leeuwen J. Serologic aspects of IgG_4 antibodies. I. Prolonged immunization results in an IgG_4-restricted response. J Immunol 1983; 130:722–726.
37. Birkner T, Rumpold H, Jarolim E, Ebner H, Breitenbach M, Skvaril T, Scheiner O, Kraft D. Evaluation of immunotherapy-induced changes in specific IgE, IgG and IgG subclasses in birch pollen allergic patients by means of immunoblotting. Correlation with clinical response. Allergy 1990; 45:418–426.
38. Secrist H, Chelen CJ, Wen Y, Marshall JD, Umetsu DT. Allergen immunotherapy decreases interleukin 4 production in $CD4^+$ T cells from allergic individuals. J Exp Med 1993; 178:2123–2130.
39. Tame A, Sakiyama Y, Kobayashi I, Terai I, Kobaysashi K. Differences in titres of IgE, IgG_4 and other IgG subclass anti-Der p 2 antibodies in allergic and non-allergic patients measured with recombinant allergen. Clin Exp Allergy 1996; 26:43–49.
40. Kobayashi I, Sakiyama Y, Tame A, Kobayashi K, Matsumoto S. IgE and IgG_4 antibodies from patients with mite allergy recognize different epitopes of *Dermatophagoides pteronyssinus* group II antigen (Der p 2). J Allergy Clin Immunol 1996; 97:638–645.
41. Witeman AM, Stapel SO, Sjamsoedin DHS, Jansen HM, Aalberse RC, Van Der Zee JS. Fel d 1-specific IgG antibodies induced by natural exposure have blocking activity in skin tests. Int Arch Allergy Immunol 1996; 109:369–375.
42. Wuse WD, Sastry L, Iverson SA, Kang AS, Alting-Mees M, Burton DR, Benkovic SJ, Lerner RA. Generation of a large combinatorial library of the immunoglobulin repertoire in phage lambda. Science 1989; 246:1275–1281.
43. McCafferty J, Griffiths AD, Winter G, Chiswell DJ. Phage antibodies: filamentous phage displaying antibody variable domains. Nature 1990; 348:552–554.
44. Barbas CF III, Kang AS, Lerner RA, Benkovic SJ. Assembly of combinatorial antibody libraries on phage surfaces: the gene III site. Proc Natl Acad Sci USA 1991; 88:7978–7982.
45. Winter G, Milstein C. Man-made antibodies. Nature 1991; 349:293–299.
46. Gram H, Marconi LA, Barbas CF III, Collet TA, Lerner RA, Kang AS. In vitro selection and affinity maturation of antibodies from a naive combinatorial immunoglobulin library. Proc Natl Acad Sci USA 1992; 89:3576–3580.
47. Steinberger P, Kraft D, Valenta R. Construction of a combinatorial IgE library from an allergic patient: isolation and characterization of human IgE Fabs with specificity for the major timothy grass pollen allergen, Phl p 5. J Biol Chem 1996; 271:10967–10972.

20

Tolerogenic Peptides
Clinical Experience in Allergy

CHRISTOPHER F. NICODEMUS

Diatide, Inc.
Londonderry, New Hampshire

GEORGE PHILIP

Merck and Company, Inc.
West Point, Pennsylvania

I. Introduction

The T-cell component of the antigen-specific immune response has become the target of various therapeutic strategies to modify diseases characterized by dysregulated immune responses. Allergy is the prototype model in which this approach has been used, but analogous efforts in autoimmune diseases, such as multiple sclerosis, have also been initiated. This chapter will focus on the scientific rationale and early clinical experience in allergy.

It is well established that the T-cell response to an antigen is fundamental to both the cellular and humoral immune responses. T cells respond in an antigen-specific manner through the T-cell receptor (TCR) that recognizes peptidic antigen fragments presented in the binding groove of the major histocompatibility complex (MHC) on antigen-presenting cells (APC). T cells provide stimulatory signals for B-cell proliferation and antibody production after the B cell binds antigen by the specific antibody expressed on the B-cell surface. Soluble peptide fragments in high doses can render T cells nonresponsive. The mechanism of this nonresponsiveness may vary according to the experimental model, but pathways of anergy, immune deviation, suppression, and deletion, all have been documented (1).

Briner and colleagues have assessed the ability of peptide fragments derived from Fel d 1, the dominant allergen in cat extract, to inhibit immune responses to this antigen (2). Soluble peptide was administered subcutaneously to primed or naive animals. In this experimental model, animals were challenged with Fel d 1 in incomplete Freund adjuvant at various time points following tolerization with peptide. The immune response to the challenge was assessed 10 days after challenge by the culture of mononuclear cells from draining lymph nodes. Data from these studies show significant downregulation of antigen-specific proliferative responses, as well as interleukin (IL)-2 production. Antibody response to antigen in culture is similarly downregulated.

Soluble peptide delivered mucosally through intranasal administration has also been documented to downregulate subsequent immune responses. Hoyne and colleagues used a peptide derived from the mite allergen Der p 1 (3). In this study, mice were tolerized with three daily administrations of solubilized peptide intranasally and then challenged with Der p 1 in adjuvant. Hoyne demonstrated early activation of T cells during tolerization, followed by subsequent unresponsiveness that peaked at day 14. Downregulation was demonstrated through proliferation assay and production of IL-2 and IL-3. Transient lymphocyte activation for several days following intranasal administration of peptide was observed in this study. The duration of tolerance was more short-lived through the mucosal route than through the subcutaneous route of Briner. Both studies demonstrated the ability of soluble peptide to moderate immune response in a consistent manner, although with differences to be anticipated based on dose and route of administration.

The effects of peptide tolerance induction on complex cellular inflammation have been elegantly modeled by McDevitt and colleagues, using a murine model of experimental allergic encephalomyelitis (EAE; 4,5). Myelin basic protein (MBP) induces a relapsing and remitting progressive encephalomyelopathy in PL/J mice. An amino terminal peptide fragment of MBP, peptide Ac1–11, contains encephalogenic potential and also ameliorates EAE when administered as a soluble peptide in a tolerizing protocol. Peptide administration can block the onset of disease, and can downregulate active disease, with suppression of an active inflammatory focus (6).

These various animal models point to the complexity of cellular immune responses, and the potential to vary the route of administration, solubility, and dose of antigen fragments to optimally modulate the immune process. Experimental models have focused on establishment of nonresponsiveness in the period several weeks following tolerance induction and, often, have not followed the early cellular events following peptide exposure. It is clear that transient T-cell activation occurs as the initial step in tolerance induction, with T-cell cytokine release occurring following peptide administration. Multiple reports have confirmed this finding (3,7,8). It is unclear what clinical manifestations this phenomenon might elicit in initial human studies.

Several strategies to identify and produce T-cell–reactive peptides are currently being pursued for therapeutic use in treatment of allergy. IgE reactivity to peptides, potentially inherent in the humoral response to the parent allergen, can be minimized through selection of non–IgE-binding peptides, demonstrating the distinction between T-cell epitope and B-cell (antibody) epitope. T-cell epitopes are generally directed to linear peptide sequences, whereas B-cell epitopes and consequent antibody specificities are generally directed to the three-dimensional antigenic structure. Although the two can overlap, these epitopes reflect very different ligand interactions and, thus, can be distinguished.

Gefter and colleagues at ImmuLogic Pharmaceutical Corporation used bulk culture methodologies to generate multiple peptide-reactive T-cell lines from large populations of allergic individuals (9). Protein fragments rich in T-cell epitopes were identified, and panels of lymphocytes from atopic donors were used to select peptide candidates that contained maximal T-cell reactivity for therapeutic use. A second method to identify T-cell epitopes was employed by Brostoff and colleagues. This group generated T-cell clones to identify T-cell epitopes for use in peptide selection for the possible treatment of grass allergy (10). Either strategy (i.e., generation of T-cell lines or of T-cell clones) can be used to identify short peptide fragments amenable to solid-phase synthesis or polypeptide regions amenable to recombinant expression, to produce therapeutic peptide candidates.

Dose selection of peptides for human trials has been guided from animal-modeling experiments and also from the doses of whole antigen administered in traditional allergen immunotherapy. A commonly used dose for optimal tolerance in murine studies is 100 μg (2,3). Multiple human studies have established that maximal treatment doses of 6–12 μg of major allergen are to be administered per injection, as tolerated, during the maintenance phase of allergen immunotherapy; this dose is continued for years at 2- to 6-week intervals to effect a therapeutic response (11–13). Extrapolating from these data, peptide doses in our initial studies have ranged from 7.5 to 1500 μg.

T-cell modulation of the allergic response is being tested in several distinct allergic syndromes. Because peptide would not be expected to modulate levels of allergen-specific antibody in the short term, early clinical effects would theoretically be derived from T-cell modulation of effector cell releasability by a change in the allergic inflammatory microenvironment that is maintained by T cells. The relevance of such changes and the strategies to achieve maximal clinical benefit may vary, depending on the allergic syndrome. Specifically, perennial allergies, such as dust mite, cockroach, and cat, are characterized by continuous immune responses and an inflammatory process that often includes the lower respiratory tract. Pulmonary–asthmatic manifestations are common. Seasonal allergy is characterized by acute upper airway pathology, most often confined to rhinoconjunctival symptoms. Seasonal immune responses have long intervening rest periods, but memory responses prevail to maintain the syndrome from season to season. The anaphylactic syndromes are also being considered for peptide immunotolerance therapy. Stinging insect venom hypersensitivity and IgE-mediated food allergy, such as peanut allergy, are clinical examples. Here exposure to antigen is sporadic, and there is no apparent inflammatory focus of disease; however, the allergic response to exposure is extremely volatile, resulting in acute anaphylaxis syndromes following trace exposures to antigen. The cause for the magnitude of this hypersensitivity is uncertain. T-cell factors are determined to contribute to the hypersensitized state, it is possible that peptide therapy might favorably alter the anaphylactic threshold and, thus, be an important therapeutic advance.

II. Experience in Perennial Allergy

Accumulated clinical experience, to date, for the use of tolerogenic peptides in the treatment of a perennial allergen has been confined to studies of Fel d 1-derived peptides in the treatment of cat allergy. Future studies for mite allergy are anticipated. A growing body of literature has established the importance of Fel d 1 as a ubiquitous allergen that is present not only in the homes of cat owners, but also in public places, such as schools and buses, and is transported in clothing and such. The familiar acute asthmatic response induced in cat allergic individuals when exposed to cats is accompanied by a more insidious chronic subclinical inflammatory state that many contribute to long-term impairment in pulmonary function and associated morbidity (14). Multiple clinical studies using Fel d 1-derived peptides have been completed; positive effects, both on immediate response to cat allergen and chronic markers of pulmonary impairment, have been established in a dose-responsive manner (15–21).

Patients selected for study have been cat allergic individuals, with histories of cat allergy and documented skin test sensitivity to cat extract. A therapeutic peptide candidate, consisting of two 27-amino acid peptides containing multiple Fel d 1 T-cell epitopes, has been formulated for subcutaneous administration. IgE reactivity to peptide is absent in most patients, despite IgE reactivity to Fel d 1, and the peptides are generally administered without evidence of a local response. An initial safety study established that 7.5–1500 μg of each peptide could be safely administered, and a program to optimize dose, dose number, and dose frequency is ongoing.

The contrast between peptide therapy and cat extract immunotherapy has been striking. Whereas small local reactions to extract are universal and large local or systemic responses requiring downward dose titration of extract immunotherapy are common, patients can be administered fixed doses of peptide without similar responses (22). Peptides are poor IgE cross-linkers and, in fact, do not contain the common B-cell epitopes encountered in an allergic population. The contrast between levels of IgE of Fel d 1 and levels of IgE to treatment peptides is illustrated in Figure 1.

The efficacy of peptide therapy appears to be a function not only of dose amount and dose number, but also of dose frequency. Twice-weekly dosing is more

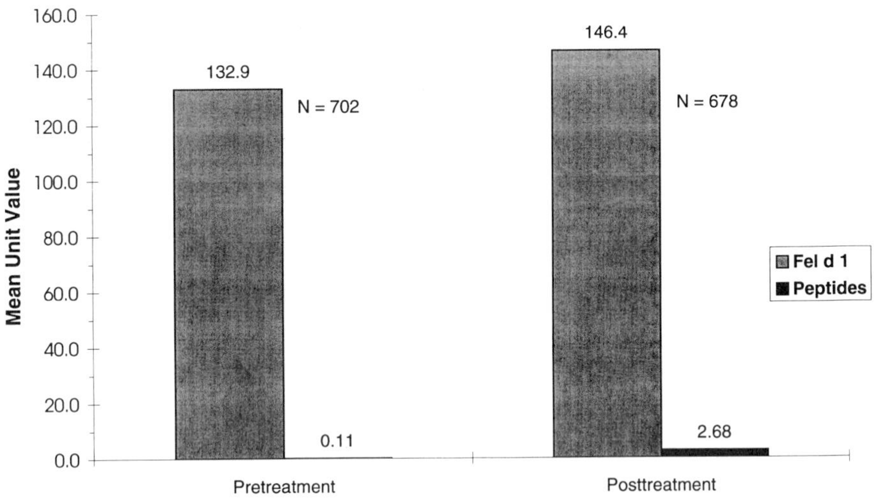

Figure 1 Relative IgE reactivity to Fel d 1 and Fel d 1-derived peptides is compared in the population treated with the ALLERVAX CAT therapeutic. Reactivity is based on an enzyme-linked immunosorbent assay (ELISA) adapted from the method of Bond (28). Data are reported as relative ELISA units. IgE reactivity to selected Fel d 1 peptides is several log units less than reactivity to native Fel d 1. (Data courtesy of N. Jones and T. Olson.)

effective than once-weekly dosing, and 750 μg is more effective than lower doses (21; Fig. 2). An initial treatment regimen of four injections given over 8–10 days has resulted in a greater than 60% reduction in symptomatic response to cat exposure in studies using the cat room model of allergen challenge (placebo reductions 20-40%). In this model, patients are placed in the presence of cats for 60 min in a small room with Fel d 1 levels higher than 50 ng/m^3. Airborne Fel d 1 is quantitated as patients' clinical responses are carefully recorded over the time of the challenge. Clinical benefit has been observed in nasal, lung, and total allergy scores; the dominant effect is on the pulmonary response, which is particularly sensitive to the levels of airborne Fel d 1 at the time of challenge (23). The effect of peptide therapy is apparent within 1 week of a treatment series, but is more pronounced at 6–8 weeks after treatment. Information on duration is as yet limited, but initial studies have suggested the effect persists for 6–9 months for most patients (16). An optimal maintenance schedule may be either tailored to the individual patient or established at a regular frequency. Studies to definitively establish approaches to maintenance dosing are being planned.

Improvements in the bronchial response to allergen challenge have also been reported with peptide therapy (17). Similar to the effects seen with corticosteroids, the shifts in airway responsiveness to allergen challenge were on the order of a twofold change and occurred in a dose-responsive manner. Twofold changes also approximate the shifts observed in acute response to allergen challenge seen in stud-

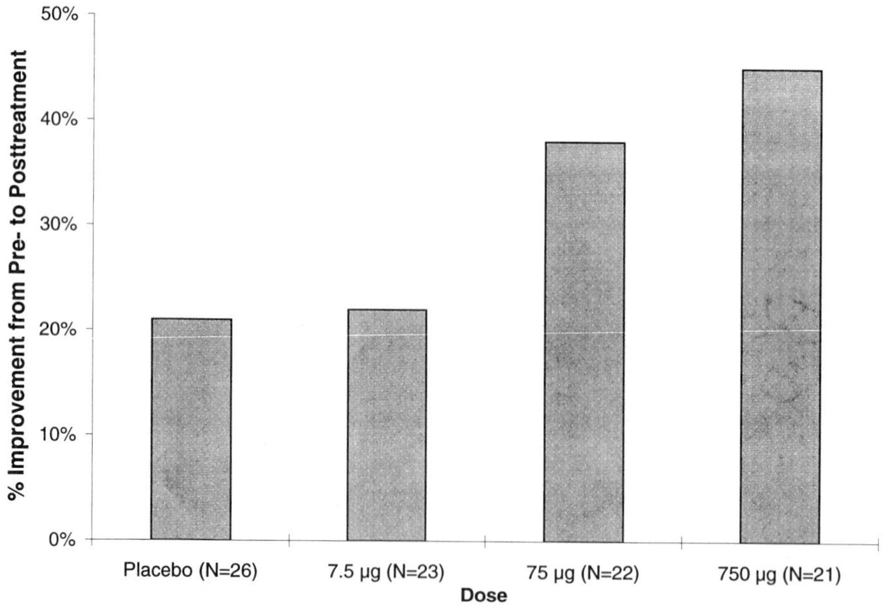

Figure 2 The dose–response relationship of four weekly injections of Fel d 1 peptides was assessed 6 weeks after completion of a treatment series. Symptomatic improvement in a cat room challenge relative to pretreatment is illustrated. Weekly dosing at 750-µg level results in significant clinical improvement ($p = 0.05$). Subsequent studies have established that more frequent dosing augments this effect. The effect is apparent within 1 week of a treatment series, is augmented at 6–8 weeks postdosing, and persists for months in the absence of any additional treatment. (Data from Ref. 18.)

ies of corticosteroids; the observed modest shifts probably reflect the lack of direct interference of both therapeutic modalities on IgE–antigen interaction. Both modalities modulate the allergic response indirectly through inflammatory pathways and not through pharmacological interference with IgE–antigen ligand interactions. Interestingly, the therapy has also been associated with more extended improvement in resting pulmonary function in patients with impaired function at baseline. The potential influence of peptide therapy on cat-associated asthma is the subject of additional ongoing research.

Effects of peptide therapy on cutaneous skin test reactivity to allergen have not been consistent in studies reported to date. Peptide therapy for cat has not been associated with significant shifts in IgE responses, perhaps explaining the lack of consistent effect on immediate cutaneous sensitivity. A single Fel d 1-derived peptide administered intravenously was associated with a decrease in the cutaneous late-phase response to cat extract 6 weeks following a treatment series (18). The mean diameter of late-phase erythema decreased from 102 ± 20 mm pretreatment to 43 ± 27 mm posttreatment ($p = 0.05$) in the small cohort of six subjects.

It has been difficult to demonstrate changes in lymphocyte function in association with peptide therapy in clinical studies for reasons that are primarily methodological. Recently, Marcotte has reported demonstration of a downregulation of IL-4 production in secondary cultures of patients treated with four doses 750 μg of cat peptides compared with a placebo-treated cohort (20). Further demonstrations of these important pharmacological observations may be shortly forthcoming.

The effects of Fel d 1-derived peptides on cat allergy appear to be anti-inflammatory and most predominant in the lower airway. As with corticosteroids, immediate skin test reactivity is not changed. Effects on acute inhaled allergen challenge can be detected, but data supporting important longer-term benefit on airway function are also emerging. The best demonstration of clinical benefit may come from long-term studies of patients with impaired airway function.

III. Experience in Seasonal Allergy

Several laboratories have been working to identify peptide structures that may be of use in treatment of seasonal allergic syndromes. By using a T-cell clone approach, peptides derived from major allergens for ryegrass allergy (10), birch tree allergy (24), and Japanese cedar allergy (25) have been identified, which appear to contain important T-cell epitopes. Vrtala and colleagues have further characterized two peptides derived from the major birch allergen, Bet v 1, which induce proliferation of human Bet v 1-specific T-cell clones, but fail to trigger basophil histamine release or to elicit skin reactions (24). Clinical experience using these peptides awaits further study.

The largest clinical experience that uses tolerogenic peptides to treat seasonal allergy has involved Amb a 1-specific peptides for treatment of ragweed allergy. Ragweed pollen is the predominant seasonal allergen in late summer and fall in central and eastern regions of North America. By using a T-cell line approach, three treatment peptides have been identified, the structure of which was derived from the major short ragweed allergen, Amb a 1. These peptides were selected for low IgE binding and low basophil histamine release in blood samples from ragweed allergic patients. An initial safety study confirmed the ability to safely administer from 7.5 to 1500 μg of each peptide (26).

Subsequent research has examined subcutaneous administration of Amb a 1-specific peptides with brief preseasonal dosing completed 2–3 weeks before ragweed season. Nine hundred and forty-four adult patients, with a history of ragweed allergy and documented skin test sensitivity to ragweed extract, were enrolled in a study that examined various dose regimens of Amb a 1-specific peptides (27). Patients completed daily symptom diaries throughout the ragweed pollen season. Three hundred twenty-four patients received 750 μg of each peptide in four injections over 2-4 weeks. These patients showed significant reduction of allergic symptoms, including rhinoconjunctival ($p < 0.04$) and total allergy ($p < 0.03$) symptom scores. Treatment was generally well tolerated, with immediate responses to peptides seen in fewer than 1% of patients; these responses were easily managed.

IV. Anaphylactic Syndromes

Efforts to characterize T-cell responses to allergens associated with anaphylactic syndromes are ongoing in multiple laboratories. Initial clinical studies have been undertaken in Switzerland under the direction of Muller and colleagues working with the honeybee venom protein phospholipase A_2. The earliest reports indicate that patients have tolerated these peptides well, but definitive assessment of efficacy is still pending. These studies will yield important insight into the role of the T cell in regulating the exquisite sensitivity exhibited by patients prone to anaphylactic syndromes.

V. Safety of Peptide Therapy

Peptides are characterized by substantially diminished antipeptide IgE reactivity relative to the IgE reactivity directed to the parent protein. Antipeptide IgE reactivity is not always absent, however, and screening methods to appropriately manage peptide-sensitive patients are being established. A response, distinct from antipeptide IgE reactivity, which occurs instead in a time course consistent with T-cell activation, has been observed in few cat-sensitive patients and, to a much more subtle degree, in ragweed-sensitive patients. The response manifests as allergic symptoms similar to the natural disease. These allergic-like symptoms are generally mild and have been reduced with coadministration of antihistamines with first dosing of the cat peptides. Interestingly, these symptoms diminish with repeat dosing; this finding is consistent with initial T-cell activation followed by induction of T-cell unresponsiveness, and follows the precedent from animal studies (3). These mild, allergic-like symptoms appear to be preventable or easily managed and are much less prevalent than side effects (local and systemic) associated with extract immunotherapy (18,19).

A growing body of data confirm that peptide therapy offers a safe and effective approach for allergen-specific disease management. Simple-dosing strategies appear to be effective, and the clinical benefit for perennial allergens may be particularly associated with pulmonary improvement. Only with additional study will the proper role of peptide therapy be established, but it appears to represent an important therapeutic alternative for the future, one that may be especially relevant for the treatment of perennial atopic asthma.

References

1. Schwartz RH. Acquisition of immunological self-tolerance. Cell 1989; 57:1073.
2. Briner TJ, Kuo M-C, Keating KM, Rogers BL, Greenstein JL. Peripheral T-cell tolerance induced in naive and primed mice by subcutaneous injection of peptides from the major cat allergen Fel d 1. Proc Natl Acad Sci USA 1993; 90:7608–7612.
3. Hoyne GF, Askonas BA, Hetzel C, Thomas WR, Lamb JR. Regulation of house dust mite responses by intranasally administered peptide: transient activation of CD4+ T cells precedes the development of tolerance in vivo. Immunol 1996; 8:335–342.
4. Gaur A, Wiers B, Lin A, Rothbard J, Fathman CG. Amelioration of autoimmune encephalomyelitis by myelin basic protein synthetic peptide-induced anergy. Science 1992; 258:1491–1494.
5. Smilek DE, Wraith DC, Hodgkinson S, Dwivedy S, Steinman L, McDevitt HO. A single amino acid change in a myelin basic protein peptide confers the capacity to prevent rather than induce experimental autoimmune encephalomyelitis. Proc Natl Acad Sci USA 1991; 88:9633–9637.
6. Karin N, Mitchell DJ, Brocke S, Ling N, Steinman L. Reversal of experimental autoimmune encephalomyelitis by a soluble peptide variant of a myelin basic protein epitope: T cell receptor antagonism and reduction of interferon γ and tumor necrosis factor α production. J Exp Med 1994; 180:2227–2237.
7. O'Hehir RE, Busch R, Rothbard JB, Lamb RJ. An in vitro model of peptide-mediated immunomodulation of the human T cell response to *Dermatophagoides* spp (house dust mite). J Allergy Clin Immunol 1991; 87:1120–1127.
8. Vidard L, Colarusso LJ, Benacerraf B. Specific T-cell tolerance may be preceded by a primary response. Proc Natl Acad Sci USA 1994; 91:5627–5631.
9. Counsell CM, Bond JF, Ohman JL, Greenstein JL, Garman RD. Definition of the human T cell epitopes of Fel d 1, the major allergen of the domestic cat. J Allergy Clin Immunol 1996; 98:884–894.
10. Bungy Poor Fard GA, Latchman Y, Rodda S, Geysen M, Roitt I, Brostoff J. T cell epitopes of the major fraction of ryegrass *Lolium perenne* (Lol p 1) defined using overlapping peptides in vitro and in vivo. I. Isoallergen clone 1A. Clin Exp Immunol 1993; 94:111–116.
11. Norman PS, Winkenwerder WL, Lichtenstein LM. Immunotherapy of hay fever with ragweed antigen E: comparisons with whole pollen extract and placebos. J Allergy 1968; 42:93–108.
12. van Metre TE, Marsh DG, Adkinson NF, Kagey-Sobotka A, Khattignavong A, Norman PS, Rosenberg GL. Immunotherapy for cat asthma. J Allergy Clin Immunol 1988; 82:1055–1068.
13. Haugaard L, Dahl R, Jacobsen L. A controlled dose–response study of immunotherapy with standardized, partially purified extract of house dust mite: clinical efficacy and side effects. J Allergy Clin Immunol 1993; 91:709–722.
14. Platts-Mills TAE, Sporik RB, Wheatley LM, Heymann PW. Is there a dose–response relationship between exposure to indoor allergens and symptoms of asthma? J Allergy Clin Immunol 1995; 96:435–440.
15. Norman PS, Ohman JL, Long AA, Creticos PS, Shaked Z, Wood R, Eggleston PA, Jones NH, Nicodemus, CF. Early clinical experience with T cell reactive peptides from cat allergen Fel d 1. J Allergy Clin Immunol 1994; 93:231.
16. Norman PS, Ohman JL, Long AA, Creticos PS, Gefter ML, Shaked Z, Wood RA, Eggleston PA, Lichtenstein LM, Jones NH, Nicodemus CF. Follow on study of the first clinical trial with T cell defined peptides from cat allergen Fel d 1. J Allergy Clin Immunol 1995; 95:259.
17. Creticos PS, Spector SL, Busse WW, Israel E, Nicodemus CF, Jones NH, Olson T, Gefter ML, Lichtenstein LM, Norman PS. Evaluation of T cell epitope defined peptides from cat allergen by bronchial challenge. J Allergy Clin Immunol 1995; 95:390.

18. Norman PS, Ohman JL, Long AA, Creticos PS, Gefter MA, Shaked Z, Wood RA, Eggleston PA, Hafner KB, Rao P, Lichtenstein LM, Jones NH, Nicodemus CF. Treatment of cat allergy with T cell reactive peptides. Am J Respir Crit Care Med 1996; 154:1623–1628.
19. Nicodemus CF. Tolerogenic peptides. In: Austen KF, Burakoff S, Rosen F, Strom T, eds. Therapeutic Immunology. Boston: Blackwell Scientific, 1996:628–635.
20. Marcotte GV, Braun CM, Norman PS, Nicodemus CF, Kagey-Sobotka A, Lichtenstein LM, Essayan DM. Effect of peptide immunotherapy (PIT) on T cell (TC) proliferation and cytokine production. J Allergy Clin Immunol 1997; 99:S405.
21. Norman PS, Nicodemus CF, the ALLERVAX CAT Study Group. Multicenter study of several doses of ALLERVAX CAT peptides in the treatment of cat allergy. J Allergy Clin Immunol 1997; 99:S127.
22. Ohman JL, Findlay SR, Leitermann KM. Immunotherapy in cat-induced asthma. Double-blind trial with evaluation of in vivo and in vitro responses. J Allergy Clin Immunol 1984; 74:230–239.
23. Ohman JL, Bennett DV, Happ MP, Settle MR, Jones NH, Hirani S, Long AA. The cat room model for associating allergen levels with asthma symptoms and evaluating treatment effects of peptide therapy. J Allergy Clin Immunol 1996; 97:387.
24. Vrtala S, Hirtenlehner K, Vangelista L, Pastore A, Eichler HG, Sperr WR, Valent P, Ebner C, Kraft D, Valenta R. Division of the major birch pollen allergen, Bet v 1, into two non-anaphylactic T-cell epitopes. Int Arch Allergy Immunol 1997; 113:246–248.
25. Ishikawa T, Ikagawa S, Matsushita S, Nishimura Y, Masuyama K. Human T cell response to antigen peptides of Japanese cedar pollen (Cry j 1). Int Arch Allergy Immunol 1997; 113:255–257.
26. Creticos PS, Norman PS, Jones NH, Settles M, Wallner B, Nicodemus CF. Initial clinical experience with T cell epitope defined peptides from ragweed allergen Amb a 1. J Allergy Clin Immunol 1995; 95:390.
27. Creticos PS, Hebert J, Philip G, the ALLERVAX RAGWEED Study Group. Efficacy of ALLERVAX RAGWEED peptides in the treatment of ragweed-induced allergy. J Clin Allergy Immunol 1997; 99:S401.
28. Bond JF, Garman RD, Keating KM, Briner TJ, Rafnar T, Klapper DG, Rogers BL. Multiple Amb a 1 allergens demonstrate specific reactivity with IgE and T cells from ragweed-allergic patients. J Immunol 1991; 146:3380–3385.

21

Manipulation of the Idiotypic Network
An Alternative Approach to Treat Allergic Asthma?

YVAN BOUTIN

Yale University School of Medicine
New Haven, Connecticut

JACQUES HÉBERT

Laval University
Centre Hospitalier de l'Université Laval
Centre Hospitalier Universitaire de Quebec
Sainte Foy, Quebec, Canada

I. Introduction

Asthma is a complex disease and the pathogenesis has not been fully elucidated. Because 40–85% of asthmatic patients have a positive skin reaction to common inhalant allergens, a role of IgE cannot be ruled out in the genesis of the disease. Indeed, levels of specific IgE are often high in those patients, and they develop acute bronchospasm on specific allergic challenge.

Immunoglobulin E, similar to other immunoglobulins, is produced by B cells, and its synthesis is controlled by T cells (1,2). An initial contact between B and T cells, which consists of the recognition of allergen peptides–major histocompatibility complex (MHC) class II molecules on B cells by the T-cell receptor (TCR) (3), results in $CD4^+$ lymphocyte activation. This event leads to the synthesis of new proteins that enable T helper (Th) cells to reciprocally deliver contact-dependent signals to B cells (4). Such interactions may involve different molecules on the surface of lymphocytes, among which are CD40 on B cells and the CD40 ligand on activated T cells (5,6). Another important signal necessarily required for synthesis of IgE is provided by interleukin (IL)-4, which is produced by a subset of Th cells, Th2. Once produced, IgE binds to specific receptors on mast cells and basophils that line up the mucosal epithelium.

The reaction of cell-bound IgE molecules with multivalent ligand stimulates the release of a variety of preformed and newly generated mediators that are involved in the acute and the late-phase reactions in allergic asthma. Therefore, it is reasonable to think that suppression of IgE response should lead to clinical improvements. It is believed that allergen immunotherapy should achieve that goal. Despite decades of use, the exact mechanism by which such a therapy works is still unknown. In allergy, symptoms are associated with the production of IL-4 and IL-5 produced by the Th2. Thus, one interesting explanation is that allergic desensitization is achieved by switching T helper type 2 (Th2)-dominated response into Th1-like pattern of cytokine expression in allergic patients. However, this approach is at a risk of systemic reactions, and it is not as effective as expected. Therefore, other approaches, such as peptide immunotherapy, anti-IgE, and anti–idiotype-based therapy are currently under evaluation to regulate IgE production.

II. Idiotypic Network

A given antibody molecule, including IgE, is specific for one target antigen. Its specificity is determined by the structure of the variable regions of the antibody. Within the variable regions, antigenic determinants are known as idiotopes, and they collectively define the idiotype (Id) of the molecule. Idiotypes are unique and specific for each antibody molecule, in the same way fingerprints are unique and specific for an individual. In the course of any immune response, this Id may become immunogenic and lead to antibody production against it. Antibodies directed against Id are called anti-idiotypic antibodies (aId), and such antibodies have been elicited by xenogenic and allogenic, as well as syngenic, immunization. It has been estimated that there are 15–20 idiotopes on the V region of a single immunoglobulin molecule (7), which may be distinguished by aId antibodies. Some of these determinants are topographically distant from the antigen-binding site (paratope). They are called nonparatopic or framework idiotopes, and the antibodies that recognized them are called Ab2α. The binding of Ab2α to Ab1 is not inhibited by the antigen. Other epitopes that overlap with the binding site are called paratopic idiotopes and the corresponding aId antibodies have been designated Ab2β. The Ab2β binding to its Ab1 is inhibited by the antigen. This aId, also called internal image, has the capacity to mimic the antigen and induce an antiantigen response.

In 1974, Jerne postulated that the interaction between Id and aId constituted an important regulatory network in the control of antibody production (8). According to this concept, an antigenic epitope induces the production of antibody (Ab1), recognizing the epitope through its paratope and expressing an Id, so called Id_1. Id_1 induces Ab2, which possesses Id_2 and recognizes Id_1. In its turn, the Id_2 induces Ab3, and so on (Fig. 1). Thus, aId antibodies are part of the normal immune response that is thought to consist of a web of interacting Id.

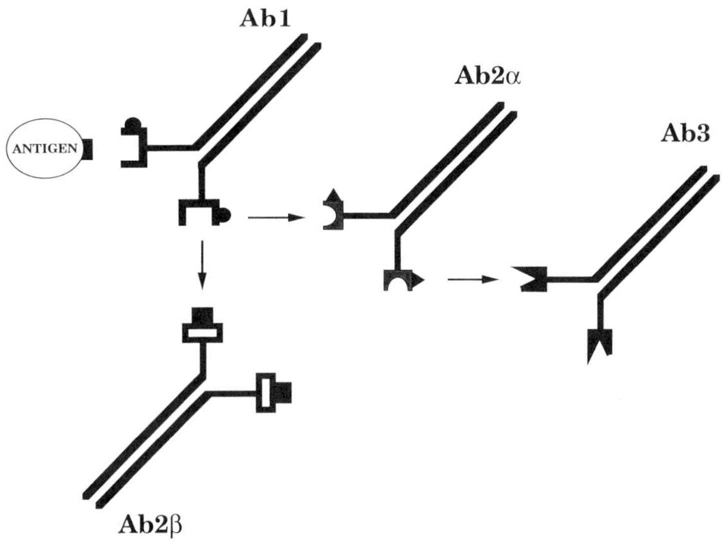

Figure 1 Idiotypic network: Interactions between antigen, Ab1, and Ab2.

One of the major problems with the original presentation of the Id network is that the T lymphocytes, which are key regulatory elements of the immune system, are not explicitly involved. Idiotypic structures have been identified on variable regions (α,β, γ, or δ) of the TCR. However, it seems rather unlikely that B and T cells that respond to the same antigen, would have common Id, because B and T cells usually recognize different epitopes. Indeed, B-cell receptors, surface immunoglobulins (sIg), recognize native epitopic structures, whereas TCR recognize processed epitopes associated with class I or class II molecules of the MHC. However, there are several reports that clearly demonstrated the existence of regulatory T-cell counterparts for Ab1 and Ab2. Helper, suppressor, or effector T cells specific for antigens can share the Id of Ab1 (9,10) and Id-specific T cells can also be identified (9–11). The mechanisms by which the Id network affects immune responses are not well understood, but it can manipulate cellular and humoral immunity.

III. Role of the Idiotypic Network in Physiopathology of Diseases

A. Autoimmune Diseases

Autoantibodies directed against nuclear antigens, intracellular components, cell membrane molecules, and circulating plasma proteins can be found in serum of healthy individuals (12,13). Some of these antigens recognized by the antibodies from healthy subjects are also targets of autoantibodies involved in the physiopathology of autoimmune diseases. Anti-idiotypic antibodies against those autoantibodies have been found in normal sera. The functions of natural autoantibodies and aId antibodies are not fully understood, but one of those functions may be to contribute to the homeostasis of autoreactivity. Disruption of the network may lead to the emergence of pathogenic autoantibodies. Production of aId antibodies that inhibit the potential harmful autoimmune repertoire may result from the activation of the Id network committed to control the secretion of natural autoantibodies.

The role of aId in the regulation of pathogenic Id is reinforced by clinical observations. The disappearance of autoantibody activity in serum is associated with the generation of aId antibodies against autoantibodies at the time of clinical remission (14–17).

B. Hypersensitivity

It is interesting to speculate that the elevated IgE levels in atopic patients are associated with impaired aId production that regulates IgE production against allergens. In fact aId antibodies have been found in sera from nonatopic patients exposed to pollen (18,19), and their levels were lower in symptomatic patients than in normal subjects. These levels were restored to normal following immunotherapy (18,20). These data suggest a role for aId in the regulation of IgE.

IV. Manipulating Immune Response with Idiotypic and Anti-Idiotypic Antibodies

For obvious reasons, there is an interest in assessing the potential ways to manipulate the immune response in an antigen-specific manner. In some instances, such as organ transplantation, autoimmune diseases, or allergic hypersensitivities, specific suppression would be desirable, whereas for other purposes, such as vaccinations or tumor rejection, a stimulation of the immune defense mechanisms is required. According to Jerne's network theory, aId antibodies might be involved in a normal event that modulates the degree and the duration of immune response. Therefore, aId reagents could be used to regulate an immune response to a specific antigen.

Indeed, many experiments have supported the Id network theory by showing that aId antibodies can enhance or suppress the immune response specific to a given epitope. Various factors influence the outcome of the Id manipulation (Table 1).

A. Regulation of Autoantibody Production

Several reports have demonstrated that experimentally induced or spontaneously occurring autoimmune diseases could be downregulated by manipulation of the Id network. For example, aId antibody administration suppresses the production of autoantibodies associated with lupus in mice (21–23) in experimental autoimmune

Table 1 Factors Influencing the Fate of Immune Response After Id Manipulation

The nature of targeted Id (private or public)
The nature of aId antibodies (monoclonal or polyclonal)
The specificity of aId antibodies (directed against nonparatopic or paratopic idiotopes)
The use of adjuvant
The coupling of aId to an immunogenic carrier
The time of aId injection (prenatal, neonatal, or adult)
The isotype of aId antibodies
The dose of antibodies given to the animal

myasthenia (24), interstitial nephritis (25), and autoimmune thyroiditis (26). Suppression of the antithyrotropin receptor antibody production using autologous aId antibodies from sera of patients with Graves' disease was demonstrated in vitro (27).

Administration of Id was also effective for the modulation of autoantibody production. De Kozak et al. (28) have demonstrated that Id immunization in rat model of uveoretinitis resulted in production of high-titer circulating auto-aId and long-lasting protection from the disease. Suppression of autoimmunity by Id pretreatment has also been reported in other experimental autoimmune diseases (22,25,29).

The most interesting finding concerning the manipulation of autoimmune responses by the Id network comes from data suggesting that the beneficial effect of therapeutic administration of high doses of IgG—prepared from large pools of normal donors—in autoimmune diseases may depend on the presence of aId antibodies in intravenous immunoglobulin preparations (IVIG). Besides its use as substitute therapy for immunodeficiencies, IVIG is increasingly being used as immunomodulating therapy in the treatment of patients with a variety of autoimmune disorders (30–37). In some cases, the efficacy of the IVIG therapy correlates with the specific content of aId antibodies to pathogenic Id of autoantibodies (38–40). However, mechanisms other than the restoration of Id network may contribute to the success of IVIG therapy in the treatment of some autoimmune diseases. Several investigators have suggested that the improved clinical autoimmunity observed in patients receiving high-dose IVIG could be due to the restoration of immune cells through their adhesion molecules (41), the cytokine network (42), or a direct effect of IVIG on T cells (43). However, the exact mechanisms by which IVIG can restore the function of cytokine network are still obscure.

B. Regulation of Immunoglobulin Production

Administration of Anti-Idiotypic Antibodies

The idiotypic regulation of primary mouse IgE response has been studied extensively by Blaser et al. (44–47). Balb/c mice were inoculated by subcutaneous or intraperitoneal route with purified isologous antibenzylpenicilloyl (BPO) antibodies. In these mice, in which active production of specific aId antibodies were detected, further immunization with BPO failed to induce IgE production (45). Passive transfer of aId antibodies has been also shown to suppress IgE response in animals. In various studies, isologous and heterologous aId antibodies have been used. Intravenous administration of anti-T15 isologous antiserum completely prevented the formation of IgE antibodies to phosphorylcholine (44).

Heterologous aId antibodies, usually from rabbit, have been used in the regulation of IgE immune response to hapten or proteins. A/J mice produce a family of Id-related IgEs in response to immunization with arsonate (48). Transfer of rabbit aId antibodies raised against antiarsonate monoclonal antibody (MAb) resulted in a complete suppression of the antiarsonate response, including IgE (49). Specific IgE raised in mice to antigen B of timothy grass pollen has been used to produce aId antibodies in rabbit. These aId antibodies, when passively transferred to recipient mice, induced a complete lack of antiantigen B IgE, despite antigen inoculation boosts (50,51). In vitro incubation of naive mouse spleen cells with rabbit aId antibodies and subsequent transfer of spleen cells to naive syngenic recipients was sufficient to induced a state of IgE unresponsiveness (51).

For the last decade we have been particularly interested in studying the role of aId–Id interactions in the modulation of immune response to Lol p 1, the major allergen of ryegrass pollen. We first produced and characterized MAbs that recognized allergenic epitopes on the allergen (52,53). We have demonstrated that the Id borne by one of these anti-Lol p 1 MAbs (290A-167) was a public Id, for it was expressed in 80% of IgE from grass-sensitive patients (54). These data suggested that the Id 290A-167 might be a preferential target for selective immunomodulation.

Because many studies have demonstrated that administration of aId antibodies before immunization suppressed IgE response in animals (44,45,55), we produced aId MAbs against the Id 290A-167 (56,57) to use them as immunoregulatory reagents. One of these aId MAbs displayed internal image properties, as assessed by its direct binding to Id and its capacity to inhibit the binding of Id to Lol p 1. It induced, in a dose-dependent fashion, histamine release by leukocytes from grass-sensitive patients. The inhibition of this histamine release by the addition of the Id (290A-167) confirmed the specificity of the reaction (57). Finally, we demonstrated that this aId MAb elicited an anti-Lol p 1 response in naive animals (56). Together these data confirmed that our aId MAb could biologically and functionally mimic the original antigen.

The effects of pretreatment with the aId MAb bearing the internal image of Lol p 1 before immunization with the antigen have been examined (58). In another study with ryegrass pollen, the administration of high doses of aId MAb bearing the internal image led to the suppression of the immune response against the allergen (55,59). In our system, administration of aId before immunization enhances the immune response to the allergen, rather than suppressing it. Surprisingly, idiotypes borne by other anti-Lol p 1 MAbs (539A-6 and 348A-6) have also been enhanced after pretreatment with the anti-290A-167 MAb. These observations suggested that the modulation of immune response by an aId MAb is not restricted to the respective Id, and it could affect the expression of other Id.

Administration of Idiotypic Antibodies

However, to achieve suppression of immune response, more encouraging results came from experiments in which Id, rather than aId was used for pretreatment in other antigenic systems (22,29,60). In our system, mice were immunized with an anti-Lol p 1 MAb (290A-167) (61). This treatment resulted in the production of aId antibodies, as evidenced by their ability to bind to the Fab fraction of 290A-167, and to inhibit the binding of rabbit polyclonal aId antibodies to 290A-167. The animals were then immunized with Lol p 1 adsorbed onto alum, and the immune response to the protein was analyzed. Antigen-specific IgG1 and IgE responses were strongly suppressed. Suppression of anti-Lol p 1 IgE was confirmed by a reduction of endpoint titers measured by passive cutaneous anaphylaxis. The suppression of antigen-specific antibody was accompanied by a reduction of anti-Lol p 1 antibody-producing spleen cells.

Our observations indicate that the administration of Id has a potential interest in therapy because this treatment has the capacity to reduce considerably the immune response to Lol p 1. However, several criteria should be considered in the choice of the Id that will be used as immunoregulatory reagent. One of the most critical parameters is the immunodominance of the epitope recognized by the Id.

Administration of Intravenous Immunoglobulin or Antigen–Antibody Complexes

The protective effect of passive transfer of plasma or IVIg has been demonstrated in the management of hypersensitivity (62–64) or asthma (65). Similar to treatment of autoimmune diseases with IVIG preparations, the clinical remission might be explained by a downregulation of IgE by Id network. Moreover, aId antibodies were found in plasma administrated to the patient (66). We had the opportunity to evaluate a patient highly allergic to honeybee venom, who experienced systemic reactions to injection therapy with bee venom (67). Because she did not tolerate sufficient amounts of venom to achieve protection against bee stings, beekeeper's plasma rich in aId antibodies was administered to the patient. After transfusion of plasma, she was immunized with increased doses of bee venom. Clinical and immunological parameters were measured along the combined immunotherapy protocol (Table 2).

Immediately after beekeeper's plasma transfer, a decrease of skin sensitivity and basophil histamine release induced by bee venom was observed. Her tolerance to bee venom was also improved, for she could receive 100 μg without reactions. No differences in specific IgG and IgE were observed. Following the modified rush immunotherapy, increased levels of aId antibodies in the serum of the patient were associated with a diminution of specific antibodies (IgG and IgE) to honeybee

Table 2 Changes in Clinical Parameters After Passive Transfer of Beekeeper's Plasma and During Rush Immunotherapy

Parameter	Before beekeeper's plasma transfer	After beekeeper's plasma transfer	76 weeks after initiation of immunotherapy
Tolerated dose (μg/mL of bee venom)	25	100	100
Endpoint titration skin test (μg/mL of bee venom)	0.1	1	n.d.
Basophil histamine release (%)	85	45	< 25
Specific IgE		No change	↓↓
Specific IgG		No change	No change
Specific aId antibodies	↑	↑↑	

n.d., not determined.

venom. These results suggest a dual role of aId: (1) an immediate action on clinical sensitivity along with a decrease of skin mast cell and basophil sensitivity, and (2) an immunoregulatory role on specific antibody production.

However the mechanisms involved in such a protection are still unknown. One may postulate that aId antibodies would bind to mast cell-bound IgE and work as blocking agents, either by competing with the antigen or by suppressing the activation of mediator release. However, such an Id–aId interaction on the mast cells may lead to the release of mediators (68), and this mast cell degranulation by aId depends on the availability of sufficient number of adjacent bound IgE molecules displaying the appropriate Id. Because it is unlikely that this situation occurs frequently, the aId are weak degranulators compared with the allergen. Moreover, we cannot rule out the possibility that other factors, such as cytokines found in beekeeper's plasma, have an effect on the reduction of hypersensitivity.

Administration of antigen–antibody complexes can also downregulate the production of IgE. This regulation is specific for the allergen of interest, and it goes with the production of aId antibodies (69–71). The mechanisms of action for this treatment remain to be clarified, but a role for aId antibodies cannot be excluded, because immune complexes increase aId responses, which are usually suppressive (72,73). Although the presence of aId antibodies may explain part of these results, it is possible that the antibody–allergen complex can alter antigen processing and presentation to the T cells (74).

V. Concluding Remarks

Several interacting factors contribute to the regulation of IgE. Although considerable evidence has accumulated on the regulation of a protective immune response to an Id–aId network, studies on allergen-specific responses are few, but support this concept. In animals, aId antibodies can be produced through repeated conventional immunization with specific antibodies. We and others have demonstrated that animals producing aId antibodies are unable to mount a specific IgE immune response on subsequent immunization. In humans, correlation was made between the levels of aId antibodies and the severity of allergic symptoms. Indeed, levels of aId antibodies are more elevated in normal subjects and patients under specific immunotherapy than in allergic patients.

The exact role of aId antibodies is still unknown. Because the balance between the T helper subsets (Th1 and Th2) is an important feature of the allergic condition, it might be interesting to speculate that aId antibodies can interact in this balance. Obviously, it is also conceivable that aId antibodies act directly on B cells. Binding of aId to surface immunoglobulin may deliver a signal to the B cells that induces tolerance. Several questions remain to be addressed concerning the role of Id network in the pathogenesis of allergic diseases, and manipulating the immune system with Id or aId reagents needs more validation.

References

1. Andersson J, Schrier MH, Melchers F. T cell-dependent B cell stimulation is H-2 restricted and antigen dependent only at the resting B cell level. Proc Natl Acad Sci USA 1980; 77:1612–1616.
2. DeFranco AL, Ashwell JD, Schwartz RH, Paul WE. Polyclonal stimulation of resting B lymphocytes by antigen-specific T lymphocytes. J Exp Med 1984; 159:861–880.
3. Tony H-P, Parker DC. Role of membrane immunoglobulin (Ig) crosslinking in membrane–Ig-mediated, major histocompatibility-restricted T cell–B cell cooperation. J Exp Med 1985; 161:223–241.
4. Noelle RJ, Daum J, Bartlett WC, McCann J, Shepherd DM. Cognate interactions between helper T cells and B cells. V. Reconstitution of T helper cell function using purified plasma membranes from activated Th1 and Th2 T helper cells and lymphokines. J Immunol 1991; 146:1118–1124.
5. Armitage RJ, Sato TA, Macduff BM, et al. Identification of a source of biologically active CD40 ligand. Eur J Immunol 1992; 22:2071–2076.
6. Noelle RJ, Ledbetter JA, Aruffo A. CD40 and its ligand, an essential ligand–receptor pair for thymus-dependent B-cell activation. Immunol Today 1992; 13:431–433.
7. Novotony J, Handschumacher M, Haber E. Location of antigenic epitopes on antibody molecules. J Mol Biol 1986; 189:715–721.
8. Jerne NK. Towards a network theory of the immune system. Ann Immunol (Paris) 1974; 125C:373–389.
9. Cerny J, Smith JS, Webb C, Tucker PW. Properties of anti-idiotypic T cell lines propagated with syngenic B lymphocytes. I. T cells bind intact idiotypes and discriminate between the somatic idiotipic variants in a manner similar to the anti-idiotypic antibodies. J Immunol 1988; 141:3718–3725.
10. Saeki Y, Chen JJ, Shi LF, Raychaudhuri S, Kohler H. Characterization of "regulatory," idiotope-specific T cell clones to a monoclonal anti-idiotypic antibody mimicking a tumor-associated antigen (TAA). J Immunol 1989; 142:1046–1052.
11. Dwyer DS, Vakil M, Bradley RJ, Oh SJ, Kearney JF. Direct receptor:receptor interactions between T and B lymphocytes: idiotypic restriction in the antibody response to a cloned helper T cell receptor. J Mol Cell Immunol 1987; 3:83–94.
12. Berneman A, Guilbert B, Eschrich S, Avrameas S. IgG auto- and polyreactivities in normal human sera. Mol Immunol 1993; 30:1499–1510.
13. Hurez V, Kaveri S, Kazatchkine MD. Expression and control of IgG autoreactivity in normal human serum. Eur J Immunol 1993; 23:783–789.
14. Abdou NI, Wall H, Lindsley HB, Suzuki T. Network theory in autoimmunity in vitro suppression of serum anti-DNA antibody binding to DNA by anti-idiotypic antibody in systemic lupus erythematous. J Clin Invest 1981; 67:1297–1304.
15. Lefvert AK. Anti-idiotypic antibodies against the receptor antibodies in myasthenia gravis. Scand J Immunol 1981; 13:493–497.
16. Sasaki T, Muryoi T, Takai O, Tamate E, Saito H, Yoshinaga K. Binding specificity of antiidiotypic autoantibodies to anti-DNA antibodies in humans. J Clin Invest 1988; 82:748–754.
17. Lundvist I, van Doorn PA, Vermeulen M, Brand A. Spontaneous recovery from Guillain–Barre syndrome is associated with anti-idiotypic antibodies recognizing a cross-reactive idiotype on anti-neuroblastoma cell line antibodies. Clin Immunol Immunopathol 1993; 67(3 pt 1):192–198.
18. Hébert J, Bernier D, Mourad W. Detection of auto-anti-idiotypic antibodies to Lol p 1 (rye I) IgE antibodies in human sera by the use of murine idiotypes: levels in atopic and non-atopic subjects and effects on immunotherapy. Clin Exp Immunol 1990; 80:413–419.
19. Bose R, Marsh DG, Delespesse G. Anti-idiotypes to anti-Lol p 1 (rye) antibodies in allergic and non-allergic individuals. Influence of immunotherapy. Clin Exp Immunol 1986; 66:231–240.

20. Castracane JM, Rocklin RE. Detection of human auto-anti-idiotypic antibodies (Ab2). I. Isolation and characterization of Ab2 in the serum of a ragweed immunotherapy-treated patient. Int Arch Allergy Appl Immunol 1988; 86:288–294.
21. Hahn BH, Ebling FM. Suppression of murine lupus nephretis by administration of an anti-idiotypic antibody anti-DNA. J Immunol 1984; 132:187–190.
22. Hahn BH, Ebling FM. Suppression of NZB/NZW murine nephritis by administration of syngenic monoclonal antibody to DNA. J Clin Invest 1983; 71:1728–1736.
23. Uner AH, Knupp CJ, Tatum AH, Gavalchin J. Treatment with antibody reactive with the nephritogenic idiotype, IdLNF1, suppresses its production and leads to prolonged survival of (NZB × SWR) F_1 mice. J Autoimmun 1994; 7:27–44.
24. Agius MA, Richman DP. Suppression of development of experimental autoimmune myasthenia gravis with isogeneic monoclonal anti-idiotopic antibody. J Immunol 1986; 137:2195–2198.
25. Neilson EG, Phillips MS. Suppression of interstitial nephritits by auto-anti-idiotypic immunity. J Exp Med 1982; 155:179–189.
26. Roubaty C, Bedin C, Charreire J. Prevention of experimental autoimmune thyroiditis through the anti-idiotypic network. J Immunol 1990; 144:2167–2172.
27. Balazs C, Molnar I. In vitro suppression of anti-TSH receptor antibody by autologous anti-idiotypic antibody in patients with Graves' disease. Acta Microbiol Immunnol Hung 1995; 42:163–169.
28. De Kozak Y, Mirshahi M. Experimental autoimmune uveoretinitis: idiotypic regulation and disease suppression. Int Ophthalmol 1990; 14:43–56.
29. Zanetti M, Glotz R, Rogers J. Perturbation of autoimmune network. II. Immunization with isologous idiotype induces autoantiidiotypic antibodies and suppresses the immune response elicited by antigen. J Immunol 1986; 137:3140–3146.
30. Dietrich G, Kazatchkine MD. Normal immunoglobulin G (IgG) for therapeutic use (intravenous Ig) contain antiidiotypic specificities against an immunodominant, disease-associated, cross-reactive idiotype of human anti-thyroglobulin autoantibodies. J Clin Invest 1990; 85:620-625.
31. Gajdos PH, Outin H, Elkharrat D, et al. High-dose intravenous immunoglobulin for myasthenia gravis. Lancet 1984; 1:406–407.
32. McGuire WA, Yong H, Bruno E, et al. Treatment of antibody-mediated pure red cell aplasia with high dose intravenous gammaglobulin. N Engl J Med 1987; 317:1004–1008.
33. Clauvel JP, Vainchenker W, Herrera A, et al. Treatment of pure red cell aplasia by high dose intravenous immunoglobulins. Br J Haematol 1983; 55:380–382.
34. Imbach P, d'Apuzzo V, Baumgartner C, et al. High doses intravenous gammaglobulin for idiopathic thrombocytopenic purpura in childhood. Lancet 198; 1:1228–1230.
35. Mc Intyre EA, Linch DC, Maccy MG, Newland AC. Successful response to intravenous immunoglobulin in autoimmune haemolitic anaemia. Br J Haematol 1985; 60:287–288.
36. Pollack S, Cunningham-Rhundles C, Smithwick EM, Barandun S, Good RA. High-dose intravenous gammaglobulin for autoimmune neutropenia. N Engl J Med 1982; 309:243–255.
37. Sany J. Intravenous immunoglobulin therapy for rheumatic diseases. Curr Opin Rheumatol 1994; 6:305–310.
38. Evans M, Abdou NI. In vitro modulation of anti-DNA secreting peripheral blood mononuclear cells of lupus patients by anti-idiotypic antibody of pooled human intravenous immune globulin. Lupus 1993; 2:371–375.
39. Silvestris F, D'Amore O, Cafforio P, Savino L, Dammacco F. Intravenous immunoglobulin therapy of lupus nephritis: use of pathogenic anti-DNA-reactive IgG. Clin Exp Immunol 1996; 104 (suppl 1):91–97.
40. Kazatchkine MD, Dietrich G, Hurez V, et al. V region-mediated selection of autoreactive repertoire by intravenous immunoglobulin. Immunol Rev 1994; 139:79–107.
41. Rigal D, Vermot-Desroches C, Heitz S, Bernaud J, Alfonsi F, Monier JC. Effects of intravenous immunoglobulins (IVIG) on peripheral blood B, NK, and T cell subpopulations in

women with recurrent spontaneous abortions: specific effects on LFA-1 and CD56 molecules. Clin Immunol Immunopathol 1994; 71:309–314.
42. Aukurst P, Froland SS, Liabakk NB, et al. Release of cytokines, soluble cytokine receptors, and interleukin-1 receptor antagonist after intravenous immunoglobulin administration in vivo. Blood 1994; 84:2136–2143.
43. Tumiati B, Casoli P, Veneziani M, Rinaldi G. High-dose immunoglobulin therapy as an immunomodulatory treatment of rheumatoid arthritis. Arthritis Rheum 1992; 35:1126–1133.
44. Blaser K, Geiser M, de Weck AL. Suppression of phosphorylcholine-specific IgE antibody formation in Balb/c mice by isologous anti-T15 antiserum. Eur J Immunol 1979; 9:1017–1020.
45. Blaser K, Nakagama T, De Weck AL. Suppression of the benzylpenicilloyl (BPO)-specific IgE formation with isologous antiidiotypic antibodies in Balb/c mice. J Immunol 1980; 125:24–30.
46. Blaser K, Nakagawa T, de Weck AL. Investigation of a syngenic murine model for the study of IgE antibody regulation with isologous aId antibodies. Int Arch Allergy Appl Immunol 1981; 64:42–50.
47. Blaser K, de Weck AL. Regulation of the IgE antibody response by idiotype–anti-idiotype network. Prog Allergy 1982; 32:203–264.
48. Hirano T, Kojima S, Hirayama N, et al. Presence of interstrain cross-reactive idiotype on A/J antibodies of the IgE class specific for *p*-azophenylarsonate group. J Immunol 1983; 130:1300–1302.
49. Hirai Y, Lamoyi E, Dohi Y, Nisonoff A. Regulation of expression of a family of cross-reactive idiotype. J Immunol 1981; 126:71–74.
50. Malley A, Brandt CJ, Deppe LB. Preparation and characterization of the anti-idiotypic properties of rabbit anti-timothy antigen B helper factor and anti-mouse timothy IgE antisera. Immunology 1982; 45:217–225.
51. Malley A, Dresser DW. Anti-idiotype regulation of timothy grass pollen IgE antibody formation. I. In vivo induction of suppressor T cells. Immunology 1982; 46:653–659.
52. Mourad W, Hébert J. Human IgG and murine monoclonal antibodies share common idiotopes as determined by competitive binding to polystyrene and nitrocellulose-bound antigens. Immunol Invest 1986; 15:801–811.
53. Mourad W, Bernier D, Hébert J. Mapping of Lol p 1 allergenic epitopes by using murine monoclonal antibodies. Mol Immunol 1989; 26:1051–1057.
54. Mécheri S, Mourad W, Lapeyre J, Jobin M, David B, Hébert J. Demonstration of idiotypes expressed on basophils-bound IgE antibodies by using anti-idiotype-induced histamine release in grass pollen-allergic patients. Immunology 1988; 64:11–15.
55. Zhou EM, Kisil FT. Regulation of levels of serum antibodies to ryegrass pollen allergen Lol p 4 by an internal image anti-idiotypic monoclonal antibody. Immunology 1995; 84:343–349.
56. Hébert J, Bernier D, Boutin Y, Jobin M, Mourad W. Generation of anti-idiotypic and anti-anti-idioptypic monoclonal antibodies in the same fusion. Support of Jerne's network theory. J Immunol 1990; 144:4256–4261.
57. Boutin Y, Jobin M, Bernier D, Hébert J. Biological activity of monoclonal anti-idiotypic antibody representing the internal image of Lol p 1. Int Arch Allergy Appl Immunol 1993; 102:10–14.
58. Boutin Y, Hébert J. Modulation of immune response to Lol p 1 by pretreatment with anti-idiotypic antibody is not restricted to the idiotypic expression. Clin Exp Immunol 1994; 96:350–356.
59. Zhou EM, Kisil FT. Antibody response to allergen Lol p 4 are suppressed following adoptive transfer of B lymphocytes from the internal image anti-idiotypic antibody-treated mice. Cell Immunol 1995; 165:77–83.
60. De Kozak Y, Mirshahi M, Boucheix C, Faure J-P. Prevention of experimentally autoimmune uveoretinitis by active immunization with autoantigen-specific monoclonasl antibodies. Eur J Immunol 1987; 17:541–554.

61. Boutin Y, Hébert J. Suppression of immune response to Lol p 1 by administration of idiotype. J Allergy Clin Immunol 1995; 95:751–758.
62. Bousquet J, Fontez A, Aznar R, Robinet-Levy M, Michel F-B. Combination of passive and active immunization in honeybee venom immunotherapy. J Allergy Clin Immunol 1987; 79:947–954.
63. Müller UR, Morris T, Bischof M, Friedli H, Skarvil F. Combined active and passive immunotherapy in honeybee-venom allergy. J Allergy Clin Immunol 1986; 78:115–122.
64. Lessof MH, Sobotka AK, Lichtenstein LM. Effect of passive antibody in bee venom anaphylaxis. Johns Hopkins Med J 1978; 142:1–7.
65. Mazer BD, Gelfand EW. An open-label study of high-dose intravenous immunoglobulin in severe childhood asthma. J Allergy Clin Immunol 1991; 87:976–983.
66. Khan RH, Szewczuck MR, Day JH. Bee venom anti-idiotypic antibody is associated with the protection in beekeepers and bee sting-sensitive patients receiving immunotherapy against allergic reaction. J Allergy Clin Immunol 1991; 88:199–208.
67. Boutin Y, Jobin M, Bédard P-M, Hébert M, Hébert J. The role of anti-idiotypic antibodies in combined passive and active immunotherapy in honeybee-sting allergy. J Allergy Clin Immunol 1994; 93:1039–1046.
68. Weyer A, Le Mao J, Etievant M, David B, Guinnepain MT, Saint-Rémy JM. Human auto-anti-idiotypic antibodies to mite-specific IgE can degranulate human basophils in vitro. Clin Exp Allergy 1995; 25:935–941.
69. Saint-Remy J-M, Lebecque SJ, Lebrun PM, Jacquemin MG. Human immune response to allergens of house dust mite, *Dermatophagoides pteronyssinus*. IV. Occurrence of natural autologous anti-idiotypic antibodies. Eur J Immunol 1988; 18:83–87.
70. Machiels JJ, Somville MA, Lebrun PM, Lebecque SJ, Jacquemin MG, Saint-Remy JMR. Allergic bronchial asthma due to *Dermatophagoides pteronyssinus* hypersensitivity can be efficiently treated by inoculation of allergen–antibody complexes. J Clin Invest 1990; 85:1024–1035.
71. Leroy BP, Boden G, Lachapelle JM, Jacquemin MG, Saint-Rémy JMR. A novel therapy for atopic dermatitis using antigen–antibody complexes: a double-blind placebo-controlled study. J Am Acad Dermatol 1993; 28:232–239.
72. Heyman B, Andrighetto G, Wigzell H. Antigen-dependent IgM-mediated enhancement of the sheep erythrocyte response in mice. Evidence for induction of B cells with specificities other than that of the injected antibodies. J Exp Med 1982; 155:994–1009.
73. Heyman B. The immune complex: possible ways of regulating the antibody response. Immunol Today 1990; 11:310–313.
74. Watts C, Lanzavecchia A. Suppressive effect of antibody on the processing of T cell epitopes. J Exp Med 1993; 178:1459–1463.

22

The Use of Allergen-Specific Antibodies for Immunotherapy

JEAN-MARIE R. SAINT-REMY

University of Leuven
Campus Gashuisberg
Leuven, Belgium

I. Introduction

Allergen-specific immunotherapies carry the obvious advantage over nonspecific methods of not altering other immune functions that can be physiologically important. One of such functions deals with the role of IgE in antigen presentation (1). On the other hand, suppressing the capacity to mount IgE toward an allergen might not be sufficient to achieve clinical efficacy: anaphylaxis can indeed occur in complete absence of IgE (2). For these reasons we chose to develop a method of treatment by which the production of antibodies toward predetermined allergens could be suppressed, independently of the isotype to which these antibodies belonged.

An allergen-specific therapy can be based on the use of allergens or derivatives, or on specific antibodies. The variable domains of an antibody are made of a series of determinants, called idiotopes. Idiotopes are located either in the antigen-binding region or between complementarity-determining regions; in the latter case, they are called framework or bystander idiotopes. The distinction between idiotopes, associated with the antigen-binding site and those making up the framework region, is important for the regulation of IgE production, as it will be fully explained later. Idiotypes, namely the ensemble of idiotopes carried by an antibody molecule, are immunogenic, and indeed, anti-idiotypic antibodies are produced as part of the normal immune response toward an antigen. Animal experiments have amply demonstrated that anti-idiotypic antibodies can suppress the production of antibodies carrying the corresponding idiotypes (3), a mechanism that is exquisitely specific for the idiotype under investigation. From animal data showing that this concept could be applied to antiallergen immune responses (see later discussion), we felt that inducing the production of anti-idiotypic antibodies to antiallergen antibodies could represent a valuable therapeutic approach for allergic diseases. It was later understood that antibodies had the capacity to alter their own production by yet another mechanism. The antigen processing and presentation to specific T cells in the context of major histocompatibility complex (MHC) can be profoundly altered whenever a specific antibody is added to the antigen (4). This was felt to be an additional potential advantage of using specific antibodies for therapy.

In the present chapter, I shall briefly review the evidence supporting a role for idiotype–anti-idiotype interactions in human immediate hypersensitivity reactions, as well as experimental data showing that an antiallergen immune response can be prevented or even downregulated by such interactions. The potential hazards of such a therapy will be considered before embarking on a more detailed description of the type of therapy we developed. Lastly, a number of open questions will be reviewed, together with current work and perspectives.

II. Antibody Idiotypes

A. Idiotypes in Human Immediate Hypersensitivity

Before describing the clinical application of idiotype–anti-idiotype interactions in human immediate hypersensitivity, it is worth summarizing a few experimental observations that establish the pertinence of such an application. To this end, four questions can basically be addressed:

1. Are anti-idiotypic antibodies produced spontaneously by atopic individuals? This would support the idea that idiotype regulation is part of a physiological mechanism of control of antibody production.
2. Are idiotypes carried by antiallergen antibodies of the IgG isotype identical with those carried by IgE of the same specificity? This would help us define whether or not IgE and IgG production can be regulated separately by the idiotypes they carry.
3. Are idiotypes carried by antiallergen antibodies shared among atopic individuals? This would help us decide whether an idiotype-based therapy could be designed to treat the ensemble of atopic individuals sensitive to a given allergen, or whether a patient-tailored therapy has to be designed.
4. Finally, does immunotherapy boost the production of anti-idiotypic antibodies?

Autoanti-Idiotypic Antibodies Are Spontaneously Produced by Atopic Individuals Toward Allergen-Specific Antibodies

Patients hypersensitive to *Dermatophagoides pteronyssinus* (*Dp*) produce anti-idiotypic antibodies that bind to purified autologous anti-*Dp* antibodies. Such anti-idiotypic antibodies bind primarily to idiotopes associated with the antigen-binding site (or paratope) of specific antibodies (5,6). Adsorption with anti-*Dp* antibody of the IgG isotype removed all anti-idiotypic antibodies toward bystander idiotopes of IgE, but not anti-idiotypic antibodies to paratope-associated idiotopes. From these results, it was concluded that bystander idiotopes are shared among specific anti-*Dp* antibody, IgG, and IgE for each individual, but paratope-associated idiotopes vary according to the isotype. The presence of autologous anti-idiotypic antibodies inhibiting the binding of IgE has also been demonstrated in ryegrass pollen allergy (7).

Idiotypes Associated with the Antigen-Binding Site Are Not Shared Between IgG and IgE

To determine whether the differences between idiotypes carried by IgE and IgG observed with autoanti-idiotypic antibodies were due to a true difference in antibody diversity, we raised heterologous anti-idiotypic antisera in rabbits. Such anti-idiotypic preparations, when adsorbed with anti-*Dp* antibodies of the IgG isotype, almost completely lost their capacity to recognize bystander idiotopes on specific IgE, indicating that the bystander idiotopes were shared between specific anti-*Dp* IgG and IgE for each individual (8). In contrast, such adsorption did not significantly reduce the binding of anti-idiotypic antibodies to paratope-associated idiotopes of IgE (9). In terms of molecular organization of the immunoglobulin genes encoding for antiallergen antibodies, the observation that bystander idiotypes are similar in IgG and IgE molecules in the same individual is consistent with the use of the same V region genes in IgG and IgE (8). The absence of cross-reactivity between the idiotopes in the antigen-binding site of IgG and IgE in a single individual may be due to allergen-driven somatic mutations of antibody complementary-determining regions. Altogether, this suggested that the production of both antiallergen IgG and IgE could be regulated either together, if bystander idiotypes were to be targeted, or separately, if idiotypes associated with the antigen-binding site were concerned.

Idiotypes Associated with the Antigen-Binding Site Are Shared Between Individuals

Cross-reactive idiotypes corresponding to antiallergen antibodies specific for ryegrass, house dust mite, or honeybee venom have been detected in atopic patients. Bose et al. have documented the presence of public idiotypic determinants expressed on human IgE and IgG antiryegrass antibodies (10). Rabbit anti-idiotypic antibodies have been produced against idiotypes of three murine anti-Lol p 1 monoclonal antibodies (MAbs) of different specificities. Idiotypes defined by such anti-idiotypic antibodies were present on IgE molecules of 30–80% of patients hypersensitive to ryegrass (11). In *Dp* hypersensitivity, the cross-reactivity of idiotypes carried by specific antibodies of unrelated individuals has been analyzed by separately examining idiotopes located close or in the antigen-binding site, or bystander idiotopes. This analysis of anti-house–dust mite-specific antibodies indicated a virtual absence of idiotype cross-reactivity at the level of framework idiotopes, whereas a remarkable degree of similarity was found when comparing idiotopes associated with the antigen-binding site (9). Human anti-idiotypic antibodies have also been used to this end, which confirmed the high degree of cross-reactivity on allergen-binding site-associated idiotopes (6). Cross-reactive idiotypes on anti-bee–venom antibodies were also detected in sting-sensitive patients, using anti-idiotypic preparations from two nonreactive beekeepers (12). Taken together, these data indicate that paratope-associated idiotypes are suitable candidates for designing a therapy applicable to most of atopic patients sensitive to a given allergen.

Conventional Desensitization Increases the Production of Anti-Idiotypic Antibodies

The influence of hyposensitization on the level of anti-idiotypic antibodies was investigated in ragweed-hypersensitive patients. Retrospective and prospective studies have suggested that the levels of anti-idiotypic antibodies in patients treated by hyposensitization was higher than in nonhyposensitized patients (13,14). In patients hypersensitive to *Lolium perenne*, immunotherapy also raised the levels of anti-idiotypic antibodies recognizing mouse MAbs directed toward Lol p 1 (15). This had also been shown by Bose et al. (16): In their groups of patients, there was an inverse relation between the changes in anti-idiotypes and those of anti-Lol p 1 antibodies. Hyperimmunization of patients allergic to honeybee stings also resulted in increased levels of anti-idiotypic antibodies in the serum and reduced specific IgG and IgE to honeybee venom (12).

B. Animal Experiments

Mice and guinea pigs are the two animal species that have been examined most thoroughly for the feasibility of suppressing IgE production (17). For the sake of clarity, one should distinguish active production of anti-idiotypic antibodies by animals immunized with isologous-specific antibodies, from passive transfer of isologous or heterologous anti-idiotypic antibodies. A further distinction should be established between the prevention of an IgE immune response and the downregulation of an ongoing IgE response. It is relatively easy to induce the production of anti-idiotypic antibodies using immunizing doses of isologous antibodies in adjuvant. This is a general property of antibody responses, and it has been amply demonstrated in systems other than that of the IgE immune response.

Broading speaking, the production of IgE can be suppressed in mice and guinea pigs either by active production of anti-idiotypic antibodies or by passive transfer of these antibodies, be they of isologous or heterologous origin (18). Animals producing anti-idiotypic antibodies are unable to mount a specific IgE immune response after subsequent immunization with alum-adsorbed proteins or hapten-carrier conjugates. This inability to produce IgE is both complete and long-lasting. The passive transfer of anti-idiotypic antibodies of isologous origin results in only a partial and short-term inhibition of IgE production, unless they are given repeatedly and at a sufficiently high dose.

However, it is much more difficult to suppress an *ongoing* IgE response. Here, active production of anti-idiotypic antibodies has not yielded convincing results. The repeated transfer of isologous anti-idiotypic antibodies or use of heterologous anti-idiotypic antibodies has perhaps been more successful. In other experiments, the production of anti-idiotypic antibodies to anticarrier antibodies (19), or the transfer of these antibodies to recipients (20) has also been attempted with some success. The state of suppression, however, frequently remains transient because subsequent exposure to antigen usually restores IgE production.

The regulation of IgE production in experimental animals by the use of antigen–antibody complexes—namely, by a procedure similar to that used in our clinical trials (see later discussion)—has been described in three recent publications. Thus, rats pretreated with complexes made from egg albumin and specific antiserum were unable to mount a primary or secondary IgE immune response toward egg albumin, provided the complexes were made at equivalence, or better, in antibody excess; in this latter case, however, the total production of antibodies to egg albumin is reduced (21). Guinea pigs can develop anaphylaxis together with bronchial hyperreactivity in response to an inhalation challenge with ovalbumin; pretreatment by regular injections of ovalbumin–antiovalbumin complexes has a transitory preventive effect on the induction of anaphylaxis, but this effect is not superior to that obtained with injections of ovalbumin alone (22). The IgE response to the same antigen can be inhibited in mice receiving intravenous injections of antigen–antibody complexes made at equivalence, provided these complexes are made of whole isologous antibodies and administered before the antigen (23).

C. From Animal Models to Patients: Risks Bound to Idiotypic Regulation

Increasing the production of anti-idiotypic antibodies carries the risk of cross-linking specific IgE at the surface of mast cells or basophils (24). Indeed, human anti-idiotypic antibodies have the capacity to degranulate human basophils in vitro in a highly specific manner (25). Whether they do so in vivo is more debatable, for the only data contained in humans have been obtained by using anti-idiotypic antibodies of rabbit origin. However, we would consider the risk of producing such an activation in vivo as very limited. Indeed, cross-linking of two IgE molecules by an anti-idiotypic antibody requires that two IgE molecules of exactly the same specificity are present at the cell surface, a situation that is definitely different from the cross-linking of IgE by allergens presenting several IgE-binding regions. Therefore, we would consider that anti-idiotypic antibodies are only weak degranulators. An intriguing hypothesis is whether such anti-idiotypic antibodies can produce a state of tachyphylaxis.

Idiotopes carried by specific antiallergen antibodies might be shared by antibodies of other specificities, which is part of the original concept of the idiotypic network (26) and has received confirmation in several experimental systems. Antibodies recognizing an idiotope would suppress the production of any antibody carrying the same idiotope, irrespective of the antibody specificity. However, anti-idiotypic antibodies raised to a set of idiotopes (an idiotype) suppress the production of antibodies carrying the same set of idiotopes (27). To the extent that we use affinity-purified antiallergen antibodies, this question might not be relevant.

III. Clinical Application

A. Methods

Allergen Preparations

Allergen preparations used in our studies were all obtained from Bencard Ltd (Epsom, Surrey, UK). Two types of extracts have been used: an extract of *Dp* and an extract containing 12 common grass pollens (B2).

The *Dp* preparations showed three main bands corresponding to Der p 2, Der p 1, and Der p 3 on sodium dodecyl sulfate–polyacrylamide gel electrophoresis (SDS–PAGE), plus two additional bands with an apparent molecular weight (MW) of 42,000 kDa and one at 60,000 kDa, respectively, not identified at the time these studies were carried out. Der p 1 and Der p 2 represented 25 and 12% of total protein content in the allergen preparation, respectively. Cyclic AMP receptor protein (CAP) inhibition assay, using an atopic serum pool, indicated that 5 ng of the *Dp* preparations inhibited 50% of the antibody binding. In vivo testing showed that 20 ng of allergens produced a wheal-and-flare reaction of a size identical with that obtained with a 1-mg/mL histamine solution. The grass pollen extract used in some studies contained 5-10% material precipitable by specific antibodies and yielded a histamine index of 25 ng.

Preparation of Specific Antibodies

Serum or plasma samples were first precipitated by addition of salt to eliminate the bulk of serum proteins, primarily albumin, which could otherwise contaminate the preparations. The samples were then submitted to chromatography over a gel filtration column to remove IgM from the other immunoglobulins. Specific antiallergen IgM was indeed detected in serum of atopic patients; the rationale for removing it from the samples was based on evidence indicating that IgM can enhance an immune response instead of the hoped-for reduction (28). The final purification step used immunoadsorption; the specific antibodies present in the samples were retained on a solid-phase column to which the allergen in question had been covalently coupled; the antibodies were subsequently removed by a dissociating agent. Sepharose was chosen as the solid phase because of its relatively low retention of nonspecific antibodies, its rigidity to mechanical pressure, and its versatility: the diversity of reactive groups available on different types of Sepharose allowed comparison of different activation and coupling methods. Carbodiimide coupling of allergen to carboxylated Sepharose was selected on the basis of its reproducibility, its capacity to retain specific IgE, and a minimal degree of antigen denaturation.

By using the foregoing method, we found a mean final yield of 14 ± 0.6 (average ± SEM) μg of specific antibodies to *Dp* per milliliter of initial serum of 80 hypersensitive patients suffering from bronchial asthma, including patients who had never been hyposensitized. We determined the isotypic distribution of specific antibodies, isolated, as just described. In asthmatic patients, IgG accounted for 85% of the total immunoglobulin content, whereas IgA represented 15% and IgE between 0.1 and 0.2%. Subclass distribution of IgG was as follows: 26.1% IgG1, 58.5% IgG2, 3.3% IgG3 and 12% IgG4. For the sake of comparison, the mean recovery of specific anti-*Dp* antibodies in atopic dermatitis reached 36 ± 1.1 μg/mL, whereas the average yield was 7 ± 0.3 μg/mL in grass pollen hypersensitivity. The presence of contaminating nonspecific proteins in the specific antibody preparations was examined by immunoephelometry, immunoelectrophoresis, and radioimmunoassay (29). No albumin, haptoglobin, α-antitrypsin, complement C3, or transferrin was detected, indicating that contamination by any of these proteins was lower than 0.1%. Anti-isotypic or antiallotypic antibodies were not found. The SDS–PAGE analysis of reduced samples showed only two bands corresponding to the MW of antibody heavy and light chains.

Antibodies recovered in the eluates retained their allergen-binding capacity. Indeed, 83% of eluted IgE was still capable of binding to the allergen (*Dp*) insolubilized on a different solid-phase (polystyrene particles). For specific anti-*Dp* IgE, the proportion reached 87% of the total IgE in the eluates. The solutions containing specific antibodies were also examined by ultracentrifugation on a 5–30% sucrose density gradient; it showed that 93.4% of the protein sedimented at 7S. When an excess of soluble *Dp* was added to antibodies, 70% of the 7S peak moved toward a higher molecular weight position, thereby confirming that the antibody preparations contained a high proportion of specific antibodies. The purified antibodies were capable of in vivo neutralization of the wheal reaction resulting from the injection of allergen; when the eluates were heated, under conditions sufficient to destroy the capacity of IgE to bind to its specific mast cell surface receptor, and mixed with allergen, there was no reaction, even when the amount of allergen was 100-fold higher than that used in skin testing with allergen alone.

Preparation of Allergen–Antibody Complexes

For several reasons we have always considered that, for therapeutic purposes, complexes of allergens with specific antibodies should be prepared in an excess of antibody. The first reason is that such complexes are efficient inducers of anti-idiotypic antibodies (30). A second reason is to ensure that all relevant (e.g., IgG-binding allergen) epitopes are masked by specific antibodies. The expected consequence of this is a significant reduction of the immediate wheal-and-flare reaction following intradermal injection. We have verified in vivo that neutralization of allergen epitopes by excess of specific antibodies was indeed obtained with both *Dp* and grass pollen; the quantity of allergen that could be administered to the patients in the form of a complex could thus be increased at least 100-fold, compared with the amount of free allergen. Third, complexes made in antibody excess are generally less soluble and of larger size than complexes made in antigen excess, which theoretically should reduce the diffusion rate after injection; complexes in antibody excess will also have altered complement-activating capacities. A "depot" effect, avoiding rapid clearance away from the injection site, was thought to be desirable to have a sustained immunogenicity of complexes.

The average ratio of allergen over antibody was 1:5 (w/w) in allergic bronchial asthma patients. Considering the differences in molecular weight of the antibody and the average molecular weight of allergen, on one hand, and the fact that allergen preparations contain molecules that are not immunogenic, on the other hand, this weight/weight ratio is very close to the actual molar ratio. This reasoning applies to *Dp* and to grass pollen allergen solutions; in the latter, the amount of material bound to specific antibodies lies between 5 and 10% of the total protein content. Both allergen and antibody solutions were diluted in 9 g/L NaCl containing 0.3% human serum albumin and 0.4% phenol as a preservative. Allergen and antibodies were mixed at the predetermined ratio and incubated for 2 h at 37°C and overnight at 4°C. Complexes were then stored at –80°C until immediately before use. Allergen–antibody complexes were analyzed by ultracentrifugation on a 5–30% sucrose gradient. At the allergen/antibody ratio used for the injections, the proportion of antibodies bound to allergens reached a mean of 57.3%. The size distribution showed that complexes containing one, two, three, four, five, or six antibody molecules represented 25.8, 30.2, 12.9, 10.1, 7.7, and 12.9% of the total amount of complexes, respectively.

Choice of a Dosage Regimen

The amount of complexes injected followed loosely the pattern normally used for allergen alone in conventional hyposensitization; that is very small initial doses, building up to a so-called maintenance dose. In the first injection, patients received a quantity of allergen equivalent to that which would have been given if allergen alone was used. However, over the whole injection schedule, these quantities usually increased by only a factor of 20, instead of 500–1000, as in conventional hyposensititization. This conservative approach was chosen for two main reasons. The first was caution: some dissociation of complexes might occur after injection, depending, among other factors, on the affinity of specific antibodies or on any denaturation during the preparation procedures. The second was that such an injection schedule might also allow the determination of a threshold dose (i.e., a minimum amount of complexes the injection of which would result in a significant biological or clinical effect).

Choice of an Injection Route

Because the aim of the therapy was the increase of the immune response toward idiotopes carried by antiallergen antibodies, it was felt that the intradermal route was preferable. The intradermal route has long been recognized as more "immunogenic" than the subcutaneous one because of the richness of immunocompetent cells in the dermis. Another important factor is that the rate of diffusion of injected material was from an intradermal site of injection is far slower than that from the subcutaneous site. Apart from further reducing the risk of immediate side effects, this fact alone also increases the immunogenicity by increasing the contact time between the material injected and the relevant immunocompetent cells.

B. Clinical Study Design

In clinical studies we have now examined the possibility of reducing the antiallergen immune response to two types of allergens, *Dp* and grass pollens. In close collaboration with Dr. Jacques Machiels (Service de Pneumologie, Clinique Saint-Pierre, Ottignies, Belgium), we designed a series of studies to evaluate the effect of allergen–antibody complex injection in patients suffering from upper or lower respiratory tract symptoms after exposure to these allergens. In addition, the clinical potential of complex injection in atopic dermatitis has also been examined in studies carried out in conjunction with Dr. Bernard Leroy (Service de Dermatologie professionnelle et de l'Environnement, Clinique Saint-Luc, Bruxelles, Belgium).

The patients who participated in the initial studies presented several characteristics that otherwise might have excluded them from conventional desensitization trials. This was particularly true for patients suffering from perennial asthma. Indeed, in the category of patients selected here, asthma could obviously be exacerbated by various factors quite distinct from allergen sensitivity. Moreover, a substantial number of patients presented a sensitivity to several allergens, unrelated to the single one used for the treatment. The patients participating in grass pollen hypersensitivity trials were those with intractable nasal symptoms and most of them also suffered from seasonal asthma. The reasons for choosing such patients were twofold. Because this type of treatment had never been used before in humans, we were confronted with an ethical issue; it was thought that the patients should have first been offered every currently available treatment, be it pharmacological or immunotherapy, and to have shown no significant benefit. Similarly, we considered it ethically justified to choose patients whose treatment required the use of drugs bearing an unacceptable risk of side effects (e.g., systemic corticotherapy). Second, our goal was to develop a therapy that would be useful to severely ill patients.

All studies carried out so far were designed as double-blind, placebo-controlled studies. The placebo group received injections of the carrier buffer alone at injection frequencies identical with those patients receiving allergen–antibody complexes. The symptoms of the patients were followed with the help of daily diary cards, on which the patients were asked to score their symptoms of asthma or rhinitis twice a day; the intensity of each symptom was evaluated on a discontinuous intensity scale. By summing each single score for each day, a mean score index was calculated, which also took into account, within the group considered, the proportion of patients suffering from the symptom. Objective assessment of the patients' physical status and appraisal of the accuracy with which they filled out their cards was made possible through regular outpatient visits, which were usually made once every-other-week for the first few months and, thereafter, monthly. The use of modification was also followed by daily recording of the quantity of drugs taken; these scores were computed in the same way as the clinical scores. The functional follow-up consisted of an evaluation of basal lung function performed at regular intervals and the daily monitoring of peak expiratory flows recorded four times a day, in the morning and at night, each time before and after medication. Nonspecific bronchial reactivity to acetylcholine inhalation was also monitored to reflect the bronchial status of the patients.

The evolution of parameters specific for the considered allergen sensitivity was also recorded. For asthma, in addition to intradermal testing with allergens, bronchial provocation tests were performed on a regular basis. These challenges, although somewhat artificial in that the quantity—and the physical form—of allergens inhaled exceeds natural exposure to the allergen, are thought to represent a reliable indicator of the bronchial reactivity of the patient. Biological parameters followed during the clinical trials included the serum concentration of specific antiallergen antibodies, corresponding anti-idiotypic antibodies and anti-isotypic antibodies.

C. Clinical Outcome

We conducted a series of clinical trials, which involved a total of about 350 patients suffering from either perennial asthma (with or without rhinitis) caused by hypersensitivity to *Dp*, or seasonal asthma with rhinitis in relation to hypersensitivity to grass pollens (31–34). More recently, we have treated several patients with atopic dermatitis and hypersensitivity to *Dp* (35,36). The salient features of these studies can be summarized as follows:

Safety of the Treatment

The injection of allergen–antibody complexes seems to be completely innocuous; no systemic or even significant local side effects were observed in a total of about 3000 injections.

Clinical Efficacy

The *Dp* hypersensitive patients showed a marked reduction in symptoms of asthma within a few weeks after the beginning of treatment and their clinical condition continued to improve progressively thereafter. Whenever present, signs of allergic rhinitis gradually disappeared over time. The treatment completely prevented the appearance of bronchial asthma related to pollen exposure, whereas 60% of placebo patients experienced regular bronchospastic reactions (Fig. 1). A significant reduction of rhinorrhea and sneezing was noted, and none of the treated patients complained of nasal obstruction.

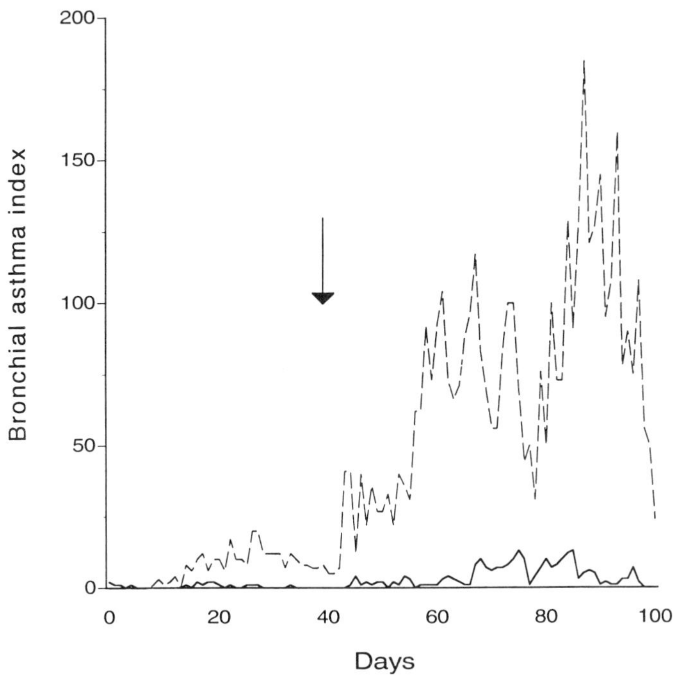

Figure 1 Evolution of bronchial asthma symptoms of patients treated by intradermal injections of allergen–antibody complexes (——) versus placebo (– – –) during the grass pollen season: Thirteen patients with sensitivity to grass pollens, as demonstrated by seasonal symptoms, positive skin-prick tests, and presence of specific serum IgE antibodies, were treated by injections of complexes made of autologus specific antibodies and of grass pollen allergens. A total cumulative amount of 5.6 μg antibodies and 0.56 μg allergen was administered during the pollen season. The 12 patients of the control group received injections of carrier buffer. Symptoms of bronchial asthma were followed with the help of diary cards, averaged daily, and the mean score was multiplied by the percentage of symptomatic patients within the group. The arrow indicates the start of the pollen season. (From Ref. 33.)

Medication

The first significant reduction in medication intake was noted after only 10 weeks of treatment of perennial asthma; a few months later one-third of the patients were able to do so without regular drug treatment, using β-adrenergic agonists only occasionally. Systemic corticosteroids were no longer used by treated patients after 3 months of treatment, whereas 60% of the placebo patients still had to use them regularly. No bronchodilators were taken for the prevention of seasonal asthma. Antihistamines were used at a significantly lower frequency in the treated group.

Parameters of Specific Reactivity

A 99% reduction in the wheal-and-flare reaction resulting from the intradermal injection of a standard amount of *Dp* allergen was observed after the second year of treatment. The amount of *Dp* that, after inhalation, induced a 35% fall in specific airway conductance gradually increase over time to reach a mean of 70 times the initial value. More than one-third of the treated patients had lost their bronchial reactivity to allergen inhalation by the second year of treatment, whereas none of the placebo patients showed any such improvement (Fig. 2).

Long-Term Effects of the Treatment

In *Dp*-hypersensitive patients, an indication that the treatment could reduce the nonspecific bronchial reactivity, in addition to its effect on inhaled allergen reactivity, was observed after the third year of follow-up. Half the treated patients had then completely lost their reactivity to inhalation of acetylcholine; the same observation was made at the end of the fourth year, even though no further injections had been administered to the patients during the previous year (Fig. 3). This unexpected and encouraging result indicates that bronchial hyperreactivity, the main characteristics of asthma, is reversible. With the possible exception of long-term avoidance of exposure to allergen—and this only with impracticably drastic avoidance measures—or perhaps, maintenance therapy on high doses of inhaled corticosteroids, this effect has never been observed with any other therapy. Injections of allergen–antibody complexes, therefore, could, carry the potential of improving forms of asthma that do not directly depend on allergen inhalation, such as exercise-induced asthma.

Overall Benefit

The overall benefit of this therapy is exemplified by the significant improvements brought to the everyday life of patients. Indeed, together with a nearly normal attendance at school or work, they resumed sports, travel, and holidays.

D. Biological Outcome

The working hypothesis behind this treatment was that the production of anti-idiotypic antibodies could be boosted by injection of antiallergen antibodies; if this

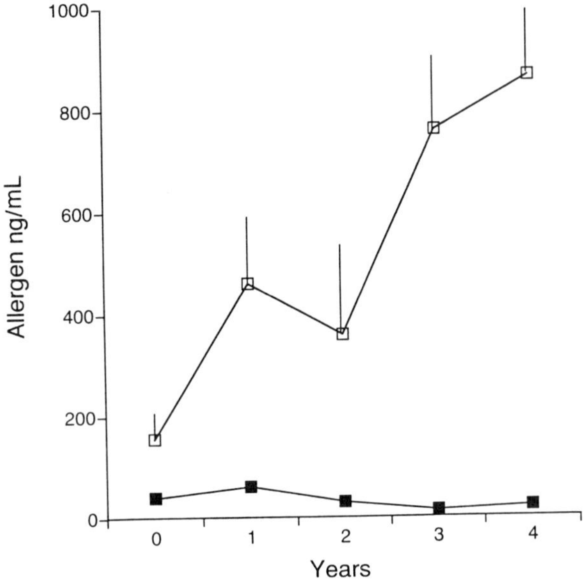

Figure 2 Bronchial reactivity to *D. pteronyssinus* allergen (*Dp*) inhalation: Variation with time of the mean concentration of *Dp,* the inhalation of which resulted in a 35% reduction of specific airway conductance. Vertical bars represent SEM. Seven patients (□) suffering from severe chronic bronchial asthma and sensitive to *Dp* were treated with intradermal injections of allergen–antibody complexes containing a total cumulative amount of 15 μg specific autologous anti-*Dp* antibodies and 3 μg of *Dp* allergens. The control group (■) consisted of seven patients treated by injections of the carrier buffer. *Dp* bronchial challenge was carried out by gradually increasing the amount of inhaled allergens until a reduction in specific airway conductance of more than 35% was achieved. The amount of allergen needed to obtain exactly 35% reduction was calculated from the dose–response curve. By years 3 and 4, the number of treated patients who had become unresponsive to the maximum administered concentration of 1 μg/mL *Dp* was five and six, respectively, versus none in the control group. Results of the treated group were significantly different from starting values at each time point except at the start of the study (Wilcoxon matched pairs analysis, $p < 0.05$ in each case). (From Ref. 32.)

turned out to be true, we wanted to examine whether this increase would result in a decrease in the production of antiallergen antibodies carrying corresponding idiotypes. Therefore, we put much emphasis on the analysis of the evolution of both specific antiallergen antibodies and anti-idiotypic antibodies (37).

Specific IgE Antibodies

Apart from minor differences, the same results were found in *Dp* and grass pollen hypersensitivity, in asthma, and in atopic dermatitis. In *Dp* hypersensitive bronchial

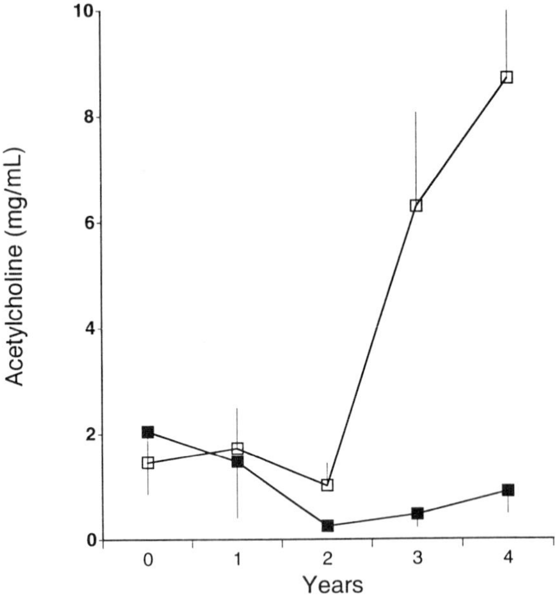

Figure 3 Bronchial reactivity to acetylcholine inhalation: Variation with time of the mean concentration of acetylcholine, the inhalation of which resulted in a 35% reduction of specific airway conductance. Vertical bars represent SEM. Patient groups are the same as in Figure 2. By the end of years 3 and 4, four and six treated patients (□), respectively, were unresponsive to the maximum administered concentration of 10 mg/mL acetylcholine, versus none in the control group (■). Results of the treated group were significantly different from starting values at the end of years 3 and 4 (Wilcoxon matched pairs analysis, $p < 0.05$ in each case). (From Ref. 32.)

asthma, a progressive decline of specific IgE was observed, becoming statistically significant at the tenth week of treatment; this decline was not preceded by an increase in IgE concentrations, as observed in conventional immunotherapy. Three months after the beginning of the treatment, IgE concentration reached a minimum value and remained at that level for at least the 2 years during which they were measured. In grass pollen hypersensitivity, the treatment was initiated shortly before the pollen season. We observed that specific IgE levels did not increase during the subsequent exposure to pollen, and that IgE levels progressively declined afterward, such that 1 year after the beginning of the treatment, they attained values significantly lower than the initial ones.

*Specific Anti-*Dp *IgG Antibodies*

The specific antibodies followed a similar initial pattern, with an early reduction in serum concentration. In grass pollen hypersensitivity, the serum concentration of specific IgG was unchanged during the pollen season, whereas, it increased steadily in placebo patients.

Antibodies Toward Affinity-Purified Dp *Allergens*

The concentration of antibodies towards Der p 1, Der p 2, and Der p 3 was assessed before and after 4 months of treatment, using specific ELISA. From Figure 4, it can be seen that a significant reduction of both IgE and IgG serum levels was obtained within this time frame.

Specificity of Antibody Suppression

By taking advantage of the sharing of epitopes between Der p 1 and Der f 1, we were able to demonstrate that administration of allergen–antibody complexes

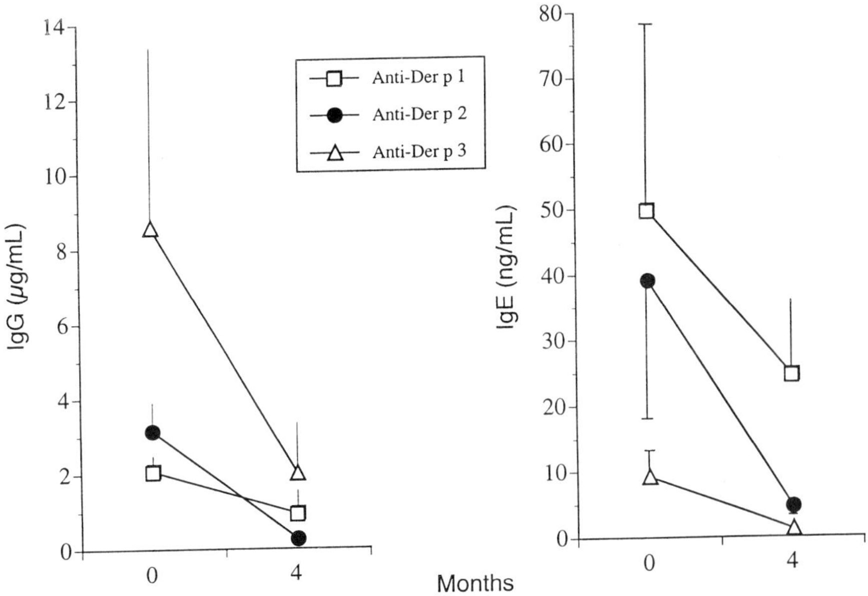

Figure 4 Evolution of the mean concentration of IgG and IgE to affinity-purified Der p 1, Der p 2, and Der p 3 allergens before and after 4 months of treatment with allergen–antibody complexes: Vertical bars represent SEM. Seventeen patients suffering from severe atopic dermatitis and sensitivity to *Dp* were treated by intradermal injections of complexes made of autologous specific anti-*Dp* antibodies and of *Dp*. A total cumulative amount of 240 μg specific antibodies and 60 μg *Dp* was administered over 4 months. The concentrations of specific IgG and IgE were measured in an ELISA system in which the binding of a predetermined concentration of anti-*Dp* antibodies to *Dp* was inhibited by an excess of the corresponding affinity-purified soluble allergen. A significant reduction of antibody titer was observed in each case (Wilcoxon matched-pairs analysis, $p < 0.02$) except for anti-Der p 1 IgE. (From Ref. 37.)

induced a suppression of the production of antibodies that were actually present in the complexes used for injection. Thus, the production of antibodies recognizing Der f 1 epitopes shared by Der p 1 was downregulated, whereas that of species-specific Der f 1 antibodies was not.

Antibodies of Unrelated Specificity

The concentration of antibodies of unrelated specificity was unaffected by the treatment. For instance, the level of IgE to allergens unrelated to those included in the allergen–antibody complexes did not change significantly. However, it was regularly observed that the level of total IgE was reduced after a few months of treatment. The level of total IgG remained constant, as did the isotypic distribution of IgG.

Anti-Idiotypic Antibodies

A rapid and sustained raise in the level of anti-idiotypic antibodies to specific anti-*Dp* antibodies was observed in both bronchial asthma and in atopic dermatitis patients. For technical reasons, the assay of anti-idiotypic antibodies was limited to those antibodies having the capacity to inhibit the binding of specific antibodies to allergens. We have recently shown, through the use of affinity-purified allergen Der p 1, that the level of anti-idiotypic antibodies was indeed very much increased after treatment. However, a few patients presenting significant clinical improvement did not show any significant increase in the level of corresponding anti-idiotypic antibodies.

IV. State of the Art

The injection of allergen–antibody complexes represents a novel approach to the treatment of IgE-mediated diseases and compares favorably with conventional immunotherapy for a number of reasons.

Safety

We have shown that allergen–antibody injections do not carry the risk of local or systemic anaphylactic reactions. This is to be expected when one considers two characteristics of the material used: first, the amount of allergen present in the complexes is at least two orders of magnitude lower than in conventional desensitization and, second, the specific antibodies mask epitopes otherwise able to bind to mastocyte-bound IgE.

Indications for Allergen–Antibody Therapy

This therapy was initially developed primarily for the treatment of allergic asthma, rather than, for example, allergic rhinitis. The reasons for this are twofold: first, upper respiratory tract symptoms are easily manageable by the use of currently available drugs, such as antihistamines or nebulized corticosteroids; second, conventional desensitization is effective in the treatment of rhinitis, whereas its efficacy in bronchial asthma is still disputed. There is no doubt that injections of allergen–antibody complexes can improve not only the symptoms evoked by exposure to allergens, but also, and most importantly, the nonspecific bronchial reactivity in bronchial asthma. Therefore, it could be speculated that, whenever an allergen—or a small number of allergens—is identified as major, on the basis of its clinical relevance, a specific treatment could be initiated that would result first in a disappearance of bronchial reactivity to that allergen and, subsequently, in an improvement of asthma in general. Apart from the fact that our treatment can be applied with success to bronchial asthma, it is obvious that it could also be applied to conditions in which conventional desensitization cannot even be envisaged. Some allergens are too dangerous to be used in free form: examples of this are food allergens, such as ovalbumin or peanut, and drug allergens, such as penicillin.

Rapidity of Action

Conventional hyposensitization usually requires several months of treatment before showing the first signs of clinical benefit. For instance, a treatment for grass pollen hypersensitivity takes a mean of 2 years before being fully effective. A prominent advantage of the current therapy is the rapidity with which the results can be obtained. As was indeed true in our studies of grass pollen hypersensitivity, the treatment can be applied during the pollen season itself, while achieving its full efficacy within a few weeks.

Material Used for Injection

It is of interest to compare the amount of material that was used during the clinical trials reported here with that used for conventional hyposensitization. The total quantity of allergen administered in the form of complex with specific antibodies is 100- to 350-fold less than that which would have been used for allergen alone, and even this does not take into account the maintenance treatment that usually follows the induction phase of conventional hyposensitization. The amount of specific antibodies administered during the treatment does not exceed 15 μg in asthma. In atopic dermatitis, however, 100–300 μg of specific antibodies had to be given. These values correspond to the quantity of antibodies contained in approximately 1 or 10 mL of serum, respectively.

Biological Alterations

The selective and parallel reduction of both specific IgE and IgG suggests that allergen–antibody complexes selectively suppress the production of antiallergen antibodies in vivo. One could, however, argue that the reduction in specific IgE per se is not sufficient to explain the clinical benefit of the treatment. We think that an important component of the therapy is the capacity to downregulate the production of specific IgG in addition to IgE.

V. Open Questions

One of the main difficulties we have encountered is related to the preparation of specific antibodies. Insolubilization of an allergen on a solid-phase column inevitably results in loss of accessibility to some epitopes, either because the three-dimentional conformation of the allergen has been altered or because the coupling procedure involves determinants that are important for antibody binding. Moreover, it can be difficult to desorb antibodies from the immunosorbent without denaturation. The overall result is that the preparation procedure can be relatively uncertain, which can severely impair the clinical outcome, for the latter would depend on the presence of a full repertoire of specific antibodies in the injection material. Novel methods for antibody purification are being evaluated.

A second limitation of the therapy is related to its autologous nature (i.e., each patient was treated with a preparation of his or her own antibodies). This restriction was dictated by ethical reasons and by the idiotype hypothesis that was at the basis of the therapy. However, some of our results on idiotype characterization (see foregoing), indicating that unrelated patients share idiotopes on antibodies directed toward a given allergen, would suggest that pools of gamma globulins could be used as a source of specific antibodies. To this end, however, we first wished to ensure that the risk of inducing an antiallotypic immune response would be limited. Therefore, we carried out a clinical trial in which patients were treated with injections of the $F(ab')_2$ fragments made from autologus antibodies (38). The favorable clinical outcome of such a study indicated not only that the Fc part of antibodies was not essential for obtaining a significant clinical outcome, but that the risk of alloimmunization could be reduced by previous digestion of specific antibodies.

A third point of concern deals with the criteria used to select patients who stand the best chance of improvement from such a therapy. Monosensitization to allergens is the exception more than the rule, and it remains sometimes difficult to identify which allergen is the most relevant in the induction of clinical symptoms. However, in most situations, one or two major allergen sensitizations are present, and one can therefore envision that a significant proportion of allergic patients could be treated with a restricted number of allergen–antibody complexes. Furthermore, there is no a priori reason why allergen–antibody complexes formed with several different allergens could not be used.

Along the same lines, one may question the validity of a therapy for which effects are limited to suppressing the production of antibodies that are used for injection. Apparently, however, it seems that in patients with an ongoing allergen sensitization, the repertoire of antibodies that are expressed at a given time point is sufficiently representative of the complete repertoire of antibodies the patients can make toward the allergen. Within the time-limited follow-up period, it does not appear as though new antibody molecules are produced. Practically, therefore, if the preparation contains antibodies representative of the full repertoire of specific antibodies made by patients, this might not be an issue.

VI. Current Work and Perspectives

Although there is convincing evidence that anti-idiotypic antibodies are produced as a result of injection of allergen–antibody complexes, the direct proof that such antibodies are playing a determining role in the successful clinical outcome is lacking. It still remains difficult to evaluate the precise function of anti-idiotypic antibodies when one has to use polyclonal anti-idiotypic antibodies. Therefore, we decided to produce human MAbs toward allergens through the transformation of peripheral B memory cells obtained from allergic individuals. This approach was preferred over alternatives, such as the use of phage-displayed libraries of antibody fragments, because we are interested in producing high-affinity specific antibodies that are part of the naturally expressed repertoire of antibodies. Monoclonal antibodies provide us with the idiotype sequences relevant to the immune response under scrutiny and, therefore, a means to obtain specific anti-idiotypic reagents to follow the titers of specific antibodies during injections with allergen–antibody complexes. In addition, such antibodies enable us to study the mechanisms by which an antibody toward an allergen can alter the way this allergen is processed and presented to T cells.

Through such an experimental approach, we can envisage several possibilities of modulating an antiallergen immune response by anti-idiotypic antibodies. Somewhat schematically, four possibilities can be outlined:

1. Anti-idiotypic antibodies carrying an internal image of the allergen could be used as a substitute for the allergen. This concept has proved to be feasible under several experimental conditions, and there is a priori no obstacle to apply such knowledge to human immediate hypersensitivity. A definite advantage would be that the degree of polymerization of such surrogate allergen epitopes could be altered, from monospecific—namely, unable to induce a cross-linking of antibodies at the surface of mast cells or basophils—to multispecific; namely, capable of inducing tolerance.
2. Anti-idiotypic antibodies could be used to modulate the production of antiallergen antibodies. Indeed, depending on the dose and route of injection, the expression of idiotypes can be up- or downregulated. A fine-tuning of specific antibody production, therefore, could be obtained. Depending on the existence of shared idiotypes on IgG and IgE, this therapy would, more or less, affect all isotypes of specific antibodies. In addition, the presence of cross-reactive idiotopes could provide a possibility of using pools of specific antibodies.

3. Anti-idiotypic antibodies could be used to modulate the reactivity of effector cells, such as basophils, mastocytes, and possibly, eosinophils, Langerhans cells, and platelets. Depending on binding affinity for idiotypes, such anti-idiotypic antibodies can compete with allergens. Activation of the cell depends on actual cross-linking of receptors, and perhaps, the functional monovalency of IgG4 could be used to avoid such an effect (39).
4. Anti-idiotypic antibodies could be used to modulate other IgE functions, such as antigen presentation by CD23, recognized as an important mechanism for allergen processing and presentation.

Clearly, the versatility of the idiotypic approach is appealing, and we think that with the advent of methodologies, such as the production of human MAbs or of genetically engineered antibodies, it should be possible to design an allergen-specific therapy that would be both safe and efficient. The results of trials in which allergen–antibody complexes were used could provided the first demonstration that such an approach is of value for allergic patients.

Acknowledgments

The author would like to thank Dr. Marc Jacquemin for the useful discussions, and Gilles Hageman for his help with the layout of the text.

References

1. Mudde GC, Hansel TT, van Reijsen FC, Osterhoff-BF, Bruijnzeel-Koomen CAFM. IgE: an immunoglobulin specialized in antigen capture? Immunol Today 1990; 11:440–443.
2. Oettgen HC, Martin TR, Wynshaw BA, Deng C, Drazen JM, Leder P. Active anaphylaxis in IgE-deficient mice. Nature 1994; 370:367–370.
3. Cerny J, Hiernaux J. Concept of idiotypic network: description and function. In: Cerny J, Hiernaux J, eds. Idiotypic Network and Diseases. Washington DC: American Society for Microbiology, 1990:13–29.
4. Watts C, Lanzavecchia A. Suppressive effect of antibody on processing of T cell epitopes. J Exp Med 1993; 178:1459–1463.
5. Saint-Remy JM, Lebecque SJ, Lebrun PM, Jacquemin MG. Human immune response to allergens of house dust mite, *Dermatophagoides pteronyssinus*. IV. Occurrence of natural autologous anti-idiotypic antibodies. Eur J Immunol 1988; 18:83–87.
6. Saint-Remy JM, Lebecque SJ, Lebrun PM, Jacquemin MG. Human immune response to allergens of house dust mite, *Dermatophagoides pteronyssinus*. V. Auto-anti-idiotypic antibody characterization and cross-reactivity. Eur J Immunol 1988; 18:1009–1014.
7. Valacer DJ, O'Reilly ME, Ilowite NT, Bonagura VR. Identification of anti-idiotypic antibodies in the sera of ryegrass-allergic and nonallergic individuals. J Allergy Clin Immunol 1991; 88:349–355.
8. Saint-Remy JM, Lebecque SJ, Lebrun SM. Human immune response to allergens of house dust mite, *Dermatophagoides pteronyssinus*. III. Cross-reactivity of bystander idiotopes on allergen-specific IgE antibodies. Eur J Immunol 1988; 18:77–81.
9. Saint-Remy JM, Lebrun PM, Lebecque SJ, Masson PL. The human immune response

against major allergens from house dust mite, *Dermatophagoides pteronyssinus*. II. Idiotypic cross-reactions of allergen-specific antibodies. Eur J Immunol 1986; 16:575–580.
10. Bose R, Marsh DG, Duchateau J, Sehon AH, Delespesse G. Demonstration of auto-anti-idiotypic antibody cross-reacting with public idiotypic determinants in the serum of rye-sensitive allergic patients. J Immunol 1984; 133:2474–2478.
11. Mecheri S, Mourad W, Lapeye J, Jobin M, David B, Hebert J. Demonstration of idiotypes expressed on basophil-bound IgE antibodies by using anti-idiotype-induced histamine release in grass pollen-allergic patients. Immunology 1988; 64:11–15.
12. Khan RH, Szewcuk MR, Day J H. J Allergy Clin Immunol 1991; 88:199–208.
13. Castracane JM, Hall TJ, Tamir R, Rocklin RE. Anti-ragweed-specific anti-idiotypic antibodies in nonatopic and atopic subjects. Trans Assoc Am Physician, 1985; 98:123–130.
14. Castracane JM, Rocklin RE. Detection of human auto-anti-idiotypic antibodies (Ab2) II. Generation of Ab2 in atopic patients undergoing allergen immunotherapy. Int Arch Allergy Appl Immunol 1988; 86:295–302.
15. Hébert J, Bernier D, Mourad W. Detection of auto-anti-idiotypic antibodies to Lol p 1 IgE antibodies in human sera by the use of murine idiotypes: levels in atopic and nonatopic subjects and effects of immunotherapy. Clin Exp Immunol 1990; 80:413–419.
16. Bose R, Marsh DG, Delespesse G. Anti-idiotypes to anti-Lol p 1 (rye) antibodies in allergic and non-allergic individuals. Influence of immunotherapy. Clin Exp Immunol 1986; 66:231–240.
17. Wetterwald A, Toffler O, de Weck AL, Blaser K. Suppression of established IgE antibody responses with isologous anti-idiotypic antibodies in guinea pigs. Mol Immunol 1986; 23:347–356.
18. Blaser K, de Weck A. Regulation of the IgE antibody response by idiotype–anti-idiotype network. Prog Allergy 1982; 32:203–264.
19. Blaser K, Nakagawa T, de Weck AL. Suppression of anti-hapten IgE and IgG antibody responses by isologous anti-idiotypic antibodies against purified anti-carrier (ovalbumin) antibodies in BALB/c mice. J Immunol 1981; 126,1180–1184.
20. Blaser K, Nakagawa T, de Weck AL. Effect of passively administered isologous anti-idiotypes directed against anti-carrier (ovalbumin) antibodies on the anti-hapten IgE and IgG antibody responses in BALB/c mice. Immunology 1983; 48:423–431.
21. Hall EP, Gault EA. Regulation of rat IgE responses by immune complexes. Immunology 1987; 61:415–419.
22. Poulsen LK, Lundberg L, Sondergaard I, Weeke B. Allergen-containing immune complexes used for immunotherapy of allergic asthma. Allergy 1988; 44:132–142.
23. da Costa PS, de Macedo MS, Perini A. Suppression of mouse IgE response by immune complexes. J Allergy Clin Immunol 1990; 86:496–502.
24. Wheeler AW, Deards MJ, Hickman BE, Spackman VM, Johanson SGO. Reactivity of mast-cell bound IgE idiotypes with anti-idiotypic antibody: mediator release or inhibition of antigen-induced mediator release? Int Arch Allergy Appl Immunol 1990; 91:192–197.
25. Weyer A, Le Mao J, Etievant M, David B, Guinnepain MT, Saint-Remy JMR. Human auto-anti-idiotypic antibodies to mite-specific IgE can degranulate human basophils in vitro. Clin Exp Allergy 1995; 25:935–941.
26. Jerne NK. Idiotypic networks and other preconceived ideas. Immunol Rev 1984; 79:5–24.
27. Müller CE, Rajewsky K. Idiotope regulation by isotype switch variants of two monoclonal antiidiotope antibodies. J Exp Med 1984; 159:758–772.
28. Enriquez-Rincon F, Klaus GGB. Differing effects of monoclonal anti-hapten antibodies on humoral responses to soluble or particulate antigens. Immunology 1984; 52:129–136.
29. Saint-Remy JMR, Lebrun PM, Lebecque SJ, Masson PL. Human immune response to allergens of house dust mite, *Dermatophagoides pteronyssinus*. Allergy 1988; 48:338–347.
30. Klaus GGB. Antigen–antibody complexes elicit anti-idiotypic antibodies to self-idiotopes. Nature 1990; 272:265–266.
31. Machiels JJ, Somville MA, Lebrun PM, Lebecque SJ, Jacquemin MG, Saint-Remy JMR.

Allergic bronchial asthma due to *D. pteronyssinus* hypersensitivity can be efficiently treated by inoculation of allergen–antibody complexes. J Clin Invest 1990; 85:1024–1035.
32. Machiels JJ, Lebrun P, Jacquemin MG, Saint-Remy JMR. Significant reduction of nonspecific bronchial reactivity in patients with *Dermatophagoides pteronyssinus*-sensitive allergic asthma under therapy with allergen–antibody complexes. Am Rev Respir Dis 1993; 147:1407–1412.
33. Machiels JJ, Somville MA, Lebrun PM, Jacquemin MG, Saint-Remy JMR. Allergen–antibody complexes can efficiently prevent seasonal rhinitis and asthma in grass pollen hypersensitive patients. Allergy 1991; 46:335–348.
34. Machiels JJ, Buche Martine, Somville MA, Jacquemin MG, Saint-Remy JMR. Complexes of grass pollen allergens and specific antibodies prevent allergic symptoms and inhibit the seasonal increase of IgE antibody. Clin Exp Allergy 1990; 20:653–660.
35. Leroy B, Lachapelle JM, Somville MM, Jacquemin MG, Saint-Remy JMR. Injection of allergen–antibody complexes is an effective treatment of atopic dermatitis. Dermatologica 1991; 182:98–106.
36. Leroy BP, Boden Griet, Lachapelle JM, Jacquemin MG, Saint-Remy JMR. A novel therapy for atopic dermatitis using antigen–antibody complexes: a double-blind placebo-controlled study. J Am Acad Dermatol 1993; 28:232–239.
37. Jacquemin M, Saint-Remy JMR. Specific down-regulation of anti-allergen IgE and IgG antibodies in man associated with injections of allergen-specific antibody complexes. Ther Immunol 1995; 2:41–52.
38. Leroy BP, Jacquemin MG, Lachapelle JM, Saint-Remy JMR. Allergen-sensitive atopic dermatitis is improved by injections of allergen combined to $F(ab')_2$ fragments of specific antibodies. Br J Dermatol 1995; 132:599–603.
39. Shakib F. Controlling allergy with anti-idiotypic antibodies. Clin Exp Allergy 1995; 10:908–909.

Part Three

REGULATION OF IgE INFLAMMATION

IMMUNOGLOBULIN

23

Anti-Immunoglobulin E Therapy for Asthma

PASCAL DEMOLY, DANY JAFFUEL, and JEAN BOUSQUET

Montpellier University and
Service des Maladies Respiratoires—INSERM U454
Montpellier University Hospital
Montpellier, France

I. Introduction

The prevalence and the severity of asthma have continually increased since 1960, despite great advances in the understanding of the physiological mechanisms of the disease and of better medical treatment. Asthma is a multifactorial and complex disease in which allergic factors and nonallergic triggers interact and result in bronchial obstruction and inflammation. Although discussed for a long time, the role of inhalant allergens in asthma has now been established. There is a strong association between exposure to indoor allergens, such as mites, and the occurrence of allergic asthma. The role of inhalant allergens in asthma exacerbations has been clearly demonstrated for indoor and outdoor allergens. Allergen avoidance is always recommended in the treatment of allergic asthma, although it is rarely completely effective.

There are unmet medical needs in asthma. Existing strategies to treat asthma consist in attempting to reduce the allergic reaction by allergen-specific immunotherapy or to improve the ongoing allergic inflammation using pharmacotherapy. The clinical efficacy of immunotherapy in asthma is debated. None of these strategies can cure the disease and many patients are still uncontrolled despite optimal pharmacological treatment. Novel immunological treatments for asthma have been recently proposed in attempting to improve IgE-mediated allergic reactions and to reduce the severity of asthma. They include allergen-specific interventions and immunomodulatory therapeutic approaches that are aimed at reducing the IgE production or the consequences of the activation by IgE antibodies.

II. Importance of Immunoglobulin E in Asthma

Asthma is a heterogeneous inflammatory disease with variable remodeling of the airways. Allergic asthma represents the most common form of the disease in childhood and early adulthood (1). Bronchial challenge with allergens can induce an airway bronchoconstrictive response, there is a strong association between exposure to indoor allergens, such as mites, and the occurrence of allergic asthma, and asthma exacerbations have been clearly associated with high levels of indoor allergens, such as house dust mites, animal danders, or insect dusts, as well as with seasonal allergens, such as grass pollens or molds. Finally, allergen avoidance reduces asthma symptoms and nonspecific bronchial hyperreactivity. Moreover, even in nonallergic asthma, an immunological basis of the disease may be proposed because the pathological features are largely similar (2,3).

Allergic asthma is essentially mediated by the triggering of IgE-bound mast cells by allergens, leading to the release of vasoactive mediators and an ongoing inflammatory reaction causing nonspecific hyperreactivity that may persist for several days. The repetition of allergen challenges leads to a complex inflammatory state, possibly followed in the long-term by airway remodeling. Allergen-specific immunotherapy improves asthma symptoms, but it is hampered by the multiple allergen sensitizations of the patients and, therefore, should be used only in selected patients. Antibodies against IgE may be of importance because they cover multiplicities of allergens (4).

Immunoglobulin E binds to the chain of the α-high-affinity IgE receptors (FcεRI) on mast cells and basophils, but also on other cells, such as dendritic cells and eosinophils, and to the low-affinity IgE receptors (FcεRII, CD23) on various inflammatory cells, including monocytes and B cells. The binding of IgE to FcεRI on the surface of mast cells and basophils primes these cells to secrete a panel of proinflammatory mediators on subsequent exposure to specific allergens. Serum IgE levels to drive basophil and mast cell IgE FcεRI display. A close relation was observed between serum IgE levels and the number of receptors for IgE on the surface of human basophils (5). IgE enhances FcεRI expression on mouse mast cell (6) and basophils (7), both in vitro and in vivo suggesting a novel amplification mechanism in IgE-dependent reactions. The finding that IgE can be a major regulator of basophil and mast cell FcεRI expression identifies a potentially important mechanism for enhancing the expression of effector cell function in IgE-dependent allergic reactions. Moreover, a monoclonal antibody (MAb) against IgE inhibits the

T-cell production of interleukin (IL)-4 and airway eosinophilia in allergen-challenged mice (8).

However, allergen-induced bronchial hyperreactivity and eosinophilic inflammation may occur in the absence of IgE in a mouse model of asthma (9), suggesting that not all asthmatic patients may respond favorably to a therapeutic strategy aimed at reducing IgE levels.

III. MAbs Against Immunoglobulin E

Two biotechnology companies, Genentech and Tanox Biosystems, have focused their efforts toward the strategy of anti-IgE therapy, and MAbs against IgE have been raised (e.g., Rhu-MAb-E25 and CGP 51901).

A MAb was raised against the domain of IgE bound to the FcεRI region involved in the binding of IgE to the receptors. The antibody (MAE11) was selected on the basis of its ability to bind circulating IgE at the same high-affinity receptor, thereby blocking the binding of IgE to mast cells and basophils and preventing subsequent release of the inflammatory agents after exposure to allergen. This antibody acts both by complexing free IgE molecules, preventing their binding to effector cells bearing FcεRI or FcεRII (10), and B-cell–bound IgE, inducing B-cell suppression. Because of its specificity, such an antibody does not affect the immune response of other antibody classes and does not activate cells bearing FcεRI or FcεRII, because the epitope on IgE against which it is directed is hidden within the receptor. Thus, the MAb does not trigger anaphylaxis nor cause lysis of cells bearing IgE receptors (11). Moreover, the administration of the anti-IgE antibody to ovalbumin-sensitized mice inhibits CD23 expression on B cells and IgE production (12). These results suggest that anti-IgE treatment suppresses IgE responses by effects on B cells, rather than on T cells. Human FcεRI–IgG and humanized anti-IgE MAb MAE11 block passive sensitization of human and rhesus monkey lung (11).

Hybridoma technology enables rodent MAbs to be created, but these have limited clinical usefulness. Nonhuman MAbs cause an immune response that both reduces their therapeutic efficacy and may induce anaphylactic reactions. There are also cleared rapidly and show only weak recruitment of effector cell functions, which leads to low efficacy. Protein engineering is now generating antibodies for the treatment of various diseases by "humanizing" rodent antibodies that significantly reduces the amount of nonhuman sequences in the molecule to less than 5% (13). Humanized antibodies have improved pharmacokinetics, have reduced immunogenicity, and have already been used during clinical trials. MAE11 was, therefore, humanized, and the best of several humanized variants, version 25 (Rhu-MAb-E25), was selected because it possessed binding affinity and biological activity comparable with MAE11 (10). From previous studies, it appeared likely that FcεRI expression on basophils and mast cells may be regulated by levels of circulating IgE. The expression of IgE and FcεRI on human basophils was examined in 15 subjects receiving humanized anti-IgE MAb intravenously (14). Treatment with the anti-IgE MAb decreased free IgE levels to 1% of pretreatment levels and also resulted in a marked downregulation of FcεRI on basophils. The responsiveness of the cells to IgE-mediated stimulation using the anti-IgE MAb was marginally decreased (approximately 40%), whereas the response of the same cells to stimulation with *Dermatophagoides farinae* antigen was reduced by approximately 90%.

Another chimeric anti-IgE antibody has been raised following the same procedure and has similar properties in animals (15). CGP 51901 is a nonanaphylactogenic mouse–human chimeric antihuman IgE that binds to free IgE and surface IgE of IgE-expressing B cells, mediating cytolysis of IgE-secreting cells, but not to IgE bound to FcεRI on mast cells and basophils or FcεRII on other cells. This antibody has shown the therapeutic potential of nonanaphylactogenic anti-IgE in murine models of skin reaction, lung function, and inflammation (16).

IV. Clinical Efficacy of MAbs Against Immunoglobulin E in Asthma and Rhinitis

A. Phase I and II Study in Allergic Rhinitis Patients

A phase I double-blind, placebo-controlled, single-dose study, with doses of 3, 10, 30, and 100 mg of CGP 51901 was conducted in 33 pollen-sensitive subjects who had raised levels of serum IgE and received either intravenous CGP 51901 or placebo (17). The administration of CGP 51901 was well tolerated and resulted in a decrease of serum free IgE levels in a dose-dependent manner, with suppression after 100 mg of CGP 51901 reaching over 93%. Time of recovery to 50% of baseline IgE correlated with the dose of administered antibody and ranged from a mean of 1.3 days for the 3-mg to 39 days for the 100-mg dose. Total IgE, comprised of free and complexed IgE, increased as stored and newly synthesized IgE bound to CGP 51901. Complexed IgE was eliminated at a rate comparable with the terminal half-life of free CGP 51901 (11–13 days at all doses). Only one subject showed a weak antibody response against CGP 51901. No significant change in histamine release or in skin-prick test reactivity to grass pollen was observed.

A phase II study in allergic rhinitis patients is ongoing with the same humanized MAb (CGP 51901). Intravenous doses ranging from 15 to 60 mg were administered serially before and during the pollen season. Free IgE was reduced by 65–80% from baseline values. Symptoms and rescue medications were significantly reduced in the actively treated patients by comparison with those under placebo.

B. Efficacy in Bronchial Allergen Challenge Studies

Two randomized, double-blind, parallel, placebo-controlled studies have examined the effects of Rhu-MAb-E25 injected intravenously in mild allergic asthmatic patients (18,19). Administration of Rhu-MAb-E25 dramatically reduced free IgE serum levels immediately after the first injection and attenuated both early- (18,19) and late-phase responses to inhaled allergens (19) after multiple injections.

Both studies were well designed, and after multiple dose injections, the early-phase reaction to bronchial allergen challenge was reduced, but not completely abrogated and this incomplete effect may be related to (1) an insufficient dose; (2) an incomplete mast cell "desensitisation" by a short course of Rhu-MAb-E25; (3) the association with non-IgE mechanisms, such as direct T-cell activation, which may participate in allergen-induced asthmatic reactions; or (4) a rapid dissociation of Rhu-MAb-E25/IgE complexes, IgE molecules thus becoming targets for allergens. However, this dissociation appears unlikely because of the usual very low K_d (0.06 nM) of antigen–antibody association (20), the pharmacokinetic studies carried out in monkeys showed a slow clearance of the complexes from the serum (21) and because at least ten times more Rhu-MAb-E25 was used by comparison with total serum IgE [mean estimated Rhu-MAb-E25/total IgE ratio was 232 (19) and 188 (18)].

The study of Fahy et al. (19) is of great interest because it also showed that the late-phase reaction to bronchial allergen challenge was reduced by about 60%. The late-phase reaction is associated with a bronchial inflammatory response, therefore, such a treatment is acting on the inflammation of the airways. Bronchial challenges in patients who received specific immunotherapy with mite extracts showed that the immediate and late-phase reactions were inhibited in many studies (for review see Ref. 22). However, the reduction of the late-phase reaction was more closely associated with improvement of asthma symptoms than that of the early-phase reaction (23), suggesting that the reduction of the late-phase reaction by Rhu-MAb-E25 may have a clinical benefit in chronic, persistent asthma.

These studies, therefore, represent the "proof of concept" of the anti-IgE therapy in asthma and suggest that targeting this pathway will likely cover multiplicities of allergens (4).

Surprisingly, Rhu-MAb-E25 (similar to CGP 51901) had no effect on allergen skin tests. The method assessing skin test reactivity was adequate and should have found changes, even if they were small. Thus, the negative results observed are clear-cut and differentiate this treatment approach from allergen-specific immunotherapy, which decreases the wheal-and-flare reaction (for review see Ref. 22). It may be argued that the late-phase skin reaction should also have been tested because specific immunotherapy is more profoundly effective on the late skin response. These results suggest that Rhu-MAb-E25 is not able to displace IgE already fixed onto cutaneous mast cells, but it is able to block passive cutaneous anaphylaxis in experimental animals (24), passive sensitization of human and rhesus monkey lung (11), and histamine release from human basophils (25). Moreover, airway mast cells appear to be more susceptible to Rhu-MAb-E25, as shown by the reduction in the early-phase reaction after allergen bronchial challenge.

The duration of efficacy of Rhu-MAb-E25 is another issue. It appeared, in these studies, that Rhu-MAb-E25 was able to diminish free IgE at least 14 days after cessation of the treatment. Pharmacokinetic studies, which are not shown [Boulet L, manuscript in preparation] have probably examined Rhu-MAb-E25 half-life, and as a consequence, the need for repeating administration, possibly with rapid induction of an immune response directed against the therapeutic proteins.

C. Usefulness in the Treatment of Chronic Persistent Asthma

Although these two challenging studies with Rhu-MAb-E25 suggest that this treatment may be beneficial for asthma (18,19), and the reduction of the late-phase reaction after bronchial allergen challenge favors this conclusion, in neither of the two studies were asthma symptoms, rescue β_2-agonist use, or FEV_1 improved, but the patients enrolled were probably too mild to observe any significant difference. However, some outcome measures of asthma severity were improved by Rhu-MAb-E25. Boulet et al. examined the evolution of methacholine challenge and found that at 76 days there was a small but significant improvement of PC_{20} methacholine (18). Fahy et al. examined both methacholine challenge and sputum inflammatory indices after allergen provocation (19). The PC_{20} methacholine 24 hr after challenge was significantly altered by Rhu-MAb-E25 treatment. Sputum eosinophil reduction was not significantly greater than the change in the placebo group. Eosinophil cationic protein levels in sputum were not significantly reduced either at baseline or after challenge in the Rhu-MAb-E25-treated group by comparison with the placebo group.

These data suggest that Rhu-MAb-E25 may have a clinical effect in chronic persistent asthma, but phase II studies in progress are needed to better appreciate the benefits of anti-IgE treatment in chronic asthma of variable severity.

V. Safety

The safety of any novel therapy for asthma and allergic diseases is critical because these diseases are rarely lethal. The short-term safety was assessed in three studies. CGP 51901 was well tolerated and only one subject had a weak antibody response against the MAb (17). Rhu-MAb-E25 appeared to be safe, with only one mild adverse reaction (transient urticarial rash) out of 21 (less than 5%) treated patients (18,19). Moreover, there was no development of antibodies against Rhu-MAb-E25. Another safety issue is the theoretical outcome of tissue damage resulting from increased serum concentrations of Rhu-MAb-E25–IgE immune complexes, which does not seem to occur in these studies. However, more patients receiving the antibody for a longer time should be studied before a definite conclusion can be raised.

The long-term safety of such an approach also needs to be carefully evaluated. Although IgE has been considered to play an essential role in host defence against parasitic helminth infections, in vivo evidence of a protective function of IgE in infected subjects is lacking. From both animal and human studies in subjects who have no detectable serum IgE, it does not seem that IgE is essential for normal immunological functions (12,15,21), even in the protection against parasites (26). However, more data are needed to ascertain the complete safety of such an approach, and mice with a targeted deletion of the IgE gene have increased worm burdens and reduced granulomatous inflammation following primary infection with *Schistosoma mansoni* (27). These data suggest that IgE participates in parasite elimination in primary infection with some parasites and in the generation of humoral immunity and cytokine responses to the parasite.

Moreover, there might be other unrecognized protective roles for IgE and mast cells (28), and each patient receiving this treatment should be carefully followed up on a long-term basis.

VI. Conclusions

The rationale for this new therapeutic approach is based on our current understanding of the role of IgE in immune function and allergic diseases. Although it represents a breakthrough of the concepts of asthma therapy, such a treatment may be effective only in allergic asthmatics. The partial reduction of some inflammatory indices is of importance, but more studies are needed in patients with a more severe form of the disease to assess the real importance of this treatment. Moreover, the route of administration probably will hamper the use of this novel treatment in patients with a milder form of the disease.

References

1. Bousquet J, Yssel H, Vignola M, Chanez P. New developments in the immunology of asthma with a focus on mechanisms and treatment. Curr Opin Pulmonary Med 1997; 3:42–50.
2. Humbert M, Grant JA, Taborda-Barata L, et al. High-affinity IgE receptor (FcεRI)-bearing cells in bronchial biopsies from atopic and nonatopic asthma. Am J Respir Crit Care Med 1996; 153:1931–1937.
3. Humbert M, Durham SR, Ying S, et al. IL-4 and IL-5 mRNA and protein in bronchial biopsies from patients with atopic and nonatopic asthma: evidence against "intrinsic" asthma being a distinct immunopathologic entity. Am J Respir Crit Care Med 1996; 154:1497–1504.
4. Jardieu P. Anti-IgE therapy. Curr Opin Immunol 1995; 7:779–782.
5. Conroy M, Adkinson N Jr, Lichtenstein L. Measurement of IgE on human basophils: relation to serum IgE and anti-IgE-induced histamine release. J Immunol 1997; 118:1317–1321.
6. Yamaguchi M, Lantz CS, Oettgen HC, et al. IgE enhances mouse mast cell FcεRI expression in vitro and in vivo: evidence for a novel amplification mechanism in IgE-dependent reactions. J Exp Med 1997; 185:663–672.
7. Lantz CS, Yamaguchi M, Oettgen HC, et al. IgE regulates mouse basophil FcεRI expression in vivo. J Immunol 1997; 158:2517–2521.

8. Coyle AJ, Wagner K, Bertrand C, Tsuyuki S, Bews J, Heusser C. Central role of immunoglobulin (Ig) E in the induction of lung eosinophil infiltration and T helper 2 cell cytokine production: inhibition by a non-anaphylactogenic anti-IgE antibody. J Exp Med 1996; 183:1303–1310.
9. Mehlhop PD, van-de-Rijn M, Goldberg AB, et al. Allergen-induced bronchial hyperreactivity and eosinophilic inflammation occur in the absence of IgE in a mouse model of asthma. Proc Natl Acad Sci USA 1997; 94:1344–1349.
10. Presta LG, Lahr SJ, Shields RL, et al. Humanization of an antibody directed against IgE. J Immunol 1993; 151: 2623–2632.
11. Saban R, Haak-Frendscho M, Zine M, et al. Human FcERI-IgG and humanized anti-IgE monoclonal antibody MaE11 block passive sensitizations of human and rhesus monkey lung. J Allergy Clin Immunol 1994; 94:836–843.
12. Haak-Frendscho M, Robbins K, Lyon R, et al. Administration of an anti-IgE antibody inhibits CD23 expression and IgE production in vivo. Immunology 1994; 82:306–313.
13. Winter G, Harris WJ. Humanized antibodies. Immunol Today 1993; 14:243–246.
14. MacGlashan D Jr, Bochner BS, Adelman DC, et al. Down-regulation of FcεRI expression on human basophils during in vivo treatment of atopic patients with anti-IgE antibody. J Immunol 1997; 158:1438–1445.
15. Davis F, Gosset L, Pinkston K, et al. Can anti-IgE be used to treat allergy? Springer Semin Immunopathol 1993; 15:51–73.
16. Heusser CH, Wagner K, Bews JP, et al. Demonstration of the therapeutic potential of non-anaphylactogenic anti-IgE antibodies in murine models of skin reaction, lung function and inflammation. Int Arch Allergy Immunol 1997; 113:231–235.
17. Corne J, Djukanovic R, Thomas L, et al. The effect of intravenous administration of a chimeric anti-IgE antibody on serum IgE levels in atopic subjects: efficacy, safety, and pharmacokinetics. J Clin Invest 1997; 99:879–887.
18. Boulet L, Chapman K, Côté J, et al. Inhibitory effects of an anti-IgE antibody E25 on allergen-induced early asthmatic response. Am J Respir Crit Care Med 1997; 155:1835–1840.
19. Fahy J, Fleming H, Wong H, et al. The effect of an anti-IgE monoclonal antibody on the early and late phase responses to allergen inhalation in asthmatic subjects. Am J Respir Crit Care Med 1997; 155:1828–1834.
20. Meng YG, Singh N, Wong WL. Binding of cynomolgus monkey IgE to a humanized anti-human IgE antibody and human high affinity IgE receptor. Mol Immunol 1996; 33:635–642.
21. Fox J, Hotaling T, Struble C, Ruppel J, Bates D, Schoenhoff M. Tissue distribution and complex formation with IgE of an anti-IgE antibody after intravenous administration in cynomolgus monkeys. J Pharmacol Exp Ther 1996; 279:1000–1008.
22. Bousquet J, Michel F. Specific immunotherapy in asthma: is it effective? J Allergy Clin Immunol 1994; 94:1–11.
23. Warner JO, Price JH, Soothill JF, Hey EN. Controlled trial of hyposensitisation to *Dermatophagoides pteronyssinus* in children with asthma. Lancet 1978; 2:912–915.
24. Haak-Frendscho M, Ridgway J, Shields R, Robbins K, Gorman C, Jardieu P. Human IgE receptor alpha-chain IgG chimera blocks passive cutaneous anaphylaxis reaction in vivo. J Immunol 1993; 151:351–358.
25. Shields RL, Whether WR, Zioncheck K, et al. Inhibition of allergic reactions with antibodies to IgE. Int Arch Allergy Immunol 1995; 107:308–312.
26. Amiri P, Haak-Frendscho M, Robbins K, McKerrow JH, Stewart T, Jardieu P. Anti-immunoglobulin E treatment decreases worm burden and egg production in *Schistosoma mansoni*-infected normal and interferon gamma knockout mice. J Exp Med 1994; 180:43–51.
27. King CL, Xianli J, Malhotra I, Liu S, Mahmoud AA, Oettgen HC. Mice with a targeted deletion of the IgE gene have increased worm burdens and reduced granulomatous inflam-

mation following primary infection with *Schistosoma mansoni*. J Immunol 1997; 158:294–300.

28. Echtenacher B, Mannel DN, Hultner L. Critical protective role of mast cells in a model of acute septic peritonitis. Nature 1996; 381:75–77.

IMMUNOGLOBULIN RECEPTORS

24

Expression and Function of the High-Affinity Receptor for Immunoglobulin E in Asthma

MARIE-HÉLÈNE JOUVIN and JEAN-PIERRE KINET

Harvard Medical School
and Beth Israel Deaconess Medical Center
Boston, Massachusetts

I. Introduction

A. Atopic and Nonatopic Asthma

There is a growing body of evidence from both human and animal studies implicating inflammatory mechanisms in the development and maintenance of asthma and airway hyperresponsiveness (1–3). However, significant controversy still persists over the factor(s) that initiate and prolong this inflammatory reaction. One classic view of the pathogenesis of atopic asthma is that allergens initiate the process by triggering IgE-bearing pulmonary mast cells (MC) to release mediators; such as histamine, leukotrienes, prostaglandins, kinins, platelet-activating factor, or others. In turn, these mediators induce bronchoconstriction and enhance vascular permeability and production of mucus. According to this model, following a type I IgE-mediated immediate allergic response, MC secrete various cytokines, including tumor necrosis factor-α (TNF-α), interleukin (IL)-4, IL-5, and IL-6, which participate in the local recruitment and activation of other inflammatory cells, such as eosinophils, basophils, T lymphocytes, platelets, and mononuclear phagocytes (4–7). These recruited cells, in turn, contribute to the development of an inflammatory response that may then become autonomous and aggravate the asthmatic symptoms.

Nonallergic stimuli, such as exercise, cold, and viral infections, can also induce asthma symptoms, and asthma can affect patients with no apparent atopy, the so-called intrinsic asthma. These observations suggest that in some patients, IgE-independent mechanisms can initiate asthma. Some studies have found differences in cell populations and mediators present in the blood, bronchoalveolar lavage (BAL) fluid, and lung biopsies between these two types (2,8,9). These differences have led some to propose that the common denominator for asthma is not a specific immunological mechanism, but instead, is the persistent airway inflammation that can be triggered by many unrelated stimuli. In this scenario, once asthma is initiated, the initial immediate response plays a minor role in sustaining the disease.

To try to answer the question of the initiating mechanisms of asthma, some studies have directly addressed the role of IgE. A correlation between IgE levels and the severity or occurrence of asthma has been reported (10,11), especially in children, for whom this correlation was independent of the presence of allergic rhinitis or eczema (12). In a carefully controlled study, taking into account the age- and sex-related variations in serum IgE levels, investigators have documented a close correlation between asthma and serum IgE levels, regardless of the atopic status of the patients. As a result, they even have questioned the existence of intrinsic asthma (13,14). Note that in these studies allergen-specific IgE levels were not measured, and the described correlations were established between total IgE and asthma. Therefore, any condition that could have resulted in elevated IL-4, IL-13, or other cytokines with a positive effect on IgE production (or in diminished levels of cytokines, such as interferon gamma [IFN-γ], that downregulate IgE) could have produced such a correlation. Nevertheless, these findings are consistent with the possibility that IgE plays a central role in asthma not only by eliciting the immediate hypersensitivity response from MC, but also by mediating antigen-dependent activation of other inflammatory cells and maintaining the inflammatory response.

B. IgE-Binding Cells in the Lung

Many cell types present in the lungs of asthmatics are capable of binding IgE through the low-affinity IgE receptor FcεRII/CD23 (15). This receptor is upregulated on eosinophils, platelets, B cells, blood monocytes, and alveolar macrophages of asthmatics, and has been shown to be functional. For example, FcεRII/CD23 mediates IgE-dependent cytotoxicity and phagocytosis of IgE-coated particles by macrophages and eosinophils (16). It has been hypothesized that IgE and antigen activate pulmonary inflammation cells through FcεRII to release inflammatory mediators. However, the combination of low IgE levels, even in atopic asthmatics, and the low affinity of FcεRII for IgE ($K_A \sim 10^7\ M^{-1}$) creates conditions in which monomeric IgE binding to FcεRII is not favored. In contrast, the avidity of FcεRII for IgE–antigen immune complexes is higher, and binding of IgE–antigen immune complexes to FcεRII could occur even at low concentrations. Therefore, in this model, one has to presume that IgE–antigen immune complexes are formed before FcεRII binding and cell activation.

The hypothesis that IgE could activate inflammatory cells other than MC has been given more weight recently by the finding that in humans the high-affinity IgE receptor (FcεRI) ($K_A \sim 10^{10}$ M^{-1}) is expressed on cells other than MC and basophils. Until recently, FcεRI was thought to be expressed exclusively on MC and basophils (17); however, in collaboration with Stingl's group in Vienna, we (18) and others (19) have now reported that FcεRI is also expressed on cutaneous Langerhans cells. This finding has led us to question the selectivity of expression of FcεRI on human cells. With the help of various collaborators, we have found that FcεRI is expressed on eosinophils of some hypereosinophilic patients (20), and on human monocytes and circulating dendritic cells (21,22). Moreover, we and other investigators (23; Jouvin M-H, Kinet J-F; unpublished) have recently found that alveolar macrophages from asthmatics can express FcεRI and that these cells have the capacity to bind IgE through FcεRI and to be activated by monomeric IgE and specific allergens. Indeed, FcεRI on circulating human monocytes is functional and is able to mediate calcium fluxes and antigen presentation (21,24). Furthermore, atopic individuals have increased levels of expression of FcεRI on their monocytes (21), arguably the most abundant cell type in the lumen of the alveoli. Thus, it appears likely that a wider variety of cells than previously recognized may be activated by IgE through FcεRI to release and secrete various enzymes, cytokines (e.g., TNF-α) and chemokines (e.g., macrophage inflammatory protein-1 [MIP-1-α]), which would act locally to produce the symptoms of asthma. Chronic challenge with antigen would then perpetuate the IgE-mediated inflammatory response.

C. The IgE–FcεRI Network

The hypothesis of an IgE–FcεRI network linking FcεRI aggregation by IgE with IgE production by B cells has been proposed based on studies showing that cross-linking FcεRI on murine MC, as well as nonspecific MC activation, stimulates the secretion of IL-4, a cytokine that promotes the isotype switch toward IgE in B cells (25) and the secretion of IL-3, a cytokine that promotes MC proliferation (26). The existence of such a network in humans (27) is suggested by the finding that, in the presence of IL-4, human mast and basophilic cell lines can provide the cell contact signals (presumably CD40L) required for IgE production by B cells (28). Some recent findings from Galli's group, in collaboration with our group, have provided additional support to the theory of the IgE–FcεRI network. We have shown that IgE upregulates FcεRI expression on MC and basophils in vivo and in vitro (see Sec. II.D; 29, 30).

D. A New Possible Mechanism for Activating Cells Through FcεRI

Although there is a general agreement that the IgE–FcεRI network, as outlined in the foregoing, plays a prominent role in the pathogenesis of atopic asthma, the question remains of whether, and how, this network might also play a role in triggering nonatopic asthmatic responses. New impetus has been given to these questions by the finding that autoantibodies (autoAb) directed against FcεRI are present in a large proportion of patients with chronic urticaria (CU), a disease caused by the release of vasoactive mediator by skin MC, but in which there is no clear evidence of allergy. These autoAb recognize the IgE binding α-chain of FcεRI (see Sec. II). Two lines of evidence suggest that these anti-FcεRI α autoAb may indeed play a role in the pathogenesis of CU and are not simply an epiphenomenon or "marker" of the disease. First, these autoAb are able to induce histamine release from human basophils in vitro (31–34) and from a rat MC line transfected with human FcεRI, but not from the control cell line (34; Fiebiger E, Kinet J-P, unpublished observations). Second, local injection of autologous serum into patient's skin induces skin lesions similar to those of CU, with the implication that a soluble factor in patient's serum is capable of inducing the disease (31). The similarity between patients with CU and patients with nonatopic asthma is that both exhibit allergic-like symptoms without clear evidence of allergy (as, for example, determined by provocation tests to a panel of allergens). This similarity has led us to investigate whether some nonatopic asthmatics may have anti-FcεRIα autoAb. Among ten such patients, anti-FcεRIα autoAbs were found in four, and in two of them they were capable of inducing histamine release in normal basophils (Fiebiger E, Jouvin H-E, Stingl G, Kinet J-P, unpublished). Based on this finding, we have formulated the hypothesis that anti-FcεRIα autoAbs similar to those found in CU, could be responsible for the symptoms of nonatopic asthma in some patients. This hypothesis is being tested in our laboratory.

The finding of anti-FcεRIα autoAbs in the serum of some patients with CU and in some patients with nonatopic asthma and the potential role of these autoAb in the pathogenesis of these diseases (as evidenced by their ability to induce MC or basophil degranulation) raise a number of interesting and important questions. Because these anti-FcεRIα autoAbs are found in the serum, why do they not trigger circulating basophils to degranulate and induce symptoms of systemic anaphylaxis? Assuming that these autoAbs are similar in both diseases (CU and asthma), why do they induce only one type of disease? In other words, what is the basis for targeting selected organs? The general question of organ selectivity is not restricted to the role of anti-FcεRIα autoAbs in asthma; as was recently reported, systemic autoreactivity can provoke an organ-specific disease involving the joints (35). This article discusses several possible mechanisms for organ selectivity, including aberrant activation of a cell population in the target organ through unknown mechanisms. Relative to the organ selectivity of anti-FcεRIα autoAbs in CU and asthma, various possible explanations need to be considered: (1) localized B-cell production of autoAb, in which case the levels found in the serum may represent only a small fraction of those present locally; (2) local alteration of the balance between the activating receptor FcεRI and the IgG receptor FcγRIIB, an inhibitory receptor to which some anti-FcεRIα autoAbs may also bind (see Sec. III.B); (3) local amplification of the FcεRI-mediated responses through the FcR β-chain or other means (see Sec. III.A.).

II. Structure and Regulation of Expression of FcεRI

A. Receptor Structure, Assembly, and Cell Distribution

FcεRI was first isolated from rat and mouse MC lines as a multimeric structure made of four subunits: one α-chain (FcεRI-α), one β-chain (FcRI-β), and two identical, disulfide-linked γ-chains (FcR γ); the α-chain is unique to FcεRI, whereas the β- and γ-chains are also present in other antigen receptors; hence, the names (36). This finding was confirmed by the observation that receptor expression at the cell surface in an heterologous cell line requires transfection of the rodent cDNAs for the three subunits (37). In contrast, when human cDNAs are used, expression of an IgE-binding receptor at the cell surface is obtained not only when the cDNAs for the three subunits are transfected, but also when only the cDNAs for α and γ are transfected (38). The requirement for the three rodent cDNAs is due to the presence of endoplasmic reticulum (ER) retention signals in the rodent α-chain that retain it in the ER where it is degraded (39,40). Assembly of the α-chain with the cotransfected β- and γ-chains renders the ER retention signals ineffective, allowing the $\alpha\beta\gamma_2$-complex to be exported to the Golgi apparatus and, from there, to the plasma membrane. When the three human cDNAs are transfected, both $\alpha\beta\gamma_2$- and $\alpha\gamma_2$-complexes are exported to the cell surface, demonstrating that human β, unlike rodent β, is not necessary for cell surface expression and that the human α-chain ER retention signals can be canceled by human γ (39). More recently, it has been shown that the two isoforms of the human receptor ($\alpha\beta\gamma_2$ and $\alpha\gamma_2$) exist in normal cells (see later discussion) and not only as a result of transfection.

The α- and the dimeric γ-chains, with or without the β-chain are maintained as a complex in the plasma membrane through a combination of hydrophobic and electrostatic noncovalent interactions, and mild detergent conditions are required to preserve the receptor multimeric structure when isolating FcεRI from cell lysates. The α-chain is a member of the immunoglobulin gene superfamily, with two extracellular immunoglobulin-related domains, one transmembrane domain, and a short cytoplasmic tail. The α-chain is heavily glycosylated at seven *N*-linked glycosylation sites (41). The extracellular domain of the α-chain is necessary and sufficient to provide the receptor with high-affinity IgE binding. This has been demonstrated by a truncation experiment in which a stop codon was inserted in the human α-chain DNA at the junction of the extracellular and transmembrane domains. Transfection of this construct into eukaryotic or bacterial cells results in the production of a truncated α-chain that is secreted as a soluble product by virtue of the presence of a leader peptide encoded in the construct and the absence of the transmembrane and cytoplasmic sequences (42,43). This soluble α-chain has the same ligand-binding characteristics as the tetrameric, plasma membrane-inserted, FcεRI complex (42,43). The β-chain crosses the plasma membrane four times and has two intracellular tails. The two γ-chains associate through a disulfide bond. They have a very short extracellular section, a transmembrane section and a cytoplasmic tail. Both β- and γ-chains are involved in signal transduction (see Sec. III). Therefore, FcεRI can be considered as a modular structure with one binding molecule, the α-chain and one signaling module, the $\beta\gamma_2$-complex.

Another feature that separates rodent and human FcεRI is cell distribution. Rodent FcεRI is expressed only on basophils and MC, whereas human FcεRI is also expressed on eosinophils in some hypereosinophilic patients (20), cutaneous Langerhans cells (18), monocytes (21), and dendritic cells (22). Importantly, in monocytes, cutaneous Langerhans cells, and dendritic cells, it is not possible to detect transcripts for the β-chain, even though α- αγ- transcripts can be detected, and the respective proteins coprecipitated and identified by Western blotting. Thus, the $\alpha\gamma_2$-isoform appears to exist in human monocytes, cutaneous Langerhans cells, and dendritic cells, whereas MC and basophils, which express the β-chain, have on their surface the classic $\alpha\beta\gamma_2$-isoform (Fig. 1). Whether human MC and basophils express only the $\alpha\beta\gamma_2$-isoform or a variable proportion of the two isoforms has not yet been determined, but, in view of the critical importance of the β-chain in signal amplification (see Sec. III), this point may become a critical question for our overall understanding of allergic responses in humans.

There are mainly two reasons why it took so long to recognize the expression of FcεRI on cells as common as human monocytes. First, specific antibodies against FcεRI have only recently become available (18). Partly for this reason, IgE binding on many of these cells, which had been previously detected, has been interpreted as binding to the low-affinity IgE receptor FcεRII (CD23). Second, the level of expression of FcεRI on monocytes, eosinophils, cutaneous Langerhans cells,

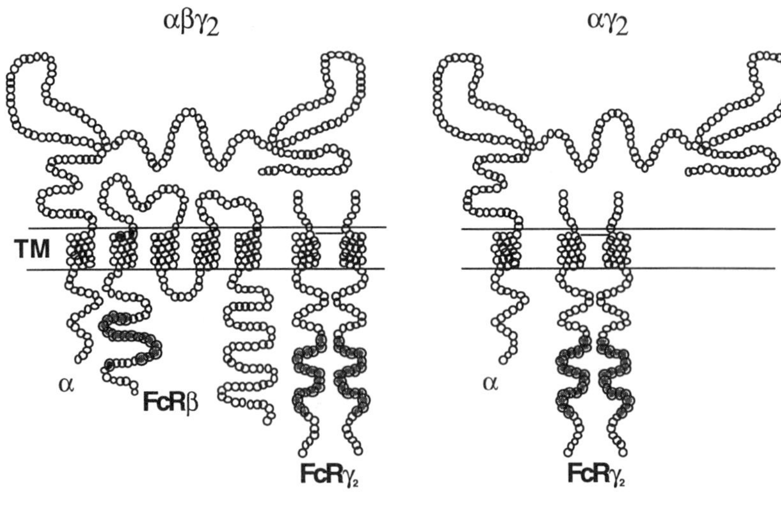

Figure 1 The two human FcεRI isoforms: Gray circles represent amino acids belonging to ITAMS; closed circles in FcRβ represent amino acids mutated in the atopy-associated genotypes.

and dendritic cells is low when compared with its level on MC and basophils (as judged by flow cytometry). For example, normal human monocytes typically express 10–100 times fewer receptors than circulating basophils. Even the upregulated levels of FcεRI on monocytes of patients with various allergic diseases (21) are lower than the levels normally expressed on MC and basophils. The basis for the difference in expression levels between these cell types, and what regulates expression levels is still unknown. However, recent progress has shed new light on how levels of FcεRI are regulated on MC and basophils (see Sec. II.B).

B. Regulation of Expression of FcεRI on Mast Cells and Basophils: Functional Consequences

Very few studies have directly addressed the question of the regulation of FcεRI expression. A correlation between IgE concentration in the serum and levels of IgE receptors on human basophils has long been recognized, but the basis for this correlation was unknown (44–46). In 1985, two concomitant studies using the MC line RBL-2H3 showed that a 1- or 2-day incubation of these cells in presence of IgE resulting in the doubling of cell surface expressed FcεRI (47,48). This FcεRI upregulation by IgE was cycloheximide-insensitive, and, therefore, judged to be independent of protein synthesis. Rather, the mechanism of this upregulation was thought to be the result of a decrease in the degradation rate of surface FcεRI "protected" by monomeric receptor-bound IgE.

Recently, Galli's group in collaboration with our group found that the level of FcεRI expression on MC and basophils of IgE knockout mice was extremely low and that normal FcεRI expression levels could be restored by in vitro incubation with IgE or injection of IgE in vivo (29,30). This upregulation was also observed after in vitro incubation with IgE of peritoneal- and bone marrow-derived MC from normal mice (29,30). Furthermore, the FcεRI upregulation of IgE resulted in enhanced IgE-mediated release of IL-4 and IL-6, thereby establishing the existence of a potential positive feedback loop. Preliminary results on human umbilical cord-derived MC show that IgE is able to upregulate human FcεRI expression (Yamaguchi M, Galli SJ, unpublished).

III. Mechanisms of FcεRI Signaling

A. FcεRI Signaling as a Result of Receptor Clustering

The binding of monovalent IgE to FcεRI is not sufficient to induce signaling. A proportion of the receptors present on circulating basophils is continuously occupied by IgE (46). The initiation of signaling requires receptor clustering, which can be induced by binding of the specific multivalent antigen to receptor-bound IgE (36,49). Receptor clustering can also be induced by chemically cross-linked IgE multimers, or by an anti-FcεRI antibody. However, the physical manner in which several receptors are brought together to form a cluster is critical. The evidence that specific physical constraints in clusters are required for cell activation has been demonstrated in a study in which some anti-FcεRI Abs induced the formation of unproductive clusters; that is, clusters incapable of inducing cell activation (50). Cluster size is one of the factors that determine the activating capacity of clusters (36).

The earliest events following receptor cross-linking are receptor tyrosine phosphorylation, which is detectable within 5 sec of receptor clustering, and inactivation of the lyn tyrosine kinase (51,52). Within a 15- to 30-sec period thereafter, activation of the syk and Btk tyrosine kinases begins concomitantly with calcium mobilization (53–56). When FcεRI is clustered on MC, release of secretory granule contents and synthesis and release of arachidonic acid metabolites begin within 1–5 min (57–59), whereas later events, such as cytokine synthesis, begin within 30–60 min (6,57,60).

B. The Concept of ITAM Motifs, and the Role of the β- and γ-Chains

Activating signals after cross-linking of antigen receptors (such as FcR, T-cell receptor, membrane immunoglobulin on B cells) involve 18-amino–acid homologous motifs found in the cytoplasmic tails of these receptors. These motifs, known as immunoreceptor tyrosine-based activation motifs (ITAMs), become tyrosine phosphorylated by the src family of kinases when receptors are engaged by clustering antigens, resulting in the recruitment to the engaged receptors of both src- and syk/zap70-family nonreceptor tyrosine kinases (61–63). Downstream propagation of the activation signal is mediated by activation of these tyrosine kinases and the resulting phosphorylation of specific substrates. The β- and γ-subunits of FcεRI each contain one ITAM (represented by shaded circles in Fig. 1). Data from our laboratory and others have established that, in the tetrameric receptor, the main early signaling events are the following: (1) The src family kinase lyn phosphorylates both FcεRI β- and γ-ITAMS (52,56); (2) β- and γ-ITAM phosphorylation by lyn causes syk to bind to γ-ITAMs (56,64,65); and (3) syk binding to γ-ITAMs leads to the lyn-dependent tyrosine phosphorylation and activation of syk (56,66; Fig. 2). This opens the question of the role played by the ITAM of β. Various studies have examined different versions of ITAMs to determine if functional differences exist and have demonstrated that individual ITAMs exhibit full cell activation capabilities when removed from their natural receptor contexts. These data have led to the widespread belief that ITAMs function redundantly or additively to increase signal strength (67,68). However, in the context of the tetrameric receptor, FcRβ functions as an amplifier: (1) it does not have autonomous cell activation capability; (2) it amplifies the cell activation signals sent by FcRγ with a gain of five- to sevenfold (as measured by syk activation and calcium mobilization); and (3) it does not qualitatively alter the FcRγ-mediated cell activation signals (69). Furthermore, we have demonstrated that the mechanism of FcRβ amplification involves the FcRβ ITAM acting as an inducible "anchor" for the lyn tyrosine kinase, resulting in enhanced

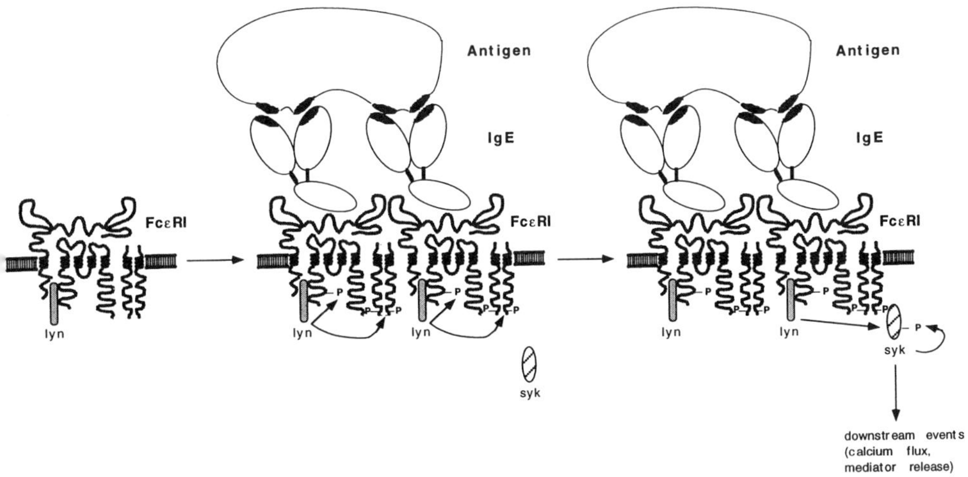

Figure 2 Tentative model for the early events in FcεRI activation.

lyn recruitment to the receptor complex after engagement, enhanced lyn-dependent phosphorylation of FcRγ, enhanced activation of the syk nonreceptor tyrosine kinase, and enhanced calcium mobilization (69). These findings represent the first clear demonstration of an alternative ITAM function. The fact that the γ-chain can function autonomously provides a rationale to explain how $\alpha\gamma_2$-complexes on human cells are capable of cell activation, as described, for example, in human monocytes (21). In addition, the amplifying function of the β-chain may help us understand the functional influence of the variants of the β-chain gene reported to be associated with an allergic phenotype (see Sec. IV; 70, 71).

Activating signals from FcεRI can be inhibited by signals sent by another cell surface receptor, in particular the low-affinity IgG receptor FcγRIIB expressed in humans on monocytes, macrophages, B lymphocytes, and possibly on mast cells and basophils (17,72). When FcεRI (occupied by IgE of a given antigen specificity) and FcγRIIB (occupied by IgG of the same antigen specificity) become co–cross-linked with multivalent antigens, the intracellular signaling and resulting cell activation is abrogated (73). The inhibitory signals originate from a 13-amino–acid sequence present in the FcγRIIB cytoplasmic tail called immunoreceptor tyrosine-based inhibitory motif (ITIM), which is also found in other inhibitory receptors. The mechanisms through which inhibitory signals are transduced are under investigation and appear to involve a protein tyrosine phosphatase, SH_2-containing phosphatase-1 (SHP-1) (74,75) or an inositol-5′-phosphatase, SH_2-containing inositol-5′-phosphatase (SHIP; 76–79). How these different phosphatases participate in the inhibitory signal remains unclear, but it is the subject of intense investigation. Nevertheless, the concept of inhibition of FcεRI signaling by FcγRIIB could be relevant to asthma if it is demonstrated that anti-FcεRIα autoAbs participate in the pathogenesis of the disease. After binding to their FcεRI α-chain target through their Fab portions, the autoAbs become part of immune complexes. This increases the avidity of the autoAbs for the low-affinity IgG receptor FcγRIIB and may allow them to bind through their Fc portions to FcγRIIB. This co–cross-linking of FcεRI and FcγRIIB would then generate an inhibitory signal. What would control the presence or absence of this cross-linking is presumably the proportion of each receptor on the cell surface. This proposed mechanism is analogous with a mechanism involving surface immunoglobulins and FcγRIIB on B cells. In some B cells, antibodies directed at surface immunoglobulins induce a negative signal in these B cells because the Fc portions of these antibodies co–cross-link the surface immunoglobulins with FcγRIIB. By contrast, incubation with $F(ab')_2$ fragments of the same antibody (lacking the Fc portion and, therefore, unable to bind and co–cross-link FcγRIIB) induces an activating signal. Thus, the extent to which these autoAbs can activate B cells is inversely proportional to their capacity to co–cross-link FcγRIIB. Similarly, anti-FcεRIα autoAbs may differ in their ability to co–cross-link FcγRIIB, because not all isotypes of IgG bind to FcγRIIB with the same affinity (17,79).

IV. Human FcRβ Polymorphism and Atopy

The FcRβ-chain amplifier function is of particular interest in view of several reports from Cookson and Hopkin's group documenting an association of variants of the FcRβ gene on chromosome 11 with atopy (80–84). Initially, the association was established with an atopic syndrome defined by the presence of one or more of the following criteria: positive skin prick tests (SPT) to common allergens, elevated total serum IgE levels, and elevated specific serum IgE levels against common allergens (81). Subsequent studies found an association with bronchial hyperresponsiveness (assessed by methacholine challenge; 85,86). The association between this region of chromosome 11 and atopy or bronchial hyperreactivity has been replicated by some, but not all, groups working with independent sets of probands, suggesting that this locus is likely to have an effect, but is not a megaphenic locus (85,87–93). One variant of the FcRβ gene on chromosome 11 is a double mutation isoleucine to leucine at position 81 and valine to leucine at position 183 (represented at filled circles in Fig. 1; 70). A second variant recently isolated consists of a glutamic acid to glycine substitution at position 237 (represented as filled circles in Fig. 1; (86). Whereas in the first variant the two mutations are located in the external part of one of the transmembrane regions of β and do not constitute a major chemical change, this last substitution introduces a significant hydrophobicity change just outside the ITAM of β. However, neither of these variants alone can account for the strength of the linkage between 11q13 and atopy, and it is likely that other variants exist in the FcRβ gene (71). Because they link the development of atopy with a receptor (FcεRI) that can be involved in generating atopic responses, and with a subunit

(FcRβ) of this receptor now known to function to enhance its signaling capacity, these reports provide an initial step toward understanding a potential immunological dysregulation that could lead to the development or enhancement of atopy. The consequences of these mutations in the β-chain on the function of FcεRI are being investigated in our laboratory through the use of mast cell lines transfected with the wild-type or mutated receptor.

References

1. Bigby TD, Nadel JA. Asthma. In: Gallin JI, Goldstein IM, R S, eds. Inflammation: Basic Principles and Clinical Correlates. New York: Raven Press, 1992:889–906.
2. McFadden ER Jr, Gilbert IA. Asthma. N Engl J Med 1992; 327:1928–1937.
3. Bochner BS, Undem BJ, Lichtenstein LM. Immunological aspects of allergic asthma. Annu Rev Immunol 1994; 12:295–335.
4. Galli SJ, Wershil BK, Gordon JR, Martin TR. Mast cells: immunologically specific effectors and potential sources of multiple cytokines during IgE-dependent responses. In: Ciba Foundation Symposium: IgE, Mast Cells and the Allergic Response. Chichester: John Wiley and Sons, 1989.
5. Metcalfe DD, Costa JJ, Burd PR. Mast cells and basophils. In: Gallin JI, Goldstein IM, Snyderman R, eds. Inflammation: Basic Principles and Clinical Correlates. New York: Raven Press, 1992:709–725.
6. Galli SJ, Gordon JR, Wershil BK. Mast cell cytokines in allergy and inflammation. Agents Actions Suppl 1993; 43:209–220.
7. Metcalfe DD. Mediators relevant in asthma and allergic diseases. Ann Intern Med, 1994; 121:701–704.
8. Jarjour NN, Calhoun WJ. Exercise-induced asthma is not associated with mast cell activation or airway inflammation. J Allergy Clin Immunol 1992; 89:60–68.
9. Walker C, Bode E, Boer L, Hansel TT, Blaser K, Virchow JC Jr. Allergic and nonallergic asthmatics have distinct patterns of T-cell activation and cytokine production in peripheral blood and bronchoalveolar lavage. Am Rev Respir Dis 1992; 146:109–115.
10. O'Hollaren MT, Yunginger JW, Offord KP, Somers MJ, O'Connell EJ, Ballard DJ, Sachs MI. Exposure to an aeroallergen as a possible precipitating factor in respiratory arrest in young patients with asthma. N Engl J Med 1991; 324:359–363.
11. Martinez FD, Wright AL, Taussig LM, Holberg CJ, Halonen M, Morgan WJ. Asthma and wheezing in the first six years of life. The Group Health Medical Associates. N Engl J Med 1995; 332:133–138.
12. Sears MR, Burrows B, Flannery EM, Herbison GP, Hewitt CJ, Holdaway MD. Relation between airway responsiveness and serum IgE in children with asthma and in apparently normal children. N Engl J Med 1991; 325:1067–1071.
13. Burrows B, Martinez FD, Halonen M, Barbee RA, Cline MG. Association of asthma with serum IgE levels and skin-test reactivity to allergens. N Engl J Med 1989; 320:271–277.
14. Adkinson NF Jr. Is asthma always an allergic disease? Trans Am Clin Climatol Assoc 1992; 103:218–227.
15. Bonnefoy JY, Aubry JP, Gauchat JF, Graber P, Life P, Flores-Romo L, Mazzei G. Receptors for IgE. Curr Opin Immunol 1993; 5:944–949.
16. Capron A, Dessaint JP, Caprin M, Joseph M, Ameisen JC, Tonnel AB. From parasites to allergy: a second receptor for IgE. Immunol Today 1986; 7:15–18.
17. Ravetch JV, Kinet J-P. Fc receptors. Annu Rev Immunol 1991; 9:457–492.
18. Wang B, Rieger A, Kilgus O, Ochiai K, Maurer D, Fodinger D, Kinet JP, Stingl G. Epidermal Langerhans cells from normal human skin bind monomeric IgE via FcεRI. J Exp Med 1992; 175:1353–1365.

19. Bieber T, de la Salle H, Wollenberg A, Hakimi J, Chizzonite R, Ring J, Hanau D, de la Salle C. Human epidermal Langerhans cells express the high affinity receptor for immunoglobulin E (FcεRI). J Exp Med 1992; 175:1285–1290.
20. Gounni AS, Lamkhioued B, Ochiai K, Tanaka Y, Delaporte E, Capron A, Kinet JP, Capron M. High-affinity IgE receptor on eosinophils is involved in defence against parasites. Nature 1994; 367:183–186.
21. Maurer D, Fiebiger E, Reininger B, Wolff-Winiski B, Jouvin MH, Kilgus O, Kinet JP, Stingl G. Expression of functional high affinity immunoglobulin E receptors (FcεRI) on monocytes of atopic individuals. J Exp Med 1994; 179:745–750.
22. Maurer D, Fiebiger E, Ebner C, Reininger B, Fischer GF, Wichlas S, Jouvin M-H, Schmitt-Egenolf M, Kraft D, Kinet J-P, Stingl G. Peripheral blood dendritic cells express FcεRI as a complex composed of FcεRIα-and FcεRIγ-chains and can use this receptor for IgE-mediated allergen presentation. J Immunol 1996; 157:607–616.
23. Ochiai K, Kagami M, Matsumura R, Kawashima T, Tomioka H. Alveolar macrophages from not only atopic patients but also non-atopic patients express high-affinity IgE receptor (FcεRI). Int Arch Allergy Immunol 1996; 111 S1:55–58.
24. Maurer D, Ebner C, Reininger B, Fiebiger E, Kraft D, Kinet JP, Stingl G. The high affinity IgE receptor (FcεRI) mediates IgE-dependent allergen presentation. J Immunol 1995; 154:6285–6290.
25. Plaut M, Pierce JH, Watson CJ, Hanley-Hyde J, Nordan RP, Paul WE. Mast cell lines produce lymphokines in response to cross-linkage of FcεRI or to calcium ionophores. Nature 1989; 339:64–67.
26. Wodnar-Filipowicz A, Heusser CH, Moroni C. Production of the haemopoietic growth factors GM-CSF and interleukin-3 by mast cells in response to IgE receptor-mediated activation. Nature 1989; 339:150–152.
27. Sutton BJ, Gould HJ. The human IgE network. Nature 1993; 366:421–428.
28. Gauchat J-F, Henchoz S, Mazzei G, Aubry J-P, Brunner T, Blasey H, Life P, Talabot D, Flores-Romo L, Thompson J, Kishl K, Butterfield J, Dahinden C, Bonnefoy J-Y. Induction of human IgE synthesis in B cells by mast cells and basophils. Nature 1993; 365:340–343.
29. Lantz CS, Yamaguchi M, Oettgen HC, Katona IM, Miyajima I, Kinet J-P, Galli SJ. IgE regulates mouse basophil FcεRI expression in vivo. J Immunol 1997; 158:2517–2521.
30. Yamaguchi M, Lantz CS, Oettgen HS, Katona IM, Fleming T, Miyamija I, Kinet J-P, Galli SJ. IgE enhances mouse mast cell FcεRI expression in vitro and in vivo. Evidence for a novel amplification mechanism in IgE-dependent reactions. J Exp Med 1997; 185:663–672.
31. Hide M, Francis DM, Grattan CEH, Hakimi J, Kochan JP, Greaves MW. Autoantibodies against the high-affinity IgE receptor as a cause of histamine release in chronic urticaria. N Engl J Med 1993; 328:1599–1604.
32. Fiebiger E, Maurer D, Holub H, Reininger B, Hartmann G, Woisetschlager M, Kinet JP, Stingl G. Serum IgG autoantibodies directed against the α chain of FcεRI : a selective marker and pathogenetic factor for a distinct subset of chronic urticaria patients? J Clin Invest 1995; 96:2606–2612.
33. Niimi N, Francis DM, Kermani F, O'Donnell BF, Hide M, Kobza-Black A, Winkelman RK, Greaves MW, Barr R. Dermal mast cell activation by autoantibodies against the high-affinity IgE receptor in chronic urticaria. J Invest Dermatol 1996; 106:1001–1006.
34. Tong LJ, Balakrishnan G, Kochan JP, Kinet J-P, Kaplan AP. Assessment of autoimmunity in chronic urticaria patients. Int Arch Allergy Immunol 1997; 99:461–465.
35. Kouskopp V, Korganow A-S, Duchatelle V, Degott C, Benoist C, Mathis D. Organ-specific disease provoked by systemic autoimmunity. Cell 1996; 87:811–822.
36. Adamczewski M, Kinet J-P. The high-affinity receptor for immunoglobulin E. In: Samelson SE, ed. Lymphocyte Activation, vol 59. Basel: S Karger, 1994:173–190.
37. Blank U, Ra C, Miller L, White K, Metzger H, Kinet JP. Complete structure and expression in transfected cells of high-affinity IgE receptor. Nature 1989; 337:187–189.

38. Miller L, Blank U, Metzger H, Kinet JP. Expression of high-affinity binding of human immunoglobulin E by transfected cells. Science 1989; 244:334–337.
39. Letourneur F, Hennecke S, Dèmollieù C, Cosson P. Steric masking of a dilysine endoplasmic reticulum retention motif during assembly of the human high-affinity receptor for immunoglobulin E. J Cell Biol 1995; 129:971–978.
40. Kurosaki T, Ravetch JV. A single amino acid in the glycosyl phosphatidylinositol attachment domain determines the membrane topology of FcγRIII. Nature 1989; 342:805–807.
41. Letourneur O, Sechi S, Willette-Brown J, Robertson MW, Kinet JP. Glycosylation of human truncated FcεRI α chain is necessary for efficient folding in the endoplasmic reticulum. J Biol Chem 1995; 270:8249–8256.
42. Blank U, Ra CS, Kinet JP. Characterization of truncated α chain products from human, rat, and mouse high affinity receptor for immunoglobulin E. J Biol Chem 1991; 266:2639–2646.
43. Robertson MW. Phage and *Escherichia coli* expression of the human high affinity immunoglobulin E receptor α-subunit ectodomain. Domain localization of the IgE-binding site. J Biol Chem 1993; 268:12736–12743.
44. Conroy MC, Adkinson NR Jr, Lichtenstein LM. Measurement of IgE on human basophils: relation to serum IgE and anti-IgE-induced histamine release. J Immunol 1977; 118:1317–1321.
45. Stallman PJ, Aalberse RC, Bruhl PC, Van Elven EH. Experiments on the passive sensitization of human basophils, using quantitative immunofluorescence microscopy. Int Arch Allergy Appl Immunol 1977; 54:364–373.
46. Malveaux FJ, Conroy MC, Adkinson NF Jr, Lichtenstein LM. IgE receptors on human basophils. Relationship to serum IgE concentration. J Clin Invest 1978; 62:176–181.
47. Quarto R, Kinet JP, Metzger H. Coordinate synthesis and degradation of the α-, β-, and γ-subunits of the receptor for immunoglobulin E. Mol Immunol 1985; 22:1045–1051.
48. Furuichi K, Rivera J, Isersky C. The receptor for immunoglobulin E on rat basophilic leukemia cells: effect of ligand binding on receptor expression. Proc Natl Acad Sci USA 1985; 82:1522–1525.
49. Scharenberg AM, Kinet J-P. Early events in mast cell signal transduction. In: Marone G, ed. Human Basophils and Mast Cells, vol. 61. Basel: S Karger, 1995:72–87.
50. Ortega E, Schweitzer-Stenner R, Pecht I. Possible orientational constraints determine secretory signals induced by aggregation of IgE receptors on mast cells. EMBO J 1988; 7:4101–4109.
51. Paolini R, Jouvin M-H, Kinet JP. Phosphorylation and dephosphorylation of the high-affinity receptor for immunoglobulin E immediately after receptor engagement and disengagement. Nature 1991; 353:855–858.
52. Eiseman E, Bolen J. Engagement of the high-affinity IgE receptor activates src protein-related tyrosine kinases. Nature 1992; 355:78–80.
53. Maeyama K, Hohman RJ, Metzger H, Beaven MA. Quantitative relationships between aggregation of IgE receptors, generation of intracellular signals, and histamine secretion in rat basophilic leukemia (2H3) cells. Enhanced responses with heavy water. J Biol Chem 1986; 261:2583–2592.
54. Benhamou M, Ryba NJ, Kihara H, Nishikata H, Siraganian RP. Protein-tyrosine kinase p72syk in high affinity IgE receptor signaling. Identification as a component of pp72 and association with the receptor γ chain after receptor aggregation. J Biol Chem 1993; 268:23318–23324.
55. Kawakami Y, Yao L, Miura T, Tsukada S, Witte ON, Kawakami T. Tyrosine phosphorylation and activation of Bruton tyrosine kinase upon FcεRI cross-linking. Mol Cell Biol 1994; 14:5108–5113.
56. Scharenberg AM, Lin S, Cuenod B, Yamamura H, Kinet JP. Reconstitution of interactions between tyrosine kinases and the high-affinity IgE receptor which are controlled by receptor clustering. EMBO J 1995; 14:3385–3394.
57. Schwartz LB. Mast cells: function and contents. Curr Opin Immunol 1994; 6:91–97.

58. Garcia-Gil M, Siraganian RP. Source of the arachidonic acid released on stimulation of rat basophilic leukemia cells. J Immunol 1986; 136:3825–3828.
59. Garcia-Gil M, Siraganian RP. Phospholipase A_2 stimulation during cell secretion in rat basophilic leukemia cells. J Immunol 1986; 136:259–263.
60. Grabbe J, Welker P, Moller A, Dippel E, Ashman LK, Czarnetzki BM. Comparative cytokine release from human monocytes, monocyte-derived immature mast cells, and a human mast cell line (HMC-1). J Invest Dermatol 1994; 103:504–508.
61. Romeo C, Seed B. Cellular immunity to HIV activated by CD4 fused to T cell or Fc receptor polypeptides. Cell 1991; 64:1037–1046.
62. Irving BA, Weiss A. The cytoplasmic domain of the T cell receptor ζ chain is sufficient to couple to receptor-associated signal transduction pathways. Cell 1991; 64:891–901.
63. Romeo C, Amiot M, Seed B. Sequence requirements for induction of cytolysis by the T cell antigen/Fc receptor ζ chain. Cell 1992; 68:889–897.
64. Jouvin MH, Adamczewski M, Numerof R, Letourneur O, Valle A, Kinet JP. Differential control of the tyrosine kinases Lyn and Syk by the two signaling chains of the high affinity immunoglobulin E receptor. J Biol Chem 1994; 269:5918–5925.
65. Kihara H, Siraganian RP. Src homology 2 domains of Syk and Lyn bind to tyrosine-phosphorylated subunits of the high affinity IgE receptor. J Biol Chem 1994; 269:22427–22432.
66. El-Hillal O, Kinet J-P, Scharenberg AM. Activation of syk by a src kinase initiated activation loop phosphorylation chain reaction. Proc Natl Acad Sci USA 1996; 94:1919–1924.
67. Weiss A, Littman DR. Signal transduction by lymphocyte antigen receptors. Cell 1994; 76:263–274.
68. Cambier JC, Johnson SA. Differential binding activity of ARH1/TAM motifs. Immunol Lett 1995; 44:77–80.
69. Lin S, Cicala C, Scharenberg AM, Kinet JP. The FcεRI β subunit functions as an amplifier of FcεRI γ-mediated cell activation signals. Cell 1996; 85:985–995.
70. Shirakawa T, Li A, Dubowitz M, Dekker JW, Shaw AE, Faux JA, Ra C, Cookson WO, Hopkin JM. Association between atopy and variants of the β subunit of the high-affinity immunoglobulin E receptor. Nature Genet 1994; 7:125–129.
71. Hill MR, James AL, Faux JA, Ryan G, Hopkin JM, le Souef P, Musk AW, Cookson WO. FcεRI-β polymorphism and risk of atopy in a general population sample. Br Med J 1995; 311:776–779.
72. Scharenberg AM, Kinet J-P. The emerging field of receptor-mediated inhibitory signaling: SHP or SHIP? Cell 1996; 87:961–954.
73. Daeron M, Malbec O, Latour S, Arock M, Fridman W. Regulation of high-affinity IgE receptor-mediated mast cell activation by murine low-affinity IgG receptors. J Clin Invest 1995; 95:577–585.
74. D'Ambrosio D, Hippen KL, Minskoff SA, Mellman I, Pani G, Siminovitch KA, Cambier JC. Recruitment and activation of PTP1C in negative regulation of antigen receptor signaling by FγRIIB1. Science 1995; 268:293–297.
75. Tonks N, Neel BG. Cell 1996; 87:365–368.
76. Lioubin MN, Algate PA, Tsai S, Carlberg K, Aebersold A, Rohrschneider LR. P150Ship, a signal transduction molecule with inositol polyphosphate-5-phosphatase activity. Genes Dev 1996; 10:1084–1095.
77. Damen JE, Liu L, Rosten P, Humphries RK, Jefferson AB, Majerus PW, Krystal G. The 145-kDa protein induced to associate with Shc by multiple cytokines is an inositol tetraphosphate and phosphatidylinositol 3,4,5-triphosphate 5-phosphatase. Proc Natl Acad Sci USA 1996; 93:1689–1693.
78. Chacko GW, Tridandapani S, Damen JS, Liu L, Krystal G, Coggeshall KM. Negative signaling in B lymphocytes induces tyrosine phosphorylation of the 145 kd inositol polyphosphate 5-phosphatase SHIP. J Immunol 1996; 157:2234–2238.
79. Ono M, Bolland S, Tempst P, Ravetch JV. Role of the inositol phosphatse SHIP in negative regulation of the immune system by the receptor FcγRIIb. Nature 1996; 383:263–265.

80. Ravetch JV, Anderson CL. FcγR family: proteins, transcripts, and genes. In: Metzger H, ed. Fc Receptors and the Action of Antibodies. Washington, DC: American Society for Microbiology, 1990:211–235.
81. Cookson WO, Sharp PA, Faux JA, Hopkin JM. Linkage between immunoglobulin E responses underlying asthma and rhinitis and chromosome 11q. Lancet 1989; 1:1292–1295.
82. Cookson WO, Young RP, Sandford AJ, Moffatt MF, Shirakawa T, Sharp PA, Faux JA, Julier C, LeSouef PN, Nakumura Y, Lathrop GM, Hopkin JM. Maternal inheritance of atopic IgE responsiveness on chromosome 11q. Lancet 1992; 340:381–384.
83. Young RP, Sharp PA, Lynch JR, Faux JA, Lathrop GM, Cookson WOCM, Hopkin JM. Confirmation of genetic linkage between atopic IgE responses and chromosome 11q13. J Med Genet 1992; 29:236–238.
84. Sandford AJ, Shirakawa T, Moffatt MF, et al. Localisation of atopy and β subunit of high-affinity IgE receptor (FcεRI) on chromosome 11q. Lancet 1993; 341:332–334.
85. Amelung PJ, Panhuysen CI, Postma DS, Levitt RC, Koeter GH, Francomano CA, Bleecker ER, Meyers DA. Atopy and bronchial hyperresponsiveness: exclusion of linkage to markers on chromosomes 11q and 6p. Clin Exp Allergy 1992; 22:1077–1084.
86. Lympany P, Welsh K, MacCochrane G, Kemeny DM, Lee TH. Genetic analysis using DNA polymorphism of the linkage between chromosome 11q13 and atopy and bronchial hyperresponsiveness to methacholine. J Allergy Clin Immunol 1992; 89:619–628.
87. Rich SS, Roitman-Johnson B, Greenberg B, Roberts S, Blumenthal MN. Genetic analysis of atopy in three large kindreds: no evidence of linkage to D11S97. Clin Exp Allergy 1992; 22:1070–1076.
88. Collee JM, ten Kate LP, de Vries HG, Kliphuis JW, Bouman K, Scheffer H, Gerritsen J. Allele sharing on chromosome 11q13 in sibs with asthma and atopy. Lancet 1993; 342:936.
89. Szepetowski P, Gaudray P. FcεRIβ, a candidate gene for atopy, is located in 11q13 between CD20 and TCN1. Genomics 1994; 19:399–400.
90. Shirakawa T, Hashimoto T, Furuyama J, Takeshita T, Morimoto K. Linkage between severe atopy and chromosome 11q13 in Japanese families. Clin Genet 1994; 46:228–232.
91. van Herwerden L, Harrap SB, Wong ZY, Abramson MJ, Kutin JJ, Forbes AB, Raven J, Lanigan A, Walters EH. Linkage of high-affinity IgE receptor gene with bronchial hyperreactivity, even in absence of atopy. Lancet 1995; 346:1262–1265.
92. Watson M, Lawrence S, Collins A, Beasley R, Doull I, Begishvili B, Lampe F, Holgate SF, Morton NE. Exclusion from proximal 11q of a common gene with megaphenic effect on atopy. Ann Hum Genet 1995; 59:403–411.
93. Hill MR, Cookson WO. A novel coding polymorphism in the C-terminus of the β subunit of the high affinity immunoglobulin E (FcεRI-β) is associated with atopy and bronchial hyper-responsiveness. Hum Mol Genet 1996; 5:959–962.

25

Factors Modulating Allergen-Induced Histamine Release

Fc-Receptors, Antibodies, and Allergens

RONALD VAN REE

Central Laboratory of the Netherlands Red Cross Blood Transfusion Service
Amsterdam, The Netherlands

I. Introduction

Histamine release from effector cells (mast cells and basophils) is the starting point of type I allergic reactions. The result is an early or immediate response in the affected target organ(s), frequently followed by a late response. The early response occurs within 15 min after allergen exposure, the late response after several hours. Mast cells play a prominent role in the immediate reaction. The late-phase response is orchestrated by several cell types, especially T cells and eosinophils, but basophils have also been implicated. Which players are pivotal in effecting release of histamine from mast cells and basophils? Three components are indispensable:

1. Allergen
2. Allergen-specific IgE antibodies
3. The high-affinity IgE receptor (FcεRI)

Clusters of several FcεRI-bound allergen-specific IgE antibodies, cross-linked by allergen are the signal for the effector cell to release its mediators. Several characteristics of the allergen–IgE–FcεRI interaction influence the efficacy of histamine release. In addition, other factors related to allergen-specific immunotherapy or autoimmune responses, potentially interfere with FcεRI-mediated histamine release:

1. Allergen-specific IgG antibodies
2. Autoanti-IgE antibodies

A complex interplay of IgE and IgG antibodies, allergens, and Fc receptors determines whether efficient histamine release occurs.

II. Interaction Between Allergen, IgE, and FcεRI

A. Basic Requirements for Histamine Release

To facilitate histamine release from effector cells, FcεRI-bound IgE molecules have to be cross-linked by allergen. This requirement was described over two decades ago by the application of haptens (1). In an in vivo situation, histamine release is the result of bridging of IgE receptors by a combination of IgE and naturally occurring allergen. Several in vitro studies have shown, that both allergen and IgE antibodies are not absolutely necessary. Histamine release without allergen can be achieved by cross-linking IgE with antibodies (2,3), or by multimers of IgE (4). When antibodies against the IgE receptors are used, even IgE antibodies can be omitted (5,6).

At the end of the 1970s, investigators tried to answer the question of how many clusters of cross-linked IgE receptors should be formed per cell, to trigger mediator release (7,8). These early studies indicated that approximately ten antigen-induced receptor clusters suffice to induce histamine release. To form enough clusters, there is a threshold density of IgE receptors loaded with specific IgE.

B. Ratio-Specific Versus Total IgE

The density of cell-bound specific IgE is not determined only by the absolute titers of these antibodies. In 1973 it was reported that high levels of total IgE of a recipient had an inhibitory effect on the Prausnitz–Küstner titer of a donor serum (9). High titers of total IgE are found in patients with helmintic infections. Several studies have demonstrated that these infections result in a lower incidence of allergic symptoms, despite the presence of allergen-specific IgE antibodies (10–12). An inverse relation between parasitic infections and allergy was confirmed in a more recent study (13). Antihelmintic treatment resulted in a decrease of total serum IgE, accompanied by an increase in skin reactivity toward common inhalant allergens. Together, these data support the model that saturation of IgE receptors with nonspecific IgE decreases the capacity to respond to specific allergens. Histamine release and skin reactivity with purified major allergens are also inversely correlated with total IgE levels in patients without extreme total IgE titers accompanying parasitic infections (14). In such "normal" allergic patients, major allergen-specific IgE ranges roughly from 0.1 to 25% of total serum IgE (15).

C. Epitope Valency

How many IgE receptors should be included in a single cluster for efficient histamine release? The first answers came from studies with multimers of IgE: Dimers of IgE are the minimum unit for facilitating histamine release (16); however, larger oligomers appear to be more efficient (17–19). In studies with rodent monoclonal IgE antibodies and dinitrophenol–human serum albumin ($DNP_{(n)}$–HSA; 20,21) or aggregated ovalbumin (21), the most efficient number of epitopes was seven. Higher degrees of substitution (or aggregation) did not result in more efficient histamine release.

The "allergens" used in the aforementioned studies are artificial. How many epitopes do we need on a natural allergen to trigger effector cells? In our laboratory this was tested for the mite allergen Der p 2. Two different chimeric antibodies directed to Der p 2 were developed, each consisting of the constant region of human IgE and the heavy and light chain variable regions derived from two different mouse monoclonal antibodies (MAbs) against Der p 2 (22). The necessity of cross-linking was confirmed by the absence of histamine release, when Der p 2 was added to basophils sensitized with just one type of chimeric antibodies (23). Histamine release was achieved after sensitization with both chimeric antibodies. Whether three or more IgE antibodies result in more efficient histamine release remains to be investigated. It is, however, unlikely that an allergen such as Der p 2 can bind more than four or five antibodies simultaneously. From the three-dimensional structures of an antigen, such as lysozyme (24) or Fab fragments (25–28), it can be calculated that an antigen of approximately 15 kDa (such as Der p 2) cannot bind many more than four antibodies at the same time. This would imply that optimal histamine release by an allergen would probably be reached after the binding of four to seven IgE molecules, depending on the actual size and shape of the allergen molecule.

D. Affinity of IgE for the Allergen

Not much is known on the role of affinity on the interaction between IgE and allergen. A study with two different mouse monoclonal IgE antibodies directed to DNP tested the influence of affinity on the degree of histamine release (21). The affinity of both antibodies for the hapten differed by one order of magnitude: for a similar degree of histamine release, IgE antibodies with lower affinity required a higher amount of $DNP_{(n)}$–HSA, or a higher ratio of specific/total IgE. These observations indicate that efficient histamine release is favored by high-affinity IgE antibodies.

E. "Irrelevant" IgE: Allergen-Specific but Biologically Inactive?

What is the relevance of the foregoing requirements for histamine release in an in vivo situation? A possible clue comes from pollen allergic subjects who demonstrate in vitro cross-reactivity of IgE antibodies directed at vegetable foods, without concordant symptomatology (29,30). Over the past decade, several cross-reactive structures were identified in pollen and vegetable foods (31): the major birch pollen allergen Bet v 1 and its homologues in fruits: profilins from a broad spectrum of plant cells; and carbohydrate determinants on glycoproteins of plants and invertebrate animals. Sensitization to these structures occurs by the inhalant route (32). Patients with birch pollinosis frequently demonstrate symptoms after consumption of fruits such as apples or peaches (33). Cross-reactive IgE antibodies to profilin can cause food-related symptoms to an even broader spectrum of vegetable foods (34). On the other hand, not every pollen allergic patient with cross-reactive IgE to Bet v1 or profilin has symptoms related to foods. Specific IgE without concordant symptomatology is most frequently observed when IgE antibodies are directed to carbohydrate determinants (35). What is the explanation of this phenomenon?

The structures of some IgE-binding carbohydrate determinants and several of the glycoproteins that carry them have been elucidated (36,37). The sugar groups involved, are *N*-linked glycans. Most allergens, described so far, have molecular weights ranging from 10 to 70 kDa. Larger proteins do not easily cross the mucosal barrier. Most glycoproteins in this molecular weight range are monoglycosylated, including major allergens such as Lol p 1 (38), Lol p 11 (39), Ara h 1 (40), PLA_2 (37) and others. Cross-reactivity between pollen and vegetable foods, exclusively based on *N*-glycan–specific IgE antibodies will not result in food-induced histamine release: food-derived glycoproteins behave as monovalent allergens. Similarly, the number of cross-reactive epitopes recognized on a pollen allergen such as Bet v 1 might determine whether fruit-reactive IgE antibodies are biologically active.

F. Concluding Remarks

Interaction between FcεRI, IgE, and allergen is the basis for mediator release from mast cells and basophils. Efficient histamine release is favored by

1. A high ratio of specific/total IgE in serum: "nonspecific" IgE saturates IgE receptors.
2. A higher number of IgE epitopes per allergen: two epitopes are the minimum, the highest release is achieved with approximately seven epitopes.
3. The high-affinity of IgE antibodies for the allergen.

The outcome of encounters between effector cells and allergens seems to be determined by a complex interplay of these three factors. There are, however, other potential factors, some of which become evident during allergen-specific immunotherapy.

III. Interference of Factors Outside the FcεRI–IgE–Allergen Complex

A. The Blocking Antibody Theory: An Obsolete Hypothesis?

A striking feature of allergen-specific immunotherapy is the induction of allergen-specific IgG (41). Early after beginning therapy, IgG1 antibodies predominate, but they are progressively replaced by IgG4. This observation led to the hypothesis that allergen-specific IgG prevents the allergen from reaching IgE on the surface of effector cells. For this reason they were designated "blocking antibodies." Passive transfer experiments with sera containing high titers of allergen-specific IgG supported the concept of blocking antibodies (42,43).

Several observations, however, have caused a decreased belief in the blocking activity of IgG as the mechanism of immunotherapy: (1) clinical outcome and allergen-specific IgG titers usually demonstrate poor correlation (41); (2) immunotherapy results in a more potent downregulation of late-phase reactions than of early-phase reactions (44); (3) the high Th1/Th2 ratio for allergen-specific T helper cells is influenced by immunotherapy in favor of Th1 (44). Together, this has resulted in another interpretation of the mechanism of immunotherapy, designating T cells as the prime target. Despite this, several lines of evidence have brought IgG back into the picture as an important factor modulating histamine release.

B. Blocking Activity of IgG: In Vitro and In Vivo

A recent study with polyclonal rabbit antibodies, obtained after immunization with a synthetic COOH-terminal peptide of the major grass pollen allergen Lol p 1, demonstrated that these antibodies can inhibit Lol p 1-induced histamine release from human basophils (45). To achieve this inhibition, allergy and blocking antibodies were added simultaneously to the basophils, thereby staying as close as possible to an in vivo situation during which IgG antibodies do not have the advantage of a preincubation with allergen.

Also, for human allergen-specific IgG, blocking activity was demonstrated in in vitro experiments. For this purpose, five different human monoclonal IgG antibodies directed at the major birch pollen allergen Bet v 1 were produced, using Epstein–Barr virus (EBV)-immortalized peripheral blood mononuclear cells (PBMC; from a donor who had undergone successful immunotherapy) and anti-CD40 antibody; 46). One of the monoclonal antibodies completely inhibited the Bet v 1-induced histamine release of several donors. With the other four MAbs this was achieved only when they were used in a mixture. Together, these data illustrate that IgG antibodies from a single donor, induced during successful immunotherapy, can block allergen-induced histamine release.

Is the blocking mechanism of relevance for an in vivo situation? Support for this comes from another field in which IgE and IgG4 play an important role: parasitic infections. A study in a community in The Gambia, West Africa, demonstrated that the odds for reinfections with *Schistosoma haematobium* are influenced in opposite directions by IgE and IgG4 (47). Patients in the lowest quintile of IgE levels had a ten times higher chance to be reinfected than those in the highest quintile. For IgG4, exactly the opposite was observed, suggesting that IgG4 blocks the beneficial effects of IgE. Several studies have confirmed this blocking mechanism in in vitro experiments (48–50).

Poor correlation between clinical outcome of immunotherapy and allergen-specific IgG4 titers seems to contradict a blocking role for IgG4. A possible explanation for the poor correlation is that, in most immunotherapy studies, IgG4 antibodies were measured with whole-allergen extracts. In this way, IgG responses to major allergens, minor allergens, and nonallergenic proteins are measured together. Relevant information, most likely, can be obtained only by measuring antibody responses to major allergens. Support for this approach comes from a study with 59 nontreated cat allergic patients (51). IgG, specific for the major cat allergen Fel d 1, induced by natural exposure, was measured and compared with skin reactivity to Fel d 1. Fel d 1-specific IgG was detected in 30 patients, ranging from less than 0.25 to 3.5 μg/mL. The Fel d 1 threshold for a positive skin test was positively correlated with Fel d 1-specific IgG titers, indicating that IgG blocks IgE-mediated skin reactivity.

C. Concluding Remarks

Both in vitro experiments and in vivo observations confirm the potential role of IgG as blocking antibodies as postulated decades ago. Ascribing the beneficial effect of immunotherapy solely to the appearance of these antibodies would be an oversimplification. The presence of blocking antibodies, however, could explain the inhibitory effect of immunotherapy on the early-phase responses. These responses are clearly IgE-mediated, without direct involvement of T cells or eosinophils.

IV. How Do IgG Antibodies Modulate Histamine Release?

A. Simple Blockade of IgE Epitopes

The simplest possible explanation of a blocking mechanism is that allergen-specific IgG prevents the allergen from binding to effector cell-bound IgE. In this scenario, efficient blockade would require overlapping epitope-specificities of IgE and IgG4. However, there are several lines of evidence showing that IgE and IgG4 recognize different sites on an allergen. In our laboratory, this was tested in a model using Fel d 1. Affinity-purified human antibodies directed to Fel d 1 were tested in an IgE radioallergosorbent test (RAST) and an IgG4 RAST with cat dander and ocelot dander extracts (52). It was demonstrated that Fel d 1-specific IgE antibodies are more cross-reactive to the related allergen of the ocelot than Fel d 1-specific IgG4 antibodies. Comparisons of the reactivity of IgE and IgG4 with recombinant chain 1 and chain 2 of Fel d 1, and with overlapping synthetic peptides spanning the complete sequence of Fel d 1, confirmed differences in specificity for both antibody isotypes (53,54). In the light of these observations, blockade of IgE epitopes by IgG4 might be too simple an explanation. On the other hand, blockade could be the result of steric hindrance caused by proximity, instead of identity, of epitopes. The aforedescribed limitation of the surface of an antigen to simultaneously bind different antibodies supports this explanation.

B. Involvement of Low-Affinity IgG Receptors

Modulation of histamine release by allergen-specific IgG might need another immunoglobulin receptor: the low-affinity IgG receptor, FcγRII. This receptor is present on mast cells and basophils (55,56). Low-affinity IgG receptors bind complexed IgG (e.g., complexes of allergen and IgG). In studies with murine mast cells and rat basophilic leukemia cells, cross-linking of FcεRI and FcγRII by IgE–allergen–IgG complexes inhibited allergen-induced histamine release (56). Cross-linking of only FcγRII receptors did not result in downregulation of IgE-mediated histamine release.

The necessity of clustering high-affinity IgE and low-affinity IgG receptors implies that overlapping epitope specificities of IgE and IgG4 would, in fact, hamper efficient blocking of IgE-mediated histamine release. Support for efficient blockade with nonoverlapping epitopes comes from the aforementioned inhibition studies with IgG directed to the COOH-terminus of Lol p 1 (45). Histamine release induced by Lol p 1 was inhibited, despite the lack of IgE reactivity of the basophil donor with the COOH-terminus of Lol p 1. Again, this could also be explained by steric hindrance of IgE binding, caused by IgG bound to the COOH-terminus of the allergen.

C. Concluding Remarks

Firm evidence is still lacking for either direct blockade of epitopes or FcγRII-mediated downregulation as the mechanism of blocking antibody activity. A combination of both mechanisms cannot be excluded. The availability of sets of allergen-specific human (46,57) or chimeric (22) monoclonal IgE and IgG enables the investigation of both proposed mechanisms.

V. Anti-IgE Antibodies

The occurrence of IgG autoantibodies directed to IgE was reported in 1972 (58). Circulating IgG–anti-IgE is usually complexed with IgE, making purification of these autoantibodies difficult (59). This has hampered the study of their role in IgE immunoregulation and modulation of allergen-induced histamine release. Recent developments in the field of repertoire cloning have enabled the isolation of human monoclonal anti-IgE antibodies (60). A high percentage of these antibodies turned out to be anti-idiotype. Only a few were found to be anti-isotype. Most knowledge on the possible pathophysiological importance of anti-isotype anti-IgE, so far, comes from studies with mouse MAbs directed at IgE (59). For the modulation of histamine release, several different effects were reported. Some antibodies were anaphylactogenic, in contrast with those recognizing the binding site of IgE to the high-affinity IgE receptor. The latter type of antibody prevents circulating IgE from binding to FcεRI. A very interesting MAb was described that recognized FcεRI-bound IgE, without being anaphylactogenic. On the contrary, the MAb promoted dissociation of bound IgE from, and prevented binding of, free IgE to FcεRI. This type of antibody could, therefore, be designated as "desensitizing." The characteristics of naturally occurring human anti-IgE, however, still largely remains to be determined.

The observations that some mouse monoclonal anti-IgE antibodies are capable of preventing binding of IgE to, or even facilitate dissociation from, its receptor has prompted several groups to investigate whether chimeric or humanized versions of such antibodies have potential as therapeutic agents (61–63). Clinical trials with these antibodies are currently underway.

VI. Summary

Immunoglobulin E-mediated histamine release is achieved by cross-linking of FcεRI-bound IgE with allergen. This reaction is favored by a high ratio of specific versus total IgE. An allergen should at least carry two IgE epitopes to facilitate release, but the optimal number probably lies between four and seven. High-affinity IgE–allergen interactions favor histamine release. Allergen-specific IgG seems to have an inhibitory effect, although the mechanism still remains unclear. Finally, autoantibodies directed to IgE potentially have both inhibitory and stimulatory effects on histamine release, depending on the epitope specificity.

References

1. Siraganian RP, Hook WA, Levine BB. Specific in vitro histamine release from basophils by bivalent haptens: evidence for activation by simple bridging of membrane bound antibody. Immunochemistry 1975; 12:149–157.
2. Ishizaka T, Ishizaka K, Johansson SG, Bennich H. Histamine release from human leukocytes by anti-gamma E antibodies. J Immunol 1969; 102:884–892.
3. Ishizaka T, Ishizaka K. Immune mechanisms of reversed type reagenic hypersensitivity. J Immunol 1969; 103:588–595.
4. Ishizaka T, Ishizaka K, Lee EH. Biologic function of the Fc fragments of E myeloma protein. Immunochemistry 1970; 7:687–702.
5. Ishizaka T, Ishizaka K. Triggering of histamine release from rat mast cells by divalent antibodies against IgE receptors. J Immunol 1978; 120:800–805.
6. Isersky C, Taurog JD, Poy G, Metzger H. Triggering of cultured neoplastic mast cells by antibodies to the receptor for IgE. J Immunol 1978; 121:549–558.
7. DeLisi C, Siraganian RP. Receptor crosslinking and histamine release I. The quantitative dependence of basophil degranulation of the number of receptor doublets. J Immunol 1979; 122:2286–2292.
8. DeLisi C, Siraganian RP. Receptor crosslinking and histamine release II. Interpretation and analysis of anomalous dose response patterns. J Immunol 1979; 122:2293–2299.
9. Bazaral M, Orgel HA, Hamburger RN. The influence of serum IgE levels of selected recipients, including patients with allergy, helminthiasis and tuberculosis, on the apparent P–K titre of a reaginic serum. Clin Exp Allergy 1973; 14:117–125.
10. Godfrey RC. Asthma and IgE levels in rural and urban communities of The Gambia. Clin Allergy 1975; 5:201–207.

11. Merrett TG, Merrett J, Cookson JB. Allergy and parasites: the measurement of total and specific IgE levels in urban and rural communities in Rhodesia. Clin Allergy 1976; 6:131–134.
12. Godfrey RC, Gradidge CF. Allergic sensitisation of human lung fragments prevented by saturation of IgE binding sites. Nature 1976; 259:484–486.
13. Lynch NR, Hagel I, Perez M, Di Prisco MC, Lopez R, Alvarez N. Effect of antihelmintic treatment on the allergic reactivity of children in a tropical slum. J Allergy Clin Immunol 1993; 92:404–411.
14. Witteman AM, Stapel SO, Perdok GJ, Sjamsoedin DHS, Jansen HM, Aalberse RC, Van der Zee JS. The relationship between RAST and skin test results in patients with asthma or rhinitis: a quantitative study with purified major allergens. J Allergy Clin Immunol 1996; 97:16–25.
15. Chapman MD, Rowntree S, Mitchell EB, Di Prisco de Fuenmajor MC, Platts-Mills TAE. Quantitative assessments of IgG and IgE antibodies to inhalent allergens in patients with atopic dermatitis. J Allergy Clin Immunol 1983; 72:27–33.
16. Segal DM, Taurog JD, Metzger H. Dimeric immunoglobulin E serves as a unit signal for mast cell degranulation. Proc Natl Acad Sci USA 1977; 74:2993–2997.
17. Fewtrell C, Metzger H. Larger oligomers of IgE are more effective than dimers in stimulating rat basophilic leukemia cells. J Immunol 1980; 125:701–710.
18. Kagey-Sobotka A, Dembo M, Goldstein B, Metzger H, Lichtenstein LM. Qualitative characteristics of histamine release from human basophils by covalently cross-linked IgE. J Immunol 1981; 127:2285–2291.
19. MacGlashan DW, Schleimer RP, Lichtenstein LM. Qualitative differences between dimeric and trimeric stimulation of human basophils. J Immunol 1983; 130:4–6.
20. Healicon RM, Foreman JC. Characteristics of histamine release from rat mast cells in relation to the valency of the stimulating ligand. Immunology 1986; 57:611–615.
21. Collins AM, Thelian D, Basil M. Antigen valency as a determinant of the responsiveness of IgE-sensitised rat basophil leukemia cells. Int Arch Allergy Immunol 1995; 107:547–556.
22. Schuurman J, Perdok GJ, Lourens TE, Parren PWHI, Chapman MD, Aalberse RC. Production of a mouse/human chimeric IgE monoclonal antibody to the housedust mite allergen Der p 2 and its use for the absolute quantification of allergen specific IgE. J Allergy Clin Immunol 1997; 99:549–550.
23. Schuurman J, Perdok, Mueller GA, Aalberse RC. Complementation of Der p 2-induced histamine release from human basophils sensitized with monoclonal IgE: Not only by IgE, but also by IgG antibodies directed to a nonoverlapping epitope of Der p 2. J Allergy Clin Immunol 1998; 101:404–409.
24. Blake CCF, Koenig DF, Mair GA, North ACT, Phillips DC, Sarma VR. Structure of hen egg-white lysozyme. A three-dimensional Fourier synthesis at 2 A resolution. Nature 1965; 206:757–761.
25. Atassa MZ. Precise determination of the entire antigenic structure of lysozyme: molecular features of protein antigenic structures and potential of "surface-simulation" synthesis—a powerful new concept for protein binding sites. Immunochemistry 1978; 15:909–936.
26. Amit AG, Mariuzza RA, Phillips SEV, Polijak RJ. Three-dimensional structure of an antigen–antibody complex at 6 A resolution. Nature 1985; 313:156–158.
27. Amit AG, Mariuzza RA, Phillips SEV, Poljak RJ. Three-dimensional structure of an antigen–antibody complex at 2.8 A resolution. Science 1986; 223:747–753.
28. Padlan EA. Anatomy of the antibody molecule. Mol Immunol 1994; 31:169–217.
29. Bircher AJ, Van Melle G, Haller E, Curty B, Frei PC. IgE to food allergens are highly prevalent in patients allergic to pollens, with and without symptoms of food allergy. Clin Exp Allergy 1994; 367–374.
30. Poor biological activity of cross-reactive IgE directed to carbohydrate determinants of glycoproteins. Van der Veen MJ, Van Ree R, Aalberse RC, Akkerdaas JH, Koppelman SJ, Jansen HM, Van der Lee JS. J Allergy Clin Immunol 1997; 100:327–334.

31. van Ree R, Aalberse RC. Pollen vegetable food crossreactivity: serological and clinical relevance of crossreactive IgE. J Clin Immunoassay 1993; 16:124–130.
32. Valenta R, Kraft D. Type I allergic reactions to plant-derived food: a consequence of primary sensitization to pollen allergens. J Allergy Clin Immunol 1996; 97:893–895.
33. Ebner C, Birkner T, Valenta R, Rumpold H, Breitenbach M, Scheiner O, Kraft D. Common epitopes of birch and apples—studies by Western and Northern blotting. J Allergy Clin Immunol 1991; 88:588–594.
34. van Ree R, Voitenko V, van Leeuwen WA, Aalberse RC. Profilin is a crossreactive allergen in pollen and vegetable foods. Int Arch Allergy Immunol 1992; 98:97–104.
35. Aalberse RC, Koshte V, Clemens JGJ. Immunoglobulin E antibodies that crossreact with vegetable foods, pollen and Hymenoptera venom. J Allergy Clin Immunol 1981; 68:356–364.
36. Faye L, Chrispeels MJ. Common antigenic determinants in the glycoproteins of plants, molluscs and insects. Glycoconjugate J 1988; 5:245–256.
37. Tretter V, Altmann F, Kubelka V, März L, Becker WM. Fucose linked α1-3 to the core-region of glycoprotein *N*-glycans forms an important epitope for IgE from honeybee venom allergic individuals. Int Arch Allergy Immunol 1993; 102:259–266.
38. Perez M, Ishioka GY, Walker LE, Chesnut RW. cDNA cloning and immunological characterization of the rye grass allergen Lol p 1. J Biol Chem 1990; 265:16210–16215.
39. van Ree R, Hoffman DR, van Dijk W, Brodard V, Mahieu K, Koeleman CAM, Grande M, van Leeuwen WA, Aalberse RC. Lol p 11, a new major grass pollen allergen, is a member of a family of soybean trypsin inhibitor-related proteins. J Allergy Clin Immunol 1995; 95:970–978.
40. Burks AW, Cockrell G, Stanley JS, Helm RM, Bannon GA. Recombinant peanut allergen Ara h 1 expression and IgE binding in patients with peanut hypersensitivity. J Clin Invest 1995; 96:1715–1721.
41. Djurup R. The subclass nature and clinical significance of the IgG antibody response in patients undergoing allergen specific immunotherapy. Allergy 1985; 40:469–486.
42. Cooke RA, Loveless M Stull A. Studies on immunity in a type of human allergy (hay fever): serologic response of non-sensitive individuals to pollen injections. J Exp Med 1937; 66:689–696.
43. Sherman WB. Changes in serological reactions and tissue-sensitivity in hay-fever patients during the early months of treatment. J Immunol 1941; 40:289–309.
44. Varney VA, Hamid QA, Gaga M, Sun Ying, Jacobson M, Frew AJ, Kay AB, Durham SR. Influence of grass pollen immunotherapy on cellular infiltration and cytokine mRNA expression during allergen-induced late-phase cutaneous responses. J Clin Invest 1993; 92:644–651.
45. van Ree R, Aalberse RC. Rabbit IgG directed to a synthetic C-terminal peptide of the major grass pollen allergen Lol p 1 inhibits human basophil histamine release induced by natural Lol p I. Int Arch Allergy Immunol 1995; 106:250–257.
46. Visco B, Dolecek C, Denepoux S, Le Mao J, Guret C, Rousset F, Guinnepain M-T, Kraft D, Valenta R, Weyer A, Banchereau J, Lebecque S. Human IgG monoclonal antibodies that modulate the binding of specific IgE to birch pollen Bet v 1. J Immunol 1996; 157:956–962.
47. Hagan P, Blumenthal UJ, Dunn D, Simpson AJG, Wilkins HA. Human IgE, IgG4 and resistance to reinfection with *Schistosoma haematobium*. Nature 1991; 349:243–245.
48. Ottesen EA, Kumaraswami V, Paranjape R, Poindexter RW, Tripathy SP. Naturally occurring blocking antibodies modulate immediate hypersensitivity responses in human filariasis. J Immunol 1981; 127:2014–2020.
49. Rihet P, Demeure Ce, Dessein AJ, Bourgois A. Strong serum inhibition of specific IgE correlated to competing IgG4, revealed by a new methodology in subjects from a *S. mansoni* endemic area. Eur J Immunol 1992; 22:2063–2070.
50. Hussain R, Poindexter RW, Ottesen EA. Control of allergic reactivity in human filariasis. J Immunol 1992; 148:2731–2737.

51. Witteman AM, Stapel SO, Sjamsoedin DHS, Jansen HM, Aalberse RC, van der Zee JS. Fel d 1-specific IgG antibodies induced by natural exposure have blocking activity in skin tests. Int Arch Allergy Immunol 1996; 109:369–375.
52. van Milligen FJ, van Swieten P, Aalberse RC. IgE and IgG4 binding to the ocelot variant of the cat (*Felis domesticus*) major allergen Fel d 1. Allergy 1994; 49:393–394.
53. van Milligen FJ, Craig S, Rogers BL, van Swieten P, Aalberse RC. Differences between specificities of IgE and IgG4 antibodies: studies using recombinant chain 1 and chain 2 of the major cat allergen *Felis domesticus* (Fel d) 1. Clin Exp Allergy 1995; 25:247–251.
54. van Milligen FJ, van 't Hof W, Aalberse RC. IgE and IgG4 binding to synthetic peptides of the cat (*Felis domesticus*) major allergen Fel d 1. Int. Arch Allergy Immunol 1994; 103:274–279.
55. Anselmino LM, Perussia B, Thomas LL. Human basophils selectively express the Fc-gamma-RII (CDw32) subtype of IgG receptor. J Allergy Clin Immunol 1989; 84:907–914.
56. Daeron M, Malbec O, Latour S, Arock M, Fridman WH. Regulation of high-affinity IgE receptor-mediated mast cell activation by murine low-affinity IgG receptors. J Clin Invest 1995; 95:577–585.
57. Steinberger P, Kraft D, Valenta R. Construction of a combinatorial IgE library from an allergic patient. Isolation and characterization of human IgE Fabs with specificity for the major timothy grass pollen allergen, *Phl p* 5. J Biol Chem 1996; 271:10967–10972.
58. Williams RC, Griffiths RW, Emmons JD, Field RC. Naturally occurring human anti-globulins with specificity for gamma-E. J Clin Invest 1972; 51:955–963.
59. Stadler BM, Rudolf PM, Zuercher AW, Miescher S, Vogel M. Anti-IgE in allergic sensitization. Immunol Cell Biol 1996; 74:195–200.
60. Vogel M, Miescher B, Biaggi C, Stadler BM. Human anti-IgE antibodies by repertoire cloning. Eur J Immunol 1994; 24:1200–1207.
61. Presta L, Lahr SJ, Shields RL, et al. Humanization of an antibody directed against IgE. J Immunol 1993; 151:2623–2632.
62. Davis FM, Gossett LA, Pinkston KL, et al. Can anti-IgE be used to treat allergy? Springer Semin Immunopathol 1993; 15:51–73.
63. Jardieu P. Anti-IgE therapy. Curr Opin Immunol 1995; 7:779–782.

26

Regulation of Immunoglobulin E–Mediated Inflammation by Soluble Fragments of the High-Affinity Immunoglobulin E Receptor

BRIAN J. SUTTON and HANNAH J. GOULD

The Randall Institute
King's College London
London, England

I. Introduction

The binding of IgE to its high-affinity receptor FcεRI on mast cells and basophils is a critical event in the allergic response. The extremely high association constant for the interaction ($K_a \approx 10^{10}\ M^{-1}$), two orders of magnitude greater than that of any other immunoglobulin for its specific receptor (1), ensures that at even low levels of circulating IgE, a large fraction of the receptors on mast cells in the tissue, or on basophils in the blood, are occupied by IgE. Following allergen challenge, however, and particularly in atopic individuals, these cells become sensitized with allergen-specific IgE, and are thus primed to respond to subsequent challenge by the allergen. The binding of multivalent allergen to receptor-bound IgE cross-links the receptors, triggering degranulation and release of molecules, such as histamine and leukotrienes, that promote an inflammatory response. Because the interaction between IgE and FcεRI is independent of the allergen, it has long been recognized as a potential target for therapeutic intervention.

The high-affinity receptor, however, is not found exclusively on mast cells and basophils as originally thought. The recent discovery that Langerhans cells (2,3), eosinophils (4), and monocytes (5) also express FcεRI implies that this reaction is involved in more than just the type I immediate hypersensitivity reaction. On Langerhans cells the receptor is clearly involved in the uptake and processing of allergen (6,7), and increased expression of FcεRI has been found in the epidermal Langerhans cells from individuals with atopic dermatitis (8). Activation of these cells by IgE-dependent cross-linking of FcεRI has also been demonstrated (8), and in some cases this culminates in the release of inflammatory mediators. Similarly, a higher proportion of dendritic cells from the airways of asthmatic patients express FcεRI compared with controls (9,10). On monocytes, the expression of FcεRI enhances presentation of allergen; when targeted to FcεRI by allergen-specific IgE, the presentation of allergen to T cells was enhanced by two to three orders of magnitude (11). Furthermore, the level of expression of FcεRI on peripheral blood monocytes has also been reported to be upregulated in atopic individuals (5), perhaps as a direct result of the increased level of IgE (12). Upregulation of FcεRI expression on eosinophils infiltrating the skin in atopic dermatitis has also been reported (13), and thus, activation of these cells by allergen–IgE complexes and mediator release may contribute to the pathogenesis of this condition (14). It is clear, therefore, that inhibitors of IgE binding to FcεRI may have effects beyond those caused by mast cells and basophils, in particular the processing and presentation of allergen to the immune system, and modulation of the inflammatory process. The targeting of these other cells, such as the Langerhans cells, may be particularly effective for certain allergic diseases in view of their accessibility to therapeutic agents.

Although interference in the binding of IgE to its receptor is potentially a very promising approach, the high affinity of the natural interaction is clearly a challenge. Progress has been made, however, in part as a result of our increasingly detailed understanding of the structures of the two components. The problem has been approached in several different ways, including the production of anti-IgE for administration as a therapeutic agent, the development of an IgE-derived vaccine to generate natural anti-IgE and the design and synthesis of inhibitors based on the structure of either the IgE molecule or the high-affinity receptor. In this review we will focus on the last of these approaches in relation to the receptor, and only briefly mention the others where information relevant to the general IgE–FcεRI inhibition strategy has been obtained. For example, it has become apparent from studies associated with the clinical trials of an anti-IgE antibody, now at an advanced stage, that this molecule has a significant inhibitory effect on IgE synthesis. Furthermore, reduction in the levels of circulating IgE can affect the level of surface expression of the receptor on basophils. Such findings clearly have an important bearing on the likely success of any strategy directed toward desensitization of mast cells and basophils by inhibition of IgE binding to FcεRI; therefore, these results will be discussed in some detail.

We begin, however, with a brief review of the structures of IgE and, more particularly, FcεRI. Our understanding of the complementary binding regions in each of these two molecules has advanced significantly in recent years, and now provides a basis not only for rational design of therapeutic agents, but also for interpretation of functional data in terms of molecular mechanisms.

II. IgE Structure

The Fc region of the IgE molecule consists of a disulfide-linked dimer of the three constant domains of the ε-heavy chain, Cε2, Cε3, and Cε4 (Fig. 1). In the absence of a crystal structure for any part of IgE, models of the Fc region have been generated (15,16), based on the known structure of IgG. However, the Cε2 domain pair, which includes the two inter–heavy-chain disulfide bridges, has no counterpart in IgG and, in effect, replaces the hinge region; consequently, the models are uncertain with respect to the disposition of the Cε2 domain pair, relative to Cε3 and Cε4. A model for the Cε3 and Cε4 domains, presumably structurally homologous to the Cγ2 and Cγ3 domains of IgG–Fc, is shown in Figure 2.

The structure of IgE and its Fc fragment is further complicated by the discovery that the IgE molecule adopts a bent structure both in solution and when bound to FcεRI. This was first detected by measuring energy transfer between fluorophores attached to each end of the molecule (17), but X-ray and neutron scattering of both IgE and IgE–Fc confirm the bent structure and suggest that the bend most probably occurs between the Cε2 and Cε3 domains in the Fc (18). This has implications for the stoichiometry of binding of IgE to FcεRI, as discussed in the following.

The consensus from numerous studies to map the FcεRI-binding site in IgE–Fc using recombinant ε-chain peptides, monoclonal anti-IgE, and chimeric IgE molecules (reviewed in Ref. 19) is that the site lies within Cε3. More recently, site-directed mutagenesis has identified several residues that constitute the binding site (20–22), which appears to be very extensive, spanning both Cε3 domains (22; see Fig. 2). Several ε-chain peptides corresponding to different parts of the Cε3 domain inhibit IgE binding to FcεRI, including a 76-residue peptide-spanning part of Cε2 and the NH_2-terminal region of Cε3, which inhibited IgE-dependent mast cell degranulation in vitro and passive sensitization of human skin mast cells in vivo

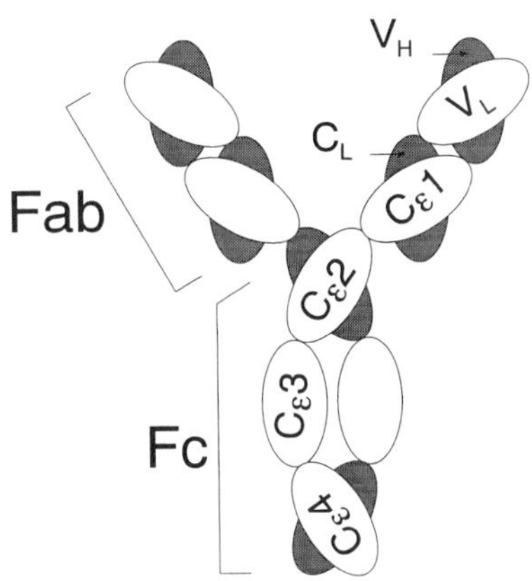

Figure 1 Schematic representation of the domain structure of the IgE molecule.

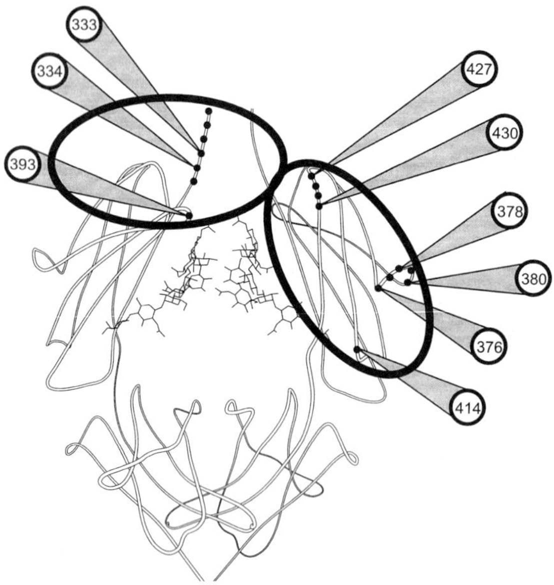

Figure 2 Modeled structure of the Cε3 and Cε4 domains of IgE–Fc, indicating the amino acid residues in Cε3 that have been implicated in binding to the high-affinity receptor by mutagenesis studies (see text). The ellipses are drawn to show the approximate extent of the two extracellular domains of the FcεRI α-chain, but the mode of interaction is unknown. The conserved carbohydrate chains, *N*-linked to residue 394 in each heavy chain, lie between the two Cε3 domains.

(23,24). A recent study employing a series of progressively truncated ε-chain peptides (25) implicated the loop region between the first two β-strands of Cε3 (the AB loop) as a critical determinant, and short peptides corresponding to this loop had earlier been shown to inhibit passive cutaneous anaphylaxis (PCA) in rats (26), and passive sensitization of human basophils (27). However, high concentrations of these peptides (in the millimolar range) were required to demonstrate activity.

An alternative approach adopted by several groups has been to generate anti-IgE antibodies. In principle, if these antibodies are directed to determinants in IgE–Fc that are accessible only in free IgE and not in the complex, then they are capable of inhibiting the binding of IgE to FcεRI, but cannot cause mast cell activation by cross-linking receptor-bound IgE. A subpopulation of naturally occurring anti-IgE antibodies in asthma patients downregulates the allergic response (28), and the production of an anti-IgE response to IgE–Fc-derived peptides in rats by a vaccine strategy has been attempted (29,30). In one study, the entire Cε2–Cε3 domains were used as immunogen (30), whereas a short peptide from the Cε4 domain, adjacent to Cε3 in the three-dimensional structure, was used in the other (29). Humanized anti-IgE antibodies for human therapy have also been generated (31–36), and clinical trials indicate that this is a very promising therapeutic approach. These strategies will not be considered further here, for they are outside the scope of this review. However, in the course of characterizing these anti-IgE monoclonal antibodies it was found that not only suppression of IgE synthesis by surface IgE on B cells was occurring (in accord with several earlier studies), but also a downregulation of FcεRI expression in response to the lowered IgE levels occurred. These phenomena will be discussed in Section IV.

III. FcεRI Structure

The receptor found on mast cells and basophils consists of four polypeptide chains with the composition $\alpha\beta\gamma_2$ and a total of seven membrane-spanning regions as indicated schematically in Figure 3 (37). The IgE-binding function is performed by the α-chain (38), and the site resides entirely within the extracellular region of this chain (39). Expression of soluble fragments corresponding to this region, sFcεRIα, in various different cell types, as described later, have since confirmed this result and shown that the extensive *N*-linked glycosylation of the native protein (there are seven potential sites) is not required for IgE binding (40–43). On antigen-presenting cells (APCs) the receptor appears to consist of a complex of only the α- and γ-chains (8,44).

The sequence of the extracellular region of the α-chain implies that it consists of two immunoglobulin-like domains (45), and the three-dimensional structures

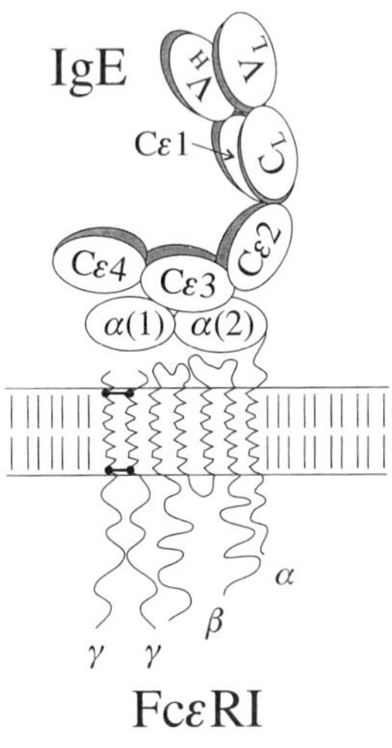

Figure 3 Schematic representation of a bent IgE molecule bound to the extracellular domains of the FcεRI α-chain, consistent with spectroscopic and binding–site-mapping studies.

of these two domains, termed α(1) and α(2), have been modeled on the basis of sequence homology either with known antibody structures (46) or the structures of other members of the immunoglobulin superfamily (47,48). The folding of the polypeptide chain within the membrane-proximal α(2) domain is shown schematically in Figure 4, and this model may be used to interpret the results of various studies to map the location of the binding site for IgE within this domain.

The first indication that the site lay principally within α(2) came from studies with monoclonal antibodies directed to defined epitopes (49), and although this was confirmed by phage display of the individual domains, which showed that α(2) alone bound IgE (41,50), both domains were required for full-binding activity. The production of chimeric receptor fragments (47,51,52) further localized the binding site to sequences within α(2), also ruling out sequences in α(1) that were distal from the α(2) domain (52). Combining these results with those from the homologous IgG–FcγR system, and the location of the glycosylation sites in sFcεRIα, the CC′FG face of α(2) was predicted to be the major IgE-binding region (reviewed in Ref. 53; see Fig. 4). This has been confirmed by recent mutagenesis studies (42,54), implicating residues in all four of these β-strands.

Although the site may lie principally in the α(2) domain, the extent of the site in IgE–Fc, spanning both Cε3 domains, implies the involvement of more than one α-chain domain as shown in Figure 2. The proximal loop regions of the α(1) domain may well be directly involved also (22). Figure 3 thus depicts a bent IgE molecule binding mainly to the FcεRI α(2) domain in an orientation, relative to the membrane, that is consistent with spectroscopic data (17). The stoichiometry of this interaction is clearly 1:1 on the cell membrane, but interestingly, the same stoichiometry was observed for sFcεRIα binding to IgE in solution (41,55), despite the presence of two potentially identical binding sites in the Fc region. Because IgE is bent, the site on the "concave" face of the IgE molecule may be inaccessible, but a 1:1 stoichiometry has also been found not only for the IgE–Fc fragment (56), but

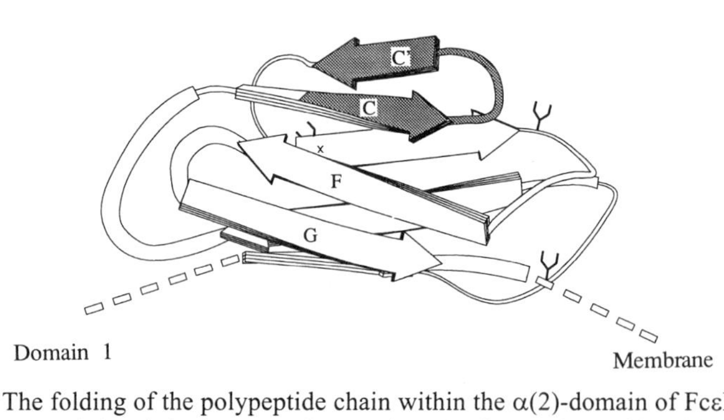

Figure 4 The folding of the polypeptide chain within the α(2)-domain of FcεRIα, showing the three potential carbohydrate attachment sites. Surface amino acid residues within β-strands C′C, F, and G have been implicated in IgE binding, and the shaded C′C loop region corresponds to the inhibitory peptide described in the text.

also for an IgE–Fc subfragment consisting of only the Cε3 and Cε4 domains (57). This suggests rather that complex formation may involve conformational changes that weaken the second site, and there is evidence to support this idea (58). If conformational change is important, then the binding of molecules to either component to prevent this change may provide another mechanism by which complex formation can be inhibited.

Before discussing the particular ways in which inhibition of IgE binding to FcεRI has been effected, it is important to take into account the concentrations of these two species that will be encountered in vivo. Furthermore, recent evidence suggests that the IgE concentration and receptor number are interdependent, with important consequences for this approach.

IV. Regulation of IgE Levels and FcεRI Expression

The relation between the serum IgE concentration and the receptor density on the mast cells or basophils is critical for determining the degree of cell degranulation and subsequent inflammatory response. In nonatopic individuals the level of IgE is close to 10 ng/mL, whereas in atopics it may lie in the range of 100–1000 ng/mL. The receptor number on basophils varies between 10^4 and 10^6 for both nonallergic and allergic individuals, but the latter typically have approximately 10^5 receptors per cell with bound IgE. However, the number of surface receptors bearing allergen-specific IgE required for a half-maximal response may typically be close to 2000, rising to about 5000 for maximal response (59 and references therein). Because about at least 10% of the IgE molecules are typically specific for the allergen in question, it may be concluded that to lower the number of receptor-bound, allergen-specific IgE molecules below the threshold for cell activation (i.e., about 100 receptor-bound IgE molecules per cell), the concentration of IgE would have to be reduced to less than 1% of its original level (59).

It is in relation to these numbers that the results of a recent analysis of the effects of a recombinant humanized anti-IgE monoclonal antibody (MAb) may be assessed. The antibody, rhuMAb-E25 (34), was administered intravenously to atopic patients in a clinical trial. The serum concentrations of free IgE fell from a mean of nearly 500 ng/mL to less than 5 ng/mL immediately, and remained at this level throughout the course of treatment (59). This dramatic reduction in IgE levels implies a downregulation of IgE synthesis, presumably by a direct effect of the anti-IgE on membrane-bound IgE (mIgE) on B cells. The same antibody inhibited antigen-specific IgE synthesis in B cells from allergic donors, and direct binding of the antibody to B cells was demonstrated (33). This is in accord with studies of another anti-IgE antibodies developed for therapeutic use (32), and yet earlier observations that administration of anti-IgE antibodies caused long-term inhibition of IgE synthesis in mice (60,61, and references therein). Thus, rather than inhibiting the binding of IgE to FcεRI, the anti-IgE antibodies were, in fact, exerting a more profound effect by suppressing IgE synthesis. It may be that the receptor-based, IgE-binding therapeutic agents, to be discussed later, also exert an effect on mIgE, rather than free IgE.

Even more striking than the reduction in the level of circulating IgE in this trial of the humanized anti-IgE MAb, however, was the consequent reduction in the surface expression of FcεRI on basophils (59). From an initial level of approximately 220,000 receptor molecules per cell (median value), after 3 months with IgE levels at about 1% of their initial level, the receptor number was close to 8,300, a reduction of 96%. In fact, this reduction occurred over a period of days (50% reduction after 3 days), but could clearly be sustained. (Upregulation of FcεRI expression on murine mast cells and basophils in response to increased levels of IgE have also been reported in vitro and in vivo (62,62); this parallels the observed upregulation of the receptor on monocytes in the aforementioned response to IgE (12)). The combined effect of this reduction in IgE levels and receptor density on basophils was assessed by measuring the degree of histamine release from patients' basophils when challenged with dust mite allergen. The average response was 90% lower after 3 months of the anti-IgE treatment, compared with that at the start of the trial, and half of the patients exhibited no response at all (59).

The conclusions from this study are of considerable significance for the development of antiallergy therapeutics. Not only does it demonstrate that IgE levels can indeed be brought to less than 1% of their initial value, but it also shows that the receptor number falls as a result, and that these two factors together can lead to a dramatic reduction in the specific response to dust mite allergen. The molecular mechanisms by which these effects are achieved are unclear, but if receptor-based inhibitors can act in a similar way to reduce IgE levels and receptor number, then the prospects for their efficacy are greatly enhanced.

V. Soluble Receptor Fragments

A soluble fragment corresponding to the two extracellular domains of the human FcεRI α-chain was first produced by Blank et al. in 1991, by expression in a stable transfected Chinese hamster ovary (CHO) cell line (40), and it displayed full IgE-binding activity. Since then, others have expressed sFcεRIα in bacterial (41), baculovirus-infected insect cells (43), and mammalian expression systems (42,64) and have confirmed this finding. The first demonstration of a biological activity relevant to allergic disease was the use of sFcεRIα expressed in CHO cells to inhibit mediator release from rat basophil leukemia (RBL) cells triggered with IgE–antigen complexes, and from human basophils sensitized with serum IgE from an atopic patient and triggered with dust mite allergen (65). (Human FcεRIα binds to rat or mouse IgE, although human IgE does not bind to the rat or mouse receptor; thus, human receptor fragments can be assayed in rodent systems, although the lower affinity of rodent IgE for human FcεRI must be taken into account when extrapolating to use in humans.) The same material also inhibited the PCA response in rats when administered *before* IgE sensitization (using mouse IgE anti-DNP, followed by challenge with dinitrophenol–bovine serum albumin [DNP–BSA] after 24 hr), and even reduced the response by up to 60% when injected *after* IgE sensitization (65). This latter result implies that the sFcεRIα is capable of causing dissociation of the cell-bound IgE, leading to desensitization, and this was also demonstrated in vitro (65).

The same recombinant sFcεRIα material was subsequently tested in an in vivo model for allergy (66). In this model, antigen-specific (anti-TNP) IgE-secreting murine hybridoma cells were transplanted into mice, and IgE was detected in the serum. These mice were then subjected to antigen challenge to the ears, and the swelling response was observed, with and without intravenous injection of sFcεRIα, 24 hr before the first challenge and periodically between the first and second antigen challenges. The treatment with sFcεRIα suppressed the response to the second challenge, but not to the first (66). The total amount of sFcεRIα injected was in excess of a molar equivalent of the possible concentration of IgE present, and the fact that sFcεRIα was indeed blocking the binding of IgE to FcεRI on mast cells in the ears was confirmed by immunohistochemical staining for IgE. However, the pretreatment with sFcεRIα only 24 hr before the first challenge was clearly insufficient to prevent sensitization of the mast cells and the first swelling response.

Further in vivo trials of the recombinant sFcεRIα confirmed the significance of this result and the timing of the dose administration. Mice were primed with anti-TNP IgE and then subsequently challenged 72 hr later with TNP–HSA, which caused anaphylactic shock in all mice, and death within 1 hr for 60% of the mice. When sFcεRIα (20 or 100 μg) was injected 24 hr before antigen challenge, survival was unaffected, whereas when the same doses were injected 48 hr before antigen challenge, the mortality rate dropped to 25% (55). The effect appeared to exhibit a dose-dependence in other experiments, but the effective doses were always in the range of 10–100 molar excess of sFcεRIα over IgE.

The conclusion from these studies is that sFcεRIα can prevent the binding of IgE to mast cell receptors, if administered before IgE sensitization (at levels at least tenfold higher than the concentration of IgE), and can even facilitate the dissociation of cell-bound IgE if administered afterward (presumably by preventing rebinding). This can occur both locally and systemically. However, the timing of the sFcεRIα dose in relation to the antigen challenge is important, and 24 hr is apparently insufficient for desensitization in these systems. The rate of dissociation of IgE from FcεRI is very slow indeed [$k_d \approx 10^{-5}\ s^{-1}$ (67)], corresponding to a period of 20 hr for loss of only half of the IgE molecules from the surface; the longer incubation time before antigen challenge, with at least a molar equivalent of sFcεRIα, is necessary to reduce the number of receptor molecules bearing IgE to below the critical threshold for cell activation. Downregulation of the receptor in response to reduced IgE levels may also be significant over these longer periods.

In addition to the purely inhibitory effect of sFcεRIα on the binding of IgE to mast cells and basophils, an alternative mode of action relevant to allergy might be the binding of this soluble receptor fragment to mIgE on B cells. It has long been known that IgE-binding molecules can affect the regulation of the IgE response (68), and recent studies with anti-IgE antibodies have confirmed that IgE synthesis can be suppressed by a direct effect on mIgE on B cells. The effect of sFcεRIα on interleukin (IL)-4–induced IgE production by human B cells was investigated (69), and dose-dependent suppression was found. Binding of sFcεRIα to the B cells was demonstrated, and the suppression was IgE class-specific. It thus appears that sFcεRIα too can inhibit IgE synthesis through a direct interaction with mIgE on B cells. The mechanism of this process is unknown, but such a molecule clearly cannot cross-link mIgE, as has been inferred from the requirement for bivalency of suppressive anti-IgE molecules (70). However, sFcεRIα might prevent co–cross-linking of two different species at the B-cell surface, such as mIgE and CD21, which may be a requirement for IgE synthesis (53).

The binding of sFcεRIα to IgE^+ B cells was also reported in a study to compare the properties of the recombinant human receptor extracellular domains expressed in both Cos and CHO cells (64). Although the IgE-binding properties of the two proteins were identical, and inhibition of the PCA reaction in rats was demonstrated, the in vivo fates of the two proteins were very different. Not only were their clearance rates in mice different (half-lives of 11 and 26 hr, respectively), but also their final localization to kidney, liver, and other tissue, and these differences were the result of alternative *N*-glycosylation states (64). It is clear that just as with other recombinant proteins, the choice of expression system may, through posttranslational modification, have a profound effect on the pharmacokinetic properties of the molecule and its efficacy as a therapeutic agent.

VI. Soluble FcεRIα–IgG "Immunoadhesin"

Following the strategy adopted in the development of a therapeutic agent to block host cell entry of human immunodeficiency virus (HIV), in which a chimeric immunoadhesin molecule was constructed with the extracellular domains of CD4 fused to the Fc region of IgG (71), an analogous molecule incorporating sFcεRIα was produced (72). The two extracellular domains of FcεRIα were fused to the γ-chain of IgG, truncated on the NH_2-terminal side of the hinge region. When secreted from mammalian cells, the molecule formed a disulfide-linked dimer of the chimeric chains, thus resembling an IgG molecule with sFcεRIα in place of each Fab arm. Such a molecule is expected to exhibit a longer half-life in vivo than the isolated sFcεRIα, on the basis of experience with the CD4 immunoadhesin. Although dimeric, and in principle capable of cross-linking IgE molecules, the chimera does not induce degranulation of mast cells sensitized with IgE (72,73) because there is no other accessible receptor-binding site on cell-bound IgE (see Fig. 3).

The molecule inhibited sensitization and subsequent histamine release from RBL cells in a dose-dependent manner when incubated with IgE, before anti-IgE antibody treatment (72); even half a molar equivalent concentration relative to IgE of the chimera caused a significant (≈ 50%) reduction in histamine release, suggesting that each molecule of the chimera binds two molecules of IgE. Its efficacy in vivo was also determined by preincubating the chimera with murine anti-DNP IgE, before intracutaneous injection into rats. The animals were challenged with DNP–HSA 4 hr later. The chimera inhibited the PCA reaction when present at equimolar or higher concentrations relative to the IgE (72). It was also effective when administered intravenously (1-mg dose) up to 30 min following sensitization, indicating that it can reach the tissue and compete with the rat mast cell receptors for the sensitizing IgE. Finally, in in vitro experiments with human and rhesus monkey lung parenchyma strips, the same chimera completely blocked antigen-induced contraction and histamine release, following passive sensitization with antigen-specific atopic patient serum (73).

There have been no reports of the effect of the chimeric immunoadhesin on IgE synthesis. Because monomeric sFcεRIα can suppress IgE synthesis, the chimera would be expected to act similarly; indeed, its bivalency might enhance its ability to inhibit IgE synthesis, for it could cross-link mIgE in the same way that anti-IgE is presumed to act.

VII. Structure-Based Design of Inhibitors

An alternative strategy to develop an inhibitor of IgE binding to FcεRIα is to use our knowledge of the structure of the receptor to design a molecule that mimics the native conformation. The advantage of this approach is that the final product may be a small, stable molecule, easier to produce and to administer than the large recombinant protein fragments just discussed, or the anti-IgE antibodies. The challenge of this approach, clearly, is to match the exceptionally high affinity of the interaction, but progress has been made in this direction with the recent report of an inhibitory peptide mimetic (48).

The starting point was the deduction that the principal component of the binding region for IgE lay within the four-stranded face of the membrane-proximal α(2)-domain of FcεRIα (see strands C′CFG in Fig. 4; 53). The C′C strands and intervening loop form a particularly prominent feature in the three-dimensional model of the domain, namely, a twisted β-hairpin loop that might be successfully mimicked by a constrained peptide. Such an approach had earlier been applied successfully to an homologous region of CD4 (74). A peptide consisting of 11 residues of the natural sequence corresponding to the CC′ loop of FcεRI α(2)-domain, cyclized by a disulfide bridge between an additional NH_2-terminal D-cysteine residue and a COOH-terminal L-cysteine residue, was synthesized (*cyclo*-L-262; Fig. 5). A second peptide consisting of the same sequence, but in the reverse order and with op-

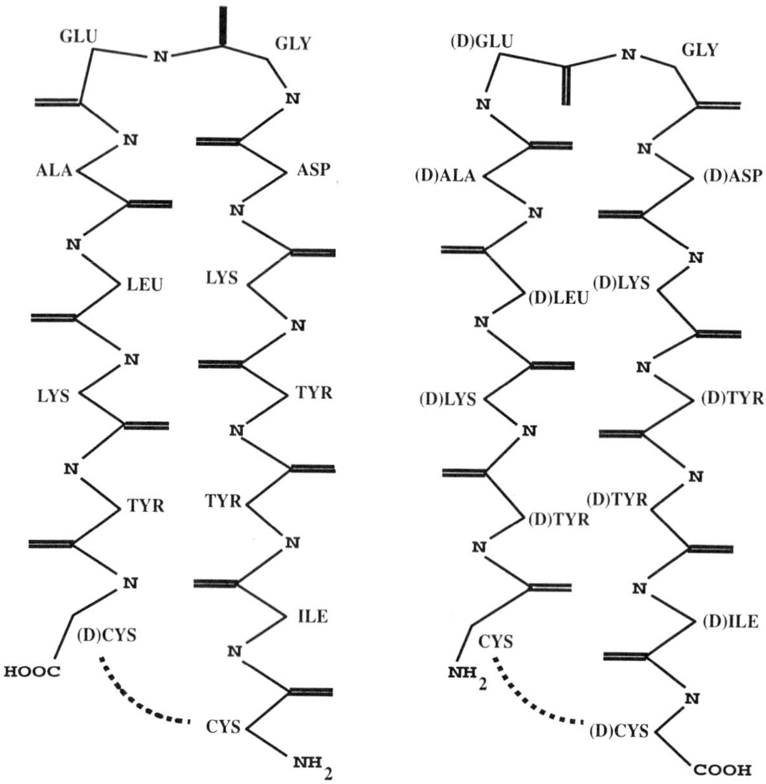

Figure 5 The structures of the cyclic peptide synthesized from L-amino acids, corresponding to the natural sequence of the CC′ loop region of FcεRI α(2)-domain, and the retro-enantiomeric form synthesized from D-amino acids.

posite chirality at each residue, was also synthesized (*cyclo*-rD-262; see Fig. 5). Such a retroenantiomeric peptide is expected to display a similar polypeptide backbone conformation and disposition of side chains (75), but may exhibit a longer half-life in vivo as a consequence of its resistance to proteolysis.

Evidence that both the *cyclo*-L- and *cyclo*-rD-peptides did indeed adopt the expected structure in solution was obtained from their circular dichroism (CD) spectra, which were not only mirror images of each other, but were characteristic of β-structure (48). Linear versions of the peptides, or cyclic peptides with scrambled sequence, displayed no such evidence for the formation of β-structure. The β-hairpin structures of both peptides have since been confirmed by nuclear magnetic resonance (NMR) analysis (76). The ability of these peptides to inhibit the binding of

IgE to FcεRIα was first assayed by surface plasmon resonance, and K_d values of 2.6 and 10.7 μM measured for the L- and rD-peptides, respectively. They also inhibited the IgE-mediated degranulation of RBL cells when incubated with IgE before sensitization. In this assay, the inhibitory activity was approximately tenfold lower, but this is consistent with the affinity of a human receptor-based peptide binding to murine IgE, which is approximately sevenfold lower than for human IgE (39,48).

These initial results are encouraging, particularly because certain key residues in the α(2)-domain identified by mutagenesis as important for IgE binding (42,54), have not yet been included in the peptide mimic. Clearly, there is scope for further rational modification of this first inhibitory peptide, but alternative approaches are available to optimize activity, such as combinatorial methods based on knowledge of the amino acid side chains of the peptide that form the binding surface. Another approach to the discovery of small-molecule inhibitors based on knowledge of protein structure is to screen libraries of preexisting compounds on the basis of their calculated complementarity to the target structure; either IgE-Fc or the FcεRI α(2)-domain. This purely computational approach has been applied successfully to identify lead compounds that bind to CD4 and inhibit binding to the major histocompatability complex (MHC) molecules (77). Alternatively, physical selection of small-molecule ligands through binding to human IgE can be combined with a random combinatorial method for generating large pools of molecules. This method has been applied using oligonucleotides and has led to the identification of several inhibitory RNA and ssDNA molecules with K_d values in the range 10–35 nM (78). These molecules also inhibit IgE-mediated degranulation of RBL cells. The search for soluble, small-molecule inhibitors of this interaction is thus not restricted to peptides and their analogues.

VIII. Summary and Future Prospects

The extracellular domains of the high-affinity receptor α-chain, or parts thereof, have been expressed in several different systems and in a variety of soluble molecular constructs. It is clear that such molecules can inhibit the binding of IgE to FcεRI, and inhibition of various manifestations of the allergic response have been demonstrated in vitro and in vivo. The production of a molecule that will compete effectively with this very high-affinity interaction, at concentrations that correspond to reasonable dose levels, and with a sufficiently long half-life in vivo, remains a challenge, but advances in our knowledge of the three-dimensional structures of the complementary binding sites in both IgE and FcεRIα will aid the design process.

However, as the studies accompanying the clinical trials of the anti-IgE therapeutics have shown, inhibition of IgE binding to FcεRIα and desensitization of mast cells and basophils may be only a part of the story. Just as anti-IgE MAbs bind to mIgE on B cells and inhibit IgE synthesis, so too does sFcεRIα (69). The molecular mechanism is unknown, but whereas the bivalent anti-IgE could, in principle, cross-link mIgE, the activity of monomeric sFcεRIα suggests that inhibition of interactions in the B-cell membrane required for IgE synthesis may be occurring, such as the postulated co-ligation of mIgE and CD21 by the soluble, oligomeric form of FcεRII/CD23, the low-affinity receptor for IgE (53,79). The receptor-binding site for FcεRII also lies within the Cε3 domain of IgE, and although distinct from the FcεRI site (see Ref. 53 for review), it is known to overlap; sFcεRII inhibits the binding of IgE to FcεRI (80). When sFcεRIα is in a bivalent form, such as the immunoadhesin described earlier, it may be even more effective, being capable of both inhibitory and cross-linking functions, if both prove to be relevant.

Although the molecular mechanisms of the up- and downregulation of IgE synthesis are not yet understood, the discovery that suppressed IgE levels lead to downregulation of FcεRIα expression on basophils (59) is very encouraging for this therapeutic approach. The simultaneous suppression of IgE synthesis, downregulation of FcεRIα expression, and desensitization of mast cells and basophils, is clearly a powerful combination. Added to this is the recent discovery that the mast cell can provide the necessary signals for B-cell proliferation and IgE synthesis—namely, IL-4 and CD40L (81); thus, inhibition of IgE binding to FcεRI may also serve to suppress local IgE synthesis.

Finally, the discovery of FcεRI on other cell types provides further encouragement that the inhibition of IgE binding may find application in the treatment of allergic disease. Such inhibitors, therefore, might interfere with the IgE-dependent uptake and processing of allergen by antigen-presenting cells, such as Langerhans cells (in the skin), monocytes (in the blood), and dendritic cells (in the airways), as well as the release of inflammatory mediators that result from the activation of these cells. Inhibition of IgE binding to FcεRI on these cells might also downregulate the receptor, as demonstrated for monocytes (12), analogous to the effect on basophils (59). This would lead to a further increase in the threshold for sensitivity to allergen. Langerhans cells and monocytes also express the low-affinity receptor for IgE, FcεRII, but because the two receptor-binding sites overlap, sFcεRIα may well inhibit antigen presentation whichever receptor is involved. Although the effects of soluble receptor-derived molecules and peptides on antigen presentation and activation by these other cell types have yet to be investigated, they constitute a very promising target, and their accessibility to allergen dictates that they must be equally accessible to such therapeutic agents.

Acknowledgments

The authors wish to thank the Medical Research Council and the National Asthma Campaign (UK) for supporting their work in this field.

References

1. Ravetch JV, Kinet J-P. Fc receptors. Annu Rev Immunol 1991; 9:457–492.
2. Bieber T, de la Salle H, Wollenberg A, Hakimi J, Chizzonite R, Ring J, Hanau D, de la Salle C. Human epidermal Langerhans cells express the high affinity receptor for immunoglobulin E (FcεRI). J Exp Med 1992; 175:1285–1290.
3. Wang B, Rieger A, Kilgus O, Ochiai K, Maurer D, Födinger D, Kinet J-P, Stingl G. Epidermal Langerhans cells from normal human skin bind monomeric IgE via FcεRI. J Exp Med 1992; 175:1353–1358.
4. Gounni AS, Lamkhioued B, Ochiai K, Tanaka Y, Delaporte E, Capron A, Kinet J-P, Capron M. High-affinity IgE receptor on eosinophils is involved in defence against parasites. Nature 1994; 367:183–186.
5. Maurer D, Fiebiger E, Reininger B, Wolff-Winiski B, Jouvin M-H, Kilgus O, Kinet J-P, Stingl G. Expression of functional high affinity immunoglobulin E receptors (FcεRI) on monocytes of atopic individuals. J Exp Med 1994; 179:745–750.
6. Bieber T. FcεRI-expressing antigen-presenting cells: new players in the atopic game. Immunol Today 1997; 18:311–313.
7. Stingl G, Maurer D. IgE-mediated allergen presentation via FcεRI on antigen-presenting cells. Int Arch Allergy Immunol 1997; 113:24–29.
8. Jurgens M, Wollenberg A, Hanau D, de la Salle H, Bieber T. Activation of human epidermal Langerhans cells by engagement of the high affinity receptor for IgE, FcεRI. J Immunol 1995; 155:5184–5189.
9. Tunon-de-Lara JM, Redington AE, Bradding P, Church MK, Hartley JA, Semper AE, Holgate ST. Dendritic cells in normal and asthmatic airways: expression of the α subunit of the high affinity immunoglobulin E receptor (FcεRI-α). Clin Exp Allergy 1996; 26:648–655.
10. Humbert M, Grant JA, Taborda-Barata L, Durham SR, Pfister R, Menz G, Barkans J, Ying S, Kay AB. High-affinity IgE receptor (FcεRI)-bearing cells in bronchial biopsies from atopic and non-atopic asthma. Am J Respir Crit Care Med 1996; 153:1931–1937.
11. Maurer D, Ebner C, Reininger B, Fiebiger E, Kraft D, Kinet J-P, Stingl G. The high affinity IgE receptor (FcεRI) mediates IgE-dependent allergen presentation. J Immunol 1995; 154:6285–6290.
12. Reischl IG, Corvaia N, Effenberger F, Wolff-Winiski B, Kromer E, Mudde GC. Function and regulation of FcεRI expression on monocytes from non-atopic donors. Clin Exp Allergy 1996; 26:630–641.
13. Tanaka Y, Takenaka M, Matsunaga Y, Okada S, Anan S, Yoshida H, Ra C. High affinity IgE receptor (FcεRI) expression on eosinophils infiltrating the lesions and mite patch tested sites in atopic dermatitis. Arch Dermatol Res 1995; 287:712–717.
14. Barata LT, Ying S, Grant JA, Humbert M, Barkans J, Meng Q, Durham SB, Kay AB. Allergen-induced recruitment of Fc epsilon RI$^+$ eosinophils in human atopic skin. Eur J Immunol 1997; 27:1236–1241.
15. Padlan EA, Davies DR. A model of the Fc of immunoglobulin E. Mol Immunol 1986; 23:1063–1075.
16. Helm BA, Ling Y, Teale C, Padlan EA, Brüggemann M. The nature and importance of the inter-ε chain disulfide bonds in human IgE. Eur J Immunol 1991; 21:1543–1548.
17. Zheng Y, Shopes B, Holowka D, Baird B. Conformations of IgE bound to its receptor FcεRI and in solution. Biochemistry 1991; 30:9125–9132.
18. Beavil AJ, Young RJ, Sutton BJ, Perkins SJ. Bent domain structure of recombinant human IgE–Fc in solution by X-ray and neutron scattering in conjunction with an automated curve fitting procedure. Biochemistry 1995; 34:14449–14461.
19. Gould HJ. The interaction between immunoglobulin E and its high-affinity receptor. In: Holgate ST, Church MK, eds. Genetics of Asthma. London: Gower, 1992:293–304.
20. Beavil AJ, Beavil RL, Chan CMW, Cook JPD, Gould HJ, Henry AJ, Owens RJ, Shi J,

Sutton BJ, Young RJ. Structural basis of the IgE–FcεRI interaction. Biochem Soc Trans 1993; 21:968–972.

21. Presta L, Shields R, O'Connell L, Lahr S, Porte J, Gorman C, Jardieu P. The binding site on human immunoglobulin E for its high affinity receptor. J Biol Chem 1994; 269:26368–26373.
22. McDonnell JM, Beavil AJ, Mackay GA, Henry AJ, Cook JPD, Gould HJ, Sutton BJ. Structure-based design of peptides that inhibit IgE binding to its high-affinity receptor FcεRI. Biochem Soc Trans 1997; 25:387–392.
23. Helm BA, Marsh P, Vercelli D, Padlan E, Gould HJ, Geha R. The mast cell binding site on human immunoglobulin E. Nature 1988; 331:180–183.
24. Helm BA, Kebo D, Vercelli D, Glovsky MM, Gould HJ, Ishizaka K, Geha R, Ishizaka T. Blocking of passive sensitization of human mast cells and basophil granulocytes with IgE antibodies by a recombinant human ε-chain fragment of 76 amino acids. Proc Natl Acad Sci USA 1989; 88:9465–9469.
24. Helm BA, Sayers I, Higginbottom A, Machado DC, Long Y, Ahmad K, Padlan EA, Wilson PM. Identification of the high affinity receptor binding region in human immunoglobulin E. J Biol Chem 1996; 271:7494–7500.
26. Nio N, Seguro K, Ariyoshi Y, Ishii K, Nakamura H. Inhibition of passive cutaneous anaphylaxis by synthetic human immunoglobulin E peptides fragments. FEBS Lett 1992; 314:229–231.
27. Nio N, Seguro K, Ariyoshi Y, Imano K, Yakuo I, Kita A, Nakamura H. Inhibition of passive sensitization of human peripheral basophils by synthetic human immunoglobulin E peptide fragments. FEBS Lett 1993; 319:225–228.
28. Shakib F, Smith SJ. In vitro basophil histamine-releasing activity of circulating IgG1 and IgG4 autoanti-IgE antibodies from asthma patients and the demonstration that anti-IgE modulates allergen-induced basophil activation. Clin Exp Allergy 1994; 24:270–275.
29. Stanworth DR, Jones VM, Lewin IV, Nayyar S. Allergy treatment with a peptide vaccine. Lancet 1990; 336:1279–1281.
30. Hellman L. Profound reduction in allergy sensitivity following treatment with a novel allergy vaccine. Eur J Immunol 1994; 24:415–420.
31. Chang TW, Davis FM, Sun N-C, Sun CRY, MacGlashan DW, Hamilton RG. Monoclonal antibodies specific for human IgE-producing B cells: a potential therapeutic for IgE-mediated allergic diseases. Biotechnology 1990; 8:122–126.
32. David FM, Gossett LA, Pinkston KL, Liou RS, Sun LK, Kim YW, Chang NT, Chang TW, Wagner K, Bews J, Brinkman V, Towbin H, Subramanian N, Heusser C. Can anti-IgE be used to treat allergy? Springer Semin Immunopathol 1993; 15:51–73.
33. Shields RL, Whether WR, Zioncheck K, O'Connell L, Fendly B, Presta LG, Thomas D, Saban R, Jardieu P. Inhibition of allergic reactions with antibodies to IgE. Int Arch Allergy Immunol 1995; 107:308–312.
34. Presta LG, Lahr SJ, Shields RL, Porter JP, Gorman CM, Fendly BM, Jardieu PM. Humanization of an antibody directed against IgE. J Immunol 1993; 151:2623–2632.
35. Kolbinger F, Saldanha J, Hardman N, Bendig MM. Humanization of a mouse antihuman anti-IgE antibody: a potential therapeutic for IgE-mediated allergies. Prot Eng 1993; 6:971–980.
36. Rudolf MP, Furukawa K, Miescher S, Vogel M, Kricek F, Stadler BM. Effect of anti-IgE antibodies on FcεRI-bound IgE. J Immunol 1996; 157:5646–5652.
37. Blank U, Ra C, Miller L, White K, Metzger H, Kinet J-P. Complete structure and expression in transfected cells of high affinity IgE receptor. Nature 1989; 337:187–189.
38. Miller L, Blank U, Metzger H, Kinet J-P. Expression of high-affinity binding of human immunoglobulin E by transfected cells. Science 1989; 244:334–337.
39. Hakimi J, Seals C, Kondas JA, Pettine L, Danho W, Kochan J. The α subunit of the human IgE receptor (FcεRI) is sufficient for high affinity IgE binding. J Biol Chem 1990; 265:22079–22081.

40. Blank U, Ra C, Kinet J-P. Characterization of truncated α chain products from human, rat and mouse high affinity receptor for IgE. J Biol Chem 1991; 266:2639–2646.
41. Robertson MW. Phage and *Escherichia coli* expression of the human high affinity immunoglobulin E receptor α-subunit ectodomain. J Biol Chem 1993; 268:12736–12743.
42. Cook JPD. Site-directed mutagenesis of the human high affinity IgE receptor α chain. Ph.D. dissertation, King's College London, London, UK 1996.
43. Yagi S, Yanagida M, Tanida I, Hasegawa A, Okumura K, Ra C. High level expression of the truncated α chain of human high-affinity receptor for IgE as a soluble form by baculovirus-infected insect cells. Eur J Biochem 1994; 220:593–598.
44. Maurer D, Fiebiger E, Ebner C, Reininger B, Fischer GF, Wichlas S, Jouvin M-H, Schmitt-Egenolf M, Kraft D, Kinet J-P, Stingl G. Peripheral blood dendritic cells express FcεRI as a complex composed of FcεRIα- and FcεRIγ-chains and can use this receptor for IgE-mediated allergen presentation. J Immunol 1996; 157:607–616.
45. Shimizu A, Tepler I, Benfey PN, Berenstein EH, Siraganian RP, Leder P. Human and rat mast cell high-affinity immunoglobulin E receptors: characterization of putative α-chain gene products. Proc Natl Acad Sci USA 1988; 85:1907–1911.
46. Padlan EA, Helm BA. A modelling study of the α-subunit of human high-affinity receptor for immunoglobulin E. Receptor 1992; 2:129–142.
47. Hogarth PM, Hulett MD, Ierino FL, Tate B, Powell MS, Brinkworth RI. Identification of the immunoglobulin binding regions (IBR) of FcγRII and FcεRI. Immunol Rev 1992; 125:21–35.
48. McDonnell JM, Beavil AJ, Mackay GA, Jameson BA, Korngold R, Gould HJ, Sutton BJ. Structure based design and characterization of peptides that inhibit IgE binding to its high-affinity receptor. Nature Struct Biol 1996; 3:419–426.
49. Riske F, Hakimi J, Mallamaci M, Griffin M, Pilson B, Tobkes N, Lin P, Danho W, Kochan J, Chizzonite R. High affinity human IgE receptor (FcεRI). Analysis of functional domains of the α-subunit with monoclonal antibodies. J Biol Chem 1991; 266:11245–11251.
50. Scarselli E, Esposito G, Traboni C. Display of functional domains of the human high affinity IgE receptor on the M13 phage surface. FEBS Lett 1993; 329:223–226.
51. Hulett MD, McKenzie IFC, Hogarth PM. Chronic Fc receptors intensify immunoglobulin-binding regions in human FcγRII and FcεRI. Eur J Immunol 1993; 23:640–645.
52. Mallamaci MA, Chizzonite R, Griffin M, Nettleton M, Hakimi J, Tsien W-H, Kochan JP. Identification of sites on the human FcεRIα subunit which are involved in binding human and rat IgE. J Biol Chem 1993; 268:22076–22083.
53. Sutton BJ, Gould HJ. The human IgE network. Nature 1993; 366:421–428.
54. Danho W, Makofske R, Swistok J, Mallamaci M, Nettleton M, Madison V, Greeley D, Fry D, Kochan J. High affinity IgE-receptor α-subunit–derived peptides as antagonists of human IgE binding. Ninth International Congress of Immunology, San Francisco, CA, July 23–29, 1995.
55. Naito K, Hirama M, Okumura K, Ra C. Recombinant soluble form of the human high-affinity receptor for IgE prevents anaphylactic shock in mice. J Allergy Clin Immunol 1996; 97:773–780.
56. Keown MB, Ghirlando R, Young RJ, Beavil AJ, Owens RJ, Perkins SJ, Sutton BJ, Gould HJ. Hydrodynamic studies of a complex between the Fc fragment of human IgE and a soluble fragment of the FcεRI α chain. Proc Natl Acad Sci USA 1995; 92:1841–1845.
57. Keown MB, Ghirlando R, Mackay GA, Sutton BJ, Gould HJ. Basis of the 1:1 stoichiometry of the high affinity receptor FcεRI–IgE complex. Eur Biophys J 1997; 25:471–476.
58. Sechi S, Roller PP, Willette-Brown J, Kinet J-P. A conformational rearrangement upon binding of IgE to its high affinity receptor. J Biol Chem 1996; 271:19256–19263.
59. MacGlashan DW, Bochner BS, Adelman DC, Jardieu PM, Togias A, McKenzie-White J, Sterbinsky SA, Hamilton RG, Lichtenstein LM. Down-regulation of FcεRI expression on human basophils during in vivo treatment of atopic patients with anti-IgE antibody. J Immunol 1997; 158:1438–1445.

60. Haba S, Nisonoff A. Inhibition of IgE synthesis by anti-IgE: role in long-term inhibition of IgE synthesis by neonatally administered soluble IgE. Proc Natl Acad Sci USA 1990; 87:3363–3367.
61. Haak-Frendscho M, Robbins K, Lyon R, Shields R, Hooley J, Schoenhoff M, Jardieu P. Administration of an anti-IgE antibody inhibits CD23 expression and IgE production in vivo. Immunology 1994; 82:306–313.
62. Yamaguchi M, Lantz CS, Oettgen HC, Katona IM, Fleming T, Miyajima I, Kinet J-P, Galli SJ. IgE enhances mouse mast cell FcεRI expression in vitro and in vivo: evidence for a novel amplification mechanism in IgE-dependent reactions. J Exp Med 1997; 185:663–672.
63. Lantz CS, Yamaguchi M, Oettgen HC, Katona IM, Miyajima I, Kinet J-P, Galli SJ. IgE regulates mouse basophil FcεRI expression in vivo. J Immunol 1997; 158:2517–2521.
64. Gavin AL, Snider J, Hulett MD, NcKenzie IFC, Hogarth PM. Expression of recombinant soluble FcεRI: function and tissue distribution studies. Immunology 1995; 86:392–398.
65. Ra C, Kuromitsu S, Hirose T, Yasuda S, Furuichi K, Okumura K. Soluble high-affinity receptor for IgE abrogates the IgE-mediated allergic reaction. Int Immunol 1993; 5:47–54.
66. Naito K, Hirama M, Okumura K, Ra C. Soluble form of the human high-affinity receptor for IgE inhibits recurrent allergic reactions in a novel mouse model of type I allergy. Eur J Immunol 1995; 25:1631–1637.
67. Wank SA, DeLisi C, Metzger H. Analysis of the rate-limiting step in a ligand–cell receptor interaction: the immunoglobulin E system. Biochemistry 1983; 22:954–959.
68. Ishizaka K. IgE-binding factors and regulation of the IgE antibody response. Annu Rev Immunol 1988; 6:513–534.
69. Yanagihara Y, Kajiwara K, Ikizawa K, Koshio T, Okumura, Ra C. Recombinant soluble form of the human high-affinity immunoglobulin E (IgE) receptor inhibits IgE production through its specific binding to IgE-bearing B cells. J Clin Invest 1994; 92:2162–2165.
70. Stampfli MR, Miescher S, Aebischer I, Zurcher AW, Stadler BM. Inhibition of human IgE synthesis by anti-IgE antibodies requires divalent recognition. Eur J Immunol 1994; 24:2161–2167.
71. Byrn RA, Mordenti J, Lucas C, Smith D, Marsters SA, Johnson JS, Cossum P, Chamow SM, Wurm FM, Gregory T, Groopman JE, Capon DJ. Biological properties of a CD4 immunoadhesin. Nature 1990; 344:667–670.
72. Haak-Frendscho M, Ridgway J, Shields R, Robbins K, Gorman C, Jardieu P. Human IgE receptor α-chain IgG chimera blocks passive cutaneous anaphylaxis reaction in vivo. J Immunol 1993; 151:351–358.
73. Saban R, Haak-Frendscho M, Zine M, Ridgway J, Gorman C, Presta LG, Bjorling D, Saban M, Jardieu P. Human FcεRI–IgG and humanized anti-IgE monoclonal antibody MaE11 block passive sensitization of human and rhesus monkey lung. J Allergy Clin Immunol 1994; 94:836–843.
74. Jameson BA, McDonnell JM, Marini JC, Korngold R. A rationally designed CD4 analogue inhibits experimental allergic encephalomyelitis. Nature 1994; 368:744–746.
75. Guichard G, Benkirane N, Zeder-Lutz G, van Regenmortel MHV, Briand J-P, Muller S. Antigenic mimicry of natural L-peptides with retro-inverso-peptidomimetics. Proc Natl Acad Sci USA 1994; 91:9765–9769.
76. McDonnell JM, Fushman D, Cahill SM, Sutton BJ, Cowburn D. Solution structures of FcεRI α-chain mimics: a β-hairpin peptide and its retroenantiomer. J Am Chem Soc 1997; 119:5321–5328.
77. Li S, Gao J, Satoh T, Friedman TM, Edling AE, Koch U, Choksi S, Han X, Korngold R, Huang Z. A computer screening approach to immunoglobulin superfamily structures and interactions: discovery of small non-peptidic CD4 inhibitors as novel immunotherapeutics. Proc Natl Acad Sci USA 1997; 94:73–78.
78. Wiegand TW, Williams PB, Dreskin SC, Jouvin M-H, Kinet J-P, Tasset D. High-affinity oligonucleotide ligands to human IgE inhibit binding to Fcε receptor I. J Immunol 1996; 157:221–230.
79. Gould HJ, Beavil RL, Reljic R, Shi J, Sutton BJ, Ghirlando R. IgE homeostasis: is CD23

the safety switch? In: Vercelli D, ed. Molecular Mechanisms of IgE Regulation. New York: John Wiley and Sons, 1997:37–59.

80. Suemura M, Kikutani H, Sugiyama K, Uchibayashi N, Aitani M, Kuritani T, Barsumian EL, Yamatodami A, Kishimoto T. Significance of soluble Fc ε receptor II (sFcεRII/CD23) in serum and possible application of sFcεRII for the prevention of allergic reactions. Allergy Proc 1991; 12:133–137.

81. Gauchat J-F, Henchoz S, Mazzei G, Aubry J-P, Brunner T, Blasey H, Life P, Talabot D, Flores-Romo L, Thompson J, Kishi K, Butterfield J, Dahinden C, Bonnefoy J-Y. Induction of human IgE synthesis in B cells by mast cells and basophils. Nature 1993; 365:340–343.

27

Regulation of Immunoglobulin E Inflammation

Anti-Immunoglobulin E Autoantibodies

BEDA M. STADLER,
MONIQUE VOGEL,
SYLVIA MARGARET MIESCHER, and
ADRIAN WALTER ZUERCHER

University of Bern
Inselspital
Bern, Switzerland

MICHAEL P. RUDOLF

Oncology Institute
Loyola University Medical Center
Maywood, Illinois

FRANZ KRICEK

Novartis Research Center
Vienna, Austria

I. Introduction

Basic research in allergy has been inspired by many different hypotheses during the last years. Different cell types have come and gone as the so-called key players in allergic reactions, and individual cytokines or patterns of cytokines produced at the same time are still en vogue as the principal regulatory moieties. Nevertheless, from the beginning of allergy research until today, the old-fashioned key player IgE has always been believed to play the most crucial role in the ontogeny of this disease.

Most allergologists are convinced that the specific IgE response has to be downregulated to treat allergic disease. Immunotherapy, still one of the often-effective treatments, is based on this hypothesis, but so far it has not been able to deliver a molecularly sound explanation for this treatment. Furthermore, we lack a stringent scientific basis for the role of certain cell types or cytokines during allergic inflammation that would explain why only some persons develop allergies and others do not.

Therefore, it is understandable that the aim of some of the newer strategies to treat IgE-mediated diseases is to eliminate IgE, the central key player. Such a strategy, as we will outline in this chapter, has basically two possible outcomes: (1)

If the elimination of IgE over a certain period in a patient results in the cure of IgE-mediated disease, we would clearly be in the position to discriminate between allergic manifestations that are caused by IgE and those that are not. The potential side effects would also finally deliver an answer concerning the true physiological role of IgE. (2) If the elimination or neutralization of IgE has no beneficial effect, then we would have to agree that IgE is not the claimed key player in IgE-mediated disease, and we would have to undertake a revision of many concepts concerning IgE-mediated diseases.

II. Anti-IgE Autoantibodies

A. Occurrence

The first observations of naturally occurring anti-IgE autoantibodies have led to speculations that such autoantibodies may have a pathophysiological role (1–7). However, the matter remained disputed, even though there have been reports showing that sera from patients containing anti-IgE autoantibodies would occasionally induce histamine release from basophils (8,9).

Additionally, we and others have shown that the occurrence of anti-IgE antibodies was not restricted only to individuals with IgE-mediated disease (10–12). Practically, it was also impossible to accurately quantify the levels of anti-IgE antibodies, and one is only able to roughly estimate that anti-IgE autoantibodies occur in quantities similar to IgE itself, except in cord blood samples, where anti-IgE autoantibodies levels are in excess.

More interesting was the finding that it was possible to induce an anti-IgE immune response in animal models (15–17). Neonatal application of IgE sometimes even led to an almost lifelong suppression of IgE synthesis in rodents (18–19). But at the time, nobody dared to follow up this concept, and it still took quite some time until the idea was taken up to eventually develop strategies for the treatment (20–22).

B. In Vitro Models for Anti-IgE Activity

Anti-IgE antibodies have always been used to trigger mediator release from basophils or mast cells in vitro; however, they never represented an agent that could be useful for therapy (23). At the time the first monoclonal anti-IgE antibodies were generated, we were interested in studying the question of whether all types of anti-IgE antibodies are actually anaphylactogenic (23). Indeed, most of the anti-IgE monoclonal antibodies (MAbs) that we have generated were anaphylactogenic, and we found only one that did not trigger histamine release (23). Similarly, others have analyzed anti-IgE antibodies, and if they used nonanaphylactogenicity as a selection criterion, they could generate a whole array of different anti-IgE antibodies that were not anaphylactogenic (Heusser C, Novartis, Basel; personal communication).

The most important question remained whether anti-IgE antibodies would be capable of influencing IgE synthesis. Interestingly, most of the anti-IgE antibodies that had been used in in vitro culture systems were strongly inhibitory for IgE synthesis (24). The inhibitory antibodies had to be present as divalent molecules, meaning that only complete antibody molecules or $F(ab)_2$, but not Fab antibodies inhibited IgE synthesis (24).

Furthermore, we could show that anti-IgE antibodies could also interfere with the binding of IgE to CD23, the low-affinity IgE receptor (25,26). Nevertheless, from all tested antibodies, only one antibody had so far all the wanted beneficial effects; namely, inhibiting IgE synthesis, not being anaphylactogenic, and interfering with IgE binding to the high- and the low-affinity receptor for IgE. This antibody, termed BSW17, was, for us, a potential candidate for human therapy. Therefore, we were interested in whether this mouse antihuman IgE specificity might also exist in humans.

C. Isolation of Anti-IgE Autoantibodies by Repertoire Cloning

Our first approach to isolate naturally occurring antibodies from serum failed primarily because antibodies could be isolated only as immune complexes and were available only in minute quantities (11,13,14). Thus, we chose the technique of phage display to express immunoglobulin light and heavy chains on the surface of the M13 phage (27). As a source of the immunoglobulin gene we chose a patient who had anti-IgE antibodies and was atopic. With this approach, we isolated numerous anti-IgE antibodies, but to our astonishment more than 99% of the antibodies we had isolated, using different IgE myelomas as the antigen, were anti-idiotypic, and less than 1% of them recognized the constant domains of the IgE molecule (27). Obviously, the variable domains of the immunoglobulins were the most "immunogenic" recognition sites for the antibody–phage display libraries, and it was not possible to generate an antibody that had the same specificity as the anti-IgE antibody BSW17 (28).

III. Mimicry of IgE Epitopes

A. Epitope Specificity and Biological Activity of Anti-IgE Antibodies

Our previous experiments had clearly demonstrated that the IgE molecule by itself contains too many different epitopes to isolate one single antibody against a rare epitope on the constant domain. Through our in vitro analysis of murine anti-IgE monoclonal antibodies (MAbs) it also became clear that only antibodies interfering directly with the binding site of IgE for its receptor, or recognize an epitope close to the binding site, were nonanaphylactogenic (29,30). Nonanaphylactogenic antibodies, as they are now known, all fulfill this criteria; namely, they recognize an epitope within the third constant domain of IgE (31–36). From these data we concluded that most naturally occurring anti-IgE antibodies are likely not to have biological activity, or have an activity that at least is not unfavorable (28). These findings were based on crisscross inhibition studies of antibodies. However, this approach did not allow us to precisely define distinct epitopes on IgE, but rather, only broader specificities within the immunoglobulin domain regions.

B. IgE Mimotopes

To further characterize the specific epitope on the IgE molecule, as recognized by the monoclonal antibody BSW17, we again used the technique of phage display. This time we used phage display libraries that on the surface expressed random peptides of nine amino acids in length (37,38). Such libraries express more than 10^8 different phages and may thereby represent a relatively large proportion of all possible epitopes that can be recognized by antibodies. We limited ourselves to the search for peptides that would bind to our model antibody BSW17. The random peptides mimic its precise epitope and, therefore, are called mimotopes.

To our astonishment, we found a mimotope within the fourth constant domain of the IgE molecule. This did not fit our previous experience with this antibody, based on the cross-inhibition experiments with other antibodies, during which we found that BSW17 is directed against an epitope within the third domain (30). Therefore, we decided to use the antibody one more time for biopanning against an new set of random peptide libraries, because theoretically, it was possible that the previously used random library did not contain the actual epitope. Furthermore, the peptide that we have found in the fourth domain did not show sequence homology with a region in the fourth IgE domain, but shared only structural homology. In this new round of biopanning, using BSW17 and random peptide phage display libraries, we used phages that expressed 6-mer, 9-mer, 10-mer, and 15-mer peptides on their surface. Again, we found a limited number of peptides that were isolated by the antibody, and this time a peptide was isolated, stretching over ten amino acids, that showed linear sequence homology within the third constant domain. These results clearly show that it is possible to isolate specific B-cell epitopes with this new technology and that, obviously, an antibody can have two binding sites on a single antigen.

IV. Anti-Idiotypic Antibodies as Epitope Mimicry

Based on Jerne's network hypothesis, and the idea of the "horror autotoxicus," it should be possible to find antibodies that express CDR loops that look like structures that already occur in our body. In other words, it should be feasible to find an anti-idiotypic antibody with structural homology to the isolated random peptides, the mimotopes of IgE. In addressing this question we used a pool of antibody-phage display libraries that had been generated from tonsils of children, adult spleen, and blood leukocytes. As template (antigen) we again used antibody BSW17 and were able to isolate antibodies that exclusively interacted with BSW17, but with no other murine antibodies, fulfilling the criteria of an anti-idiotypic antibody. Interestingly, these antibodies were indeed inhibited by the presence of the previously isolated IgE mimotopes. Furthermore, sequence analysis of the isolated anti-idiotypic antibodies showed sequence homology with the mimotopes (Vogel M, manuscript in preparation).

Work that is now in progress should answer the last question: Will it be possible by using the IgE mimotope, or the anti-idiotypic antibodies, to induce an antibody that has the same specificity and the same structure as the murine monoclonal antibody BSW17?

V. Therapeutic Strategies Based on Anti-IgE Antibodies

A. Passive Immunization with Humanized Antibodies

Several anti-IgE antibodies have been selected for therapy in patients. The approach of Genentech was to generate an antibody that interferes with the binding site for IgE to its high-affinity receptor, thereby warranting that the application of the antibody would not lead to an immediate anaphylactic reaction (33). There is abundant literature on this antibody stating its efficacy in different in vitro and animal models (34–36,39,40). Moreover, this antibody is in phase II trials and preliminary experiments indicate that it may become a therapeutic reagent. The strategy chosen by Novartis/Tannox was first based on antibodies that would recognize only membrane IgE on B cells, but later an antibody was chosen that was selected for its in vitro absence of anaphylactogenicity (21). Also this antibody is in clinical trials, and a decrease of IgE levels with a concomitant increase in IgE complexes, as has also been observed with autoantibodies, could be demonstrated (41). This reagent inhibited in vivo IgE-mediated skin reactions, bronchial constriction, and pulmonary eosinophil infiltration in different animal models (42,43). However, unless we do analyze the results from phase III clinical trials, the final clinical efficacy of both types of antibodies cannot be judged.

B. Active Immunization

There may be an alternate strategy: that is, active immunization with small IgE epitopes to induce a natural autoimmune response, resulting in the formation of autoantibodies that may have the same effect as passively administered anti-IgE antibodies.

We have already shown that our isolated IgE mimotopes induce an anti-IgE immune response in rabbits, and experiments are under way to address the option of whether or not it is possible to induce such a beneficial autoimmune response in dogs and primates. In addition, the availability of anti-idiotypic antibodies, representing IgE structures, makes it feasible to consider an alternative vaccination procedure. These anti-idiotypic antibodies may eventually be better tolerated than peptides that have to be coupled to immunogenic carriers.

VI. Conclusion

Modern gene technological tools have provided a way to dissect the natural anti-IgE response. Further clinical trials will show whether it is possible to treat allergies either by passive or active immunization. For an understanding of allergic disease it can also be envisaged that the radical approach to eliminate or neutralize IgE will finally be the proof of how important this molecule is during the ontogeny and pathophysiology of the so-called IgE-mediated diseases.

References

1. Williams RC, Griffiths RW, Emmons JD, Field RC. Naturally occurring human antiglobulins with specificity for gamma-E. J Clin Invest 1972; 51:955.
2. Inganäs M, Johansson SG, Bennich H. Anti-IgE antibodies in human serum: occurrence and specificity. Int Arch Allergy Appl Immunol 1981; 65:51–61.
3. Carini C, Brostoff J. An antiglobulin: IgG anti-IgE. Occurrence and specificity. Ann Allergy 1983; 51:251–254.
4. Stevens WJ, Bridts CH. IgG-containing and IgE-containing circulating immune complexes in patients with asthma and rhinitis. J Allergy Clin Immunol 1984; 73:276.
5. Nawata Y, Koike T, Hosokawa H, Tomioka Y, Yoshida S. Anti-IgE autoantibody in patients with atopic dermatitis. J Immunol 1985; 135:478–482.
6. Paganelli R, Quinti I, Carbonari M, Pontesilli O, D'Offizi GP, Letta T, Aiuti F. IgG anti-IgE in circulating immune complexes in the hyper-IgE syndrome. Clin Allergy 1986; 16:513–521.
7. Carini C, Fratazzi C, Barbato M. IgG autoantibody to IgE in atopic patients. Ann Allergy 1988; 60:48–52.
8. Marone G, Casolaro V, Paganelli R, Quinti. IgG anti-IgE from atopic dermatitis induces mediator release from basophils and mast cells. J Invest Dermatol 1989; 93:246–252.
9. Shakib F, Smith SJ. In vitro basophil histamine-releasing activity of circulating IgG1 and IgG4 autoanti-IgE antibodies from asthma patients and the demonstration that anti-IgE modulates allergen-induced basophil activation. Clin Exp Allergy 1994; 24:270.
10. Wilson PB, Fairfield JE, Beech N. Detection of IgG subclass-specific anti-IgE antibodies in normal and atopic individuals. Int Archs Allergy Appl Immunol 1987; 84:198–204.
11. Ritter C, Bättig M, Kraemer R, Stadler BM. IgE hidden in immune complexes with anti-IgE autoantibodies in children with asthma. J Allergy Clin Immunol 1991; 88:793–801.
12. Magnusson CGM, Johansson SGO. Clinical significance of anti-IgE autoantibodies and immune complexes containing IgE. Clin Rev Allergy 1989; 7:73.
13. Vassella CC, de Weck AL, Stadler BM. Natural anti-IgE auto-antibodies interfere with diagnostic IgE determination. Clin Exp Allergy 1990; 20:295–303.
14. Jensen-Jarolim E, Vogel M, de Weck AL, Stadler BM. Anti-IgE autoantibodies mistaken for specific IgG. J Allergy Clin Immunol 1992; 89:31–43.
15. Marshall JS, Bell EB. Induction of an auto-anti-IgE response in rats. I. Effects on serum IgE concentrations. Eur J Immunol 1985; 15:272–277.
16. Marshall JS, Bell EB. Induction of an auto-anti-IgE response in rats. III. Inhibition of a specific IgE response. Immunology 1989; 66:428–433.
17. Jaffery G, Bell EB, Coleman JW. Induction of an auto-anti-IgE response in rats. IV. Effects

on mast cell degranulation. Immunology 1993; 78:635–642.
18. Haba S, Nisonoff A. Inhibition of IgE synthesis by anti-IgE. Role in long-term inhibition of IgE synthesis by neonatally administered soluble IgE. Proc Natl Acad Sci USA 1990; 87:3363–3367.
19. Haba S, Nisonov A. Effects of synergistic anti-IgE antibodies on the development of IgE memory and on the secondary IgE response. J Immunol 1994; 152:51.
20. Stadler BM, Gang Q, Vogel M, Jarolim E, Miescher S, Aebischer I, de Weck AL. IgG anti-IgE autoantibodies in immunoregulation. Int Arch Allergy Appl Immunol 1991; 94:83–86.
22. Davis FM, Gossett LA, Pinkston KL, Liou RS, Sun LK, Kim YW, Chang NT, Wagner K, Bews J, Brinkmann V, Towbin H, Subramanian N, Heusser C. Can anti-IgE be used to treat allergy. Springer Semin Immunopathol 1993; 15:51–73.
22. Kolbinger J, Saldanha J, Hardman N, Bendig MM. Humanization of a mouse anti-human IgE antibody: a potential therapeutic for IgE-mediated allergies. Protein Eng 1993; 6:971–980.
23. Kings MA, Conroy MA, Stadler BM, Magnusson CG, Skvaril F, de Weck AL. Histamine release from human leukocytes by anti-IgE antibodies: influence of multiple or single epitope recognition. Diagn Immunol 1986; 4:89–96.
24. Stämpfli MR, Miescher S, Aebischer I, Stadler BM. Modulation of IgE synthesis by anti-IgE antibody. Eur J Immunol 1994; 24:2161–2167.
25. Nakajima K, de Weck AL, Stadler BM. Effect of anti-IgE antibodies on IgE binding to CD23. Allergy 1989; 44:187–191.
26. Miescher S, Vogel M, Stämpfli MR, Holzner ME, Wasserbauer E, Kricek F, Vorburger S, Stadler BM. Domain specific anti-IgE antibodies interfere with IgE binding to FcεRII. Int Arch Allergy Immunol 1994; 105:75–82.
27. Vogel M, Miescher S, Stadler BM, Human anti-IgE antibodies by repertoire cloning. Eur J Immunol 1993; 24:1200–1207.
28. Stadler BM, Stämpfli MR, Miescher S, Furukawa K, Vogel M. Biological activities of anti-IgE antibodies. Int Arch Allergy Immunol 1993; 102:121–126.
29. Stämpfli RM, Rudolf MP, Miescher S, Pachlopnik JM, Stadler BM. Antigen-specific inhibition of IgE binding to the high-affinity receptor. J Immunol 1995; 155:2948.
30. Rudolf M, Furukawa K, Miescher S, Vogel M, Stadler BM. Apparant removal of IgE from human FcεRI mediated by monoclonal anti-IgE antibodies. J Immunol 1996; 157:5646–5652.
31. Helm B, Marsh P, Vercelli D, Padlan E, Gould H, Geha R. The mast cell binding site on human immunoglobulin E. Nature 1988; 331:180–183.
32. Nissim A, Jouvin M, Eshhar Z. Mapping of the high affinity Fce receptor binding site to the third constant domain of IgE. EMBO J 1991; 10:101.
33. Presta L, Shields R, O'Connel L, Lahr S, Porter J, Gorman C, Jardieu P. The binding site on human immunoglobulin E for its high affinity receptor. J Biol Chem 1994; 269:26368–26373.
34. Shields RL, Whether WR, O'Connell L, Fendly B, Presta LG, Thomas D, Saban R, Jardieu P. Inhibition of allergic reactions with antibodies to IgE. Int Arch Allergy Immunol 1995; 107:308–312.
35. Saban R, Haak-Frendscho M, Zine M, Ridgway J, Gorman C, Presta LG, Bjorling D, Saban M, Jardieu P. Human FcεRI–IgG and humanized anti-IgE monoclonal antibody MaE11 block passive sensitization of human and rhesus monkey lung. J Allergy Clin Immunol 1994; 94:836–843.
36. Tai Wai Fei D, Lowe J, Jardieu P. A novel bioactivity assay for monoclonal antibodies directed against IgE. J Immunol Methods 1994; 171:189–199.
37. Luzzago A, Felici F, Tramontano A, Pessi A, Cortese R. Mimicking of discontinuous epitopes by phage-displayed peptides. I. Epitope mapping of human H ferritin using a phase library of constrained peptides. Gene 1993; 128:51–57.
38. Felici F, Castagnoli L, Musacchio A, Jappelli R, Cesareni G. Selection of antibody ligands from a large library of oligopeptides expressed on a multivalent exposition vector. J Mol

Biol 1991; 222:301–310.

39. Amiri P, Haak-Frendscho M, Robbins K, McKerrow JH, Stewart T, Jardieu P. Anti-immunoglobulin E treatment decreases worm burden and egg production in *Schistosoma mansoni*-infected normal and interferon γ knockout mice. J Exp Med 1994; 180:43–51.
40. Haak-Frendscho M, Robbins K, Lyon R, Shields R, Hooley J, Schoenhoff M, Jardieu P. Administration of an anti-IgE antibody inhibits CD23 expression and IgE production in vivo. Immunology 1994; 82:306–313.
41. Corne J, Djukanovic R, Thomas L, Warner J, Botta L, Grandordy B, Gygax D, Heusser CH, Patalano F, Richardson W, Kilcherr E, Staehelin T, Davis F, Gordon W, Sun L, Liou R, Wang G, Chang T-W, Holgate S. The effect of intravenous administration of a chimaeric anti-IgE antibody on serum IgE levels in atopic subjects—efficacy, safety and pharmakokinetics. J Clin Invest 1997; 99:879–887.
42. Coyle AJ, Wagner K, Betrand C, Tsuyuki S, Bews J, Heussser C. Central role of immunoglobulin (Ig) E in the induction of lung eosinophil infiltration and T helper 2 cell cytokine production: inhibition by a non-anaphylactogenic anti-IgR antibody. J Exp Med 1996; 183:1303–1310.
43. Heusser CH, Wagner K, Bews JPA, Coyle A, Bertrand C, Einsle K, Kips J, Eum S-Y, Lefort J, Vargaftig B. Demonstration of the therapeutic potential of nonanaphylactogenic anti-IgE antibodies in murine models of skin reaction and lung function and inflammation. Int Arch Allergy Immunol 1997; 113:231–235.

Part Four

NON–IgE-DEPENDENT IMMUNOTHERAPY

28

Non–Immunoglobulin E-Dependent Immunotherapy

Treatment of Asthma with Inhaled Interferon Gamma

GIDEON LACK

Imperial College
St. Mary's Medical School
London, England

DONALD Y. M. LEUNG and ERWIN W. GELFAND

National Jewish Medical and Research Center
and the University of Colorado Health Sciences Center
Denver, Colorado

I. Introduction

The past decade has witnessed a remarkable increase in our understanding of IgE regulation and allergic inflammation. Perhaps the most important observations have been the role of T cells and inflammatory cytokines in these disease processes. Consequently, it is now possible to develop new strategies to target different sites in the allergic inflammatory cascade, particulary to modulate T- and B-lymphocyte function. Advances in the molecular cloning of allergens and recognition of immunodominant T-cell epitopes offer possibilities of inhibiting allergic responses and improving on the safety and efficacy of conventional allergic desensitization. Recognition of the tight control of IgE production by cytokines has led to consideration of immunomodulatory agents, such as the soluble interleukin (IL)-4 receptor, and anti-IL-4 monoclonal antibody (Mab), interferon gamma (IFN-γ, IFN-α), and IL-12 for the treatment of allergic disease.

Human allergic diseases are characterized by high levels of circulating IgE, allergen-specific IgE, and allergic inflammation (eosinophils and mast cells) in specific target organs. IgE is critical in the pathogenesis of early- and late-phase allergic responses (1–3). In vitro work on animal and human tracheal smooth muscle indicates that IgE may play an important role in the pathogenesis of increased airways responsiveness (AR; 4,5). Indeed, a prospective study (6) has shown that increased airways responsiveness in children is positively correlated with serum IgE levels, even in subjects without clinical evidence of allergy; also, in the elderly, an increased serum IgE level correlates with a greater likelihood of acquiring asthma.

Cytokines produced mainly by $CD4^+$ T cells are critically involved in immunoglobulin (Ig) isotype switching and in the regulation of allergic inflammation. IL-4 causes both murine and human B cells to undergo isotype switching to IgE synthesis (8–12); IL-4 also induces IgG1 and IgG4 production by murine and human B cells, respectively (13,14). IL-13 also induces immunoglobulin isotype switching to IgE synthesis (15).

Interferon-γ has an inhibitory effect on in vitro IgE production by murine and human lymphocytes (8,16–19). Although the mechanism of action is not entirely defined, IFN-γ antagonizes the effect of IL-4 on IgE synthesis in the presence of $CD4^+$ T cells (7,17). At the transcriptional level, IFN-γ reduces the level of IL-4–induced germline ε-mRNA by more than 50% and the productive ε-transcript by more than 80% (20). Additionally, IFN-γ inhibits IL-13–driven IgE synthesis by human B cells (15).

$CD4^+$ cells are believed to be critical in determining the allergic inflammatory response. T helper type 2 (Th2) lymphocytes that produce IL-4 and IL-5 in bronchial biopsy specimens appear to be important in the development of the late-phase allergic response and recruitment of eosinophils into the airways (21). In vitro, IFN-γ selectively inhibits the proliferation of Th2 cells and favors the differentiation of precursor Th0 cells into cells with a Th1 phenotype (22,23). An alteration of the cytokine profile of lymphocytes by IFN-γ from a Th2 profile to a Th1 profile could potentially alter the allergic inflammatory response and prevent the migration of eosinophils into inflamed tissue. There is evidence in the mouse that in vivo, IFN-γ prevents the IL-5–dependent migration of eosinophils into the airways by inhibiting $CD4^+$ T-cell infiltration (24).

In addition to modulating allergic inflammation through the T cell, IFN-γ may act directly on the eosinophil and other inflammatory cells. In vitro IFN-γ inhibits eosinophil degranulation (25). Furthermore, by inhibiting mast cell functions, IFN-γ could also modulate allergic inflammation. IFN-γ has inhibitory effects on mast cell precursors (26), and it also prevents the proliferation of connective tissue mast cells in the mouse (27). Both the sensitization of murine peritoneal mast cells with IgE (28) and the release of serotonin (29) have been blocked in vitro by the addition of IFN-γ. Basophil function is also affected by IFN-γ (30). Thus, there is a complexity of biological interactions through which IFN-γ may modulate allergic inflammation and airway responsiveness, in addition to its effects on IgE and T-cell function.

Importantly, there is evidence to suggest that allergic patients are deficient in IFN-γ production (31–34). We recently showed, in human atopic peripheral blood mononuclear cells (PBMC), that there is deficient IFN-γ production, and localized this defect to the CD4 subset of T cells (35). Furthermore, following allergic desensitization, atopic patients who previously had reduced IFN-γ production developed an increase in IFN-γ production that correlated with a decline in cutaneous and nasal reactivity to house dust mite (36).

These data provide a rationale for treating allergic disease with IFN-γ based on achieving two objectives: first, the inhibition of IgE production; second, the correction of the cytokine imbalance, with consequent reduction of allergic inflammation.

II. Clinical Trials

There have been several clinical trials aimed at treating allergic diseases with recombinant (r)IFN-γ. In the following sections we will summarize the important findings in these trials, discuss their limitations, and attempt to define the problems in rIFN-γ–based cytokine therapy, at least in the light of recent animal work. In particular, emphasis is placed on the need to target rIFN-γ to the site of allergic disease; namely, the airways and lungs in asthma. These studies of IFN-γ therapy may serve as a prototype for effective delivery of other cytokines and experimental immunomodulatory agents for treatment of allergic responses.

A. Atopic Dermatitis

The first case report on the use of the rIFN-γ in atopic dermatitis was published in 1990 (37). Three patients with unremitting severe atopic dermatitis and high serum IgE levels were treated with subcutaneous IFN-γ, initially receiving injections of 0.1 mg daily for 5 days, followed by three injections a week for a further 3 weeks. Marked improvement in the dermatitis was noted after 2 weeks of therapy. Serum total IgE levels decreased during treatment, and spontaneous IgE production in vitro was also reduced.

Subsequently, in an open study that included 22 patients with chronic severe atopic dermatitis, rIFN-γ administered subcutaneously resulted in a significant reduction in the severity of skin disease (38). There was no change in total serum IgE levels, but there was a variable and incomplete inhibition of IgE synthesis by PBMC. Additionally, this study found that patients were able to tolerate doses of 0.05 mg/m^2, whereas the high dose of 0.1 mg/m^2 produced side effects in 25% of patients (tension headache, malaise, fever, chills, myalgia, or nausea). Given these promising results, a double-blind, placebo-controlled study was carried out in a group of 83 patients with atopic dermatitis (39). They received 0.05 mg/m^2 rIFN-γ daily by subcutaneous injection for 12 weeks. Two patients receiving rIFN-γ dropped out owing to constitutional side effects. Forty-five percent of the rIFN-γ–treated patients and 21% of the placebo-treated patients achieved more than a 50% improvement in their atopic dermatitis ($p = 0.016$). Occasional constitutional symptoms were effectively prevented by pretreatment with acetaminophen. Importantly, clinical improvement in skin disease was associated with a significant reduction in mean eosinophil count ($p = 0.003$). Interestingly, there was no significant change in serum total IgE levels; however, allergen-specific IgE was not determined.

B. Allergic Rhinitis

There has been one study examining rIFN-γ treatment in allergic rhinitis (40). Forty-five adults, with a history of ragweed allergic rhinitis for more than 2 years, serum IgE antibody to short ragweed, and skin test reactivity to ragweed, participated in a randomized double-blind, two-period design study. Each subject was treated with rIFN-γ or placebo by subcutaneous injections three times a week for 4 weeks during the off season and for 6 weeks during the ragweed season. Therefore, this study included treatment both during the off season, when patients were not exposed to allergen, and during the ragweed season when patients were exposed to high levels of ragweed allergen. Importantly, this is the only clinical study that compared the effects of IFN-γ treatment during a period of allergen exposure with a period of no allergen exposure.

Subjects were divided into three groups to receive either 0.2 mg of IFN-γ, 0.02 mg IFN-γ, or placebo. There was no significant difference in hay fever scores during spring and summer among the three treatment groups after the ragweed season. All three groups experienced an increase in ragweed-specific IgE during the ragweed season, and there were no significant differences among the groups. Similarly, neither was there a difference in total IgE. The authors noted that, in mice, only very large doses of IFN-γ administered systemically suppressed IgE responses. The doses of IFN-γ required to significantly suppress IgE responses in vivo in mice were approximately 1000-fold higher than the largest dose of IFN-γ administered in the allergic rhinitis study. However, at a 0.2-mg dose of IFN-γ, humans were already suffering side effects, and there was no ability to increase the dosage.

C. Asthma

IFN-γ Treatment of Steroid-Dependent Asthma

A two-center, double-blind, placebo-randomized trial was conducted with 20 steroid-dependent asthmatics to determine the safety and efficacy of parenteral IFN-γ treatment in steroid-dependent asthma (41). Nine patients were treated with rIFN-γ at a dose of 0.05 mg/m^2 and 11 received placebo, both given daily by subcutaneous injection for 90 days. All patients received acetaminophen 1 hr before and 4 hr after injections. Prednisolone dose was constant for the first few weeks of the study and, then, was reduced at 2-week intervals if the patient had no symptoms and the forced 1-sec expiratory volume (FEV_1) and peak expiratory flow rate (PEFR) remained stable.

All patients tolerated rIFN-γ given daily at a dose of 0.05 mg/m^2. Only one patient required a dose reduction for transient granulocytopenia. However, the regimen was not effective in treating steroid-dependent asthma, as assessed by failure to achieve corticosteroid dose reduction, compared with placebo and a lack of improvement in pulmonary function. As in previous study with IFN-γ, there was no change in serum IgE levels. However, there was a selective decrease in the peripheral blood eosinophil count in the rIFN-γ treatment group when compared with the placebo-treated group. The authors commented that higher doses of IFN-γ than those used in this study would have resulted in unacceptable levels of side effects.

Aerosolized IFN-γ in Asthma

One possible explanation for the failure of subcutaneous rIFN-γ administration in the treatment of asthma was that it did not reach the airways. Indeed, subcutaneously administered rIFN-γ, given over a 3-day period, does not reach the respiratory epithelial cell surface (42). Therefore, a study was undertaken to examine the effects of inhaled rIFN-γ in normal human airways (43). Importantly, 60% of the aerosol droplets produced were demonstrated by laser nephelometry to have a diameter between 1 and 5 μm. The effectiveness of inhaled rIFN-γ demonstrated by the recovery of free rIFN-γ in bronchoalveolar lavage fluid (BAL) and also by the upregulation of macrophage expression of IP10, an IFN-γ–inducible molecule, after IFN-γ therapy. Therefore, the particles were (1) in the respirable range, (2) bioavailable to the airways, and (3) bioactive on the local inflammatory cells.

The same group examined, in a small open-labeled study, effects of nebulized rIFN-γ on patients with chronic asthma (44). Five adults with atopic asthma received nebulized rIFN-γ at regular intervals over a 19-day period. All patients tolerated the nebulized rIFN-γ well. Symptoms scores, methacholine challenges, and pulmonary function did not significantly change before or after treatment. Nebulized rIFN-γ was recoverable in the BAL, and upregulation of mRNA for IP10 was demonstrated after IFN-γ therapy. Importantly, four out of five patients had a significant decrease in the percent of BAL eosinophils. The authors concluded that future studies are needed to examine the potential role of nebulized rIFN-γ in asthma.

D. Limitations in Study Design

These studies, carried out in patients, were unable to address certain important issues. Their interpretation and conclusions, therefore, are limited for the following reasons:

First, parenteral treatment was the sole route employed in most clinical trials. There is murine data showing that local delivery of rIFN-γ is more effective than distal delivery in enhancing local killing of *Listeria monocytogenes* by tissue macrophages (45). Additionally, there is evidence in humans showing that the local delivery of IFN-γ by nebulization is more bioavailable to the lungs than is systemic treatment (42). Second, the important element of timing of IFN-γ treatment was not studied. There are data showing that the late addition of IFN-γ treatment to PBMC cultured with IL-4 does not inhibit IgE synthesis (18). Third, most of the studies did not differentiate between polyclonal and allergen-specific IgE production. Allergic disease is characterized by both elevated total serum IgE and allergen-specific IgE, as well as by allergen-specific cutaneous reactivity. Indeed, cutaneous reactivity may be a far more important and sensitive readout. In allergen immunotherapy, a decline in cutaneous reactivity is not generally paralleled by a decrease in allergen-specific IgE (36). Finally, clinical studies do not permit comparison of the effect of IFN-γ treatment on primary allergic sensitization with secondary and subsequent allergic responses. Patients who present with allergic disease generally have well-established ongoing IgE production, resulting from many months or years of exposure to allergen.

III. Treatment with IFN-γ in a Murine Model of Allergic Sensitization

To address these important issues, we employed a murine model that allowed analysis of these critical variables (46–48). IgE high-responder Balb/c mice were sensitized via the airways and lungs by ultrasonic nebulization of ovalbumin (OVA). Mice exposed to daily OVA (20 min) over a 10-day period developed high anti-OVA IgE responses in the serum and immediate cutaneous reactivity to OVA. Exposure of tracheal smooth muscle to electrical field stimulation showed that OVA-exposed mice developed altered airway function. Increased airway responsiveness (AR) was observed in sensitized compared with nonsensitized controls. This correlated with increased acetylcholine release and impaired muscarinic M_2 receptor function (49). To evaluate the ability of IFN-γ to modify these responses, mice were treated with rIFN-γ using different routes of administration, dosages, and timing schedules (50).

A. Parenteral IFN-γ Decreases Total, but not Allergen-Specific IgE

Mice were treated with 25,000 units of IFN-γ by the intraperitoneal route daily for 3 days before and during the 10-day course of ovalbumin sensitization. The use of higher doses was abandoned because of toxicity and no apparent benefits over the lower doses. Mice sensitized to OVA developed a twofold increase in serum total IgE levels (50; Table 1). IFN-γ treatment given by the intraperitoneal route caused a 50% decrease in total serum IgE to levels equivalent to those seen in phosphate-buffered saline (PBS)-treated controls. In contrast, intraperitoneal IFN-γ failed to decrease anti-OVA IgE responses that followed OVA sensitization through the airways. These mice had persistently elevated anti-OVA IgE levels, cutaneous reactivity to OVA, and increased AR, similar to untreated animals that had received OVA alone (see Table 1). Even employing different treatment routes, such as intradermal or intravenous IFN-γ failed to inhibit anti-OVA IgE responses.

B. Bioavailability of Nebulized, but not Intraperitonal IFN-γ to the Local Airway Lymphoid Tissues

When given intraperitoneally, IFN-γ actively inhibited systemic polyclonal IgE production, but may not have been available to the local lymphoid tissue of the air-

Table 1 Comparison of the Effects of Nebulized (neb) and Intraperitoneal (ip) IFN-γ[a]

Treatment	OVA	OVA–IFN-γ neb	OVA–IFN-γ ip
Total IgE	↑	↑	↓
Anti-OVA IgE	↑↑	↓↓	↑↑
Anti-OVA IgG2a	—	↑↑	↑
Airway responsiveness	↑↑	↓↓	↑↑
Cutaneous reactivity to OVA	↑↑	↓↓	↑↑

[a]Recombinant IFN-γ was administered ip or by nebulization to BALB/c animals for 3 days before and during the 10-day period of OVA sensitization through the airways. On day 12, serum for IgE levels was obtained; immediate cutaneous reactivity and airway function were also determined.

ways, where allergen-specific IgE production was occurring. We hypothesized that the local delivery of nebulized IFN-γ, unlike intraperitoneal IFN-γ, would be active in the airways and thus modulate the local production of anti-OVA IgE. We first established by laser nephelometry that more than 60% of the IFN-γ particles were in the respirable range for mice (0.5–2 μm) and bioavailable to the airways and lungs. Second, we showed that nebulized IFN-γ (250,000 units dissolved in 7 mL PBS) retained its bioactivity (50). Aerosolized particles were collected by condensation, and the condensate effectively inhibited IgE production by IL-4–stimulated mononuclear cells (MNC) in 14-day cultures.

After having established that nebulized IFN-γ was bioactive and in the desirable range for particle diameter, we compared the bioavailability of nebulized versus intraperitoneal IFN-γ to the peribronchial lymphoid tissue (PBLN) draining the trachea and upper airways. The nebulized IFN-γ increased class II major histocompatibility complex antigen (Ia) expression in PBLN-derived MNC but to a lesser extent in the spleen, as determined by surface staining and flow cytometry (50). By contrast, intraperitoneal IFN-γ induced a significant increase of Ia expression in the spleen, but did not induce Ia expression in the PBLN. These data demonstrate that, whereas nebulized IFN-γ was effective in the local environment of the airways where sensitization to ovalbumin was occurring, systemic IFN-γ was unable to modulate local allergic sensitization. As further confirmation of these results, nebulized IFN-γ, but not intraperitoneal IFN-γ, was able to inhibit subsequent in vitro IgE production by PBLN-derived MNC (50).

C. Inhibition of Allergic Sensitization to Ovalbumin by Nebulized IFN-γ

Nebulized IFN-γ treatment for 13 days, 3 days before sensitization and daily during the 10-day period of OVA exposure, decreased anti-OVA IgE by more than 60%

compared with OVA-treated controls (Fig. 1). The dosage of 250,000 units IFN-γ per nebulization was optimal, and it was estimated that each mouse received a maximum of 5000 units per nebulization. Treatment regimens that continued for 13 days and included pretreatment produced the greatest decline in anti-OVA IgE. With this treatment regimen, IFN-γ also prevented the development of cutaneous reactivity to OVA (see Table 1). This resulted from allergen-triggered mast cell degranulation and the responses correlated with allergen-specific IgE in the serum (47).

Airways responsiveness was measured to electrical field stimulation of tracheal smooth muscle preparations in tissue baths. Mice sensitized to OVA showed increased AR, compared with controls, as measured by a decrease in the mean ES_{50} (electrical stimulation in hertz required to produce 50% of the maximal contraction). Mice exposed to nebulized IFN-γ alone had normal AR compared with controls. However, 13 days of nebulized IFN-γ prevented the development of increased AR in mice sensitized to OVA (50; Fig. 2). Shorter IFN-γ treatments that started on the first day of OVA sensitization or were delayed further after OVA sensitization had started were less effective than the 13-day course of IFN-γ treatment in inhibiting anti-OVA IgE. Initiation of IFN-γ treatment after day 6 of OVA sensitization failed to inhibit anti-OVA IgE.

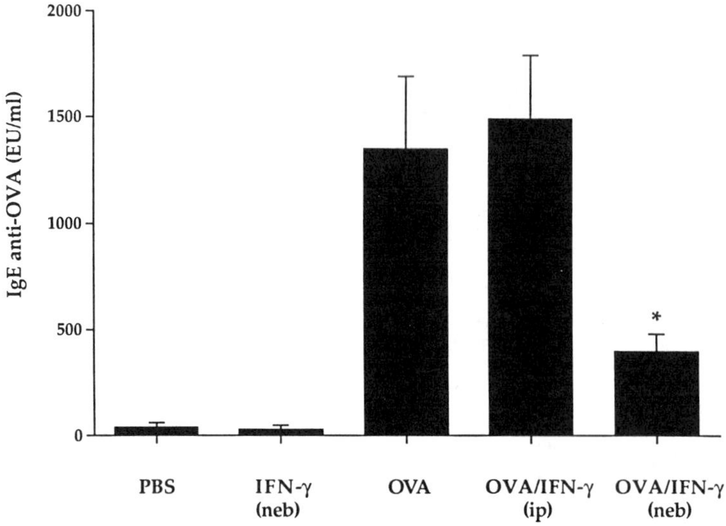

Figure 1 Nebulized, but not intraperitoneal (ip) rIFN-γ decreases serum anti-OVA IgE: Serum was obtained from the different treatment groups as indicated, 2 days after completion of the sensitization protocol. Antibody levels were determined by enzyme-linked immunosorbent assay (ELISA). Shown are the mean (±SEM) for anti-OVA IgE expressed as ELISA units/mL.

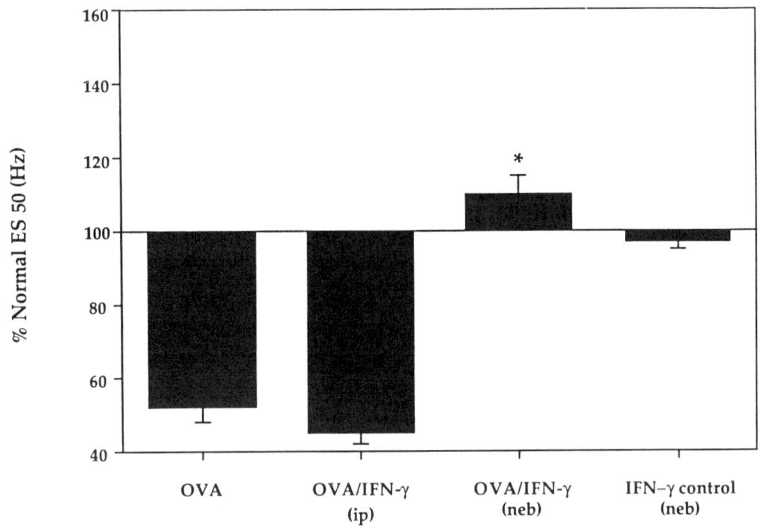

Figure 2 Nebulized, but not intraperitoneal, rIFN-γ normalizes AR: Groups of mice received the following treatments: PBS ($n = 20$); rIFN-γ ($n = 12$); OVA ($n = 24$); OVA and ip rIFN-γ ($n = 10$); and OVA and nebulized rIFN-γ ($n = 12$). On day 12, 2 days after completion of sensitization, AR was determined by electrical field stimulation (ES) of individual tracheal smooth muscle preparations. Expressed along the y-axis is the percentage deviation from normal airways responsiveness represented by ES_{50} (± SEM). A low ES_{50} (<100% of the value for control mice) represents increased AR.

D. Reciprocal Regulation of Anti-OVA IgE and Anti-OVA IgG2a Production by Nebulized IFN-γ

The inhibitory effects of IFN-γ on anti-OVA IgE, airway hyperresponsiveness, and cutaneous reactivity can be explained either in terms of its immunomodulatory effects on lymphocytes or, alternatively, by nonspecific blocking or inhibitory mechanisms. Because there is evidence that IFN-γ reciprocally regulates IgE and IgG2a production both in vitro and in vivo (8,19), we examined the effects of nebulized IFN-γ on anti-OVA IgG2a production. IFN-γ–treated mice developed a significant anti-OVA IgG2a response, not observed in OVA-treated animals and nonsensitized controls. There was a significant inverse correlation between anti-OVA IgE and anti-OVA IgG2a, confirming the reciprocal regulation of these isotypes by IFN-γ (Fig. 3). Therefore, nebulized IFN-γ exerted its inhibitory actions on allergic sensitization through immunomodulatory effects on the B cell, rather than through nonspecific blocking effects. It did not prevent sensitization to antigen, but shifted the response from IgE production toward IgG2a production.

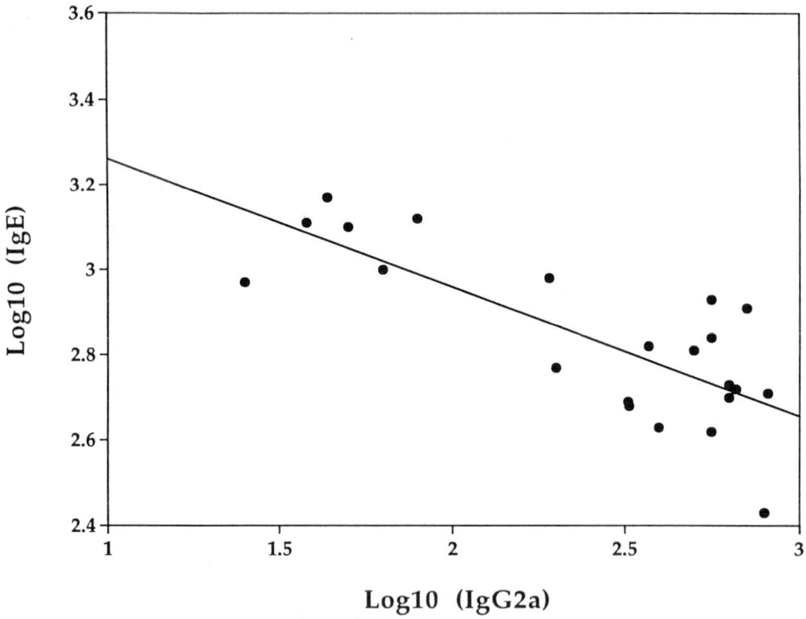

Figure 3 Nebulized rIFN-γ reciprocally regulates anti-OVA IgE and anti-OVA IgG2a production: OVA-sensitized mice received rIFN-γ treatment for different time periods. On day 12, 2 days after completion of sensitization, serum was obtained and analyzed by ELISA for anti-OVA IgE and anti-OVA IgG2a. The relation between both isotypes for all groups of treated mice was described by plotting $\log_{10}$ (IgE) against $\log_{10}$ (IgG2a) for each serum sample ($n = 22$). The correlation coefficient was –0.81 ($p < 0.0001$).

E. Inhibition of Secondary IgE Responses by IFN-γ

Whether or not IFN-γ is able to prevent IgE responses to secondary allergen challenge and subsequent allergen exposure has important implications for the treatment of human allergic disease. The answer partly depends on the cellular interactions and signaling requirements for secondary IgE production by B cells. If secondary IgE production is derived from a pool of IgE-committed memory B cells, then it is likely too late for IFN-γ to prevent immunoglobulin isotype switching to IgE. If, on the other hand, the secondary response is derived from IgM^+ memory B cells that undergo de novo isotype switching to IgE, there is a window of opportunity for IFN-γ to inhibit IgE production. In the mouse, there is evidence that B cells require IL-4 and a signal from $CD4^+$ cells to generate both primary and secondary IgE responses in vivo (51). This suggests that de novo isotype switching to IgE is also necessary for the generation of a secondary IgE response.

To examine the control of secondary IgE responses in vivo, mice that had been initially sensitized to OVA received a secondary OVA challenge (52). Following 10 days of OVA sensitization, serum anti-OVA IgE levels declined to less than 30% of the peak response (days 12–18) by day 30. At that point, animals lost their cutaneous reactivity to OVA and had reacquired normal airway function. Secondary OVA challenge on days 30 and 31 induced a secondary anti-OVA IgE response, measured on day 37, which was accompanied by cutaneous reactivity (ST) to OVA and increased AR. Nebulized IFN-γ administered for 13 days during primary ovalbumin sensitization, as well as inhibiting the primary allergic response, prevented the development of a secondary IgE response, cutaneous reactivity to OVA, and increased airway responsiveness following secondary OVA challenge. If nebulized IFN-γ was administered for shorter periods (days 26–30), even after normal allergen sensitization had been achieved, it prevented the development of secondary IgE and immediate hypersensitivity responses following secondary ovalbumin challenge. Therefore, treatment with nebulized IFN-γ was able to prevent the development of secondary allergic responses, even if treatment was initiated after normal primary allergic responses were established.

F. Nebulized IFN-γ Treatment

Treatment with nebulized IFN-γ modulates T-cell function and alters cytokine production from a Th2- to a Th1-like pattern. Lymphocytes from the PBLN of mice sensitized to OVA develop in vitro proliferative responses to OVA (Fig. 4). Treatment of mice with nebulized IFN-γ significantly inhibited the proliferative responses and shifted the dose–response curve to the right (52). These inhibitory effects on T-cell function persisted even after secondary OVA challenge in mice that had received only rIFN-γ early during initial OVA exposure. This indicated that IFN-γ was able to modulate T-cell function for many weeks beyond the course of treatment. A likely explanation for this antiproliferative effect is that IFN-γ was able to selectively inhibit the proliferative response of Th2-like OVA-reactive T cells. IFN-γ treatment did not affect the proliferative response to nonspecific mitogen stimulation.

To examine the effect of IFN-γ on the profile of cytokine production by T cells, we examined in situ production of IL-4 and IFN-γ in T cells obtained from PBLN and spleen. The naive animals had very low frequencies of IL-4– and IFN-γ–producing cells following mitogen stimulation. OVA sensitization caused a large increase in the frequency of IL-4– and IFN-γ–producing T cells, both in the spleen and PBLN. IL-4 was produced almost entirely by $CD4^+$ and $CD8^+$ T-cell subsets. Nebulized IFN-γ markedly decreased the frequency of IL-4–producing T cells, both in the PBLN and in the spleen. Therefore, in vivo treatment with IFN-γ was able to decrease the capacity of T cells to produce Th2-type cytokines as measured at the single-cell level and shifted the T-cell response toward a Th1 pattern of cytokine production.

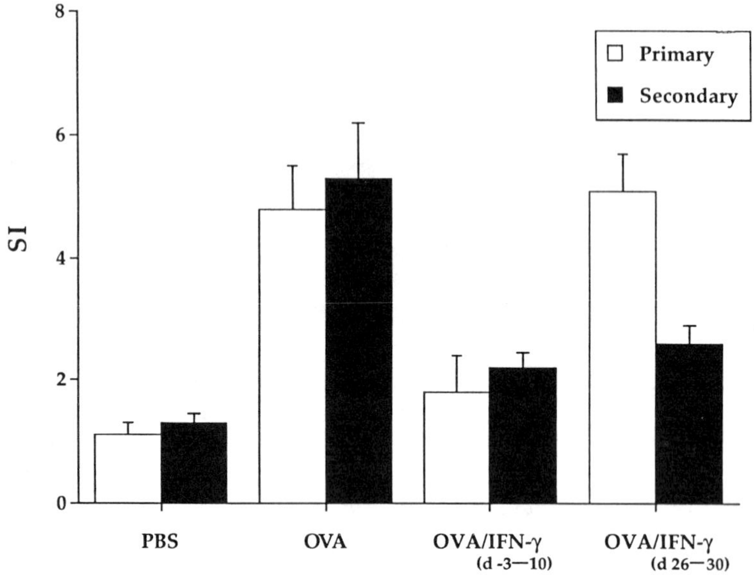

Figure 4 Nebulized IFN-γ inhibits T-cell proliferation: One group of mice was treated with OVA, or OVA and IFN-γ (day –3 through day 10) and sacrificed on day 12 (primary). A second group of mice was sensitized to OVA through day 10 and again on days 30 and 31; one set of mice received IFN-γ on days –3 to 10, and the other IFN-γ from days 26 to 30. These animals were sacrificed on day 37 (secondary). PBLN-derived MNC were stimulated in vitro with OVA and [^{3}H]thymidine uptake was assessed after 5 days of in vitro stimulation. Expressed is the stimulation index (SI) from a representative experiment (of three similar experiments) using PBLN pooled from three to four mice in each set, carried out in triplicate.

G. Inhibition of Allergic Responses by IFN-γ

There are data showing that IFN-γ inhibits IgE production through its action on B cells, and conflicting data showing that IFN-γ acts on T cells as well (10,16,20). For IFN-γ to influence lymphocyte function, it must bind to the IFN-γ receptor (IFN-γR) on the cell surface. Constitutive IFN-γR expression is very low on B cells (53), and it is only expressed on 5% of resting T cells (54). IFN-γ is only able to alter lymphocyte function once lymphocytes have been preactivated and expression of IFN-γR is upregulated (55). There are several different lines of evidence in our model that point to a requirement for the presence of allergen for the response to IFN-γ to be expressed.

First, there was no reduction in IL-4 production by lymphocytes from animals that were treated with IFN-γ alone. Inhibition of IL-4 production by $CD4^+$ T cells occurred only in mice that had the combination of IFN-γ and OVA exposure. Second, $CD4^+$ T cells from OVA-sensitized, and IFN-γ–treated mice were able to inhibit polyclonal and anti-OVA IgE production in vitro, whereas $CD4^+$ T cells from mice that had been exposed to IFN-γ alone did not inhibit IgE production.

There is also supportive evidence in humans that immunotherapy with an allergen induces IFN-γ production and allergen-specific IgE, but results in the inhibition of in vitro lymphocyte proliferation to the injected allergen, but not to an irrelevant allergen (36). These specific changes may similarly be explained in terms of the antiproliferative effects of IFN-γ on Th2 type cells and its ability to prevent IgE isotype switching. That these changes are allergen-specific suggests that IFN-γ, produced during immunotherapy, influences only allergen-specific T cells and B cells that have been specifically activated by allergen. This may explain why human clinical studies of IFN-γ in allergic disease showed demonstrable effects only on macrophages and eosinophils and did not alter lymphocyte function. It may also explain why rIFN-γ has been successfully used to treat chronic granulomatous disease (56), in which the target cells—namely, granulocytes—express the IFN-γ receptor constitutively.

IV. Summary and Future Directions

In a murine model of allergen sensitization through the airways, nebulized IFN-γ successfully prevents the development of both primary and secondary IgE responses as well as immediate hypersensitivity reactions. Three important conditions are necessary for successful immunomodulation by IFN-γ: (1) IFN-γ must be delivered early during the course of a primary or secondary response to allergen. (2) It must be delivered locally to the site of allergic sensitization (i.e., by nebulization into the lungs in the case of asthma) to inhibit allergen-specific IgE production induced by aeroallergen. (3) It must be delivered together with allergen to influence antigen-specific lymphocyte cell function.

In light of these observations, the relative lack of success with parenteral IFN-γ treatment in clinical trials, particular for asthma, may not be surprising. The important clinical findings that nebulized IFN-γ is both bioavailable and bioactive in the lungs, and decreases eosinophil numbers in BAL from asthmatics suggest that, in the presence of allergen, it may successfully reduce local allergic responses, as in the murine model. The critical requirement for organ-targeted delivery is also likely applicable to other therapeutic agents that modulate the local immune response in asthma. The soluble IL-4R for example, has similarly been shown in a murine model to normalize AR and inhibit allergic responses more effectively in the nebulized form when compared with parenteral delivery (57). Recognition of these requirements in the design of subsequent trials may reveal the therapeutic potential of IFN-γ and other important regulatory cytokines with antiallergic potential.

References

1. Ishizaka T. Analysis of triggering events in mast cells for immunoglobulin E-mediated histamine release. J Allergy Clin Immunol 1981; 67:90–96.
2. Nagy L, Lee TH, Kay AB. Neutrophil chemotactic activity in antigen-induced late asthmatic reaction. N Engl J Med 1982; 306:497–501.
3. MacGlashan DW, Schleimer RP, Peters S, Chulman ES, Adams GK III, Newball HH, Lichtenstein LM. Generation of leukotrienes by purified human lung mast cells. J Clin Invest 1982; 70:747.
4. Norel X, Haye-Legrand I, Labat C, Benveniste J, Brink FC. Antigen-induced contraction of human isolated lung preparations passively sensitized with monoclonal IgE: effects of indomethacin. Int Arch Allergy Appl Immunol 1991; 96:368–375.
5. Haye-Legrand I, Norel X, Labat C, Benviste J, Brink C. Antigenic contraction of guinea pig tracheal preparations passively sensitized with monoclonal IgE: pharmacological modulation. Int Arch Allergy Appl Immunol 1988; 87:342–348.
6. Sears MR, Burrows B, Flannery EM, Herbison GP, Hewitt CJ, Holdaway MD. Relation between airways responsiveness and serum IgE in children with asthma and in apparently normal children. N Engl J Med 1991; 235:1067–1071.
7. Burrows B, Lebowitz MD, Barbee RB, Cline MG. Findings before diagnosis of asthma among the elderly in a longitudinal study of a general population sample. J Allergy Clin Immunol 1991; 88:870–877.
8. Snapper CM, Paul WE, Interferon-γ and B-cell stimulatory factor-1 reciprocally regulate Ig isotype production. Science 1987; 236:944–947.
9. Rousset FE, Garcia E, Banchereau J. Cytokine induced proliferation and immunoglobulin production of human B lymphocytes triggered through their CD40 antigen. J Exp Med 1991; 173:705–710.
10. Thyphronitis G, Tosokos GC, June CH, Levine AD, Finkelman FD. IgE secretion by Epstein–Barr virus-infected purified human B lymphocytes is stimulated by interleukin 4 and suppressed by interferon gamma. Proc Natl Acad Sci USA 1989; 86:5580–5584.
11. Sarfti M, Luo H, Delespesse H. IgE synthesis by chronic lymphocytic leukemia cells. J Exp Med 1989; 170:1775–1780.
12. Jabara HH, Fu SM, Geha RS, Vercelli DC. CD40 and IgE: synergism between anti-CD40 monoclonal antibody and interleukin 4 in the induction of IgE synthesis by highly purified human B cells. J Exp Med 1990; 172:1861–1864.
13. Finkelman FD, Holmes J, Katona IM, Urban JF Jr, Beckman MP, Park LS, Schooley KA, Coffman RL, Mosmann TR, Paul WE. Lymphokine control of in vivo immunoglobulin isotype selection. Annu Rev Immunol 1990; 8:303–333.
14. Gascan H, Gauchat JF, Aversa G, Van Vlasselaer P, de Vries JE. Anti-CD40 monoclonal antibodies of $CD4^+$ T cell clones and IL-4 induce IgG4 and IgE switching in purified human B cells via different signaling pathways. J Immunol 1991; 147:8–11.
15. de Vries JE, Zurawski G. Immunoregulatory properties of IL-13: its potential role in atopic disease. Int Arch Allergy Immunol 1995; 106:175–179.
16. Coffman RL, Carty J. A T cell activity that enhances polyclonal IgE production and its inhibition by interferon-gamma. J Immunol 1986; 136:949–954.
17. Péne J, Rousset F, Brière F, Chrétien I, Bonnefoy JY, Spits H, Yokota T, Arai N, Arai K, Banchereau J. IgE production by normal human lymphocytes is induced by interleukin 4 and suppressed by interferons gamma and alpha and prostaglandin E_2. Proc Natl Acad Sci USA 1988; 85:6880–6884.
18. Chrétien I, Péne J, Brière F, De Waal Malefijt R, Rousset F, de Vries JE. Regulation of human IgE synthesis. I. Human IgE synthesis in vitro is determined by the reciprocal antagonistic effects of interleukin 4 and interferon-gamma. Eur J Immunol 1990; 20:243–251.

19. Finkelman FD, Katona IM, Mosmann TR, Coffman RL. IFN-gamma regulates the isotypes of Ig secreted during in vivo humoral immune responses. J Immunol 1988; 140:1022–1027.
20. Gauchat JF, Lebman DA, Coffman RL, Gascan H, de Vries JE. Structure and expression of germline epsilon transcripts in human B cells induced by interleukin 4 to switch to IgE production. J Exp Med 1990; 172:463–467.
21. Bentley AM, Meng Q, Robinson DS, Hamid Q, Kay AB, Durham SR. Increases in activated T lymphocytes, eosinophils, and cytokine mRNA expression for interleukin-5 and granulocyte/macrophage colony-stimulating factor in bronchial biopsies after allergen inhalation challenge in atopic asthmatics. Am J Respir Cell Mol Biol 1993; 8:35–42.
22. Maggi E, Parronchi P, Manetti R, Simonelli C, Piccinni MP, Rugiu S, Carli M, Ricci M, Romagnani S. Reciprocal regulatory effects of IFN-γ and IL-4 on the in vitro development of human Th1 and Th2 clones. J Immunol 1992; 48:2142–2147.
23. Bradley LM, Yoshimoto K, Swain SL. The cytokines IL-4, IFN-γ, and IL-12 regulate the development of subsets of memory effector/helper T cells in vitro. J Immunol 1995; 155:1713–1724.
24. Iwamoto I, Nakajima H, Endo H, Yoshida S. Interferon gamma regulates antigen-induced eosinophil recruitment into the mouse airways by inhibiting the infiltration of $CD4^+$ T cells. J Exp Med 1993; 177:573–536.
25. Fujisawa T, Abu-Ghazaleh R, Kita H, Sanderson CJ, Gleich GJ. Regulatory effect of cytokines on eosinophil degranulation. J Immunol 1990; 144:642–646.
26. Nafziger J, Arock M, Guillosson J, Wietzerbin J. Specific high-affinity receptors for interferon-gamma on mouse bone marrow-derived mast cells: inhibitory effect of interferon-gamma on mast cell precursors. Eur J Immunol 1990; 20:113–117.
27. Takagi M, Kenichi K, Nahahata T. Antiproliferative effect of IFN-gamma on proliferation of mouse connective tissue-type mast cells. J Clin Immunol 1990; 145:1880–1884.
28. Coleman JW, Morris AG. Identification of a spleen cell-derived factor that inhibits sensitisation of murine peritoneal mast cells as interferon-gamma. Int Arch Allergy Appl Immunol 1991; 94:179–180.
29. Coleman JW, Buckeley MG, Holliday MR, Morris AG. Interferon-gamma inhibits serotonin release from mouse peritoneal mast cells. Eur J Immunol 1991; 21:2559–2564.
30. Schleimer RP, Derse CP, Friedman B, Gillis CS, Plaut MP, Lichtenstein LM, MacGlashan DW Jr. Regulation of human basophil mediator release by cytokines. I. Interaction with antiinflammatory steroids. J Immunol 1989; 143:1310–1317.
31. Reinhold U, Pawelec G, Wehrmann W, Kukel S, Oehr P, Kreysel HW. Cytokine release from cultured peripheral blood mononuclear cells of patients with severe atopic dermatitis. Acta Derm Venereol 1989; 69:497–502.
32. Jujo K, Renz H, Abe J, Gelfand EW, Leung DYM. Decreased gamma interferon and increased interleukin-4 production promote IgE synthesis in atopic dermatitis. J Allergy Clin Immunol 1992; 90:323–330.
33. Rousset F, Robert J, Andary M, Bonni JP, Souillet G, Chrétien I, Brière F, Péne J, de Vries JE. Shifts in interleukin-4 and interferon-gamma production by T cells of patients with elevated serum IgE levels and the modulatory effects of these lymphokines on spontaneous IgE synthesis. J Allergy Clin Immunol 1991; 87:58–69.
34. Tang M, Kemp A, Varigos G. IL-4 and interferon-gamma production in children with atopic disease. Clin Exp Immunol 1993; 92:120–124.
35. Jung T, Lack G, Schauer U, Uberück W, Renz H, Gelfand EW, Reiger CHL. Decreased frequency of interferon-γ and interleukin-2-producing cells in patients with atopic diseases measured at the single cell level. J Allergy Clin Immunol 1995; 96:515–527.
36. Lack G, Nelson HS, Amran D, Oshiba A, Jung T, Bradley KL, Giclas PC, Gelfand EW. Rush immunotherapy results in allergen-specific alterations in lymphocyte function and IFN-γ production in $CD4^+$ T cells. J Allergy Clin Immunol 1997; 99:530–538.
37. Reinhold U, Wehrmann W, Kukel S, Kreysel HW. Recombinant interferon-gamma in severe atopic dermatitis [letter]. Lancet 1990; 335:1282.

38. Boguniewicz M, Jaffe HS, Izu A, Sullivan MJ, York D, Geha RS, Leung DYM. Recombinant gamma interferon in treatment of patients with atopic dermatitis and elevated IgE levels. Am J Med 1990; 88:365–370.
39. Hanifin JM, Schneider LC, Leung DY, Ellis CN, Jaffe HS, Izu AE, Bucalo LR, Hirabayashi SE, Tofte SJ, Cantu-Gonzales G. Recombinant interferon gamma therapy for atopic dermatitis. J Am Acad Dermatol 1993; 28:189–197.
40. Li JT, Yunginger JW, Reed CE, Jaffe HS, Nelson DR, Gleich GJ. Lack of suppression of IgE production by recombinant interferon gamma: a controlled trial in patients with allergic rhinitis. J Allergy Clin Immunol 1990; 85:934–940.
41. Boguniewicz M, Schneider LC, Milgrom H, Newell D, Tam P, Izu AE, Jaffe HS, Bucalo Lr, Leung DYM. Treatment of steroid-dependent asthma with recombinant interferon-gamma. Clin Exp Allergy 1993; 23:785–790.
42. Jaffe HA, Buhl R, Mastrangeli A, Holroyd KJ, Saltini C, Czerski D, Jaffe HS, Kramer S, Sherwin S, Crystal RG. Organ specific cytokine therapy. Local activation of mononuclear phagocytes by delivery of an aerosol of recombinant interferon-γ to the human lung. J Clin Invest 1991; 88:297–302.
43. Martin RJ, Boguniewicz M, Henson JE, Celniker AC, Williams, M, Giorno RC, Leung DYM. The effects of inhaled interferon gamma in normal human airways. Am Rev Respir Dis 1993; 148:1677–1682.
44. Boguniewicz M, Martin RJ, Martin D, Gibson U, Celniker A, Williams, M, Leung DYM. The effects of nebulized recombinant interferon-gamma in asthmatic airways. J Clin Immunol 1995; 95:133–135.
45. Kiderlen AF, Kaufmann SHE, Lohmann-Matthes ML. Protection of mice against the intracellular bacterium *Listeria monocytogenes* by recombinant immune interferon. Eur J Immunol 1984; 14:964–967.
46. Renz H, Smith HR, Henson JE, Ray BS, Irvin CG, Gelfand EW. Aerosolized antigen exposure with adjuvant cause increased IgE production and increased airway responsiveness in the mouse. J Allergy Clin Immunol 1992; 89:1127–1138.
47. Saloga JH, Renz H, Lack G, Bradley KL, Greenstein JL, Larsen G, Gelfand EW. Development and transfer of immediate cutaneous hypersensitivity in mice exposed to aerosolized antigen. J Clin Invest 1993; 91:133–140.
48. Larsen GL, Renz H, Loader JE, Bradley KL, Gelfand EW. Airway response to electrical field stimulation in sensitized inbred mice. J Clin Invest 1992; 89:747–752.
49. Larsen GL, Fame TM, Renz H, Loader JE, Graves J, Hill M, Gelfand EW. Increased acetylcholine release in tracheas from allergen-exposed IgE-immune mice. Am J Physiol 1994; 266:L263–L270.
50. Lack G, Renz H, Saloga J, Bradley KL, Loader J, Leung DYM, Larsen G, Gelfand EW. Nebulised but not parenteral IFN-γ decreases IgE production and normalizes airways function in a murine model of allergen sensitisation. J Immunol 1994; 152:2546–2554.
51. Finkelman FD, Katona IM, Urban JF Jr, Holmes J, O'Hara J, Tung AS, Sample JG, Paul WE. IL-4 is required to generate and sustain in vivo IgE responses. J Immunol 1988; 252:2335–2341.
52. Lack G, Bradley KL, Hamelmann E, Renz H, Loader J, Leung DYM, Larsen G, Gelfand EW. Nebulized IFN-γ inhibits the development of secondary allergic responses in mice. J Immunol 1996; 157:1432–1439.
53. Valente G, Ozmen L, Novelli F, Geuna M, Palestro G, Forni G, Garrotta G. Distribution of interferon-γ receptor in human tissues. Eur J Immunol 1992; 22:2403–2412.
54. Nashwa SA, Chace JH, Fleming AL, Cowdery JS. Interferon-gamma regulation of B lymphocyte differentiation: activation of B cells is a prerequisite for interferon-gamma mediated inhibition of B cell differentiation. Cell Immunol 1994; 153:356–366.
55. Novelli F, Giovarelli M, Gentz R, Zucca M, di Pierro F, Garotta G, Forni G. Modulation of interferon-γ receptor during human T lymphocyte alloactivation. Eur J Immunol 1993; 23:1226–1231.

56. Ezekowitz RA, Dinauer MC, Jaffe HS, Orkin SH, Newburger PE. Partial correction of the phagocyte defect in patients with X-linked chronic granulomatous disease by subcutaneous interferon gamma. N Engl J Med 1988; 319:146–151.
57. Renz H, Enssel K, Lauffer L, Kurrle R, Gelfand EW. Inhibition of allergen-induced IgE and IgG1 production by soluble IL-4 receptor. Int Arch Allergy Immunol 1995; 106:46–54.

29

Role of Interleukin-5 in Eosinophil-Based Diseases

FRANCIS M. CUSS, RICHARD W. CHAPMAN, SHELBY P. UMLAND, MICHAEL MINNICOZZI, and ROBERT W. EGAN

Schering–Plough Research Institute
Kenilworth, New Jersey

I. Introduction

There is strong, but still circumstantial, evidence for a role of interleukin-5 (IL-5) in asthma and other eosinophilic disorders. This evidence has arisen from animal models, measurements of IL-5 in human and animal tissue, and the essential role of IL-5 in the maturation of eosinophil precursor cells to eosinophils in the bone marrow. Following their release from the bone marrow, eosinophils accumulate in certain inflamed tissues, including the lungs in persons with asthma, the nasal cavity in persons with allergic rhinitis, and in the skin of persons with atopic dermatitis. Inhibition of the action of IL-5's action by decreasing its circulating levels, or by blocking the association with its receptor, should provide therapy for eosinophilic diseases. Furthermore, in the human, the IL-5 receptor exists only on eosinophils and basophils, so inhibiting the action of IL-5 would not be expected to cause the severe immunosuppressive consequences that would arise from inhibiting effector functions of other leukocytes, such as T cells, macrophages, or neutrophils. This chapter describes the role of IL-5 in a variety of eosinophilic diseases and the various mechanisms for curtailing its actions.

II. Biochemical Regulation of IL-5

Interleukin-5 is produced by several cell types, including T cells, mast cells, and eosinophils, each being triggered by cell type-specific ligands. An association of allergic inflammation with elevated expression of Th2 cytokines, in particular IL-4 and IL-5, has been noted in allergic diseases of the lungs, nose, skin, and gastrointestinal tract. For example, there is the preferential activation of cells expressing a Th2 pattern of cytokines (IL-3, IL-4, IL-5, and granulocyte–macrophage colony-stimulating factor [GM-CSF]), but not Th1 cytokines (IL-2 and interferon [IFN]-γ) in allergen-induced late-phase cutaneous reactions (1). Furthermore, in the lung, increased activation of $CD4^+$ T cells and increased T-cell expression of IL-4 and IL-5, but not IFN-γ mRNA has been demonstrated in bronchial biopsies and in bronchoalveolar lavage (BAL) fluid of allergen-challenged atopic asthmatics (2,3) and nonatopic asthmatics (4,5). Increased levels of IL-5 have also been demonstrated in the BAL fluid of allergic individuals following segmental antigen challenge, and this correlated with levels of eosinophil-derived cationic proteins (6).

The major source of IL-5 in allergic disorders is likely to be the T cell (7,8), although immunohistochemical and in situ hybridization studies from a variety of tissues, including airways, have shown that numerous cells, including mast cells and eosinophils, can synthesize IL-5 (9–10). In some animal models of asthma, mast cells contribute substantially to the recruitment of eosinophils into the lungs (11,12), suggesting that mast cell products, such as IL-5, are essential for the early recruitment of eosinophils. The finding that eosinophils can synthesize IL-5 raises the possibility of an autocrine production of IL-5 by these cells. This may contribute to the recruitment and activation of eosinophils, and to the chronicity of eosinophilic inflammation. Interestingly, cytokine production by mast cells and eosinophils may be regulated differently from that in T cells, because in the former cell types, intracellular preformed protein (i.e., IL-5) is localized in granules (9,10). In contrast, initiation of IL-5 production in T cells occurs through activation of gene transcription and does not involve release of stored cytokines (13).

Strategies aimed at inhibiting IL-5 biosynthesis in allergic disease must take into account the contributions of different IL-5–producing cell types and the major mechanisms regulating IL-5 production in each cell type. The regulation of IL-5 gene induction during T-cell activation is controlled primarily at the level of transcription, although IL-5 mRNA is noted to be highly stable in activated mouse (14) and human T cells (13). Protein kinase C (PKC) activation is obligatory and sufficient for IL-5 mRNA induction (15), although IL-5 gene expression in response to PKC activation is enhanced by stimuli that increase intracellular calcium (11). The cytokine inhibitor and immunosuppressant, cyclosporine, inhibits the cytoplasmic to nuclear translocation of nuclear factor of activated T cells (NF-AT), by inhibiting the Ca^{2+}–calmodulin-dependent phosphatase, calcineurin (16). IL-5 induction by T-cell receptor (TCR) activation is sensitive to cyclosporine (14). However, similar to other cytokines, maximal IL-5 production requires signals contributed to the

T-cell receptor pathway, as well as a costimulatory pathway provided by CD28 signaling (14,17). The CD28-mediated costimulation for IL-5 synthesis confers significant resistance to the inhibitory effects of cyclopsorine (17). Although differences in the regulation of mast cell and T-cell synthesis of IL-5 most likely exist, cyclosporine also blocks the induction of IL-5 mRNA in stimulated mouse mast cell lines (18). Importantly, it is moderately beneficial in some individuals with severe asthma (19).

The IL-5 gene expression in mouse (14) and human T cells (Umland S, unpublished observations) requires de novo protein synthesis. This requirement may distinguish signaling in T cells and mast cells, because IL-5 mRNA was observed in anti-IgE–stimulated human lung fragments in the absence of protein synthesis (20). Collectively, studies of cytokine synthesis in the presence of cyclosporine or protein synthesis inhibitors indicate that cytokines are independently regulated, and opportunities exist for the development of selective small-molecule inhibitors of IL-5 synthesis for treatment of allergic disease.

Glucocorticoids are potent inhibitors of cytokine production and act pre- and posttranscriptionally (21). By modulating cytokine and T-cell involvement in asthma, glucocorticoids are effective drugs for the treatment of the inflammatory component of allergic responses (22). Interestingly, although IL-4 and IL-5 secretion in vitro is highly sensitive to the effects of glucocorticoids, IFN-γ is less inhibited (23,24). The mechanism for this differential efficacy of steroids against various cytokines is unknown, yet in the treatment of asthma, it would serve to reverse the exaggerated Th2 response (25,26), including IL-5-induced eosinophilia, that contributes to pathophysiology.

Interleukin-5 exists as a glycosylated homodimer (45–60 kDa), with dimerization (27), but not glycosylation (28), being required for full activity. It induces its multiple functions through interaction with a two-chain receptor (R) composed of a unique transmembrane α-subunit and a common transmembrane β-subunit, shared with the IL-3 and GM-CSFR (29). Interaction of the β-subunit, which alone does not bind ligand, with the α-subunit, which alone can bind IL-5, creates a high-affinity (K_d = 300 pM) receptor (30). The restricted expression of the α-subunit to human eosinophils and basophils, explains the limited range of functions that IL-5 exerts on human cells (31) and suggests that an antagonist of IL-5–IL-5R interaction has potential as a selective therapy for allergic disease. However, identification of a small-molecule inhibitor of a high-affinity protein–protein interaction is difficult.

Transcripts of the human IL-5R α-subunit lacking a transmembrane region have been identified, and expressed protein has demonstrated antagonistic activity in vitro (32). Although the existence of soluble IL-5R α-chains in serum has not been shown, such an endogenous or administered entity could antagonize the activity of IL-5 and protect against excessive eosinophil recruitment and activation. However, development of protein-based therapeutics, although potentially able to disrupt high-affinity ligand–receptor binding, must take into account issues of delivery and short half-life.

The β-subunit of IL-5R is critical for high-affinity binding and signal transduction, resulting in biological responsiveness (30). The cytoplasmic domain of the β-subunit lacks a consensus sequence for either tyrosine kinase or phosphatase domains, although IL-5 interaction with its receptor induces rapid tyrosine phosphorylation of multiple proteins (33,34). IL-5, similar to IL-3 and GM-CSF receptors, primarily activates Jak2 kinases (a subset of protein tyrosine kinases physically associated with cytokine receptors) in response to ligand binding, with subsequent activation of the signal transducer and activator of transcription (STAT)5, a member of a family of transcriptional regulatory proteins (35,36). The mechanisms by which these cytokines generate different cellular responses while sharing a common receptor-signaling subunit and activating the same JAK–STAT pathway remain to be elucidated.

III. Eosinophilic Diseases and IL-5

A. Asthma

Eosinophilic infiltration into the airways is a consistent finding after antigen administration in sensitive subjects (37–40). The most prominent cytokine seen in BAL fluid of subjects with late antigen responses is IL-5 (2,6,41). IL-5 is not seen immediately after antigen administration (6), but is increased after 24 hr and returns to baseline concentrations after 1–2 weeks (42). Interestingly, increased concentrations of IL-5 and eosinophils in BAL fluid are seen only in subjects who exhibit late antigen responses, but not in those with early responses alone (6), suggesting that IL-5 is an important element of the late response. When recombinant human (rh)IL-5 is delivered as an aerosol to the airways of atopic subjects, eosinophilia is seen in bronchial biopsies and BAL fluid (43).

In patients with asthma, BAL fluid and tissues from bronchial biopsies show increased expression of IL-5, compared with samples from nonasthmatic subjects (5,44–47). Furthermore, in samples from asthmatic patients, IL-5 protein and mRNA is predominantly localized to T cells (48–51). Additionally, several studies have found a correlation between the activation of T cells, IL-5 concentrations in serum and BAL fluid, and asthma symptoms (50,52–54). Specifically, there is a strong positive relation between the number of BAL cells expressing IL-5 mRNA, the patient's baseline forced 1-sec expiratory volume (FEV_1) and the degree of airway responsiveness to methacholine challenge (48). Serum concentrations of IL-5 are significantly higher during asthma exacerbations than during remissions (52); in symptomatic, rather than asymptomatic, patients (55); and in patients with severe asthma, compared with those without asthma, or with only mild asthma (52). Over a 3-year period, increases in serum IL-5 concentrations are correlated with lung function decline (56). Therapeutically, the treatment of asthma symptoms with theophylline or corticosteroids is associated with lower IL-5 concentrations (25,53,57). Eosinophilia is more prominent during the nighttime hours in patients with nocturnal asthma (58), but the relation to IL-5 concentrations is unclear. In one study of nocturnal asthma, eosinophil survival-enhancing activity in BAL fluid was not detectable (59), whereas in another IL-5 immunoreactivity in bronchial biopsy tissues changed in phase with the diurnal cycle of asthma symptoms (60). Immunoreactivity for IL-5, along with other proinflammatory cytokines, such as IL-3 and GM-CSF, is often present in the intestinal mucosa of asthmatics, suggesting that the whole mucosal immune system is activated in pulmonary inflammatory diseases (61).

The mechanisms by which IL-5 produces its pathophysiology have been investigated extensively in animal models of asthma. Antigen challenge to sensitized mice (62–67), guinea pigs (68–70), and monkeys (71) produces pulmonary eosinophilia and airway hyperresponsiveness, and these effects are blocked by treatment with monoclonal antibodies (MAbs) to IL-5 (72). In some studies, the presence of a pulmonary eosinophilia does not correlate with the development of bronchial hyperresponsiveness, suggesting that accumulation of eosinophils in the lungs is not sufficient to induce airway hyperreactivity (67,73–77). The importance of IL-5 and of eosinophils in general for allergen-induced hyperreactivity and for protection against parasitic infections has been evaluated in IL-5 knockout mice (64,78). In the former study (64), IL-5–deficient mice did not generate BAL eosinophilia or hyperreactivity following allergic challenge, whereas their normal counterparts did. When IL-5–deficient mice were reconstituted with the IL-5 gene, they exhibited allergen-induced BAL eosinophilia and hyperreactivity. In the latter study (78), IL-5–deficient mice did not mount an eosinophilic response to *M. corti* (a helminthic parasite infection). However, baseline levels of circulating eosinophils were maintained. Furthermore, the worm burden in IL-5–deficient mice and their normal counterparts was the same, suggesting that eosinophils were not involved in controlling the infection. The IL-5–deficient mice were healthy and fertile and had normal circulating IgE levels as well as normal T- and B-cell function (78).

Eosinophil activation with release of granule proteins, such as major basic protein (MBP), is probably the most important factor inducing the airway hyperresponsiveness (37,79). MBP is toxic to airway epithelium, and when instilled into the airways of cynomolgus monkeys, it produced bronchial hyperresponsiveness (80). Similar results were demonstrated in experiments performed on rodents (81–83). Furthermore, neutralization of major basic protein with an antibody directed against this protein inhibited the development of antigen-induced bronchial hyperreactivity in guinea pigs (84). Eosinophils also release large amounts of leukotriene C_4, which can cause bronchial hyperresponsiveness (85–87), and this mediator probably contributes to the bronchial hyperresponsiveness to antigen challenge in animal models of asthma and, possibly also in human asthma. Major basic protein and eosinophil peroxidase are both allosteric antagonists of muscarinic M_2 receptors and produce a condition of augmented cholinergic bronchoconstrictor responsiveness in guinea pigs (82). The critical role for IL-5 in augmented cholinergic hyperresponsiveness in allergic guinea pigs has now been identified (88). IL-5 primes eosinophils for activation and migration by other mediators (70,89), and this may be an important mechanism by which IL-5 is linked to bronchial hyperresponsiveness. It is unlikely that IL-5, per se, has any direct effect on airway function because instillation of recombinant human or guinea pig IL-5 to normal guinea pig airways had no effect on basal airway function, bronchoconstrictor reactivity, or airway microvascular leakage induced by substance P (77).

Interleukin-5 is important in the terminal differentiation of eosinophil precursors in the bone marrow (90,91), especially in response to an antigen challenge. Pulmonary challenge with antigen also triggers the release of eosinophils from the bone marrow into the blood, and IL-5 is important for the mobilization of bone marrow eosinophils into the blood in response to inflammatory stimuli (62,92). Several eosinophil-active cytokines, such as IL-3, GM-CSF, and possibly IL-5, are released from the lungs into the circulation after antigen challenge (93,94), and they may trigger the release of eosinophils from bone marrow in response to the antigen stimulus. It appears that expression of IL-5 in lung tissue is critical for the recruitment of eosinophils into the lungs during inflammatory conditions, and this effect may work in conjunction with eosinophil-active chemokines, such as eotaxin (92). Airway eosinophilia does not appear as a passive consequence of an increase in the number of blood eosinophils, but rather, as a result of other IL-5–dependent processes, such as upregulation of adhesion molecules, augmented chemotaxis, and possibly, delayed apoptosis of lung eosinophils.

B. Allergic Rhinitis

In many ways, the nasal cavity responds to allergic challenge in a manner similar to that of the pulmonary airways. For example, mast cell activation, eosinophil infiltration into nasal tissues, and altered physiology are often seen after antigen provocation. Nasal eosinophilia is also correlated with pathophysiology, such as sneezing, rhinorrhea, congestion, and nasal hyperreactivity (95,96). Furthermore, eosinophils collected during seasonal allergic rhinitis by nasal lavage show enhanced luminal-dependent chemiluminescence, suggesting that eosinophil activation had occurred (97). Stored granule enzymes and proteins, such as eosinophil peroxidase, MBP, and eosinophil-derived neurotoxin, are increased in nasal secretions after nasal antigen challenge (98), as are the sulfidopeptide leukotrienes, such as leukotriene C_4 (99).

It is likely that IL-5 is important in the nasal eosinophilia observed in nasal allergies. In patients with a history of allergic rhinitis who have antigen administered nasally, IL-5 concentrations in the nasal lavage fluid increase and peak at 6 hr (95,100,101). Furthermore, immunohistological evaluation of biopsy specimens in the nasal mucosa of patients with allergic rhinitis revealed increased expression of IL-5 along with other Th2-dependent cytokines, such as IL-3, IL-4, and GM-CSF, after nasal antigen challenge (102,103). IL-5 has been localized to CD45RO$^+$ cells (T cells), EG2-positive cells (eosinophils), and metachromatic positive cells (mast cells) in nasal fluids and tissues, suggesting that IL-5 is synthesized and released from a variety of sources in the nose. Most of the IL-5 in nasal allergies is probably derived from T cells (104–106), although Bradding et al. (9) performed immunohistochemical staining of sections from the inferior turbinates in patients with perennial allergic rhinitis and found that approximately 50% of the IL-5 immunoreactive cells were mast cells. Increased levels of IL-5 in the nasal secretions have been correlated with clinical responses in allergic rhinitis (101,107). Furthermore, symptomatic patients treated with a topical corticosteroid have lower concentrations of IL-5 in nasal lavage fluid than nontreated patients (108), and this effect is associated with improved symptom score (109). Topical corticosteroid treatment did not reduce IL-5 mRNA in biopsy specimens of the nasal mucosa of allergic rhinitics, even though there was a marked reduction in the number of cells expressing IL-4 mRNA (109,110). This may reflect a differential sensitivity to inhibition by corticosteroids of IL-4– and IL-5–containing cells in the nasal mucosal relative to that in nasal fluids.

C. Nasal Polyps

Eosinophils are a prominent inflammatory cell in nasal polyps (111). The proliferation of the epithelial layer, the hyperplasia of glands, edema, and the thickening the basement layer, all hallmarks of a nasal polyp, are directly related to the growth factors and mediators released by eosinophils (112,113). Specifically, there are many cells present that contain IL-5 protein, as shown by immunohistochemistry (114), and IL-5 mRNA, as shown by reverse transcription–polymerase chain reaction (RT-PCR; 114–117). Supernatants from nasal polyps contain significant eosinophil survival activity (118), and IL-5 protein concentrations are increased in nasal polyp tissue compared with normal mucosa (118). Proteins with chronic hyperplastic sinusitis and nasal polyps show increased IL-5 mRNA and protein expression (119).

D. Skin Diseases

Late antigen responses can be elicited in sensitive individuals in the skin, as well as in the lungs and the nose, and here also IL-5 appears to be an important mediator. In most of 14 patients who exhibited late responses to injected antigen, IL-5 mRNA and protein were elevated 6 and 24 hr after injection (1,120,121). IL-5 also may be important in atopic dermatitis and other cutaneous disorders that display eosinophilic inflammation, such as episodic angioedema, urticaria, and IL-2 capillary leak syndrome (122,124). Biopsies of the skin lesions of atopic dermatitis have significantly higher number of cells positive for IL-5 mRNA than does skin from unaffected areas or from normal subjects (125–127). Chronic lesions have more IL-5–expressing cells than acute lesions (128). In an anecdotal case of a 6-month-old child with severe eczema and hypereosinophilia, significantly raised serum concentrations of IL-5 were observed, which dropped with clinical improvements (129). Furthermore, peripheral blood mononuclear cells isolated from a severe atopic pediatric patient with atopic dermatitis displayed production of IL-5 that was suppressed after treatment with cyclosporine (129a).

E. Gastrointestinal Disorders

There are several gastrointestinal tract diseases that are associated with the infiltration of eosinophils (e.g., hypereosinophilic syndrome, Crohn's disease, eosinophilic granuloma, parasitic infections, and eosinophilic gastroenteritis; 122). Of these gastrointestinal disorders, eosinophilic gastroenteritis is a condition that probably involves IL-5. In a corticosteroid-resistant patient with eosinophilic gastroenteritis, Quan et al. showed an increase in the in vitro survival of blood eosinophils (130), which was blocked by the preaddition of a MAb to human IL-5. Jaffe et al. (131) examined the possible direct contribution of Th2 cytokines to the processes of eosinophilic gastroenteritis and found that in vitro mitogen stimulation of gastroenteritis-derived T cells induced higher levels of IL-4 and IL-5 than did similarly treated T cells from normal individuals. Lymphocytes from several of these gastroenteritis patients spontaneously produced IL-5. Furthermore, IL-5 mRNA, but not IL-4, IL-2, or IFN-γ mRNA, was found in mucosal biopsies from patients with the gastroenteritis. By using immunohistochemical techniques to identify the cytokine profile in mucosal biopsies from eosinophilic gastroenteritis patients, increased levels of IL-3, GM-CSF, and IL-5 were localized to the matrix of the eosinophil granule (132). Therefore, IL-5, and perhaps other cytokines, contribute to the disease process of eosinophilic gastroenteritis. More importantly, it appears that IL-5 acts not only to recruit eosinophils, but also promotes propagation or retention of the eosinophils at the site of inflammation.

F. Other Conditions

Interleukin-5 has been implicated in several other disease states. In acute eosinophilic pneumonia, high concentrations of IL-5 are found in the BAL fluid, but not in serum, during an exacerbation and, as in other conditions, these fall with treatment and reduction of symptoms (133). Increases in serum IL-5 concentrations in episodic angioedema precede development of eosinophilia (134). Cigarette smoking in normal subjects is associated with a significant decrease in serum IL-5 concentrations (135), and in patients with chronic bronchitis there was no increase in IL-5–positive cells seen during an exacerbation (136). Infusion of IL-2 in cancer patients induces an increase in IL-5 (137,138), and this may explain the increases in circulating eosinophils and reduction in lung function observed in some of these patients. In a murine model of bleomycin-induced pulmonary fibrosis, an increased number of cells expressing mRNA for IL-5 were found in the lungs (139).

It is clear that IL-5 production is seen in response to antigen administration in sensitive individuals, whether the site is the lung, the nose, or the skin. The increased expression takes several hours to be measurable and may last for several days. In clinical situations in which IL-5 is elevated, there is a good correlation between degree of disease severity and IL-5 concentrations, with reductions in IL-5 being observed when treatment is effective and symptoms regress. Thus, in allergic inflammation and other diseases for which IL-5 is an inflammatory mediator, removing it or blocking its action may be a very effective therapeutically.

IV. Therapeutic Potential of IL-5 Inhibition

The mechanisms that underlie IL-5 production, release, receptor activation, and cell signaling, all are possible targets for therapeutic intervention. IL-5 biosynthesis is effectively inhibited by glucocorticosteroids (24,140) and, to a somewhat lesser degree, by cyclosporine (112). Therefore, it should be possible to identify other small-molecule inhibitors of IL-5 biosynthesis, particularly if IL-5–specific transcription factors or regulatory elements in the gene promoter can be identified. In a similar manner, biosynthesis inhibitors of the expression of the α-chain of the IL-5 receptor would also be a means of inhibiting IL-5 action.

Once released from the cell, IL-5 can be neutralized with anti-IL-5 MAbs or soluble IL-5 receptors (141,142). This approach selectively inhibits the effects of IL-5 and, for anti-IL-5 antibodies, can have a very long duration of action (71). The longevity of immunoglobulins, which normally remain in the systemic circulation for many days, most likely explains their extended action (143). Monoclonal antibodies and soluble receptors that inhibit specific cytokines, such as tumor necrosis factor (TNF), have had impressive therapeutic effects in the treatment of inflammatory diseases in clinical trials (144–146).

Cytokine receptor antagonists have been developed by mutagenesis whereby the mutant protein binds to its receptor with high affinity, but does not signal. An IL-4 receptor antagonist has been produced by this method (147), and this approach is reportedly successful for IL-5. Although it should also be possible to find small-molecule, nonpeptidic antagonists, this has proved very difficult in practice, perhaps because the area of protein–protein interaction is too large for "small" molecules to be effective antagonists. Rather than targeting ligand–receptor interactions, the IL-5–signaling pathway is now becoming better elucidated, and in the future, it may be possible to find inhibitors of specific tyrosine kinases or transcription factors induced by IL-5.

Although there are several possible targets for inhibition of the IL-5 pathway, the most practical and specific and the most likely to provide "proof of principle" is currently neutralization of IL-5 by a MAb. The IL-5 pathway is a relatively difficult one to approach for medicinal chemistry, but there are other areas of eosinophil biology, such as chemokines (148) and integrins (149) that are involved in chemotaxis and activation, that may offer more feasible targets.

Two major criteria will determine the exact place of an IL-5 inhibitor in the treatment of human disease, or whether it has any role at all. The first is how critical IL-5 is in the pathogenesis of the particular disease or how effective an IL-5 inhibitor is in clinical trials. The second is how important is IL-5 in normal immune homeostasis and what effect its inhibition may have on host defenses. Practical considerations, such as the severity of the disease, the availability and relative efficacy of treatment options, and the characteristics of the therapeutic (e.g., oral or parenteral dosing, duration of effect, and such) will also determine the value of an IL-5 inhibitor in any particular disease.

Production of IL-5 has clearly been demonstrated in asthma and is reduced after treatment or during remission. It is likely that in some, if not all asthmatic patients (150), IL-5 plays a significant role in their disease, and its inhibition will have a beneficial effect on symptoms and lung function. Glucocorticosteroids are the mainstay of asthma treatment and suppresses IL-5 biosynthesis in vitro. To inhibit eosinophil infiltration to the same extent as anti-IL-5 MAbs, much larger doses of corticosteroids are required in animal models (151) than are used in treatment of human diseases. Therefore, it is possible that anti-IL-5 therapeutics either alone or in combination with glucocorticosteroids may be more effective in suppressing IL-5 action than present therapy, particularly in severe or steroid-unresponsive asthma. IL-5 inhibitors would be expected to be effective in some patients with allergic rhinitis and particularly in those with nasal polyps. In other diseases in which IL-5 is thought to be involved, especially in those for which relatively ineffective or no treatment is available, anti-IL-5 therapeutics could provide significant benefit and be rapidly adopted. Additionally, it may be possible in the future to identify those patients who are likely to respond to anti-IL-5 therapeutics by characterizing their genotype or gene expression profile.

The inhibition of any element of the immune systems may result in impairment of host defenses, and it is possible that this could occur if the activity of IL-5 is blocked. Although the effects of IL-5 inhibition on host defenses can be properly assessed only in clinical trials, there are several pieces of evidence that suggest that this could be of clinical significance. Raised IgE levels and eosinophilia are prominent features of parasitic infestation, both in animals and humans, and in mice IL-4 and IL-5 production, respectively, have been increased (152,153). In most studies, administration of an anti-IL-5 MAb suppresses parasite-induced eosinophilia without having an effect on protective immunity (152–155). In one study, the survival of a nematode parasite in mice was prolonged by blocking IL-5 (156). IL-5 knockout mice, as described earlier, have normal humoral and cytotoxic T-cell responses, have normal baseline levels of eosinophils, lack an eosinophilic response after worm infestation, but do not manifest an excessive worm load. In studies of parasitic infestation in IL-5 knockout mice and in most studies of administration of anti-IL-5 MAbs in normal mice, it is possible to completely abolish allergic responses, without significantly impairing responses to parasites. It is reasonable to hope, therefore, that clinical use of anti-IL-5 therapeutics should improve allergic inflammation without a major effect on host responses to parasites; however, it would seem sensible to limit the early clinical trials of anti-IL-5 medication to patients in areas where parasite infestation is uncommon.

Data from some murine models suggest that local production of cytokines such as IL-5 and IL-4 may have antitumor effects under certain circumstances, but their importance in tumor surveillance is unclear. For example, transfection of murine colon cancer cells with an IL-5 gene, and their transfer into mice leads to increased eosinophil infiltration into the subsequent tumors and reduced tumor colony growth compared with unchanged tumor cells (157). Neutralization of IL-5 by a MAb only partially reversed this tumor inhibition. In contrast, IL-5 gene transfection of plasmacytoma or mammary tumor cells, had no effect on tumor growth, despite eosinophil infiltration of the tumors. Also in mice, Tepper reported an eosinophil-dependent antitumor effect with administration of IL-4, which could be partially reversed by an anti-IL-5 MAb (158). These data may indicate that local IL-5 production, perhaps through the action of eosinophils, which have antitumor effects in vitro (159), may be important in tumor growth inhibition under some circumstances. Alternatively, these data may indicate that therapeutically enhanced production of IL-5 by transfection of tumor cells would be a novel approach to cancer therapy, or even that there is a considerable degree of redundancy in the action of locally produced cytokines on tumor cells. Although the clinical data are conflicting, suppression of the immune system in humans, particularly when profound and prolonged, such as in organ transplantation or treatment of severe autoimmune diseases, seems to be associated with an increase risk of neoplasia. Studies in renal transplant recipients, who are continuously and significantly immunosuppressed, suggest there is a small, but cumulatively, increased incidence of de novo tumors (160–162). However, in the treatment of rheumatic diseases, long-term use of immunosuppressive drugs, such as methotrexate, does not carry the same risk (162). Overall, although immunosuppression sufficient to ensure successful transplantation may be associated with a modest increase in tumor incidence, it is unlikely that milder or more selective immunosuppression inhibition of IL-5, even over several months, would have a significant clinical effect on tumor surveillance in humans.

References

1. Kay AB, Ying S, Varney V, Gaga M, Durham SR, Moqbel R, Wardlaw AJ, Hamid Q. Messenger RNA expression of the cytokine gene cluster, interleukin 3 (IL-3), IL-4, IL-5, and granulocyte/macrophage colony-stimulating factor, in allergen-induced late-phase cutaneous reactions in atopic subjects. J Exp Med 1991; 173:775–778.
2. Robinson DS, Hamid Q, Ying S, Tsicopoulos A, Barkans J, Bentley AM, Corrigan C, Durham S, Kay AB. Predominant Th2-like bronchoalveolar T-lymphocyte population in atopic asthma. N Engl J Med 1992; 326:298–304.
3. Robinson DS, Hamid Q, Bentley A, Ying S, Kay AB, Durham SR. Activation of $CD4^+$ T cells, increased Th2-type cytokine mRNA expression and eosinophil recruitment in bronchoalveolar lavage after allergen inhalation challenge in patients with atopic asthma. J Allergy Clin Immunol 1993; 92:313–324.

4. Marini M, Avoni E, Hollemborg J, Mattoli S. Cytokine mRNA profile and cell activation in bronchoalveolar lavage fluid from nonatopic patients with symptomatic asthma. Chest 1992; 102:661–669.
5. Hamid Q, Azzaw M, Ying S, Moqbel R, Wardlaw AJ, Corrigan CJ, Bradley B, Durham SR, Collins JV, Jefrey PK, Quint DJ, Kay AB. Expression of mRNA for interleukin-5 in mucosal bronchial biopsies from asthma. J Clin Invest 1991; 87:1541–1546.
6. Sedgwick JB, Calhoun WC, Gleich GJ, Kita H, Abrams JS, Schwartz LB, Volovitz B, Ben-Yaakov M, Busse WW. Immediate and late airway response of allergic rhinitis patients to segmental antigen challenge. Characterization of eosinophil and mast cell mediators. Am Rev Respir Dis 1991; 144:1274–1281.
7. Garlisi CG, Falcone A, Kung TT, Stelts D, Pennline KJ, Beavis AJ, Smith SR, Egan RW, Umland SP. T cells are necessary for Th2 cytokine production and eosinophil accumulation in airways of antigen-challenged allergic mice. Clin Immunol Immunopathol 1995; 75:75–83.
8. Garlisi CG, Falcone A, Billah MM, Egan RW, Umland SP. T cells are the predominant source of interleukin-5 but not interleukin-4 mRNA in the lungs of antigen-challenged allergic mice. Am J Respir Cell Mol Biol 1996; 15:420–428.
9. Bradding P, Feather IH, Wilson S, Bardin PG, Heusser C, Holgate ST, Howarth PH. Immunolocalization of cytokines in the nasal mucosa of normal and perennial rhinitic subjects. J Immunol 1993; 151:3853–3865.
10. Dubucquoi S, Desreumaux P, Janin A, Klein O, Goldman M, Tavernier J, Capron A, Capron M. Interleukin 5 synthesis by eosinophils: association with granules and immunoglobulin-dependent secretion. J Exp Med 1994; 179:703–708.
11. Kung TT, Stelts D, Zurcher J, Jones H, Umland S, Kreutner W, Egan RW, Chapman RW. Mast cells modulate allergic pulmonary eosinophilia in mice. Am J Respir Cell Mol Biol 1995; 12:401–409.
12. Ohkawara Y, Lei Y-F, Stämpfli MR, Marshall JS, Xing Z, Jordana M. Cytokine and eosinophil responses in the lung, peripheral blood, and bone marrow compartments in a murine model of allergen-induced airways inflammation. Am J Respir Cell Mol Biol 1997; 16:510–520.
13. Umland SP, Razac S, Shah H, Nahrebne DK, Egan RW, Billah MM. Interleukin-5 mRNA stability in human T cells is regulated differently than interleukin-2, interleukin-3, interleukin-4, granulocyte/macrophage colony-stimulating factor and interferon-γ. Am J Respir Cell Mol Biol 1998; 18:631–642.
14. Naora H, Altin JG, Young IG. TCR-dependent and -independent signaling mechanisms differentially regulate lymphokine gene expression in the murine T helper clone D10.64.1. J Immunol 1994; 152:5691–5702.
15. Staynov DZ, Lee TH. Expression of interleukin-5 and granulocyte–macrophage colony-stimulating factor in human peripheral blood mononuclear cells after activation with phorbol myristate acetate. Immunology 1992; 75:196–201.
16. Northrop JP, Ho SN, Chen L, Thomas DJ, Timmerman LA, Nolan GP, Admon A, Crabtree GR. NF-AT components define a family of transcription factors targeted in T-cell activation. Nature 1994; 369:497–501.
17. Shandene L, Alonso-Vega C, Willems F, Gerard C, Delvaux A, Velu T, Devos R, de Boer M, Goldman M. B7/CD28-dependent IL-5 production by human resting T cells is inhibited by IL-10. J Immunol 1994; 152:4368–4374.
18. Hatfield SM, Roehm NW. Cyclosporin and FK506 inhibition of murine mast cell cytokine production. J Pharmacol Exp Ther 1992; 260:680–688.
19. Alexander AG, Barnes NC, Kay AB. Trial of cyclosporin in corticosteroid-dependent chronic severe asthma. Lancet 1992; 339:324–328.
20. Glaum MC, Jaffe JS, Gillespie DH, Raible DG, Post TJ, Wang Y, Dimitry E, Shulman ES. IgE-dependent expression of interleukin-5 mRNA and protein in human lung: modulation of dexamethasone. Clin Immunol Immunopathol 1995; 75:171–178.

21. Vaca F, Felli MP, Farina AR, Martinotti S, Maroder M, Screpanti I, Meco D, Petrangeli E, Frati L, Gulina A. Glucocorticoid receptor-mediated suppression of the interleukin-2 gene expression through impairment of the cooperativity between nuclear factor of activated T cells and AP-1 enhancer elements. J Exp Med 1992; 175:637–646.
22. Barnes PJ, Pederson S. Efficacy and safety of inhaled corticosteroids in asthma. Am Rev Respir Dis 1993; 148 (suppl 4):1–26.
23. Brinkmann V, Kristofic C. Regulation by corticosteroids of Th1 and Th2 cytokine production in human $CD4^+$ effector T cells generated from $CD45RO^-$ and $CD45RO^+$ subsets. J Immunol 1995; 155:3332–3328.
24. Umland SP, Nahrebne DK, Razac S, Beavis A, Pennline KJ, Egan RW, Billah MM. The inhibitory effects of topically active glucocorticoids on IL-4, IL-5 and IFN-γ production by cultured primary $CD4^+$ T cells. J Allergy Clin Immunol 1997; 100:511–519.
25. Robinson D, Hamid Q, Ying S, Bentley A, Assoufi B, Durham S, Kay AB. Prednisolone treatment in asthma in association with modulation of bronchoalveolar lavage cell interleukin-4, interleukin-5, and interferon-γ cytokine gene expression. Am Rev Respir Dis 1993; 148:401–406.
26. Krouwels FH, van der Heijden JF, Lutter R, van Neerven J, Jansen HM, Out TA. Glucocorticosteroids affect functions of airway- and blood-derived human T-cell clones, favoring the Th1 profile through two mechanisms. Am J Respir Cell Mol Biol 1996; 14:388–397.
27. Takahashi T, Yamaguchi N, Mita S, Yamaguchi Y, Suda T, Tominaga A, Kikuchi Y, Miura Y, Takatsu K. Structural comparison of murine T-cell (B151K12)-derived T-cell-replacing factor (IL-5) with rIL-5: dimer formation is essential for the expression of biological activity. Mol Immunol 1990; 27:911–920.
28. Tominaga A, Takahashi T, Kikuchi Y, Mita S, Naomi S, Harada N, Yamaguchi Y, Miura Y, Takatsu K. Role of carbohydrate moiety of IL-5. J Immunol 1990; 144:1345–1352.
29. Tavernier J, Devos R, Cornellia S, Tuypens T, van der Heyden J, Fiers W, Plaetinck G. A human high affinity interleukin-5 receptor (IL-5R) is composed of an IL-5 specific α chain and β chain shared with the receptor for GM-CSF. Cell 1991; 66:1175–1184.
30. Murata Y, Takaki S, Migita M, Kikuchi Y, Tominaga A, Takatsu K. Molecular cloning and expression of the human interleukin 5 receptor. J Exp Med 1992; 175:341–351.
31. Miyajima A, Kitamura T, Harada N, Yokota T, Aria KI. Cytokine receptors and signal transduction. Annu Rev Immunol 1992; 10:295–331.
32. Tavernier J, Tuypens T, Plaetinck G, Verhee A, Fiers W, Devos R. Molecular basis of the membrane-anchored and two soluble isoforms of the human interleukin-5 receptor α subunit. Proc Natl Acad Sci USA 1992; 89:7041–7045.
33. Sakamaki K, Miyajima I, Kitamura T, Miyajima A. Critical cytoplasmic domains of the common β subunit of the human GM-CSF, IL-3 and IL-5 receptors for growth signal transduction and tyrosine phosphorylation. EMBO J 1992; 11:3541–3549.
34. Murata Y, Yamaguchi N, Hitoshi Y, Tominga A, Takatsu K. Interleukin 5 and interleukin 3 induce serine and tyrosine phosphorylations of several cellular proteins in an interleukin 5 dependent cell line. Biochem Biophys Res 1990; 173:1102–1108.
35. Silvennoinen O, Witthuhn BA, Quelle FW, Cleveland JL, Taolin Y, Ihle JN. Structure of the murine Jak2 protein-tyrosine kinase and its role in interleukin 3 signal transduction. Proc Natl Acad Sci USA 1993; 90:8429–8433.
36. Mui AL-F, Wakao H, O'Farrell A-M, Harada N, Miyajima A. Interleukin-3, granulocyte–macrophage colony stimulating factor and interleukin-5 transduce signals through two STATS homologues. EMBO J 1995; 14:1116–1175.
37. Gleich GJ, Kita H, Adolphson CR. Eosinophils. In: Frank MN, Austen KF, Cloman HN, Unanue ER, eds. Samsters Immunologic Diseases, 5th ed. Boston: Little, Brown, 1995:205–245.
38. Kay AB. Asthma and inflammation. J Allergy Clin Immunol 1991; 87:893–910.

39. Durham SR, Kay AB. Eosinophils, bronchial hyperreactivity and late phase asthmatic reactions. Clin Allergy 1985; 13:411–418.
40. Wardlaw AJ, Dunnett S, Gleich GJ, Collins JV, Kay AB. Eosinophils and mast cells in bronchoalveolar lavage in subjects with mild asthma: relationship to bronchial hyperreactivity. Am Rev Respir Dis 1988; 137:62–69.
41. Ohnishi T, Kita, H, Weiler D, Sur S, Sedgwick JB, Calhoun WJ, Busse WW, Abrams JS, Gleich GJ. IL-5 is the predominant eosinophil-active cytokine in the antigen-induced pulmonary late-phase reaction. Am Rev Respir Dis 1993; 147:901–907.
42. Shaver JR, Zangrilli J, Cho SK, Pollice M, Cirelli RA, Hastie AT, Everts KB, Fish JE, Peters SP. IL-3, IL-5 and GM-CSF have different patterns of production during recovery from IgE-mediated inflammation in allergic asthmatics. Am J Respir Crit Care Med 1996; 153:A793.
43. Shi H, Qin S, Huang G, Chen Y, Xiao C, Xu H, Liang G, Xie Z, Qin X, Wu J, Li G, Zhang C. Infiltration of eosinophils into the asthmatic airways caused by interleukin 5. Am J Respir Cell Mol Biol 1997; 16:220–224.
44. Broide DH, Pain MM, Firestein GS. Eosinophils express interleukin 5 and granulocyte–macrophage colony-stimulating factor mRNA at sites of allergic inflammation in asthmatics. J Clin Invest 1992; 90:1414–1424.
45. Fukuda T, Nakajima H, Fukushima Y, Akutsu I, Numao T, Majima K, Motojima S, Sato Y, Takatsu K, Makino S. Detection of interleukin-5 messenger RNA and interleukin-5 protein in bronchial biopsies from asthma by nonradioactive in situ hybridization and immunohistochemistry. J Allergy Clin Immunol 1994; 94:584–593.
46. Hamid Q, Azzawi M, Ying S, Moqbel R, Wardlaw AJ, Corrigan CJ, Bradley B, Durham SR, Collins JV, Jeffery PK. Interleukin-5 mRNA in mucosal bronchial biopsies from asthmatic subjects. Int Arch Allergy Appl Immunol 1991; 94:169–170.
47. Humbert M, Durham SR, Ying S, Kimmitt P, Barkans J, Assoufi B, Pfister R, Menz G, Robinson DS, Kay AB, Corrigan CJ. IL-4 and IL-5 mRNA and protein in bronchial biopsies from patients with atopic and nonatopic asthma: evidence against "intrinsic" asthma being a distinct immunopathologic entity. Am J Respir Crit Care Med 1996; 154:1497–1504.
48. Robinson DS, Ying S, Bently AM, Meng Q, North J, Durham SR, Kay AB, Hamid Q. Relationships among numbers of bronchoalveolar lavage cells expressing messenger ribonucleic acid for cytokines, asthma symptoms, and airway methacholine responsiveness in asthma. J Allergy Clin Immunol 1993; 92:397–403.
49. Bentley AM, Qiu Meng DS, Robinson DS, Hamid Q, Kay AB, Durham SR. Increases in activated T lymphocytes, eosinophils and cytokine mRNA expression for interleukin-5 and granulocyte/macrophage colony-stimulating factor in bronchial biopsies after allergen inhalation challenge in atopic asthmatics. Am J Respir Cell Mol Biol 1993; 8:35–42.
50. Walker C, Bauer W, Braun RK, Menz G, Braun P, Schwarz F, Hansel TT, Villiger B. Activated T cells and cytokines in bronchoalveolar lavages from patients with various lung diseases associated with eosinophilia. Am J Respir Crit Care Med 1994; 150:1030–1048.
51. Ying S, Durham SR, Corrigan CJ, Hamid Q, Kay AB. Phenotype of cells expressing mRNA for Th2-type (interleukin-4 and interleukin-5) and Th1-type (interleukin 2 and interferon-γ) cytokines in bronchoalveolar lavage and bronchial biopsies from atopic asthmatic and normal control subjects. Am J Respir Cell Mol Biol 1995; 12:477–487.
52. Motojima S, Akutsu I, Fukuda T, Makino S, Takatsu K. Clinical significance of measuring levels of sputum and serum ECP and serum IL-5 in bronchial asthma. Allergy 1993; 48:98–106.
53. Corrigan CJ, Haczku A, Gemou-Engesaeth V, Doi S, Kikuchi Y, Takatsu K, Durham SR, Kay AB. CD4 T-lymphocyte activation in asthma is accompanied by increased serum concentrations of interleukin-5. Am Rev Respir Dis 1993; 147:540–547.
54. Walker C, Bode E, Baer L, Hansel TT, Blaser K, Virchow JC Jr. Allergic and nonallergic asthmatics have distinct patterns of T cell activation and cytokine production in peripheral blood and bronchoalveolar lavage. Am Rev Respir Dis 1992; 146:109–115.

55. Sur S, Gleich GJ, Swanson MC, Bartemes KR, Broide DH. Eosinophilic inflammation is associated with the elevation of interleukin-5 in the airways of patients with spontaneous symptomatic asthma. J Allergy Clin Immunol 1995; 96:661–668.
56. Tollerud DJ, Sparrow DW, Guevarra L, O'Connor GT, Weiss ST. Relationships of serum IL-5 level to longitudinal rate of FEV_1 decline among asthmatics. Am J Respir Crit Care Med 1994; 149:A913.
57. Kosmas EN, Polychronaki A, Adamidou A, Demertzis P, Michaelides S, Polychonopoulos V, Baxevanis CN. Theophylline-induced down-regulation of circulating cytokines in young asymptomatic asthmatics. Am J Respir Crit Care Med 1996; 153:A805.
58. Martin RJ, Cicutto LC, Smith HR, Ballard RD, Szefler SJ. Airways inflammation in nocturnal asthma. Am Rev Respir Dis 1991; 143:351–357.
59. Jarjour NN, Busse WW. Cytokines in bronchoalveolar lavage fluid of patients with nocturnal asthma. Am J Respir Crit Care Med 1995; 152:1474–1477.
60. Wilson SJ, Kraft M, Martin R, Holgate ST, Djukanovic R. Lung immunostaining for IL-4 and IL-5 in nocturnal asthma. Am J Respir Crit Care Med 1996; 153:A879.
61. Wallaert B, Desreumaux P, Copin MC, Tillie I, Bernard A, Colombel JF, Gosselin B, Tonnel AB, Janin A. Immunoreactivity for interleukin 3 and 5 and granulocyte/macrophage colony-stimulating factor of intestinal mucosa in bronchial asthma. J Exp Med 1995; 182:1897–1904.
62. Kung TT, Stelts DM, Zurcher JA, Adams GK III, Egan RW, Kreutner W, Watnick AS, Jones H, Chapman RW. Involvement of IL-5 in a murine model of allergic pulmonary inflammation: prophylactic and therapeutic effect of an anti-IL-5 antibody. Am J Respir Cell Mol Biol 1995; 13:360–365.
63. Nagai H, Yamaguchi S, Inagaki N, Tsuruoka N, Hitoshi Y, Takatsu K. Effect of anti-IL-5 monoclonal antibody on allergic bronchial eosinophilia and airway hyperresponsiveness in mice. Life Sci 1993; 53:243–247.
64. Foster PS, Hogan SP, Ramsay AJ, Matthaei KI, Young IG. Interleukin 5 deficiency abolishes eosinophilia, airway hyperreactivity, and lung damage in a mouse model. J Exp Med 1996; 183:195–201.
65. Eum S-Y, Hailé S, Lefort J, Huerre M, Vargaftig BB. Eosinophil recruitment into the respiratory epithelium following antigenic challenge in hyper-IgE mice is accompanied by interleukin-5 dependent bronchial hyperresponsiveness. Proc Natl Acad Sci USA 1995; 92:12290–12294.
66. Hamelmann E, Oshiba A, Loader J, Larsen GL, Gleich G, Lee J, Gelfand EW. Anti-interleukin-5 antibody prevents airway hyperresponsiveness in a murine model of airway sensitization. Am J Respir Crit Care Med 1997; 155:819–825.
67. Hessel EM, van Oosterhout AJM, van Ark I, van Esch B, Hofman G, van Loveren H, Savelkoul HFJ, Nijkamp FP. Development of airway hyperresponsiveness is dependent on interferon-γ and independent of eosinophil infiltration. Am J Respir Cell Mol Biol 1997; 16:325–334.
68. Mauser PJ, Pitman A, Witt A, Fernandez X, Zurcher J, Kung T, Jones H, Watnick AS, Egan RW, Kreutner W, Adams GK III. Inhibitory effect of the TRFK-5 anti-IL-5 antibody in a guinea pig model of asthma. Am Rev Respir Dis 1993; 148:1623–1627.
69. van Oosterhout AJM, Ladenius ARC, Savelkoul HFJ, van Ark I, Delsman KC, Nijkamp FP. Effect of anti-IL-5 and IL-5 on airway hyperreactivity and eosinophils in guinea pigs. Am Rev Respir Dis 1993; 147:548–552.
70. Coëffier E, Joseph D, Vargaftig BB. Role of interleukin-5 in enhanced migration of eosinophils from airways of immunized guinea pigs. Br J Pharmacol 1994; 113:749–756.
71. Mauser PJ, Pitman AM, Fernandez X, Foran SK, Adams GK III, Kreutner W, Egan RW, Chapman RW. Effects of an antibody to interleukin-5 in a monkey model of asthma. Am J Respir Crit Care Med 1995; 152:467–472.
72. Egan RW, Umland SP, Cuss FM, Chapman RW. Biology of interleukin-5 and its relevance to allergic disease Allergy 1996; 51:71–81.
73. Nagai H, Yamaguchi S, Maeda Y, Tanaka H. Role of mast cells, eosinophils and IL-5 in

the development of airway hyperresponsiveness in sensitized mice. Clin Exp Allergy 1996; 26:642–647.
74. Lefort J, Bachelet C-M, Leduc D, Vargaftig BB. Effect of antigen provocation of IL-5 transgenic mice on eosinophil mobilization and bronchial hyperresponsiveness. J Allergy Clin Immunol 1996; 97:758–799.
75. van Oosterhout AJM, Fattah D, van Ark I, Hofman G, Buckley TL, Nijkamp FP. Eosinophil precedes development of airway hyperreactivity and mucosal exudation after intranasal administration of interleukin-5 to mice. J Allergy Clin Immunol 1995; 96:104–112.
76. Corry DB, Folkesson HG, Warnock ML, Erle DJ, Mathay MA, Wiener-Kronish JP, Locksley RM. Interleukin 4, but not interleukin 5 or eosinophils, is required in a murine model of acute airway hyperreactivity. J Exp Med 1996; 183:109–117.
77. Lilly CM, Chapman RW, Sehring SJ, Mauser PJ, Egan RW, Drazen JM. Effects of interleukin-5-induced pulmonary eosinophilia on airway reactivity in the guinea pig. Am J Physiol 1996; 270:L368–L375.
78. Kopf M, Brombacher F, Hodgkin P, Ramsay AJ, Milbourne EA, Dai WJ, Ovington KS, Behm CA, Kohler G, Young IG, Matthaei KI. IL-5 deficient mice have a developmental defect in $CD5^+$ B-1 cells and lack eosinophilia but have normal antibody and cytotoxic T cell responses. Immunity 1996; 5:81–89.
79. Frigas E, Loegering DA, Gleich GJ. Cytotoxic effects of the guinea pig eosinophil major basic protein on tracheal epithelium. Lab Invest 1980; 42:35–43.
80. Gundel RH, Letts LG, Gleich GJ. Human eosinophil major basic protein induces airway constriction and airway hyperresponsiveness in primates. J Clin Invest 1991; 87:1470–1473.
81. Uchida DA, Ackerman SJ, Coyle AJ, Larsen GL, Weller PF, Freed J, Irvin CG. The effect of human eosinophil granule major basic protein on airway responsiveness in the rat in vivo. Am Rev Respir Dis 1993; 147:982–988.
82. Jacoby DB, Gleich GJ, Fryer AD. Human eosinophil major basic protein is an endogenous allosteric antagonist at the inhibitory muscarinic M_2 receptor. J Clin Immunol 1993; 91:1314–1318.
83. White SR, Ohno S, Munoz NM, Gleich GJ, Abrahams C, Solway J, Leff AR. Epithelium-dependent contraction of airway smooth muscle caused by eosinophil MBP. Am J Physiol 1990; 259:L294–L303.
84. Lefort J, Nahori M-A, Ruffié C, Vargaftig BB, Pretolani M. In vivo neutralization of eosinophil-derived major basic protein inhibits antigen-induced bronchial hyperreactivity in sensitized guinea pigs. J Clin Invest 1996; 97:1117–1121.
85. Hamann KJ, Strek ME, Baranowski SL, Munoz NM, Williams FC, White SR, Vita A, Leff AR. Effects of activated eosinophils cultured from human umbilical cord blood on guinea-pig trachealis. Am J Physiol 1993; 265:L301–L307.
86. Strek ME, White SR, Hsiue WTR, Kulp GVP, Williams FS, Leff AR. Effect of mode of activation of human eosinophils on tracheal smooth muscle contraction in guinea pigs. Am J Physiol 1993; 264:L475–L481.
87. Aizawa T, Sekizawa K, Aikawa T, Maruyama N, Itabashi S, Tamura G, Sasaki H, Takishima T. Eosinophil supernatant 9 causes hyperresponsiveness of airway smooth muscle in guinea-pig trachea. Am Rev Respir Dis 1990; 142:133–137.
88. Elbon CL, Jacoby DB, Fryer AD. Pretreatment with an antibody to interleukin-5 prevents loss of pulmonary M_2 muscarinic receptor function in antigen-challenged guinea pigs. Am J Respir Cell Mol Biol 1995; 12:320–328.
89. Coëffier E, Joseph D, Vargaftig BB. Activation by human recombinant IL-5 of guinea pig eosinophils. Selective priming to PAF and interference of its antagonists. J Immunol 1991; 174:2595–2602.
90. Clutterbuck EK, Hirst EMA, Sanderson CJ. Human interleukin-5 (IL-5) regulates the production of eosinophils in human bone marrow cultures: comparison and interaction with IL-1, IL-3, IL-6 and GM-CSF. Blood 1989; 73:1504–1512.
91. Yamaguchi Y, Suda T, Suda J, Eguchi M, Miura Y, Harad N, Taminaga A, Takatsu K.

Purified interleukin-5 supports the terminal differentiation and proliferation of murine eosinophilic precursor. J Exp Med 1988; 167:43–56.
92. Mould AW, Matthaei KI, Young IG, Foster PS. Relationship between interleukin-5 and eotaxin in regulating blood and tissue eosinophilia in mice. Am J Respir Cell Mol Biol 1997; 99:1064–1071.
93. Wooley MJ, Denburg JA, Ellis R, Dahlbäck M, O'Byrne P. Allergen-induced changes in bone marrow progenitors and airway responsiveness in dogs and the effect of inhaled budesonide on these parameters. Am J Respir Cell Mol Biol 1994; 11:600–606.
94. Inman MD, Denburg JA, Ellis R, Dahlbäck M, O'Byrne PM. Allergen-induced increase in bone marrow progenitors in airway hyperresponsive dogs: regulation by a serum hemopoietic factor. Am J Respir Cell Mol Biol 1996; 15:305–311.
95. Terada N, Konno A, Togawa K. Biochemical properties of eosinophils and their preferential accumulation mechanism in nasal allergy. J Allergy Clin Immunol 194; 94:629–642.
96. Murray AB, Anderson DO. The epidemiologic relationship of clinical nasal allergy to eosinophils and to goblet cells in the nasal smear. J Allergy 1969; 43:1–8.
97. Shult PA, Graziano FM, Busse WW. Enhanced eosinophil luminol-dependent chemiluminescence in allergic rhinitis. J Allergy Clin Immunol 1986; 77:702–708.
98. Bascom R, Pipkorn U, Proud D, Dunnett S, Gleich GJ, Lichtenstein LM, Naclerio RM. Major basic protein and eosinophil-derived neurotoxin concentrations in nasal-lavage fluid after antigen challenge: effect of systemic corticosteroids and relationship to eosinophil influx. J Allergy Clin Immunol 1989; 84:338–346.
99. Volovitz B, Osur SL, Bernstein JM, Ogra PL. Leukotriene C_4 release in upper respiratory mucosa during natural exposure to ragweed in ragweed-sensitive children. J Allergy Clin Immunol 1988; 82:414–418.
100. Rasp G, Thomas P. Interleukin-5 release in late antigen-induced nasal secretion is associated with eosinophil activation. J Allergy Clin Immunol 1995; 95:258.
101. Sim TC, Grant JA, Hilsmeir KA, Fukuda Y, Alam R. Detection of proinflammatory cytokines in the nasal secretions of allergic subjects following antigen challenge. Am J Respir Crit Care Med 1994; 149:339–344.
102. Saito H, Asakura K, Kataura A. Study on the IL-5 expression in allergic nasal mucosa. Int Arch Allergy Immunol 1994; 104(suppl 1):39–40.
103. Durham SR, Ying S, Varney VA, Jacobson MR, Sudderick RM, Mackay IS, Kay AB, Hamid QA. Cytokine messenger RNA expression for IL-3, IL-4, IL-5, and granulocyte/macrophage-colony-stimulating factor in the nasal mucosa after local allergen provocation: relationship to tissue eosinophilia. J Immunol 1992; 148:2390–2394.
104. Pawankar RU, Okuda M, Suzuki K, Okumura K, Ra C. Phenotypic and molecular characteristics of nasal mucosal gamma delta T cells in allergic and infectious rhinitis. Am J Respir Crit Care Med 1996; 153:1655–1665.
105. Ying S, Durham SR, Barkans J, Masuyama K, Jacobson M, Rak S, Lowhagen O, Moqbel R, Kay AB, Hamid QA. T cells are the principal source of interleukin-5 mRNA in allergen-induced rhinitis. Am J Respir Cell Mol Biol 1993; 9:356–361.
106. Kay AB, Ying S, Durham SR. Phenotype of cells positive for interleukin-4 and interleukin-5 mRNA in allergic tissue reactions. Int Arch Allergy Immunol 1995; 107:208–210.
107. Dunnette SL, Kita H, Reed CE, Gleich GJ. Topical glucocorticoid treatment of ragweed hay fever. II. Relationship of eosinophil-derived neurotoxin (EDN) and IL-5 to disease severity. J Allergy Clin Immunol 1997; 99:S124.
108. Jorgensen RK, Gleich GJ, Kita H, Reed CE. Topical glucocorticoid treatment of ragweed hay fever. I. Effects of IgE and IgA antibody production. J Allergy Clin Immunol 1997; 99:S360.
109. Garrelds IM, DeGraaf-in't Veld T, Nahori MA, Vargaftig BB, Gerth van Wijk R, Zijlstra FJ. Interleukin-5 and eosinophil cationic protein in nasal lavages of rhinitis patients. Eur J Pharmacol 1995; 275:392–300.
110. Bradding P, Feather IH, Wilson S, Holgate ST, Howarth PH Cytokine immunoreactivity

in seasonal rhinitis: regulation by a topical corticosteroid. Am J Respir Crit Care Med 1995; 151:1900–1906.
111. Djukanovic R. Nasal polyps—a model of chronic respiratory mucosal inflammation. Clin Exp Allergy 1995; 25:582–585.
112. Weller PF. The immunobiology of eosinophils. N Engl J Med 1991; 324:1110–1114.
113. Ohno I, Nitta Y, Yamauchi K, Hoshi H, Honma M, Woolley K, O'Byrne P, Dolovich J, Jordana M, Tamura G. Eosinophils as a potential source of platelet-derived growth factor B-chain (PDGF-B) in nasal polyps and bronchial asthma. Am J Respir Cell Mol Biol 1995; 13:639–647.
114. Dater I, Bachert C. Localization of interleukin-5 (IL-5) in RNA in eosinophils of nasal polyps by in situ hybridization. J Allergy Clin Immunol 1996; 97:276.
115. Wagenmann M, Dater I, Rudack C, Ganzer U, Bachert C. Interleukin-5 protein and mRNA are increased in nasal polyps. J Allergy Clin Immunol 1996; 97:300.
116. Simon HU, Yousefi S, Weber M, Schapowal A, Schmitz M, Blaser K. Direct demonstration of delayed eosinophil apoptosis as a mechanism to cause tissue eosinophilia. Am J Respir Crit Care Med 1996; 153:A56.
117. Lee CH, Rhee CS, Min YG. Cytokine gene expression in nasal polyp. J Allergy Clin Immunol 1996; 97:192.
118. Xaubet A, Mullol J, Lopez E, Roca-Ferrer J, Rozman M, Carrion T, Fabra JM, Picado C. Comparison of the role of nasal polyps and normal nasal mucosal epithelial cells on in vitro eosinophil survival mediation by GM-CSF and inhibition by dexamethasone. Clin Exp Allergy 1994; 24:307–317.
119. Hamilos DL, Plout M, Leung DYM, Huston DP, Hamid QA. GM-CSF, IL-5 and RANTES mRNA expression and protein levels in chronic hyperplastic sinusitis with nasal polyposis. J Allergy Clin Immunol 1997; 99:S130.
120. Vowels BR, Rook AH, Cassin M, Zweiman B. Expression of interleukin-4 and interleukin-5 mRNA in developing cutaneous late-phase reactions. J Allergy Clin Immunol 1995; 96:92–96.
121. Parrott CM, Graif Y, Lessin SR, Zweiman B. Quantitative analysis of cytokines in cutaneous late phase (LPR) allergic reactions: a role for IL-5 in the developing LPR. J Allergy Clin Immunol 1997; 99:S170.
122. Nutman TB, Ottesen EA, Cohen SG. The eosinophil, eosinophilia, and eosinophil-related disorders. Allergy Proc 1989; 10:33–46.
123. Leiferman KM, Peters MS, Gleich GJ. The eosinophil and cutaneous edema. J Am Acad Dermatol 1986; 15:513–517.
124. van Haelst Pisani C, Kovach JS, Kita H, Leiferman KM, Gleich GJ, Silver JR, Abrams JS. Administration of interleukin 2 (IL-2) results in increased plasma concentrations of IL-5 and eosinophilia in patients with cancer. Blood 1991; 78:1538–1544.
125. Kagi MK, Wuthrich B, Montano E, Barandun J, Blaser K, Walker C. Differential cytokines profiles in peripheral blood lymphocyte supernatants and skin biopsies from patients with different forms of atopic dermatitis, psoriasis and normal individuals. Int Arch Allergy Immunol 1994; 103:332–340.
126. Hamid Q, Boguniewicz M, Leung DYM. Differential in situ cytokine gene expression in acute versus chronic atopic dermatitis. J Clin Invest 1994; 94:870–876.
127. Tanaka Y, Delaporte E, Dubucquoi S, Gounni A.S, Porchet E, Capron A, Capron M. Interleukin-5 messenger RNA and immunoreactive protein expression by activated eosinophils in lesional atopic dermatitis skin. J Invest Dermatol 1994; 103:589–592.
128. Taka RA, Leung DYM, Boguniewicz M, Minshall E, Hamid Q. IL-4 and IL-5 receptor mRNA expression in acute and chronic atopic dermatitis. J Allergy Clin Immunol 1997; 99:S331.
129. Spergel JM, Boyce J, Schneider LC. Hypereosinophilia, elevated IgE and interleukin-5 levels in neonatal atopic dermatitis. J Allergy Clin Immunol 1997; 99:S322.
129a. Ishii E, Yamamoto S, Sakai R, Hamasaki Y, Miyazaki S. Production of interleukin-5 and the suppressive effect of cyclosporin A in childhood severe atopic dermatitis. J Pediatrics 1996; 128:152–155.

130. Quan SF, Sedgwick JB, Nelson MV, Busse WW. Corticosteroid resistance in eosinophilic gastritis—relation to in vitro eosinophil survival and interleukin 5. Ann Allergy 1993; 70:256–260.
131. Jaffe JS, James SP, Mullins GE, Braun-Elwert L, Lubensky I, Metcalfe DD. Evidence for an abnormal profile of interleukin-4, IL-5, and γ-interferon in peripheral blood T cells from patients with allergic eosinophilic gastroenteritis. J Clin Immunol 1994; 14:299–309.
132. Desreumaux P, Bloget F, Seguy D, Capron M, Corto A, Colombel J-F, Janin A. Interleukin 3, granulocyte–macrophage colony stimulating factor, and interleukin 5 in eosinophilic gastroenteritis. Gastroenterology 1996; 110:768–774.
133. Allen JN, Liao Z, Wewers MD, Altenberger EA, Moore SA, Allen ED. Detection of IL-5 and IL-1 receptor antagonist in bronchoalveolar lavage fluid in acute eosinophilic pneumonia. J Allergy Clin Immunol 1996; 97:1366–1374.
134. Butterfield JH, Leiferman KM, Abrams J, Silver JE, Bower J, Gonchoroff N, Gleich GJ. Elevated serum levels of interleukin-5 in patients with the syndrome of episodic angioedema and eosinophilia. Blood 1992; 79:688–692.
135. Tsunoda M, Guevarra L, Tollerud DJ. Serum cytokine levels, cigarette smoking and ethnicity among healthy men. Am J Respir Crit Care Med 1996; 153:A103.
136. Saetta M, DiStefano A, Maestrelli P, Turato G, Mapp CE, Pieno M, Zanguochi G, Del Prete G, Fabbri LM. Airway eosinophilia and expression of interleukin-5 protein in asthma and in exacerbations of chronic bronchitis. Clin Exp Allergy 1996; 26:766–774.
137. Pisano CVH, Korvach JS, Kita H, Leiferman KM, Gleich GJ, Silver JE, Dennin R, Abrams JS. Administration of interleukin-2 (IL-2) results in increased plasma concentrations of IL-5 and eosinophilia in patients with cancer. Blood 1991; 78:1538–1544.
138. Lazarus DS, Kurnick JT, Kradin RL. Alterations in pulmonary function in cancer patients receiving adoptive immunotherapy with tumor-infiltrating lymphocytes and interleukin-2. Am Rev Respir Dis 1990; 141:193–198.
139. Gharaee-Kermani M, Phan SH. Lung interleukin-5 expression in murine bleomycin-induced pulmonary fibrosis. Am J Respir Cell Mol Biol 1997; 16:438–447.
140. Rolfe FG, Hughes JM, Armour CL, Sewell WA. Inhibition of interleukin-5 gene expression by dexamethasone. Immunology 1992; 77:494–499.
141. Tavernier J, Devos R, Cornelis S, Tuypens T, van der Heyden J, Flers W, Plaetinck G. A human high affinity interleukin-5 receptor (IL-5R) is composed of an IL-5 specified chain and chain shared with the receptor for GMCSF. Cell 1991; 66:1175–1184.
142. Yamaguchi S, Nagai H, Tanaka H, Tsujimoto M, Tsuruoka N. Time course study for antigen-induced airway hyperreactivity and the effect of soluble IL-5 receptor. Life Sci 1994; 54:PL471–475.
143. Garlisi CG, Kung TT, Wang P, Minnicozzi M, Umland SP, Chapman RW, Stelts D, Crawley Y, Falcone A, Myers JC, Jones H, Billah MM, Kreutner W, Egan RW. Effects of chronic anti-interleukin-5 monoclonal antibody treatment in a murine model of pulmonary inflammation. Am J Respir Cell Mol Biol 1999; 20:248–255.
144. Wee S, Pascual M, Eason JD, Schoenfeld DA, Phelan J, Boskovic S, Blosch C, Mohler K, Cosimi AB. Biological effects and fate of a soluble, dimeric, 80-kDa tumor necrosis factor receptor in renal transplant recipients who receive OKT3 therapy. Transplantation.1997; 63:570–577.
145. Elliott MJ, Maini RN, Feldmann M, Kalden JR, Antoni C, Smolen JS, Leeb B, Breedveld FC, Macfarlane JD, Bijl H, Woody JN. Randomized double-blind comparison of chimeric monoclonal antibody to tumour necrosis factor A (CA2) versus placebo in rheumatoid arthritis. Lancet 1994; 344:1105–1110.
146. Stack WA, Mann SD, Roy AJ, Heath P, Sopwith M, Freeman J, Holmes G, Long R, Forbes A, Kamm MA. Randomized controlled trial of CDP571 antibody to tumour necrosis factor–α—in Crohn's disease. Lancet 1997; 349:521–524.
147. Kruse N, Tony HP, Sebald W. Conversion of human interleukin-4 into a high affinity antagonist by a single amino acid replacement. EMBO J 1992; 11:3237–3244.
148. Lukacs NW, Standiford TJ, Chensue SW, Kunkel RG, Strieter RM, Kunkel SL. C–C

chemokine-induced eosinophil chemotaxis during allergic airway inflammation. J Leukoc Biol 1996; 60:573–578.

149. Bloemen P, Henricks P, Nijkamp F. Cell adhesion molecules and asthma. Clin Exp Allergy 1997; 27:128–141.

150. Zangrilli JG, Shaver JR, Cirelli RA, Cho SK, Garlisi CG, Falcone A, Cuss FM, Fish JE, Peters SP. sVCAM-1 levels after segmental antigen challenge correlate with eosinophil influx, IL-4 and IL-5 production, and the late phase response. Am J Respir Crit Care Med 1995; 151:1346–1353.

151. Kung TT, Jones H, Adams KG III, Umland SP, Kreutner W, Egan RW, Chapman RW, Watnick AS. Characterization of a murine model of allergic pulmonary inflammation. Int Arch Allergy Immunol 1994; 105:83–90.

152. Coffman R, Seymour B, Hudak Jackson S, Rennick D. Antibody to interleukin 5 inhibits helminth induced eosinophilia in mice. Science 1989; 245:308–310.

153. Sher A, Coffman R, Hieny S, Cheever AW. Ablation of eosinophil and IgE responses with anti-IL-5 or anti-IL-4 antibodies fails to affect immunity against *Schistosoma mansoni* in the mouse. J Immunol 1990; 145:3911–3916.

154. Sher A, Coffman R, Hieny S, Scott P, Cheever AW. Interleukin-5 is required for blood and tissue eosinophilia but not granuloma formation induced by infection with *Schistosoma mansoni*. Proc Natl Acad Sci USA 1990; 87:61–65.

155. Korenaga M, Hitoshi Y, Yamaguchi N, Soto Y, Takatsu K, Tada I. The role of interleukin-5 in protective immunity to *Strongyloides venezuelensis* infection in mice. Immunology 1991; 72:502–507.

156. Sasaki O, Sugaya H, Ishida K, Yoshimura K. Ablation of eosinophils with anti-IL-5 antibody enhances the survival of intracranial worms of *Angiostrongylus cantonensis* in the mouse. Parasite Immunol 1993; 15:349–354.

157. Masuda Y, Mita S, Sakamoto K, Ishiko T, Ogawa M. Suppression of in vivo tumor growth by the transfection of the interleukin-5 gene into colon tumor cells. Cancer Immunol Immunother 1995; 41:325–330.

158. Tepper RI, Coffman RL, Leder P. An eosinophil-dependent mechanism for the anti-tumor effect of interleukin-4. Science 1992; 257:548–551.

159. Rivoltini L, Viggiano V, Spinazze S, Santoro A, Colombo MP, Takatsu K, Pamiani G. In vitro anti-tumor activity of eosinophils from cancer patients treated with subcutaneous administration of interleukin 2. Role of interleukin 5. Int J Cancer 1993; 54:8.

160. Walz MK, Albrecht KH, Niebel W, Eigler FW. De novo malignant tumors during drug immunosuppression. The findings following 1245 cadaveric kidney transplants in 1080 patients. Dtsch Med Wochenschr 1992; 117:927–934.

161. Bouwes Bavinck JN, Hardie DR, Green A, Cutmore S, MacNaught A, O'Sullivan B, Siskind V, van Der Woude FJ, Hardie IR. The risk of skin cancer in renal transplant recipients in Queensland, Australia. A follow-up study. Transplantation 1996; 6:715–721.

162. Balint G, Gergely P Jr. Clinical immunotoxicity of antirheumatic drugs. Inflamm Res 1996; 45(suppl 2):S91–S95.

Part Five

PREVENTION OF ALLERGIC ASTHMA: IS IT POSSIBLE?

30

Primary Prevention of Atopic Asthma

Prophylactic Strategies Based on Immunomodulation of Host Responses During Childhood

PATRICK G. HOLT

TVW Telethon Institute for Child Health Research
Perth, Western Australia, Australia

I. Introduction

It is now clear that active immunity against common inhalant allergens is essentially universal among the adult population, and is polarized toward the Th1 cytokine phenotype in normal individuals, as opposed to the Th2 phenotype in atopic patients (1–5). It is also becoming evident that T helper (Th)-cell memory often becomes imprinted in the immune system during childhood (reviewed in Ref. 6), thereby determining allergen-specific responder phenotype in subsequent adult life. The cellular and molecular basis for this process is the subject of intensive study in many centers, and the information rapidly accumulating provides the theoretical basis for a range of prophylactic strategies for primary prevention of atopic disease by manipulation of the underlying mechanisms. The key recent findings on perinatal allergen-specific T-cell immunity, and the prophylactic strategies suggested by the latter, are discussed in this chapter.

II. Regulation of T-Cell Immunity in Experimental Animals to Allergens Presented at Mucosal Surfaces: Pointers to Studies in Humans

The phenomenon of oral tolerance to dietary antigens was first described over 80 years ago (7). These early studies in guinea pigs indicated that initial exposure commonly provoked immediate hypersensitivity responses, which on continuing exposure waned, leaving the animals in a state of longer-term antigen-specific unresponsiveness that was described as "tolerance." Subsequent studies indicated that the process was more complex and rather than classic tolerance, it involved the selective downregulation of IgE and delayed-type hypersensitivity (DTH), with concomitant sparing of secretory IgA and certain IgG subclass responses (8).

More recently, the nature of the underlying regulatory processes has been demonstrated to be a function of the intensity and duration of antigen exposure. Thus, short-term oral exposure to a small number of moderate-high antigen doses induces classic high-zone tolerance involving T-cell deletion or anergy, whereas prolonged exposure to low concentrations of antigen induces low-zone tolerance, or immune deviation (9,10).

Exposure through the respiratory tract also results in selective elimination of IgE and DTH responses (6). In low-level passive exposure to aerosolized allergens at dosages that approximate the physiological (i.e., environmental) range, the regulatory process involves selective elimination of Th2 immunity by immune deviation, which is mediated by allergen-specific $CD8^+$ T cells (11,12), whereas the use of higher dosages, delivered as intranasal drops, achieves the same result, but appears dependent on $CD4^+$ Th1 cells (13).

Three sets of observations from these studies are of particular relevance to the studies in humans detailed in the following. First, the efficiency of these tolerance processes in both organ systems is genetically determined, being manyfold less effective in rat and mouse strains that express the high-IgE–responder phenotype (14,15). Second, although static high-dose intranasal exposures are partially effective in terminating ongoing IgE responses (e.g., 16), aerosols that mimic normal (low-dose) environmental exposures only serve to further boost antibody production (17), and similar findings have been reported for oral tolerance (18). This suggests that once the Th-cell memory compartment is stabilized, it is relatively refractory to regulation by immune deviation. Third, both oral tolerance and its respiratory tract equivalent are inoperative during the early postnatal period, and early exposure during infancy can lead to T-cell priming as opposed to tolerance (19–21). Moreover, these mechanisms do not become fully functional postnatally until approaching the time of weaning.

Collectively, in relation to applicability to the human situation, these observations underscore (1) the potential importance of the initial response to allergens in immunologically naive individuals (i.e., during early life), (2) the likely relevance of genetic background, and (3) the likelihood that very early postnatal exposures may elicit outcomes that are qualitatively different from those resulting from exposures that are not initiated until later during infancy.

III. Initiation of Allergen-Specific Antibody Responses in Humans: Prospective Seroepidemiological Studies

The central question of "when" do these responses commence has been answered definitively by studies on IgG subclass antibodies to house dust mite (HDM) (22). These studies demonstrated, first, that most infants are born with relatively high titers of maternally derived HDM-specific IgG that is cleared within a few weeks of birth, at which time the infants commence production of their own antibodies (22). IgG responses against food allergens are also initiated at this time and are maintained throughout later life (23).

Parallel IgE production against dietary antigens is also demonstrable at this early time point in infants of the atopic genotype (i.e., with positive family history; FH^+), and typically peaks within the first year of life, before declining in the vast majority of subjects to below levels of detection by age 2 years. These transient responses also occur in family history negative (FH^-) infants, albeit at much lower titers (24–26). This pattern is reminiscent of the situation described earlier for oral tolerance in animals.

The situation for early IgE production against inhalants is more complex. These responses are often not initiated until 1.5–2 years of age (24,26,27), and commonly wax and wane repeatedly in a cyclic fashion for several years before termination (24,27). Moreover, a subset of these responses in a significant (and increasing) proportion of children are not switched off, but instead, continue to climb and become persistent, and are eventually associated with respiratory (atopic) symptoms (24,27). It can thus be postulated that the development of clinical atopic sensitization in these subjects is the result of a failure of the immunoregulatory mechanisms that successfully terminate IgE responses in their nonatopic counterparts.

IV. Allergen-Specific T-Cell Reactivity During the Perinatal Period: In Vitro Lymphoproliferation Studies

The issue of when initial T-cell priming of these responses occurs has been resolved by a series of studies on cord blood mononuclear cells (CBMCs). Several laboratories have recently reported that CBMCs from a high proportion of subjects demonstrate small, but significant, lymphoproliferative responses to both dietary and inhalant allergens (28–31). Considerable scepticism surrounds these reports, owing to the possibility of contamination of CBMCs with T cells of maternal origin during collection. However, we have recently cloned allergen-specific CBMC T cells from a series of subjects, and performed DNA fingerprinting on the latter, in parallel with DNA from maternal cells, and have definitively demonstrated the fetal origin of the responding CBMCs (32).

As part of the latter studies, we also demonstrated that the CBMCs failed to respond to the classic vaccine antigen tetanus toxoid (31), which infants do not normally encounter until their first postnatal vaccination, given that the mothers in our studies were not vaccinated during pregnancy. This suggests that in utero T-cell priming is likely to be the result of transplacental transfer of allergens to which the mothers are exposed at low levels during pregnancy, possibly in combination with IgG antibodies, which (as noted earlier) also cross the placenta. There is also a trend for these responses to be higher in CBMCs from subjects with an atopic family history (32,33), but the differences between the latter and family history negative subjects are inconsistent.

We have additionally performed a series of cross-sectional studies spanning the period from birth to age 2.5 years, paralleled by cross-sectional studies involving young children and adults (31,34). Collectively, these indicate markedly different patterns of age-dependent antigen-specific lymphoproliferative activity, comparing food with inhalant allergens. Thus, responses to the archetypal food allergen ovalbumin (OVA) increase in frequency from approximately 40% of CBMC to in the order of 70% during infancy, but decline thereafter, such that less than 20% of samples from 5 year olds or adults respond, and the latter positive responses are extremely weak. In contrast, responses to the archetypal inhalant allergen, house dust mite (HDM), increase slowly in frequency and magnitude between infancy and early childhood, and expand further into adulthood, such that virtually 100% of subjects (both atopic and nonatopic) respond vigorously (31,34), and these are polarized toward either the Th1 (in normals) or Th2 (in atopics) cytokine profile. We have accordingly hypothesized that the underlying regulation of responses to inhalants is dominated by low-zone tolerance (immune deviation) mechanisms that result in selection for Th1-dominant versus Th2-dominant T-cell memory, as opposed to high-zone tolerance mechanisms (T-cell deletion or anergy) for dietary allergens. This general hypothesis is consistent with reports from the animal models cited earlier on the significance of antigen dosage in "selection" of respective control mechanisms for low- versus high-level exposures.

In indirect support of the role of high-zone tolerance mechanisms in regulation of responses to dietary allergens, we have shown a marked age-dependent reduction in the number of OVA epitopes recognized during early childhood (34). Additionally, earlier reports have provided evidence for a form of T-cell anergy in relation to anti-OVA responses in children, characterized by allergen-induced expression of the interleukin-2 receptor (IL-2R) on T-cells in the absence of responsiveness to exogenous IL-2 (35,36).

V. Allergen-Specific Cytokine Responses During Childhood

There is limited information available in this area, but nevertheless, some broad principles have been established. Our recent cross-sectional studies (34,36a) involving cohorts of up to 60 subjects indicate that by median age 1.5 years, FH^+ children typically respond to either OVA or HDM by production of IL-4, IL-5, as well as interferon gamma (IFN-γ), whereas FH^- subjects express weak responsiveness by IFN-γ secretion; cytokine responses correlated poorly with symptoms. However, at the age of 5 years we were able to segregate children into HDM-response positive, versus nonresponsive by the skin prick test (SPT), the latter correlating strongly with personal history of symptoms; SPT^+ subjects responded consistently in vitro to HDM by secretion of IL-4, IL-5, IL-9, IL-13, and IFN-γ, whereas SPT^- subjects produced only low levels of IFN-γ. Very few weak responses to OVA were observed in either group.

These findings indicate that as early as 5 years of age, the pattern of Th2-polarized allergen-specific immunity associated with adult atopic respiratory disease, is already firmly entrenched in immunological memory in susceptible children (34).

VI. Transplacental T-Cell Priming and the Immunology of Pregnancy

Ongoing studies in our laboratory (32,37) are focusing on the nature of the cytokine responses that precede those described in the foregoing (i.e., during fetal life). Because of the T-cell low precursor frequencies in these early responses, detection of allergen-specific cytokine production is generally restricted to the use of semiquantitative reverse transcription–polymerase chain reaction (sqRT–PCR) analysis of mRNA. Employing this technique to examine RNA extracts from allergen-stimulated CBMCs, we have observed almost universal reactivity to both OVA and HDM, typically characterized by coproduction of message for IL-4, IL-5, and IL-9; corresponding IFN-γ signals are much weaker or absent.

However, two cytokines are produced in sufficient amounts for detection of protein by conventional enzyme-linked immunosorbent assay (ELISA), IL-13 and IL-10, the latter being secreted at extremely high levels in culture (up to 3000 pg/mL supernatant at the 24-hr time point in allergen-stimulated microcultures). These responses (in particular to OVA) were often more intense in samples from FH^+ subjects, but nevertheless, virtually all subjects display Th2-polarized responses to both classes of allergens, regardless of family history.

This provides a logical explanation for the sensitization "window" in infancy, associated with early postnatal exposure to high levels of inhalant allergens (38,39); i.e., this early exposure facilitates rapid expansion of weakly primed allergen-specific Th2 cells, leading to development and consolidation of long-term Th2 memory (further discussion follows).

There is additionally a plausible explanation at hand for this enigmatic finding, as a result of recent research developments relating to the immunology of pregnancy. A large body of evidence (e.g., see Refs. 40–44) indicates that the cytokine milieu at the fetomaternal interface is constitutively polarized away from Th1, to protect the placenta from the highly toxic effects of Th1 Cytokines (especially IFN–γ). This appears to be orchestrated at the level of the placenta, in which trophoblasts produce and secrete large amounts of IL-4, together with the Th1-antagonistic cytokine IL-10 (45); the resulting Th2 polarization of fetal immune responses may be further enhanced by local production of progesterone, which is also tropic for Th2 cells (46).

VII. Kinetics of Postnatal Maturation of Th1-Associated Immune Functions as a "Risk Factor" for Atopy

Although it is clear that in utero expression of Th1 immunity requires tight negative control to ensure fetal survival by preservation of the integrity of the placental unit, it is equally clear that postnatal survival requires effective Th1 immunity to survive challenge from microbial pathogens. Hence, it is axiomatic that Th1 functions must mature progressively during early infancy to a significant level to maintain homeostasis, as protection mediated by maternally derived immunoglobulins declines. However, it may be expected that a "window period" exists postnatally during which maturing Th1 functions are relatively ineffective, possibly spanning the period up to weaning, at which time maternal-derived protection terminates.

This indeed appears to be true in experimental animals, in which parenteral antigen challenge during infancy leads to preferential expansion of Th2 cells, effectively "locking out" Th1 immunity (47–53). A similar situation occurs in humans, as peripheral blood mononuclear cells (PBMC) from children younger than 5 years display a marked deficit in IFN-γ production relative to adults (54–57). There is additionally accumulating evidence that this deficit may be more marked in association with the atopic genotype, given that production of IFN-γ by polyclonally stimulated mononuclear cells from FH^+ cord blood (29,58–61) and also from T-cell clones from FH^+ 2 year olds (62), are significantly reduced relative to FH^- donors.

The strongest supporting evidence for a maturational defect in Th1-associated immune function in atopics has been provided by a recent retrospective study on BCG vaccination history in Japanese school children (63). These children were given initial BCG vaccinations at 3 months of age, and skin tested for tuberculin responses at age 6; nonresponders were revaccinated, and all subjects were retested at entry into the study at age 12, enabling identification of those who had again failed to respond at age 6. Significantly, those who failed to develop Th1-dependent tuberculin reactivity at ages 3 months and 6 years exhibited 32% prevalence of atopy and 13% asthma, in marked contrast with those who responded to first or second vaccination in whom prevalence rates of atopy or asthma were, respectively, only 8 and 4% (63).

VIII. Regulation of Neonatal Th1 Immunity: The Key Role of Antigen-Presenting Cells

A recent series of reports on the phenomenon of neonatal tolerance (51–53), a process characterized by the apparent "tolerance" of adult mice to exogenous antigens to which they were exposed during infancy, has revealed that the underlying mechanism does not involve classic tolerance (T-cell deletion or anergy), but instead, immune deviation. Thus, owing to the postnatal persistence of the fetal "skewing" of immune responses away from the Th1 phenotype, antigen challenge in infancy generates covert low-level Th2 memory; after rechallenge with the same antigen in adulthood, Th2 memory cells are activated and deviate immune responses away from Th1, thereby inhibiting the development of the Th1-dependent responses (especially the DTH and IgG subclass antibody production) classically employed to assess immune reactivity in these experimental models.

Additionally, if endogenous antigen-presenting cells (APC) in the infant mice were bypassed by challenging them with antigen-pulsed syngeneic dendritic cells (DC; the principal APC responsible for priming naive T cells) instead of free antigen, they generated normal Th1 responses (52). The latter finding is consistent with current notions that competent DC are specialized for polarization of T-cell responses towards the Th1 cytokine phenotype (64), in keeping with their role in the generation of primary antimicrobial immunity (65), particularly at mucosal surfaces (66,67).

We have recently demonstrated that airway intraepithelial DC populations, which are highly likely to play a determining role in Th1 to Th2 switch regulation in responses to inhalant allergens, develop very slowly postnatally, and they do not attain adult-equivalent functional capacity until after weaning (68,69). These studies were restricted to rodents. Although there is as yet no formal evidence for a similar DC defect in human infants, indirect evidence strongly suggests that this is true both for DC and other APC populations. Thus, a significant proportion (but not all) of the human infants' deficit in IFN-γ production following polyclonal T-cell stimulation can be restored by addition of small numbers of maternal T-cell–depleted mononuclear cells, indicating that part of the defect is due to poor costimulator activity infant APC (55,56; see also Ref. 70).

IX. Postnatal Maturation of Adaptive Immune Functions: Evidence of Widespread Developmental Deficiencies During Infancy

As well as likely deficiencies in DC function, infants appear to manifest varying levels of functional incapacity in several cellular compartments. The most significant of these in relation to allergy is the T-cell compartment itself. As noted in a recent review (57), infant human T cells display diminished responsiveness to a variety of polyclonal stimuli, including anti-CD2 and anti-CD3, and also to a variety of cytokines including IL-2; the latter may be a consequence of underexpression of cytokine receptors, a recently reported example being the IL-2Rγ chain (71). These infant T cells also underproduce cytokines such as IL-4 and, particularly, IFN-γ, both in bulk culture and after cloning, suggesting that the differences between infants and adults in this context are not due to variations in respective T-memory compartments, but instead, are due to intrinsic differences between naive infant T cells and adult naive T cells (57). The notion that a phenotypically immature fetal T-cell population persists at the periphery into postnatal life is also consistent with recent studies on the responses of infant T cells to bacterial superantigens, which demonstrate that they are much more susceptible to anergy induction than their functionally mature adult counterparts (72).

Of particular relevance to the role of APC in Th1–Th2 switch regulation during infancy, are recent findings relevant to IL-12 regulation. It is recognized that the principal mechanism employed by DC to skew primary immune responses toward Th1 is by secretion of IL-12 (73,74). However, DCs do not produce IL-12 constitutively, and require an activation stimulus, the most potent being CD40L expressed on the surface of activated T cells (75). Recent studies indicate that CD40L is underexpressed on human neonatal T cells (76–78) and, moreover, that this deficiency persists into infancy (78), and the rapidity with which this function matures postnatally may be a significant rate-limiting factor in the overall kinetics of development of immunocompetence. In addition, naive neonatal T cells are hyporesponsive to IL-12 relative to adult naive T cells (79).

Interestingly, responsiveness to lipopolysaccharide (LPS), the second most potent stimulant for IL-12 production by DCs (and other APCs), is also reduced during infancy, principally owing to hypoproduction of the LPS-carrier protein that engages the low-affinity LPS-receptor on human mononuclear cells (80).

X. Induction and Expression of Atopic Respiratory Disease: A Working Hypothesis

The scheme depicted in Figure 1 represents an attempt to integrate the foregoing findings into a broad, working model that describes the key immunological events underlying the postnatal development of susceptibility of resistance to respiratory allergy.

Thus, initial T-cell priming commonly occurs in utero, resulting in development of weak Th2-polarized allergen-specific immunological memory. This Th2 polarization appears likely to be due (at least partly) to the inability of fetal APC to deliver an accompanying Th1-deviating signal to fetal T cells, when they present incoming (maternally-derived) allergen; in the absence of such a signal, ensuing T-cell responses will theoretically default toward the Th2 phenotype under the influence of IL-4 produced by naive T cells (81,82). Consequently, if high levels of inhalant allergen are encountered during the immediate postnatal period, it is

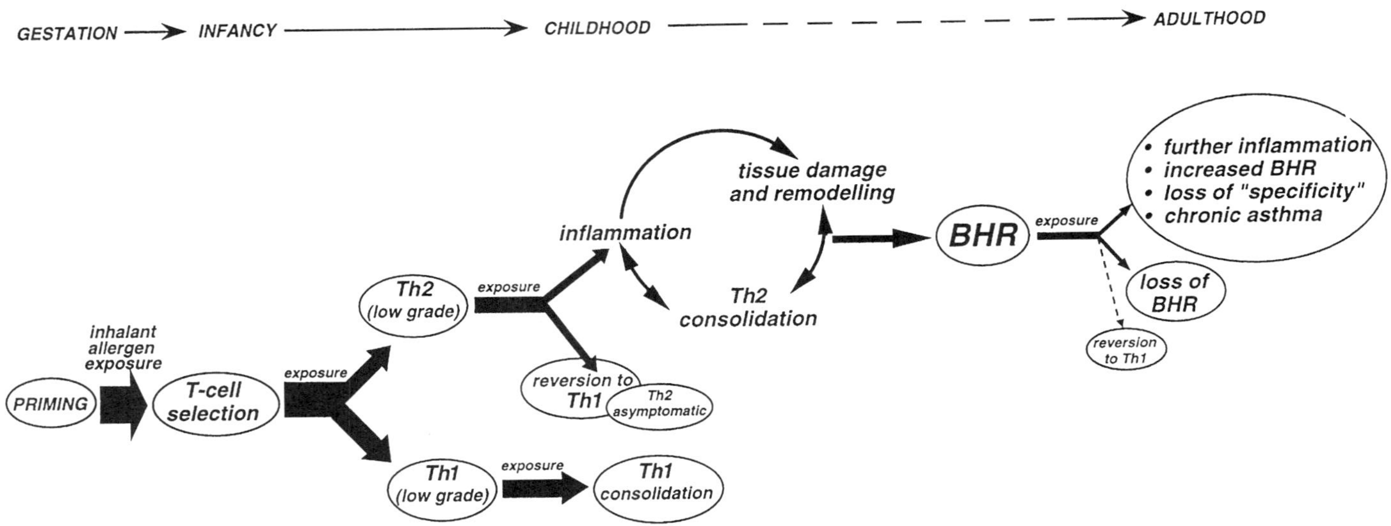

Figure 1 The natural history of allergic respiratory disease—the immunological perspective. (From Ref. 114.)

reasonable to propose that weakly primed Th2 responses are rapidly amplified, potentially leading to consolidation of Th2 memory, which could permanently lock these responses into the Th2 phenotype; such a scenario may explain the well-known sensitization window in infancy.

However, as the airway mucosal DC population matures, it will presumably deliver increasingly potent allergen-specific Th1-deviating signals, which should progressively select against Th2. Clearly, this fails in a subset of children, as shown in our in vitro studies (34) and by recent epidemiology (83), which indicates that up to 40% of young children express Th2-dependent SPT-reactivity to one or more inhalant allergens. Nevertheless, expression of Th2-polarized reactivity to inhalants during childhood does not of itself, connote susceptibility to chronic respiratory allergy, for the frequency of suffers among the adult population is considerably less than this initial 40%. This infers an inherent capacity of the immune system to spontaneously redeviate Th2 responses in children back to Th1, consistent with observed age-dependent patterns of serum IgE antibody and SPT reactivity (84). It is also clear that a significant subset of adult subjects with positive SPT responses to inhalants either remain asymptomatic or manifest only mild disease, as opposed to chronic asthma, suggesting that allergy to inhalants is not necessarily sufficient by itself for the induction of severe airways disease.

The scheme in Figure 1 echoes an increasingly widely held view in this field, that the "missing link" is local inflammation in the airways. It is evident that a hallmark of atopic asthma is local activation of $CD4^+$ Th2 cells in the airway mucosa, and this local T-cell activation is believed to be the key factor in triggering repeated cycles of cell-mediated inflammation, involving eosinophils and a variety of other effector cells (85–87). This results in a vicious circle of tissue damage, wound-healing responses, and progressive amplification of Th2 reactivity by the inherent "adjuvant" effects of the inflammation itself, ultimately leading to the phenotypic changes in the local tissue milieu that manifest as hyperresponsiveness to irritant stimuli (BHR).

Why does this occur in some Th2-responsive subjects, but not in others? Although the answer is unclear, it is pertinent that a series of control mechanisms normally operate in lung and airway tissues to dampen local T-cell activation, including those targeted at local APC (in particular DC; 88) as well as responding T cells (89–92), and it is possible that these may fail in severe atopics.

This model also provides a useful framework for systematic analysis of the effects of respiratory virus infection on the pathogenesis of atopic asthma. It is reasonable to speculate that, in addition to their immediate effects in precipitating asthma attacks in children with preexisting BHR (93), virus infections may act synergistically with allergen-responsive Th2 cells in the vicious cycle phase of the process outlined in Figure 1. However, it is also conceivable, given the effects of virus infection in triggering large natural killer (NK)-cell–mediated and $CD8^+$–T-cell–mediated Th1-like responses in both the airway mucosa and downstream draining lymph nodes, that virus infections during the period of allergen-driven Th1–Th2 cross-regulation in infancy preceding commitment to a particular cytokine phenotype, may actually be protective (i.e., by production of Th1-selective "bystander" IFN-γ signals; 94). This thesis is consistent with recent suggestions (e.g., see Refs. 95,96) that respiratory infections in the first year of life are negatively associated with atopic respiratory disease beyond the age of 5 years, whereas infections occurring later appear to have the opposite effect (93). The frequency of these early infections (95,96) may be a factor in the East–West gradient in allergy prevalence (96,97), and in the inverse relation between prevalence and family size (98) and social class (99).

XI. Theoretical Options for Early Intervention

Given the foregoing model, five major types of strategy appear to be worthy of further exploration, as follows.

A. Environmental Control Measures Especially in the Nursery

It is clear that reduction of levels of exposure to inhalant allergens should have a beneficial effect on disease development, at a variety of levels. There is increasing evidence that the intensity of allergic respiratory disease in SPT^+ atopics is positively correlated with domestic levels of the major allergen(s) to which they respond (100), and there is justifiably increasing interest in the use of allergen reduction techniques as an adjunct to treatment of established disease with anti-inflammatory drugs. Nevertheless, there are clearly limitations to how well such procedures can work, given that many inhalant allergens come from sources outside the home, and it is not yet clear as to the precise thresholds that need to be met for each allergen. In addition, to be effective in established disease, the measures need to be rigorously and continuously applied, with attendant problems of compliance as well as cost.

However, a more cogent case can be made for the period preceding development of disease. The epidemiology linking maximal risk of primary allergic sensitization to very early postnatal exposure to inhalant allergens is clear-cut (39,40), particularly in infants with positive atopic family history (101), and this phenomenon is now cogently explicable on the basis of intrauterine Th2-skewed priming against allergens to which the mother is exposed. Thus, a case can be made for focusing on the first 3–6 months of life, particularly in genetically at-risk infants, with an extremely aggressive program of environmental allergen reduction, which could then be progressively eased to procedures that are less taxing on the parents. Such a two-phase approach may have considerably greater long-term benefits than the currently practiced single-level eradication procedures. Given the increasingly high prevalence of atopy among children, a case could also be made for the formal (and mandatory) introduction of allergen-reduction procedures in obstetric and neonatal wards in hospitals.

B. The Early Use of Anti-inflammatory Drugs

A central element in the model in Figure 1 is the vicious cycle of chronic inflammation that underlies the changes in the local tissue milieu in the airway mucosa, that ultimately results in BHR. The intrinsic propensity of DC throughout the body to skew immune responses toward the Th1 phenotype, as argued in the foregoing, provides a potent mechanism for the immune system to ultimately rectify the "mistake" of Th2 sensitization, and although this clearly occurs in a large proportion of SPT^+ children, it must fail in those who develop chronic atopy. The population dynamics of airway mucosal DC is markedly upregulated in response to virtually all allergenic–antigenic and microbial stimuli (66,67), and indirect evidence of similar changes is accumulating in relation to atopic human adults (102,103). These changes are likely to be accompanied by variations in both quantitative and qualitative aspects of their APC activity, both in situ and after migration to draining lymph nodes (DLN); the latter are highly likely to include IL-10–mediated downregulation of IL-12 production (104), given that recruitment of monocytes into airway mucosal tissue is also an integral part of this inflammatory cycle (86).

In principle if the cycle can be broken long enough to permit reestablishment of local immunological homeostasis in the airway mucosa—which, by definition, includes (1) maintenance of local DC in an antigen "surveillance" as opposed to "presentation" mode (88); (2) absence locally of significant numbers of alternative APCs, such as B cells and monocytes; and (3) continual translation of incoming inhalant allergen into a Th1-skewing signals by DC after they migrate to DLN—the process leading to establishment of BHR may be permanently terminated.

Accordingly, a logical case can be made for the early use of topical steroids in children, at a stage before they manifest full-blown allergic respiratory disease, and several such trials targeting different age groups are currently in progress in different parts of Europe and the United States. However, concern has been raised over possible growth retardation effects of these drugs; hence, such trials need to be approached with caution.

The recruitment of DC into the airway mucosa in rats during the steady-state and also during acute inflammation is highly sensitive to steroids (105), and evidence has recently been presented of similar effects in atopic humans (103). However, we have also shown that steroids do not prevent resident DC from presenting preprocessed antigen to T cells, provided a source of granulocyte–macrophage colony-stimulating factor (GM-CSF) is present (106), which it is in the atopic airway epithelium (107). It is unclear, therefore, what the net effects of topical steroids would be in the context of the foregoing model—it is conceivable that they may be efficacious in minimizing in situ T-cell activation, but by interfering with DC communication between the airway mucosa and T cells in the DLN, they may at the same time inhibit the "self-curing" element of the host immune response by diminution of incoming DC-borne allergen-specific Th1-polarizing signals. Whether a beneficial balance between these two opposing possibilities can be struck, remains to be determined.

It is possible that these considerations may not apply to nonsteroidal anti-inflammatories, which may open up further possibilities. Of particular theoretical interest are mast cell stabilizing agents such as cromolyn sodium (Intal), which has been used for many years in pediatric practice, but generally with older age groups in whom disease is already established.

C. Active "Vaccination" Strategies

An active vaccination strategy (6,108) is based on the notion that the process underlying Th1 or Th2 selection in these responses during early childhood should be highly susceptible to exogenous Th1-selective immune-deviating signals. Several approaches are theoretically possible, including the very early use of conventional immunotherapy, which in adults generates strong Th1-selection signals (109,110), antigen feeding in an effort to harness the potent combination of high- and low-zone tolerance mechanisms that appears to underlie the effectiveness of oral tolerance (6), or administration of tolerogenic doses of allergen by intranasal drops, which generates potential Th1-selective signals in mice (13,16).

Preliminary trials using these principles are currently in the planning phase in several centers.

D. The "Adjuvant" Approach

Sluggish postnatal maturation of immunocompetence, particularly in the APC compartment, appears to be a major risk factor for development of allergy. I have argued previously that the principal signal for the postnatal development of Th1-switching capacity in DC is likely to be contact with the microbial world, in particular by the LPS "signature" of bacteria, for which a series of high- and low-affinity receptors exist on bone marrow-derived cells (95). The clearest illustration of this principle comes from the gnotobiology literature that indicates that animals maintained in a germ-free state fail to develop Th1-dependent immune function postnatally (e.g., see Ref. 111). The most potent stimulus in this context is provided by the bacterial flora of the gastrointestinal tract, which are normally established during early postnatal life.

Thus, it may be possible to hasten the postnatal maturation of immunocompetence by either actively promoting the establishment of a "normal" gastrointestinal flora (for example, by dietary means), or by the use of oral or parenteral microbial-based stimulants that mimic the natural effects of the normal flora. Several such oral preparations are employed currently around the world for enhancing general immune function in immunocompromised adults and children, but they have not yet been tested in the context of atopic disease.

It is intriguing to contemplate the possible effects of overuse of antibiotics in pediatric practice, which is a worldwide problem.

E. Treating the Mother

The emerging picture of virtually universal selective Th2-priming of allergen-specific immune responses in utero, taken with the epidemiology indicating that this process may be amplified in persons who are atopic, raises the obvious question of whether it may be possible to manipulate the priming process in the developing fetus by the transplacental route.

Formal proof that fetal immune responses can be generated by active immunization of mothers has been recently supplied by studies on tetanus vaccination (112); however, there is no evidence that such an approach with allergens would do anything to modulate the overall Th2 bias at the fetomaternal interface.

Perhaps of more direct relevance to this discussion, a study on 14 subjects has shown that specific immunotherapy during pregnancy had a small, but nonsignificant, effect on levels of allergen-specific IgE and IgG in their offspring in later life (113). However, the small sample size, and marginal nature of the effects, makes it difficult to conclude anything from the study.

There are tantalizing (but as yet indefinitive) indications that the degree of Th2 polarization of allergen-specific responses at birth may be greatest in children genetically predisposed to atopy. If so, a case could be made (and is being made in some circles) for promoting allergen avoidance during pregnancy, particularly for atopic mothers. Although this may prove to be useful, it is a loaded issue that must be approached with great caution. The ramifications of providing advice to pregnant women that might be extrapolated or misconstrued in such a way that it could limit intake of essential nutrients present in dietary items known to contain allergens, are potentially serious. Moreover, given the virtually universal nature of this neonatal Th2-skewed priming, it may yet prove to be part of the normal "education" process by which the developing immune system is instructed about the antigenic nature of the normal extrauterine environment.

It is not unreasonable to speculate that this initial Th2 polarization, at least for dietary allergens, may in fact protect against the postnatal development of strong Th1-polarized immunity of these agents, which might have much more severe pathogenic consequences than the discomforts of transient Th2 immunity.

References

1. Wierenga EA, Snoek M, de Groot C, Chrétien I, Bos JD, Jansen HM, Kapsenberg ML. Evidence for compartmentalization of functional subsets of $CD2^+$ T lymphocytes in atopic patients. J Immunol 1990; 144:4651–4656.
2. Romagnani S. Induction of T_H1 and T_H2 responses: a key role for the "natural" immune response? Immunol Today 1992; 13:379–381.

3. O'Hehir RE, Hoyne GF, Thomas WR, Lamb JR. House dust mite allergy: from T cell epitopes to immunotherapy. Eur J Clin Invest 1993; 23:763–772.
4. Upham JW, Holt BJ, Baron-Hay MJ, Yabuhara A, Hales BJ, Thomas WR, Loh RKS, O'Keeffe P, Palmer P, Le Souef P. Inhalant allergen-specific T-cell reactivity is detectable in close to 100% of atopic and normal individuals: covert responses are unmasked for serum-free medium. Clin Exp Allergy 1995; 25:634–642.
5. Imada M, Estelle F, Simons R, Jay FT, Hayglass KT. Allergen-stimulated interleukin-4 and interferon-γ production in primary culture: responses of subjects with allergic rhinitis and normal controls. Immunology 1995; 85:373–380.
6. Holt PG. Immunoprophylaxis of atopy: light at the end of the tunnel? Immunol Today 1994; 15:484–489.
7. Wells HG, Osborne TB. The biological reactions of the vegetable proteins. I. Anaphylaxis. J Infect Dis 1911: 8:66–124.
8. Mowat AM. The regulation of immune responses to dietary protein antigens. Immunol Today 1987; 8:93–98.
9. Gregerson DS, Obritsch WF, Donoso LA. Oral tolerance in experimental autoimmune uveoretinitis. J Immunol 1993; 151:5751–5761.
10. Friedman A, Weiner HL. Induction of anergy or active suppression following oral tolerance is determined by antigen dosage. Proc Natl Acad Sci USA 1994; 91:6688–6692.
11. McMenamin C, Holt PG. The natural immune response to inhaled soluble protein antigens involves major histocompatibility complex (MHC) class I-restricted $CD8^+$ T cell-mediated by MHC class II-restricted $CD4^+$ T cell-dependent immune deviation resulting in selective suppression of IgE production. J Exp Med 1993; 178:889–899.
12. McMenamin C, Pimm C, McKersey M, Holt PG. Regulation of IgE responses to inhaled antigen in mice by antigen-specific gamma delta T cells. Science 1994; 265:1869–1871.
13. Hoyne GF, Asknonas BA, Hetzel C, Thomas WR, Lamb JR. Regulation of house dust mite responses by inhaled peptides: transient activation precedes the development of tolerance in vivo. Int Immunol 1996; 8:335–342.
14. Sedgwick JD, Holt PG. Suppression of IgE responses in inbred rats by repeated respiratory tract exposure to antigen: responder phenotype influences isotype specificity of induced tolerance. Eur J Immunol 1984; 14:893–897.
15. Holt PG, Britten D, Sedgwick JD. Suppression of IgE responses by antigen inhalation: studies on the role of genetic and environmental factors. Immunology 1987; 60:97–102.
16. Hoyne GF, O'Hehir RE, Wraith DC, Thomas WR, Lamb JR. Inhibition of T-cell and antibody responses to house dust mite allergen by inhalation or the dominant epitope in naive and sensitised mice. J Exp Med 1993; 178:1783–1788.
17. Holt PG, Leivers S. Tolerance induction via antigen inhalation: isotype specificity, stability, and involvement of suppressor T cells. Int Arch Allergy Appl Immunol 1982; 67:155–160.
18. Hanson DG, Vaz NM, Rawlings LA, Lynch JM. Inhibition of specific immune responses by feeding protein antigens. II. Effects of prior passive and active immunization. J Immunol 1979; 122:2261–2265.
19. Strobel S, Ferguson A. Immune responses to fed protein antigens in mice. 3. Systemic tolerance or priming is related to age at which antigen is first encountered. Pediatr Res 1984; 18:588–594.
20. Hanson DG. Ontogeny of orally induced tolerance to soluble proteins in mice. I. Priming and tolerance in newborns. J Immunol 1981; 127:1518–1524.
21. Nelson D, McMenamin C, Wilkes L, Holt PG. Postnatal development of respiratory mucosal immune function in the rat: regulation of IgE responses to inhaled allergen. Pediatr Allergy Immunol 1991; 4:170–177.
22. Mariani F, Price JF, Kemeny DM. The IgG subclass antibody response to an inhalant antigen (*Dermatophagoides pteronyssinus*) during the first year of life: evidence for early stimulation of the immune system following natural exposure. Clin Exp Allergy 1992; 22:29–33.

23. Devey ME, Beckman S, Kemeny DM. The functional affinities of antibodies of different IgG subclass to dietary antigens in mothers and their babies. Clin Exp Immunol 1993; 94:117–121.
24. Hattevig G, Kjellman B, Björkstén B. Clinical symptoms and IgE responses to common proteins and inhalants in the first 7 years of life. Clin Allergy 1987; 17:571–578.
25. Van Asperen PP, Kemp AS. The natural history of IgE sensitisation and atopic disease in early childhood. Acta Paediatr Scand 1989; 78:239–245.
26. Hattevig G, Kjellman B, Björkstén B. Appearance IgE antibodies to ingested and inhaled allergens during the first 12 years of life in atopic and non-atopic children. Pediatr Allergy Immunol 1993; 4:182–186.
27. Rowntree S, Cogswell JJ, Platts-Mills TAE, Mitchell EB. Development of IgE and IgG antibodies to food and inhalant allergens in children at risk of allergic disease. Arch Dis Child 1985; 60:727–735.
28. Kondo N, Kobayashi Y, Shinodoa S, Kasahara K, Kameyama T, Iwasa S, Orri T. Cord blood lymphocyte responses to food antigens for the prediction of allergic disorders. Arch Dis Child 1992; 67:1003–1007.
29. Piastra M, Stabile A, Fioravanti G, Castagnola M, Pani G, Ria F. Cord blood mononuclear cell responsiveness to beta-lactoglobulin: T-cell activity in "atopy-prone" and "non–atopy-prone" newborns. Int Arch Allergy Immunol 1994; 104:358–365.
30. Piccini M-P, Mecacci F, Sampognaro S, Manetti R, Parronchi P, Maggi E, Romagnani S. Aeroallergen sensitization can occur during fetal life. Int Arch Allergy Immunol 1993; 102:301–303.
31. Holt PG, O'Keeffe PO, Holt BJ, Upham JW, Baron-Hay MJ, Suphioglu C, Knox B, Stewart GA, Thomas WR, Sly PD. T-cell "priming" against environmental allergens in human neonates: sequential deletion of food antigen specificities during infancy with concomitant expansion of responses to ubiquitous inhalant allergens. Pediatr Allergy Immunol 1995; 6:85–90.
32. Prescott SL, Macaubas C, Holt BJ, Smallacombe T, Loh R, Sly PD, Holt PG. Transplacental priming of the human immune system to environmental allergens: universal skewing of initial T-cell responses towards the Th-2 cytokine profile. J Immunol 1998; 160:4730–4737.
33. Warner JA, Miles EA, Jones AC, Quint DJ, Colwell BM, Warner JO. Is deficiency of interferon gamma production by allergen triggered cord blood cells a predictor of atopic eczema? Clin Exp Allergy 1994; 24:423–430.
34. Yabuhara A, Macaubas C, Prescott SL, Venaille T, Holt BJ, Habre W, Sly PD, Holt PG. Th-2-polarised immunological memory to inhalant allergens in atopics is established during infancy and early childhood. Clin Exp Allergy. 1997; 27:1261–1269.
35. Noma T, Yoshizawa I, Maeda K, Ichikawa K, Baba M, Yata J. Allergen-specific induction of interleukin-2 (IL-2) responsiveness in lymphocytes from children with asthma. J Allergy Clin Immunol 1989; 84:255–262.
36. Noma T, Kawano Y, Yoshizawa I, Itoh M, Mukouyama T, Baba M, Yata J. Ovalbumin-specific induction of IL-2 responsiveness in lymphocytes from patients with hen egg allergy and its regulation by the culture supernatant of normal lymphocytes. Ann Allergy 1990; 64:33–41.
36a. Macaubas C, Sly PD, Burton P, Tiller K, Yabuhara A, Holt BJ, Smallacombe TB, Kendall G, Jenmalm M, Holt PG. Regulation of Th-cell responses to inhalant allergens during early childhood. Submitted.
37. Prescott SL, Macaubas C, Yabuhara A, Venaille TJ, Holt BJ, Habre W, Loh R, Sly PD, Holt PG. Development patterns of T cell memory to environmental allergens in the first two years of life. Int Arch Allergy Immunol 1997; 113:75–79.
38. Holt PG, McMenamin C, Nelson D. Primary sensitisation to inhalant allergens during infancy. Pediatr Allergy Immunol 1990; 1:3–13.
39. Björkstén B. Risk factors in early childhood for the development of atopic diseases. Allergy 1994; 49:400–407.

40. Wegmann TG, Lin H, Guilbert L, Mosmann TR. Bidirectional cytokine interactions in the maternal–fetal relationship: is successful pregnancy a Th2 phenomenon? Immunol Today 1993; 14:353–356.
41. Krishnan L, Guilbert LJ, Russell AS, Wegmann TG, Mosmann TR, Belosevic M. Pregnancy impairs resistance of C57BL/6 mice to *Leishmania major* infection and causes decreased antigen-specific IFN-γ responses and increased production of T helper 2 cytokines. J Immunol 1996; 156:644–652.
42. Krishnan L, Guilbert LJ, Wegmann TG, Belosevic M, Mosmann TR. T helper 1 response against *Leishmania major* in pregnant C57BL/6 mice increases implantation failure and fetal resorptions. J Immunol 1996; 156:653–662.
43. Lin H, Mosmann TR, Guilbert L, Tuntipopipat S, Segmann TG. Synthesis of T helper 2-type cytokines at the maternal–fetal interface. J Immunol 1993; 151:4562–4573.
44. Mosmann TR, Sad S. The expanding universe of T-cell subsets: Th1, Th2 and more. Immunol Today 1996; 17:138–146.
45. Roth MD, Golub SH. Human pulmonary macrophages utilize prostaglandins and transforming growth factor β_1 to suppress lymphocyte activation. J Leukoc Biol 1993; 53:366–371.
46. Piccinni M-P, Giudizi M-G, Biagiotti R, Beloni L, Giannarini L, Sampognaro S, Parronchi P, Manetti R, Annunziato F, Livi C. Progesterone favours the development of human T helper cells producing Th2-type cytokines and promotes both IL-4 production and membrane CD30 expression in established Th1 cell clones. J Immunol 1995; 155:128–133.
47. Chen N, Gao Q, Field EH. Expansion of memory Th2 cells over Th1 cells in neonatal primed mice. Transplantation 1995; 60:1187–1193.
48. Chen N, Field EH. Enhanced type 2 and diminished type 1 cytokines in neonatal tolerance. Transplantation 1995; 59:933–941.
49. Barrios C, Brawand P, Berney M, Brandt C, Lambert P-H, Siegrist C-A. Neonatal and early life immune responses to various forms of vaccine antigens qualitatively differ from adult responses: predominance of a Th2-biased pattern which persists after adult boosting. Eur J Immunol 1996; 26:1489–1496.
50. Barrios C, Brandt C, Berney M, Lambert P-H, Siegrist C-A. Partial correction of the Th2/Th1 imbalance in neonatal murine responses to vaccine antigens through selective adjuvant effects. Eur J Immunol 1996; 26:2666–2670.
51. Singh RR, Hahn BH, Sercarz EE. Neonatal peptide exposure can prime T cells, and upon subsequent immunization induce their immune deviation: implications for antibody vs. T cell-mediated autoimmunity. J Exp Med 1996; 183:1613–1622.
52. Ridge JP, Fuchs EJ, Matzinger P. Neonatal tolerance revisited: turning on newborn T cells with dendritic cells. Science 1996; 271:1723–1726.
53. Forsthuber T, Yip HC, Lehmann PV. Induction of T_h1 and T_h2 immunity in neonatal mice. Science 1996; 271:1728–1730.
54. Miyawaki T, Seki H, Taga K, Sato H, Taniguchi N. Dissociated production of interleukin-2 and immune (γ) interferon by phytohaemaglutinin stimulated lymphocytes in healthy infants. Clin Exp Immunol 1985; 59:505–511.
55. Taylor S, Bryson YJ. Impaired production of γ-interferon by newborn cells in vitro is due to a functionally immature macrophage. J Immunol 1985; 134:1493–1498.
56. Wilson CB, Westall J, Johnston L, Lewis DB, Dover SK, Apert AR. Decreased production of interferon gamma by human neonatal cells. Intrinsic and regulatory deficiencies. J Clin Invest 1986; 77:860–867.
57. Holt PG. Postnatal maturation of immune competence during infancy and early childhood. Pediatr Allergy Immunol 1995; 6:59–70.
58. Rinas U, Horneff G, Wahn V. Interferon-γ production by cord-blood mononuclear cells is reduced in newborns with a family history of atopic disease and is independent from cord blood IgE-levels. Pediatr Allergy Immunol 1993; 4:60–64.
59. Tang MLK, Kemp AS, Thorburn J, Hill DJ. Reduced interferon-γ secretion in neonates and subsequent atopy. Lancet 1994; 344:983–986.
60. Martinez FD, Stern DA, Wright AL, Holberg CJ, Taussig LM, Halonen M. Association of

interleukin-2 and interferon-γ production by blood mononuclear cells in infancy with parental allergy skin tests and with subsequent development of atopy. J Allergy Clin Immunol 1995; 96:652–660.

61. Liao SY, Liao TN, Chiang BL, Huang MS, Chen CC, Chou CC, Hsieh KH. Decreased production of IFNγ and decreased production of IL-6 by cord blood mononuclear cells of newborns with a high risk of allergy. Clin Exp Allergy 1996; 26:397–405.
62. Holt PG, Clough JB, Holt BJ, Baron-Hay MJ, Rose AH, Robinson BWS, Thomas WR. Genetic "risk" for atopy is associated with delayed postnatal maturation of T-cell competence. Clin Exp Allergy 1992; 22:1093–1099.
63. Shirakawa T, Enomoto T, Shimazu S, Hopkin JM. Inverse association between tuberculin responses and atopic disorder. Science 1997; 275:77–79.
64. De Becker G, Sornasse T, Nabavi N, Bazin H, Tielemans F, Urbain J, Leo O, Moser M. Immunoglobulin isotype regulation by antigen-presenting cells in vivo. Eur J Immunol 1994; 24:1523–1528.
65. Janeway CA. The immune response evolved to discriminate infectious nonself from noninfectious self. Immunol Today 1992; 13:11–16.
66. McWilliam AS, Nelson D, Thomas JA, Holt PG. Rapid dendritic cell recruitment is a hallmark of the acute inflammatory response at mucosal surfaces. J Exp Med 1994; 179:1331–1336.
67. McWilliam AS, Napoli S, Marsh AM, Pemper FL, Nelson DJ, Pimm CL, Stumbles PA, Wells TNC, Holt PG. Dendritic cells are recruited into the airway epithelium during the inflammatory response to a broad spectrum of stimuli. J Exp Med 1996; 184:2429–2432.
68. Nelson DJ, McMenamin C, McWilliam AS, Brenan M, Holt PG. Development of the airway intraepithelial dendritic cell network in the rat from class II MHC (Ia) negative precursors: differential regulation of Ia expression at different levels of the respiratory tract. J Exp Med 1994; 179:203–212.
69. Nelson DJ, Holt PG. Defective regional immunity in the respiratory tract of neonates is attributable to hyporesponsiveness of local dendritic cells to activation signals. J Immunol 1995; 155:3517–3524.
70. Stiehm ER, Sztein MB, Oppenheim JJ. Deficient DR antigen expression on human cord blood monocytes: reversal with lymphokines. Clin Immunol Immunopathol 1984; 30:430–436.
71. Zola H, Fusco M, Weedon H, MacArdle PJ, Ridings J, Roberton DM. Reduced expression of the interleukin-2-receptor γ chain on cord blood lymphocytes: relationship to functional immaturity of the neonatal immune response. Immunology 1996; 87:86–91.
72. Takahashi N, Imanishi K, Nishida H, Uciyama T. Evidence for immunologic immaturity of cord blood T cells. J Immunol 1995; 155:5213–5219.
73. Macatonia SE, Hosken NA, Litton M, Vieira P, Hsieh C-S, Culpepper JA, Wysocka M, Trinchieri G, Murphy KM, O'Garra A. Dendritic cells produce IL-12 and direct the development of Th1 cells from native $CD4^+$ T cells. J Immunol 1995; 154:5071–5079.
74. Heufler C, Koch F, Stanzl U, Topar G, Wysocka M, Trinchieri G, Enk A, Steinman RM, Romani N, Schuler G. Interleukin-12 is produced by dendritic cells and mediates T helper 1 development as well as interferon-γ production by T helper 1 cells. Eur J Immunol 1996; 26:659–668.
75. Cella M, Scheidegger D, Palmer-Lehmann K, Lane P, Lanzavecchia A, Alber G. Ligation of CD40 on dendritic cells triggers production of high levels of interleukin-12 and enhances T cell stimulatory capacity: T–T help via APC activation. J Exp Med 1996; 184:747–752.
76. Brugnoni D, Airo P, Graf D, Marconi M, Lebowitz M, Plebani A, Giliani S, Malcarne F, Cattaneo R, Ugazio AG. Ineffective expression of CD40 ligand on cord blood T cells may contribute to poor immunoglobulin production in the newborn. Eur J Immunol 1994; 24:1919–1924.
77. Fuleihan R, Ahern D, Geha RS. Decreased expression of the ligand for CD40 in newborn lymphocytes. Eur J Immunol 1994; 24:1925–1928.
78. Durandy A, De Saint Basile G, Lisowska-Grospierre B, Gauchat J-F, Forveille M, Kroczek

RA, Bonnefoy J-Y, Fischer A. Undetectable CD40 ligand expression on T cells and low B cell responses to CD40 binding antagonists in human newborns. J Immunol 1995; 154:1560–1568.

79. Shu U, Demeure CE, Byun D-G, Podlaski F, Stern AS, Delespesse G. Interleukin 12 exerts a differential effect on the maturation of neonatal and adult human CD45RO$^-$ CD4 T cells. J Clin Invest 1994; 94:1352–1358.
80. Cohen L, Haziot A, Shen DR, Lin X-Y, Sia C, Harper R, Silver J, Goyert SM. CD14-independent responses to LPS require a serum factor that is absent from neonates. J Immunol 1995; 155:5337–5342.
81. Demeure CE, Yang L-P, Byun DG, Ishihara H, Vezzio N, Delespesse G. Human naive CD4 T cells produce interleukin-4 at priming and acquire a Th2 phenotype upon repetitive stimulations in neutral conditions. Eur J Immunol 1995; 25:2722–2725.
82. Yang L-P, Byun D-G, Demeure CE, Vezzio N, Delespesse G. Default development of cloned human naive CD4 T cells into interleukin-4– and interleukin-5–producing effector cells. Eur J Immunol 1995; 25:3517–3520.
83. Peat JK, Gray EJ, Mellis CM, Leeder SR, Woolcock AJ. Differences in airway responsiveness between children and adults living in the same environment: an epidemiological study in two regions of New South Wales. Eur Respir J 1994; 7:1805–1813.
84. Cline MG, Burrows B. Distribution of allergy in a population sample residing in Tucson, Arizona. Thorax 1989; 44:425–431.
85. Corrigan CJ, Kay AB. T-cells and eosinophils in the pathogenesis of asthma. Immunol Today 1992; 13:501–507.
86. Beasley R, Roche WR, Roberts JA, Holgate ST. Cellular events in the bronchi of mild asthmatics after bronchial provocation. Am Rev Respir Dis 1989; 139:806–817.
87. Wallaert B, Desreumaux P, Copin MC, Tillie I, Benard A, Colombel JF, Gosselin B, Tonnel AB, Janin A. Immunoreactivity for interleukin 3 and 5 and granulocyte/macrophage colony-stimulating factor of intestinal mucosa in bronchial asthma. J Exp Med 1995; 182:1897–1904.
88. Holt PG, Oliver J, Bilyk N, McMenamin C, McMenamin PG, Kraal G, Thepen T. Downregulation of the antigen presenting cell function(s) of pulmonary dendritic cells in vivo by resident alveolar macrophages. J Exp Med 1993; 177:397–407.
89. Strickland DH, Kees UR, Holt PG. Regulation of T-cell activation in the lung: alveolar macrophages induce reversible T-cell anergy in vivo associated with inhibition of IL-2R signal transduction. Immunology 1996; 87:250–258.
90. Upham JW, Strickland DH, Bilyk N, Robinson BWS, Holt PG. Alveolar macrophages from humans and rodents selectively inhibit T-cell proliferation but permit T-cell activation and cytokine secretion. Immunology 1995; 84:142–147.
91. Bilyk N, Holt PG. Cytokine modulation of the immunosuppressive phenotype of pulmonary alveolar macrophages via regulation of nitric oxide production. Immunology 1995; 86:231–237.
92. Poulter LW, Janossy G, Power C, Sreenan S, Burke C. Immunological/physiological relationships in asthma: potential regulation by lung macrophages. Immunol Today 1994; 15:258–261.
93. Johnston SL, Pattemore PK, Sanderson G, Smith S, Campbell MJ, Josephs LK, Cunningham A, Robinson BS, Myint SH, Ward ME. The relationship between upper respiratory infections and hospital admissions for asthma: a time–trend analysis. Am J Respir Crit Care Med 1996; 155:654–660.
94. Holt PG. Infections and the development of allergy. Toxicol Lett 1996; 86:205–210.
95. Holt PG. Environmental factors and primary T-cell sensitisation to inhalant allergens in infancy: reappraisal of the role of infections and air pollution. Pediatr Allergy Immunodl 1995; 6:1–10.
96. Von Mutius E, Martinez FD, Fritzsch C, Nicolai T, Roell G, Theimann H-H. Prevalence of asthma and atopy in two areas of West and East Germany. Am J Respir Crit Care Med 1994; 149:358–364.

97. Bråbäck L, Breborwciz A, Dreborg S, Knutsson A, Pieklik H, Björkstén B. Atopic sensitisation and respiratory symptoms among Polish and Swedish school children. Clin Exp Allergy 1994; 24:826–835.
98. Von Mutius E, Martinez FD, Fritzsch C, Nicolai T, Reitmeir P, Theimann H-H. Skin test reactivity and number of siblings. Br Med J 1994; 308:692–695.
99. Strachan D. Socioeconomic factors and the development of allergy. Toxicol Lett 1996; 86:199–203.
100. Peat JK, Tovey E, Toelle GB, Haby MM, Gray EJ, Mahmic A, Woolcock AJ. House dust mite allergens: a major risk factor for childhood asthma in Australia. Am J Respir Crit Care Med 1996; 153:141–146.
101. Croner S, Kjellman N-I. Predictors of atopic disease: cord blood IgE and month of birth. Allergy 1986; 41:68–70.
102. Semper AE, Hartley JA. Dendritic cells in the lung: what is their relevance to asthma? Clin Exp Allergy 1996; 26:485–490.
103. Möller GM, Overbeek SE, Van Helden-Meeuwsen CG, Van Haarst JMW, Prens EP, Mulder PG, Postma DS, Hoogsteden HC. Increased numbers of dendritic cells in the bronchial mucosa of atopic asthmatic patients: downregulation by inhaled corticosteroids. Clin Exp Allergy 1996; 26:517–524.
104. D'Andrea A, Aste-Amezaga M, Valiante NM, Ma X, Kubin M, Trinchieri G. Interleukin 10 (IL-10) inhibits human lymphocyte interferon γ-production by suppressing natural killer cell stimulatory factor/IL-12 synthesis in accessory cells. J Exp Med 1993; 178:1041–1048.
105. Nelson DJ, McWilliam AS, Haining S, Holt PG. Modulation of airway intraepithelial dendritic cells following exposure to steroids. Am J Respir Crit Care Med 1995; 151:475–481.
106. Holt PG, Thomas JA. Steroids inhibit uptake and/or processing but not presentation of antigen by airway dendritic cells. Immunology 1997; 91:145–150.
107. Poston RN, Chanez P, Lacoste JY, Litchfield T, Lee TH, Bousquet J. Immunohistochemical characterisation of the cellular infiltration in asthmatic bronchi. Am Rev Respir Dis 1992; 145:918–921.
108. Holt PG. A potential vaccine strategy for asthma and allied atopic diseases in early childhood. Lancet 1994; 344:456–458.
109. Varney VA, Hamid QA, Gaga M, Sun Ying M, Jacobson AJ, Frew AB, Kay AB, Durham SR. Influence of grass pollen immunotherapy on cellular infiltration and cytokine mRNA expression during allergen-induced late-phase cutaneous responses. J Clin Invest 1993; 92:644–651.
110. McHugh SM, Deighton J, Stewart AG, Lachmann PJ, Ewan PW. Bee venom immunotherapy induces a shift in cytokine responses from as Th-2 to a Th-1 dominant pattern: comparison of rush and conventional therapy. Clin Exp Allergy 1995; 25:828–838.
111. Inagaki H, Suzuki T, Nomoto K, Yoskikai Y. Increased susceptibility to primary infection with *Listeria monocytogenes* in germfree mice may be due to lack of accumulation of L-selectin$^+$ CD44^{++} T cells in sites of inflammation. Infect Immun 1996; 64:3280–3287.
112. Datsur FD, Shastry P, Iyer E, Awatramani V, Raut S, Mehta SD, Irani SF. The foetal immune response to maternal tetanus toxoid immunization. J Assoc Physicians India 1993; 41:94–96.
113. Glovsky MM, Ghekiere L, Rejzek E. Effect of maternal immunotherapy on immediate skin test reactivity, specific rye I IgG and IgE antibody, and total IgE of the children. Ann Allergy 1991; 67:21–26.
114. Holt PG, Sly PD. Allergic respiratory disease—strategic targets for primary prevention during childhood. Thorax 1996; 52:1–4.

31

Outdoor Air Pollution and Asthma

ERIKA von MUTIUS

University Children's Hospital
Munich, Germany

I. Introduction

Asthma and wheezing respiratory illnesses are a leading cause of acute and chronic illness from childhood to adulthood. Because of its frequent occurrence, it would seem that asthma should be easily characterized and defined. There is, however, no universally accepted definition of this disease. In clinical practice asthma may be considered an obstructive lung disease, with hyperreactivity of the airways to a variety of stimuli, and a high degree of reversibility of the obstructive process, either spontaneously or as a result of treatment. Numerous studies have additionally described a variety of parameters that are related to the asthma complex, such as elevated total IgE, the production of specific IgE antibodies to environmental allergens, airway inflammation, and various measures of lung volumes and airflow limitation. But there is not always a clear relation between the results of these measurements and the clinical expression of the disease. Furthermore, confusion about the asthmatic phenotype has arisen because of different clinical outcomes, such as frequent wheeze, shortness of breath with exercise, or persistent night cough.

In epidemiology further methodological problems arise. Questionnaires are the most widely used method for classifying subjects as affected. At present, there are only two standardized respiratory symptoms questionnaires available for children, one developed by the American Thoracic Society (1), the other by ISAAC, the International Study of Asthma and Allergies in Childhood (2). When considering a parent's report of asthma as affirmative evidence, one must bear in mind that this type of estimate is affected by patterns of use of medical care and the choice of diagnostic labels by individual physicians. Estimates based on parents' reports of wheeze may be affected by linguistic particularities. In some languages there is no term for "wheeze." Surveys that refer solely to a physician's diagnosis of asthma may pick out subjects with more severe illness and, therefore, may skew the reported characteristics of the condition. Conversely, studies that use the presence of wheezing as an indicator of asthma may overestimate the prevalence of the disease because of the poor specificity of wheezing symptoms for asthma. Similar difficulties are encountered in studies among adults.

A. Is all that wheezes asthma?

In early childhood, wheeze is a very common respiratory symptom. About half of a random sample of children enrolled as newborns in a prospective, population-based survey, the Tucson Children's Respiratory Study in the United States, wheezed at some time from birth up to the age of 6 years (3). European population studies estimated that 15–32% of children wheezed in the first 5 years of life (4,5). In a subgroup of wheezy children, diminished lung function is a predisposing factor for the development of a subsequent wheezing illness in infancy (6–8). Results of the Tucson cohort suggest that these infants start wheezing early in life, but stop at about their third birthday. This benign course of disease showed neither an association with a parental history of asthma nor with atopic symptoms or the production of IgE in the child. These findings are in agreement with results of a British birth cohort study enrolling 67 babies born to parents with a history of hay fever or asthma (9). These children were followed up prospectively for 11 years. The yearly period prevalence of wheeze showed a bimodal distribution, with a peak before the age of 2 years, and a gradual increase thereafter. Of the 21 children who wheezed before their second birthday, most never wheezed again and did not show increased risks of airway hyperresponsiveness and atopy at age 11.

A major determinant of reduced pulmonary function at birth is maternal smoking during pregnancy (10). In female offsprings of smoking mothers neonatal lung function was reduced to approximately half the control value (8). Furthermore, in several other studies (11,12), maternal smoking was associated with the occurrence of wheezing lower respiratory infections (LRIs) in infancy. To what extent this relation reflects prenatal or postnatal exposure is difficult to establish, because mothers who smoke during pregnancy usually continue after delivery.

Few studies have measured bronchial responsiveness in infants and preschool children. Airway responsiveness to inhaled histamine is present in many normal, healthy infants soon after birth (13,14) and is not related to the previous occurrence of lower respiratory tract symptoms, including wheeze in 6-month-old infants (14).

Results of an Australian study of 19 recurrently wheezing infants corroborate these findings (15). No difference in bronchial responsiveness to histamine was found for the cases when compared with a control group matched for age, height, weight, gender, and presence of a first-degree relative with asthma or a parent who smoked.

Thus, a distinct subgroup of recurrent wheezy lower respiratory tract illnesses in infancy can be identified. This transient benign condition is related to diminished lung function in the neonatal period, maternal smoking during pregnancy, and low birth weight. Bronchial hyperresponsiveness at birth and atopy are not risk factors, and these children do not have increased risks of asthma or allergies later in life.

Apart from the benign condition of transient early wheezing, the clinical presentation of children with recurrent or chronic bronchitis may be confused with asthma. An airway that suffers an insult responds in a limited number of ways (16). Inflammation, edema, increased sputum production, and disordered clearance of mucus occur in varying degrees and produce cough. Depending on the severity of the airway damage and the resulting increase in airflow resistance, wheezing may also be present. Thus, cough as well as wheezing are nonspecific symptoms that reflect airway damage and narrowing, regardless of mechanism and etiology.

B. Asthma

In a substantial minority of infants wheezing episodes early in life are related to a predisposition to childhood asthma. In the Tucson cohort, a subgroup of children showed recurrent episodes of wheeze from birth up to the age of 6 years. These infants had normal lung function and cord-blood serum IgE levels at birth, but developed significantly higher IgE levels at 9 months of age and skin test reactivity to a panel of aeroallergens at the age of 6 years. Furthermore, this condition was associated with a maternal history of asthma and the occurrence of eczema in the child (3). Pulmonary function that had been within normal limits in the first year of life decreased by the age of 6 years in these persistent wheezers, pointing toward a more severe form of the disease or to long-term consequences of recurrent airway obstruction. More boys than girls were affected.

It has long been recognized that asthma is associated with immunological processes that induce an increased production of total IgE. Burrows and co-workers (17) showed that the prevalence of physician-diagnosed asthma after the age of 6 years was closely related to serum IgE levels in the population, and that no asthma was present in the subjects with the lowest IgE levels. Sears et al. (18) reported that, even in children who have been asymptomatic throughout their lives, airway responsiveness was closely linked to serum IgE.

Many studies have consistently shown that atopy (i.e., the production of specific IgE antibodies to environmental allergens) is strongly associated with childhood asthma. In cross-sectional and clinical studies, atopic sensitization was related to an increased prevalence of asthma, airway hyperresponsiveness, and a greater severity of respiratory symptoms, compared with the absence of atopy (19–21).

Moreover, the strength of atopic sensitization, as assessed by increasing numbers of positive skin prick test results (22) or increasing wheal sizes (23), was linearly related to the severity of childhood asthma and bronchial hyperresponsiveness (BHR). Early sensitization developing before the age of 6–8 years was a stronger predictor for asthma than sensitization, being detectable only thereafter (23,24). Thus, factors enhancing the production of specific IgE antibodies or the lack of protective mechanisms to induce tolerance toward environmental allergens early in life might also increase the risk for asthma.

Unlike in infants and preschool children, airway hyperresponsiveness is strongly associated with asthma and active wheezing in older children and adults. In clinical studies, the presence and degree of BHR correlated well with the physician's diagnosis and the severity of the disease. The mechanisms underlying BHR are still not fully understood. After allergen exposure, an acute airway obstruction occurs within 15 min in almost all atopic asthmatics (5). In a significant proportion of these subjects (25,26), allergen inhalation not only initiates an immediate reaction, but also the reappearance of airway obstruction 3–8 hr later, the late asthmatic reaction. This dual response is characterized by features typical of chronic asthma, such as decreased responsiveness to bronchodilator therapy, increased airway responsiveness, and the development of bronchial inflammation (27,28).

The acute allergic airway response is initiated by the release, from pulmonary mast cells of preformed, or generated, intragranular or membrane-derived mediators and factors. Some of these factors are involved in the acute bronchospasm occurring after allergen inhalation because of their airway smooth-muscle contractile properties (29). The reaction subsides within 30–60 min. With the reappearance of bronchial obstruction 4–6 hr later, recruitment of a variety of inflammatory cells, such as eosinophils, lymphocytes, neutrophils, macrophages, monocytes, and basophils occurs. Eosinophils and lymphocytes are considered the most important effector cells in this late asthmatic reaction, with a potentially pivotal role in the generation of airway inflammation that is associated with asthma (5,30,31). All these findings suggest that airway inflammation might play an important role in the pathogenesis of airway responsiveness and asthma.

There is ample evidence to suggest that the prevalence of childhood asthma and atopic diseases is increasing over the last decades. Several studies in developed countries, using identical measures of disease, have reported increased prevalences of wheeze, BHR, hay fever, and atopic dermatitis in recent years (33–42). Because of the short time period in which these changes occurred, environmental, rather than genetic, influences may cause these rising trends. Exposure to outdoor air pollutants such as SO_2, particulate matter, vehicle exhausts, and ozone has been incriminated as a potential risk factor for the development of asthma, atopy, and airway hyperresponsiveness, particularly because a significant proportion of citizens in the United States and other Western countries still live in areas with air quality levels that are higher than those of the United States primary National Ambient Air Quality Standards, 1991 (43). Besides the concern that atmospheric pollution may be causally related to the initiation of new cases of asthma, the importance of environmental pollutants in aggravating existing disease has been matter of debate.

C. Atmospheric Pollution

Air pollution is felt by many to be one of the more pressing problems toward the end of this century, posing a potential threat to the health and well-being of entire populations. Several severe air pollution episodes in the Meuse Valley in 1930, in Donora, Pennsylvania in 1948, and in London in 1952 with excessive death rates, have shown the potential hazard associated with uncommonly high air pollution levels. Moreover, widespread concern has arisen because by-products of industrialization have increasingly been released into the environment by constructing buildings and creating infrastructure and transportation to raise the comfort of living in the more-developed societies. In the United States and in European countries increasing awareness of these problems has led to legislation of air pollution in the 1950s and 1960s. At about 1970, the U.S. Environmental Protection Agency (EPA) was commissioned to identify all air pollutants that ". . . may reasonably be anticipated to endanger public health" (43). The six pollutants currently identified by the Clean Air Act Amendments of 1990 are ozone (O_3), sulfur dioxide (SO_2), respirable particulate matter (PM_{10}), nitrogen dioxide (NO_2), carbon monoxide, and lead.

Ozone is a powerful oxidizing agent and is generated by photochemical reactions driven by the action of ultraviolet light on precursor pollutants, such as NO_x and volatile organic compounds. In late spring to early autumn, oxides of nitrogen that are released from car exhausts are converted to O_3 in the presence of sunlight. However, close to busy traffic, ozone is again removed by nitric oxide (NO) from car exhausts, which explains why ozone levels are often highest in suburban regions downwind from large cities. Ozone levels typically begin to rise in midmorning, several hours after the morning rush-hour, and peak in the late afternoon.

Airborne particulates are made up of a complex mixture of organic and inorganic substances of varying size. Particles derived from combustion sources are usually more acidic, smaller, and therefore, more likely to be in the respirable range than particles originating from abrasion, such as road dust or windblown soil. The toxicity of particles varies with size and physicochemical composition, which are highly variable. Particles with a diameter less than 10 μm (PM_{10}) can penetrate into the lungs, whereas larger particles are deposited in the extrathoracic airways. Within the respirable range, fine (< 2.5 μm) and ultrafine (< 0.1 μm) particles can be distinguished that may affect airways in different ways. Furthermore, two fractions of fine particles can be measured: the particle mass that is mostly attributable to particles in the size range of 0.1–0.5 μm, and the number of particles that most of the particles are in: the ultrafine fraction.

Sulfur is a natural contaminant of fossil fuels, and SO_2 is thus released into the environment by coal- and oil-fired power plants and by industrial processes involving fossil fuel combustion. Because particles are also produced during combustion of sulfur-containing fuels, the concentrations of SO_2 and particles often vary in a parallel fashion. Before the 1970s, sulfur oxides were mostly emitted from smoke stacks at relatively low heights, resulting in a quick deposition on the ground and reaction of SO_2 with different surfaces. In response to federal regulation of SO_2 levels, power plants and other SO_2 emission sources constructed tall stacks to reduce local ambient SO_2 concentrations. These tall stacks, however, resulted in less mixing of SO_2 to the ground and subsequent local removal. Instead, emissions reach higher altitudes and have longer residence times in the air. If SO_2 is then dissolved in liquids or adheres to surfaces of particles, various oxidation reactions occur, depending on the concentration and mix of pollutants, temperature, sunlight intensity, and other physical factors. These transformations yield acid particles containing sulfate species, mainly sulfuric acid (H_2SO_4) and its partial neutralization product ammonium bisulfate.

Where car exhausts contribute most acid precursors, nitrate species of acidic particles prevail, as on the West Coast of the United States. Other strong acids, as nitric acid and hydrochloric acid can become incorporated into fog droplets. The concentration of acid in the air is difficult to measure and has not been widely documented. Acidic particles can be neutralized by ground level ammonia and by alkaline particles. Therefore, concentrations of strong acidity tend to be higher in communities away from agricultural and urban sources of ammonia. Acid events occur more frequently during the spring and summer, mainly in the 4 months from May through August (44).

Nitrogen oxides are gaseous products of combustion of fossil fuels in power generation and cars. Indoor sources of NO_2 include cigarette smoke, gas and oil heaters and cookers, which often result in high indoor concentrations. NO_2 is a strong oxidant. In contrast with sulfur dioxide, the total direct emissions of nitrogen dioxides have not declined in the past decades in Western countries and the United States.

The air quality standards in Table 1 have been set in Europe and the United States:

Table 1 Air Quality Standards as Set in Europe and the United States

	Reference period	SO_2 (ppm)	TSP (μg/m^3)	NO_2 (ppm)	O_3 (ppm)
WHO					
Europe	10 min	0.175			
	1 hr	0.122		0.21	0.08–0.10
	24 hr	0.04	120	0.078	0.05–0.06 (8h)
	1 yr	0.017			
USA	1 hr				0.12
	24 hr	0.127	150		
	1 yr	0.027	50	0.053	

Source: Ref. 45.

The conversion of units (ppm and mg/m^3) at 25°C, 101.3 kPa follows.

Ozone	1 mg/m^3 = 0.5 ppm	1 ppm = 2 mg/m^3
Nitrogen dioxide	1 mg/m^3 = 0.56 ppm	1 ppm = 1.8 mg/m^3
Sulfur dioxide	1 mg/m^3 = 0.38 ppm	1 ppm = 2.62 mg/m^3

Source: Ref. 45.

D. How Are the Effects of Air Pollution Assessed?

An understanding of the potential adverse health effects of air pollution exposure requires the interpretation and integration of different disciplines: namely, toxicology, with animal, in vitro, and human exposure studies, and epidemiology. Each approach has its strengths and limitations.

Animal studies are used to investigate pathogenetic mechanisms of pollutant injury. Ideally, a selected animal model would closely resemble the human response. Then, methods can be used that would not be practical or ethical in human, such as tissue collection, high-dose exposure, long-term exposure, and comparison of the response in multiple species. However, the most important and unavoidable limitation of animal studies is the qualitative and quantitative extrapolation from these animal models to humans. Some confidence in the qualitative aspects of findings from animal studies may be justified when consistency of results across more than one species is found. Then, the underlying mechanism may be generic and applied to studies of human risk assessment. However, quantitative extrapolation from animal models to humans is not warranted because uncertainties about target tissue dose and relative test sensitivity of different species exist. No prediction of dose–response relations in humans can be deduced from air pollutant studies in animals.

In vitro studies have been used extensively to investigate chemical reactions of pollutants with substrates of interest. Airway epithelial cells and macrophages can both be studied immediately after brushing or lavaging their airways, and be grown in cell culture techniques. It has thus become possible to expose specific types of human and animal cells to pollutants in vitro. However, results of these studies must be cautiously interpreted, given the artificial experimental models involved. For example, cell–cell interactions cannot occur, the influx of other cells in the model is impossible, and the presence of overlying culture medium may hamper the direct access of gases to the cultured cells. Furthermore, because of the limited duration of viability of cultured cells, the investigation of effects of long-term exposure to air pollutants is impossible.

Human exposure studies are useful to study the responses of normal subjects and of patients with asthma or chronic obstructive pulmonary disease (COPD) to carefully controlled concentrations of single pollutants or defined mixtures of pollutants. An immediate health effect caused by a specific pollutant or a specific component of a pollution mixture can convincingly be demonstrated by such type of study. Furthermore, sensitive human subjects can be identified. Apart from subjective symptoms, physiological endpoints, such as spirometry or airway reactivity, can be assessed, and through bronchoscopy and nasal lavage, biological markers of inflammation can be measured. But controlled human exposure studies also have limitations. Most studies have been performed involving young patients with mild disease. Yet, the most susceptible population may involve patients with more severe or progressive disease and young children. Effects of prolonged exposure cannot be studied, because ethical considerations and compliance of volunteers limit the duration of exposure. A subject's exposure to ambient air pollution before being involved in a chamber study cannot be standardized, and responses in the chamber might be influenced by variations of ambient air pollution levels.

Epidemiological studies examine the relation between actual environmental exposure to air pollution and health effects in representative human populations. In contrast with controlled human exposure studies, epidemiological surveys can estimate irreversible health effects, such as mortality or loss of lung function, and effects relevant to public health concerns, such as hospital admission rates or frequency of emergency room visits. Furthermore, the effects can be studied among the most sensitive individuals, such as patients with severe asthma or young children. Epidemiological air pollution studies can take a variety of forms, mainly addressing effects of changing air pollution concentrations over time, as in panel studies or time–trend analyses, or by comparing areas with different pollution profiles. Careful design and analysis is required to control for other factors that may also influence health outcomes. Furthermore, erroneous measurement and classification of exposure may introduce significant bias in air pollution studies. Personal exposure of enrolled study participants who spend most of their time indoors may differ substantially from estimates derived from measurements of centrally sited outdoor monitors. This may especially apply to ozone, for which indoor concentrations are generally lower than outdoor levels. However, random misclassification always results in an underestimate of the true relative risk. Thus, weak associations that have been reported in many epidemiological air pollution studies using outdoor monitors for exposure assessment may be strengthened with the use of personal monitors that are now available for particles, NO_2, CO, and volatile organic compounds (VOCs; 43).

In recent years, significant progress has been achieved in methods and tools of environmental epidemiology that has substantially contributed to the ability to study air pollution health effects. Epidemiological studies can identify risks for broad groups of people, consider the full range of exposures, and the many combinations of environmental and social factors that determine the development of disease in exposed and unexposed individuals. Thus, the results of epidemiological studies substantially complement those of in vitro studies and controlled human exposure studies for predicting risk in a given community.

II. Human Exposure Studies

A. Ozone

Ozone is a potent oxidant, capable of reacting with a variety of biomolecules. Its cytotoxicity may be attributable to its interactions with unsaturated lipids that generate damaging free radicals or toxic intermediate products (46,47). These injure resident lung cells (48), trigger further inflammation (49), and stimulate neural afferents in the airways. Zone is a relatively soluble, but highly reactive, gas that is mostly removed by the nasal epithelium and along the larger lower airways (50). According to theoretical predictions, the highest tissue dose of ozone occurs at the bronchoalveolar junction (51). These predictions have been confirmed by histopathological studies in primates and lower mammals (52,53). Nevertheless, there is some evidence from animal and human studies that inspired ozone also has significant access to the distal lung and the alveolar regions.

Acute Exposure

Single ozone exposure has been shown to evoke cough, breathlessness, and chest pain on inspiration, to result in a restrictive ventilatory defect with decrements in forced vital capacity (FVC) and forced 1-sec expiratory volume (FEV_1), to induce neutrophilic inflammation of the airway submucosa, and to increase airway reactivity.

The response to ozone shows large intersubject variability, even among a homogeneous study populations of carefully selected healthy volunteers (54–58). A proportion of approximately 10–20% of the population is sensitive and will develop reductions in lung function after ozone exposure, whereas others are nonsensitive (59,60). Increased symptoms and larger lung function decrements in subgroups of study subjects are relatively reproducible (61,62). Why certain subjects are at risk remains largely unknown. No clear relation was found between the level of reduction in lung function, airway responsiveness, and various cellular and biochemical markers of inflammation. It has, however, been shown that cigarette smokers do not respond to ozone in chamber studies (63). Furthermore, a decreasing susceptibility toward adverse effects of ozone has been demonstrated with increasing age (64). These findings may partly explain why patients with COPD do not respond to ozone exposure (65,66). Atopic and asthmatic subjects are as susceptible to the effects of ozone as healthy nonsmoking subjects, but in contrast to exposure to SO_2 or NO_2 do not show enhanced or modified responsiveness (67–71).

In controlled human exposure studies, an increase in ozone concentrations up to 0.4 ppm did not result in strong effects if subject were at rest. However, FVC and FEV_1 were reduced when study participants performed intermittent moderate to heavy exercise. The extent to which exercise affects the response to ozone has been very clearly shown in a retrospective analysis by Hazucha (72; Fig. 1).

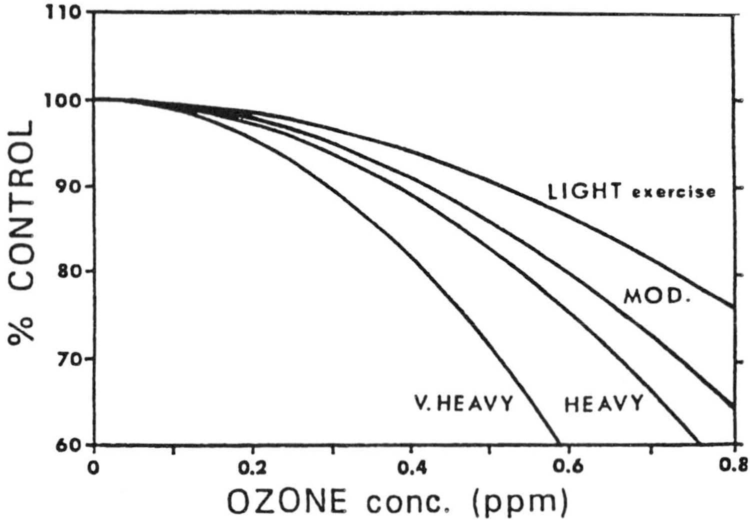

Figure 1 Effects of intermittent exercise on O_3 concentration-forced expiratory volume at 1s regression curves.

To mimic ambient peak exposure levels several protocols exposed subjects for a duration of 1–2 hr to varying ozone levels and found consistent reductions of lung function parameters with increasing pollutant concentrations in the 0.21–0.4 ppm range (73–76). Because the response is widely variable among subjects, only a small shift in group mean value may occur, whereas a much greater effect and individually significant shift will appear in a few susceptible individuals. In some urban areas, however, ozone levels may remain elevated for several hours a day. Studies using a longer exposure duration of 6–8 hr with intermittent exercise demonstrated effects at exposure levels as low as 0.08 ppm (77–79). Horstman and colleagues also reported that ozone concentration was slightly more influential than exposure duration for inducing FEV_1 response (79), which is in agreement with results of other studies (80,81).

Several studies have shown an increase in airway responsiveness to methacholine, histamine, and allergens, but no exercise, after exposure to ozone concentrations ranging from 0.12 to 0.6 ppm. Golden and co-workers studied the effect of a 2-hr exposure to 0.6 ppm ozone in eight healthy, nonsmoking subjects by measuring the increase in airway resistance produced by histamine (82). The mean response to histamine immediately after exposure was significantly greater than the preozone response. The group value returned to baseline after 1 day, but two subjects still had a significantly increased histamine responsiveness for more than 1 week after exposure. These results were confirmed in 16 healthy volunteers using a similar protocol (2-hr exposure to 0.6 ppm ozone) and bronchial challenge with methacholine and histamine (70). In this study, the increase in SR_{aw} after ozone exposure returned to control values in all subjects by the following day. In both studies, baseline SR_{aw} was not altered significantly by exposure to the pollutant. Pretreatment with atropine blocked ozone-induced airway hyperresponsiveness, suggesting that cholinergic postganglionic pathways may be involved in the causal mechanisms. The presence of atopic sensitization did not change the findings. Likewise, Jörres and co-workers demonstrated that, in mild asthmatics, the $PC_{20}FEV_1$ of methacholine decreased by 0.9-doubling concentrations after exposure to 0.25 ppm ozone for 3 hr of intermittent exercise (83). No difference in ozone-induced bronchial responsiveness ($PC_{100}SR_{aw}$) between asthmatics and healthy subjects was found (73).

In contrast, two studies investigating the effect of ozone on exercise-induced airway hyperresponsiveness in mild asthmatics have failed to show any adverse effect in patients undergoing 1-hr exposure to ozone concentrations of 0.12, 0.25, and 0.4 ppm, respectively (84,85). Exercise-induced airway hyperresponsiveness was considered present if a FEV_1 decrease of 15% (84) and 20% or more (85) occurred after a standardized exercise challenge on a treadmill. Changes in SR_{aw} were not reported.

Molfino and co-workers reported an increased responsiveness to inhaled pollen allergen after short-term exposure for 1 hr to 0.12 ppm ozone in asthmatics at rest (86). These results have been much discussed and criticized for the small number of subjects ($n = 7$), the nonrandomized design that was used for allocation of study days, the application of a lower significance level of hyperresponsiveness (PC_{15} and not PC_{20}) and the short time interval between different exposures that might enhance responses in subsequent challenges. However, Jörres and colleagues confirmed these results when investigating 24 subjects with mild, stable asthma (83). After exposure to 0.25 ppm ozone for 3 hr of intermittent exercise the $PD_{20}FEV_1$ of allergen fell by 1.7-doubling doses. The concomitant postexposure changes in lung function and airway response to methacholine challenge did not correlate with allergen responsiveness. Moreover, in 12 subjects with allergic rhinitis, without asthma, ozone induced a similar, although slighter increase in allergen responsiveness of the lower airways, suggesting that short-term exposure to ozone can increase bronchial allergen responsiveness in subjects with mild allergic asthma or rhinitis.

Repeated Exposures

Linn and co-workers demonstrated that responsiveness to ozone varied with the season in Los Angeles Basin residents (87). The residents were less sensitive to ozone following high exposure in the summer. After the winter season, when ozone levels were low, they had regained the responsiveness of the previous spring. Further animal and human studies have revealed development of tolerance, or adaptation, to the adverse effects of ozone with repeated exposure (88,89). Studies repeating ozone exposure over 4–5 days have shown that the greatest decrement in FVC and FEV_1 occurs on the second day, with the effect on symptoms, spirometric changes, and neutrophilia in bronchoalveolar lavage fluid becoming negligible by day 5. In the absence of further ozone exposure, this attenuation of responsiveness to ozone persists for 4–7 days and then regresses.

It remains unclear whether ozone-induced airway hyperresponsiveness persists after repeated exposure (90–93). Dimeo and co-workers studied seven healthy adult subjects on 3 consecutive days of 2-hr exposures to 0.4 ppm of ozone (91). As in previous studies, a stronger rise in posthistamine SR_{aw} was found after ozone exposure than with filtered air, but returned to preexposure values after the third day. Folinsbee and colleagues, using a slightly different index of airway responsiveness (i.e., the ratio of SR_{aw} postmethacholine to SR_{aw} postsaline aerosol) did not find a full attenuation of increased airway responsiveness after 5 days of repeated exposure to 0.12 ppm ozone for 6.6 hr (92). In 11 of the 17 study subjects a persistent increase in responsiveness for all 5 days of exposure was seen, whereas in the remaining individuals the methacholine response returned to control levels on days 4 and 5. Kulle and co-workers studied methacholine-induced airway responsiveness during 5 days of daily 2-hr exposures to 0.4 ppm ozone (93). The greatest increase in airway responsiveness was during the first 3 days of exposure and a gradual decrease thereafter, with values returning toward baseline on day 5. These findings suggest that with repeated ozone exposure pulmonary function responses and airway responsiveness change are not closely correlated and do not follow the same time course. A subgroup of individuals may be at risk of developing prolonged increases in airway responsiveness after exposure to ozone, but this unresolved question needs further careful investigation.

Potential Mechanisms of Ozone Toxicity

The mechanisms involved in lung function changes secondary to ozone exposure are not fully understood. A reduction in inspiratory capacity has been suggested to underlie the ozone-induced decrease in FVC and FEV_1, because the FRC is not appreciably altered (94,95). Reflex mechanisms may limit the ability to perform deep inspiration during exposure, whereas respiratory muscle force and mechanical properties of the lung remain unchanged (94). Atropine pretreatment prevents the increase in airway resistance with ozone exposure, but does not hinder a significant fall in FVC or abate the frequency of reported respiratory symptoms (95). Thus, mechanisms dependent on muscarinic cholinergic receptors of the parasympathetic nervous system may play a prominent role in the postexposure increase in airway resistance, whereas changes in other measured variables may be mediated differently. Immediate spirometric responses in healthy subjects have been reported to be significantly diminished by pretreatment with indomethacin, suggesting that changes in lung function are partly mediated by cyclo-oxygenase products (96,97). Conversely, pretreatment with indomethacin did not alter the ozone-induced increase in bronchial responsiveness to methacholine (97). Thus, different mechanisms may be involved in adverse effects of ozone exposure on the respiratory system, partly explaining the apparent dissociation of effects on lung function, airway responsiveness, and various cellular and biochemical markers of inflammation.

Inflammation of the respiratory tract after ozone exposure occurs in all species that have been studied and has been observed as redness and swelling through bronchoscopy in animals and humans, and as pain in exposed individuals. Bronchoscopies with biopsies and bronchoalveolar lavage (BAL) studies have recently been used to complement investigations of adverse effects of air pollutants on the human respiratory system. After exposure to ozone, most studies have found significant increases in numbers of neutrophils, but not eosinophils in BAL fluid (98–102) nor in large-airways mucosal biopsies (101). Further increases in several markers of inflammation, such as neutrophil elastase, prostaglandin (PG)E_2, interleukin (IL)-6, IL-8, lactate dehydrogenase (LDH), fibronectin, plasminogen activator, and leukotriens C_4–E_4 have been reported (98–101). Asthmatics develop greater inflammatory responses after ozone exposure than do healthy subjects (98,102). The type of airway inflammation seen after ozone exposure differs, however, substantially from inflammatory changes occurring in the airways of asthmatics.

B. Sulfur Dioxide

In contrast with ozone and nitrogen dioxide, sulfur dioxide is a highly water-soluble gas that is mostly absorbed in the upper airways in subjects at rest. With increasing ventilation, absorption occurs in deeper portions of the lung (103). At ambient concentrations sulfur dioxide does not cause significant acute or chronic toxicity in animals and healthy subjects (104–108). Levels above 5 ppm SO_2 that may be encountered in some heavily polluted industrial workrooms can result in increased airway resistance in healthy subjects (45).

Controlled exposure studies, however, have clearly shown that asthmatics are more sensitive than healthy subjects and respond with airway obstruction and respiratory symptoms to lower levels of SO_2 exposure (0.25–0.5 ppm) than asymptomatic individuals (109–113). When asthmatics are briefly exposed to SO_2 levels as low as 0.25 ppm, increases in airway resistance are found in many exercising subjects. A reduction in FEV_1 occurs at higher concentrations, above 0.4 ppm SO_2. Both SO_2 concentration and minute ventilation affect the magnitude of the response. When exposing an asthmatic subject to SO_2, the response can be detected within 2 min. It increases further with exposure up to 10–30 min, remains relatively stable as long as the exposure continues, and resolves within 1 hr after the end of exposure (109,114–119). Late reactions or repetitive nocturnal attacks have not been found, with the possible exception of a few subjects in one study (120). The symptoms occurring with SO_2 exposure are usually mild and include nose irritation, an unpleasant smell of sulfur, throat irritation, shortness of breath, and wheeze (121,122). The SO_2-induced bronchoconstriction and symptoms are rapidly reversed by inhalation of β-adrenergic agonists (112).

Sulfur dioxide may cause bronchoconstriction in asthmatics at concentrations of less than 0.25 ppm when inhaled by increased minute ventilation in dry air (123). Conversely, high temperature and high humidity tend to mitigate the bronchoconstriction produced by 0.6 ppm SO_2 (124). Levels higher than 0.25 ppm SO_2, however, seldom occur in ambient air over large areas, except in periods of heavy air pollution. Downwind of certain point sources sulfur dioxide may peak toward levels higher than 0.25 ppm during short time periods (45).

Pretreatment with atropine, ipratropium bromide, cromolyn, or a selective H_1-receptor antagonist all block, at least partially, the SO_2-induced bronchial obstruction (112,113,125). Cromolyn has been suggested to act on sensory receptors (126). Atropine plus cromolyn was more effective than either drug alone, suggesting that several mechanisms involving vagal afferent and cholinergic efferent reflexes may be involved in eliciting the SO_2-induced bronchoconstriction (127,128).

With high SO_2 exposure to 8 ppm, a level that greatly exceeds ambient concentrations, but may be encountered as peak exposures in industrial indoor environments, inflammatory changes occur. In eight healthy, nonsmoking men significant increases in the numbers of macrophages, lymphocytes, and mast cells in BAL fluid 24 hr after exposure were found (129); 72 hr after exposure the cell numbers had returned to normal. It is unknown whether similar inflammatory responses occur at the much lower ambient concentrations, and whether asthmatics are at higher risk of aggravating airway inflammation subsequent to SO_2 exposure.

C. Acid Aerosols

The predominant acid aerosols are sulfate (SO_4^{2-}) and bisulfate (HSO_4^-) ions, which coexist with ammonium (NH_4^+), the counterion in the atmosphere (43). Much of the irritant potential of sulfate aerosols appears to lie in the acidity or H^+ concentration of that aerosol. Thus, H_2SO_4, which at ambient relative humidities has a pH of less than 1.0, appears to be more irritative than ammonium bisulfate (NH_4HSO_4) and ammonium sulfate ($[NH_4]^2SO_4$) which are formed by neutralization by trace ammonia in the atmosphere or in the respiratory tract, and are less acidic (130,131). H_2SO_4 and its partially or fully neutralized salts are generally smaller than 1 μm in aerodynamic diameter and constitute a major fraction of the smaller respirable particles found in ambient air (43).

Endogenous respiratory gaseous ammonia (NH_3), which is present in the upper respiratory tract, can neutralize inhaled H_2SO_4 (132). Indeed, high respiratory levels of NH_3 inhibit H_2SO_4-induced bronchoconstriction in exercising asthmatics (133). The buffering capacity of mucus and surfactant may further influence the response. In addition, the rate of neutralization is a function of NH_3 concentration and droplet size (i.e., the smaller the droplets the faster is neutralization).

In several controlled exposure studies no effect of exposure to H_2SO_4 aerosols at levels below 500 μg/m^3 was found in healthy subjects at rest or with intermittent exercise (134–139). Inconsistent evidence exists about adverse effects at higher concentrations, over 500 μg/m^3 up to 1000 μg/m^3 H_2SO_4 in healthy subjects; some authors reporting no effects (133,136,140,141), others throat irritation, cough, and slight decrements of lung function (138,139).

In contrast to sulfur dioxide, there is no clear evidence that asthmatics are more sensitive to exposure to acid aerosols than healthy individuals. Some short-term controlled exposure studies have found that decrements of pulmonary function occur in asthmatics at H_2SO_4 concentrations equivalent to ambient levels in the United

States (131,142–144). Other studies failed to confirm an increased susceptibility of asthmatics to acid aerosol exposure (136,137,145). These widely varying results remain largely unexplained. In asthmatics, the degree of preexisting nonspecific airway hyperreactivity may predict the magnitude of the response (146). Alternatively, the size of generated particles may differ between different laboratories and may exert different effects in exposed individuals.

Likewise, asthmatics appear to be no more reactive to H_2SO_4 fog aerosols than are healthy individuals. Extremely high levels of large-droplet acid fog were required to increase specific airway resistance in asthmatics, and even higher concentrations were needed to cause a degree of airway obstruction comparable with that resulting from exposure to submicron aerosols of H_2SO_4 (147,148). Other components of acid fog failed to cause reductions in lung function in asthmatics (149). No influx of inflammatory cells was found after exposure to 1000 μg/m^3 H_2SO_4 in the BAL fluid of healthy subjects (150).

D. Nitrogen Dioxide

The principal source of NO and NO_2 in outdoor air is motor vehicle emissions, but power plants and fossil fuel–burning industries also contribute. Ambient levels of NO_2 vary with traffic density. Annual average concentrations range from 0.015 to 0.035 ppm in the United States (151). When measuring 48-hr integrated mean concentrations by passive diffusion samplers in outdoor air at homes in Low Angeles, NO_2 levels ranged from 0.007 to 0.040 ppm in areas with low traffic density, and from 0.011 to 0.065 ppm in the more urbanized regions. Exposure during travel in motor vehicles may, however, considerably surpass levels measured at nearby ambient sites. In a recent air pollution episode in London, England, NO_2 concentrations went above 0.40 ppm for 8 hr on 2 consecutive days (152).

Nitrogen dioxide contaminates both outdoor and indoor air. In fact, indoor levels can exceed those found outdoors. Indoor concentrations are determined by the infiltration of NO_2 from the outside, the air-exchange rate, and the emission from indoor sources, such as gas cooking ranges and kerosene space heaters. Because most people spend the largest proportion of their time indoors (153), the residential environment is generally the most important contributor to the population's exposure to NO_2 (151). The physical and chemical characteristics of nitrogen dioxide found in outdoor and indoor air differ. In outdoor air, a complex mixture of pollutants including NO_2 and other products of combustion is present that may enhance transformation of NO_2 to acidic nitrates. Indoors, gas cooking stoves emit other nitrogen oxides in addition to NO_2, and adverse health effects to combustion appliances may not necessarily be attributable to NO_2 alone.

Nitrogen dioxide is a poorly water-soluble gas, in contrast to the insoluble ozone and the highly soluble sulfur dioxide. Therefore, NO_2 is deposited far more peripherally in the airways than SO_2 (i.e., in the conducting airways and the terminal bronchioli), but may not reach the alveolar space, except at extremely high concentrations (154). NO_2 is considerably less dependent on the breathing mode than SO_2, but exercise may enhance adverse effects by increasing deposition (155). NO_2 is a potent, though slightly less reactive, oxidant than ozone, but surface reactivity appears to be the most important determinant of uptake (156). Lipid peroxidation in cell membranes and various actions of free radicals on structural and functional molecules (157–160) may contribute to the toxicity of NO_2. The formation of nitric and nitrous acids in aqueous solution on moist surfaces of the airspaces may added to the averse effects of NO_2 (161).

In healthy subjects, most studies examining responses to NO_2 at levels as high as 4.0 ppm have not shown alteration of airway mechanics (i.e., spirometry and flow resistance; 162–168). However, two authors have reported increases in airway resistance at low exposure levels (169,170). Curiously, Bylin and co-workers found an elevated airway resistance in healthy volunteers exposed for 20 min to 0.25 ppm at rest, a decreased resistance after exposure to 0.5 ppm, but no change in bronchial responsiveness to histamine in the same subjects. Beil and Ulmer found an increase in airway resistance. At high exposure levels an increase in airway reactivity was found by some investigators. Mohsenin (165) reported increased responsiveness to methacholine, as measured by changes in specific airway conductance, in healthy subjects exposed to 2.0 ppm NO_2 for 1 hr, which could be prevented by pretreatment with ascorbic acid. Similarly, a mild increase in responsiveness to carbachol was observed after a 3-hr exposure to 1.5 ppm NO_2 (171). Low-dose studies with 0.1 ppm (167), 0.48 ppm (170), and 0.05 ppm with three, 15-min peaks of 2.0 ppm NO_2 (171) failed to show any effect on airway reactivity. Thus, at ambient levels there is little evidence of adverse effects of NO_2 on airway reactivity in healthy subjects.

In asthmatics, a wide range of responses have been reported, and a clear understanding of effects of nitrogen dioxide exposure on pulmonary function in asthmatics has not been reached. Orehek and colleagues first suggested that a relatively brief exposure of asthmatics to low concentrations of NO_2 (1 hr to 0.1 ppm at rest) might enhance subsequent responsiveness to a nonspecific challenge (172). In their study, using a much-discussed stratification of subjects into "responder" and "nonresponder," 13 of the 20 asthmatics showed increased airway responsiveness to carbachol after NO_2 exposure. Others were unable to confirm these findings in asthmatic adolescents or adults at levels of 0.1–4.0 ppm NO_2 (167,170,173–177). In contrast, Kleinman and co-workers exposed 30 slightly exercising asthmatics to 0.2 ppm NO_2 and showed that approximately two-thirds of the subjects experienced increased reactivity to methacholine, as assessed by specific airway resistance (173). Bauer and colleagues evaluated the response of 15 asthmatics to inhalation of 0.3 ppm NO_2 (178). At this level, NO_2 exposure produced significant decrements in FEV_1 after exercise, but not at rest. Furthermore, response to inhalation of cold air, in three successive rates of increasing isocapnic hyperventilation, increased after NO_2 exposure. Others found slight increases of airway reactivity in asthmatics exposed to 0.5 ppm NO_2 (170). However, even within-laboratories positive results of enhanced airway responsiveness in groups of asthmatics at levels of 0.3 ppm NO_2 could not be reproduced (175,179,180), although within-subjects reproducibility of findings was observed (175,179). The inconsistency of the results of these different studies has not been satisfactorily explained, but may reflect differences in selection of subjects and study protocols, or differences in intrinsic susceptibility of some asthmatics to adverse health effects of NO_2 exposure.

The findings of two recent studies suggest that similarly to ozone, exposure to nitrogen dioxide can potentiate the specific airway response of patients with mild asthma to inhaled allergens. Tunicliffe and co-workers reported on ten nonsmoking asthmatics were exposed to 0.10 or 0.40 ppm NO_2 and then immediately underwent allergen challenge with house dust mites (181). Baseline FEV_1 was not affected by NO_2 exposure, but the early and late asthmatic response to allergen challenge was significantly enhanced after the higher exposure level of 0.4 ppm NO_2. Devalia and colleagues failed to reproduce the findings with exposure to 0.40 ppm NO_2. However, exposure to a mixture of 0.40 ppm NO_2 and 0.20 ppm SO_2 enhanced the airway response to inhaled allergen (182).

Unlike exposure to ozone, NO_2 inhalation at near ambient levels of less than 0.2 ppm does not cause a significant influx of polymorphonuclear leukocytes into the airways and alveoli (183). However, when analyzing cells from the first proximal lavage aliquot using a modified BAL technique, a mild neutrophilic inflammatory response was observed after high exposures to 3.5 ppm NO_2 in healthy subjects (184). No neutrophils were found in peripheral BAL fluid samples. In all, NO_2 appears to be much less potent than ozone in inducing a neutrophilic inflammatory response. However, a significant, dose-related increase in lymphocytes and mast cells has been found after exposure of healthy nonsmoking individuals to levels ranging from 0.6 to 7.75 ppm NO_2 (185–187).

E. Combined Exposures

Environmental exposures do not involve one single pollutant, rather complex mixtures of many pollutant compounds occur simultaneously or sequentially in ambient outdoor and indoor air. Failure to consider the presence of other pollutants may confuse the interpretation of the observed results because of potential synergistic, additive, or antagonistic effects.

The influence of NO_2 exposure on SO_2-induced bronchoconstriction has been investigated in two studies, with inconsistent results. Whereas Jörres and colleagues found an enhanced response to SO_2 in asthmatics following inhalation of 0.25 ppm NO_2 for 30 min (188), Rubinstein and co-workers did not see any effect at similar exposure levels (0.30 ppm NO_2; 189). No interactive effects have been found for mixtures of nitrogen dioxide and ozone (190–192). The combination of the two gases did not produce a more pronounced effect than the individual gases alone.

There is little evidence to support the notion that prior exposure to ozone potentiates the pulmonary response to subsequent exposure to sulfur dioxide and sulfuric or nitric acid. Only one study reported that preexposure to ozone (0.120 ppm) promotes bronchoconstriction after exposure to a subthreshold concentration of SO_2 (0.100 ppm; 193). Others failed to show that the admixture of ozone to either SO_2, sulfuric, or nitric acid enhances effects produced by these pollutants alone (194–198). Antagonistic effects may also occur when mixing different pollutants. Aris and co-workers (198) showed that exposure to nitric acid fog reduce the subsequent response to ozone, an effect that might be attributable to the nitric acid or to the fog itself.

III. Exacerbation of Asthma

A. Studies of Emergency Room Visits and Hospital Admissions for Asthma

Asthma has been defined as a highly reversible obstructive lung disease with hyperreactivity of the airways. Thus, by definition asthma is an illness that is characterized by considerable short-term variability attributable to a variety of causes, such as allergen exposure, epidemics of virus infection, climatic changes, and exercise. The effects of fluctuations in air pollution levels are, by comparison, subtle and difficult to quantify with certainty.

Time series analyses have been applied to studies of hospital admissions or emergency room visits for asthma in relation to short-term fluctuations in air pollution levels. Simple correlations of daily asthma attack rates and concentrations of air pollutants are, however, prone to statistical artifacts that may tend to overestimate the true relation (199). Both, asthma incidence and exposure exhibit cyclical fluctuations throughout the year. These cycles may exaggerate or obscure correlations between asthma incidence and pollution levels. To overcome these problems more advanced statistical methods, using autoregressive modeling and thus taking account of serial correlation of the observations from adjacent days have been applied. Moreover, in most studies the number of daily asthma admissions or visits is small. Therefore, Poisson regression models appear more suitable than conventional regression models, which assume a statistically normal distribution of asthma incidence.

The induction period (i.e., the period of time from causal action of pollution exposure until disease exacerbation) is unknown. Many studies, therefore, have analyzed correlations between daily asthma attack rates and pollution levels 1 to several days before the event. Although this procedure appears biologically plausible, the opportunity of multiple comparisons and thereby attaining a significant positive result by chance alone, is increased. The problem of multiple statistical comparisons may further be aggravated by including into the analyses several pollutants and several health outcomes, and by stratifying the data set by age, season, area of residence, or other.

Finally, problems in exposure assessment arise because most analyses rely on measurements from a small number of fixed outdoor monitoring stations. Although daily mean concentrations of regionally dispersed pollutants may correlate over a wide area, peaks of exposure that may be more relevant to the occurrence of adverse health effects may vary more significantly over space. Furthermore, within a single area, several pollutants may display similar fluctuations and levels may be highly intercorrelated. Thus, even when including each pollutant separately into a regression model, the resulting coefficient indicates the effect of a pollution mixture, rather than the independent effect of a single pollutant species.

Several studies have shown an increased frequency of emergency room visits and hospital admission rates for both acute respiratory illnesses and asthma with increasing levels of air pollution. The evidence appears strongest for the type of summer haze pollution that affects Canada and the eastern part of the United States, whereas most of the episodes of increased SO_2 exposure in winter have not been shown to induce exacerbations in asthmatic patients. However, particulate pollution was found by several authors to affect asthma hospital admissions or emergency room visits.

Hospital admission rates were studied by Bates and colleagues in two periods, January to February and July to August over the years 1974 and 1976–1983 in southern Ontario, Canada (200–202). No relation between asthma admissions and pollutant concentrations was found in the winter period. In the summer months, however, positive correlations of asthma admissions with levels of SO_2 (lagged 2 days); ozone (lagged 1 day); and sulfates (lagged 1 day) were found. All pollutants were cross-correlated with each other and temperature on the same day, thus the independent effect of each pollutant could not be identified with certainty. Nevertheless, increases in ozone concentrations appeared to have the strongest effects. A 0.050 ppm increase in maximum hourly concentration of ozone during July and August was associated with a significant 8.3% increase in admissions for childhood asthma on the following day (203). Aerolized sulfuric acids, which might alternatively or synergistically be relevant for the effects of summer haze pollution, had not been measured.

In Toronto, hospital admission rates for asthma during the summers of 1986, 1987, and 1988 were recorded and acid aerosol levels were measured (204). When controlling for temperature, significant positive correlations between asthma admissions and both ozone and acid aerosol levels on the same day were found. However, in two-pollutant models, ozone remained a significant predictor of admission rates when controlling for other pollutants, whereas after adjustment for ozone, airborne acid, sulfates, and particulates became nonsignificant. The independent effect of ozone was estimated as a 32% increase in asthma admission rate on days of maximum ozone levels (0.159 ppm) compared with days of average ozone concentration (0.070 ppm).

In New Jersey, where summer ozone levels are generally higher than in Canada, emergency room visits for asthma were studied during two summer periods (May to August 1988 and 1989; 205). Ozone (lagged by 1 day) emerged as a significant predictor of asthma attacks after adjusting for temperature. The effect was estimated as a 2.4% increase in asthma visits per 0.010 ppm increase in ozone concentration on the previous day. Over the same two summers a second study was performed in New York City and Buffalo, New York (204). Levels of maximum daily ozone, daily sulfates, and daily acid aerosol were highly cross-correlated in this area, and the independent effect of a single pollutant could not be identified with certainty. Each was positively correlated with asthma attendances on the same or following day. The effect of ozone was estimated as a 1.7% increase in asthma visits per 0.010 ppm increase in hourly maximum ozone on the previous day. In other words, a 23% relative increase in asthma visits was found on days of maximal ozone concentrations (0.206 ppm) as compared with days of average ozone levels (0.069 ppm). Effects of similar magnitude were found for airborne acid (32% increase) and sulfates (19% increase). Another Canadian study investigating emergency room visits for asthma in Vancouver, British Columbia, failed to demonstrate a significant relation between ambient ozone concentration and asthma attack rates (206). In contrast, airborne sulfates were significantly and positively associated with asthma in the summer in all age groups, and with asthma in the elderly in the winter months.

Early studies of adverse effects of SO_2 and particles on the frequency of emergency room visits for asthma in New York did not find any relation between pollution levels and asthma attendances (207,208). Because the analyses were based on daily average SO_2 concentrations, effects of short-term peak exposures of SO_2 may have been missed. This question was specifically addressed in further studies in Harlem and Brooklyn, New York, during 1969–1972 (209–210). No acute effects on asthma emergency room visits were seen for high short-term SO_2 exposure, even at maximum hourly concentrations well in excess of 0.123 ppm, the current WHO guideline.

Several recent studies have carefully investigated the effects of particulate pollution on asthma hospital admissions. In Birmingham, United Kingdom, a significant association with black smoke levels (lagged 2 days) during two winter periods from April 1988 to March 1990 was observed (211). The risk was estimated as a 19% increase in asthma admissions per day per 20 $\mu g/m^3$ increase in winter smoke level. Similarly, in the Seattle, Washington, area, a significant positive correlation between asthma emergency room visits and PM_{10} levels was found over one winter season from September 1989 to September 1990 (212). The association was strongest for the averae PM_{10} concentration over the previous 4 days and was seen for children and adults younger than 65. The risk was estimated as a 12% increase in asthma attendances per 30 $\mu g/m^3$ increase in PM_{10} (4-day average). Over the observed concentration range (10–60 $\mu g/m^3$ PM_{10}), no threshold level could be identified. Further evidence for adverse effects of exposure to particles arises from another Canadian study. Thurston and co-workers found a significant effect of summertime pollution on asthma admissions, the relative strengths of association being generally $H^+ > SO_4^- > FP > PM_{10} > TSP$, indicating that particle size and composition might be of central importance for the occurrence of adverse health effects of pollution (204). Likewise, Delfino and colleagues in Canada demonstrated an increase in admission rates by 2.7% for each 12 μg/m^3 increase in PM_{10} levels (lagged by 3 days) and a slightly stronger association with SO_4^{2-} levels that exceeded 8.1 μg/m^3 4 days before admission (*RR* = 1.1; 95% CI, 1.05–1.19) (213). Others have confirmed these findings showing a significant positive relation between asthma admissions and particulate pollution in subjects younger than age 65, but not in the elderly (214,211,215–218).

Few studies have addressed the effect of exposure to nitrogen dioxide on severe asthma attacks requiring hospital admission or emergency room treatment. In Spain, Castellsague and colleagues reported an association between asthma attendances and increasing NO_2 levels in both summer and winter (*RR* = 1.05) (217). In the United Kingdom, hospital admission rates for asthma in children younger than 5 years of age have been associated with background urban NO_2 concentrations in the ward of residence (219). Neither study satisfactorily adjusted for autocorrelation and confounding factors. Exceptionally high levels of NO_2 (0.423 ppm) occurred in London, England, in December 1991 (152). Concomitantly, levels of black smoke were elevated, but SO_2 and ozone were low. A very small 3% increase in asthma admissions in Greater London and the surrounding hospitals was found, whereas chronic bronchitis and emphysema in the elderly was affected to a greater extent.

C. Panel Studies

Panel studies are prospective studies enrolling subjects selected for the specific purpose of the study. Daily symptoms and peak flow are usually measured as response variables in asthmatic subjects. Each subject is used as his or her own control. The use of medication may have a masking effect on recorded symptoms and peak flow measurements, particularly in mild asthma. This can be assessed and, in itself, be used as an outcome variable. As the responses are generally small, other contributing factors such as meteorological conditions, exposure to infections or allergens, and the presence or absence of an attack on the previous day may be of greater importance. Furthermore, levels of pollutants and meteorological conditions often change together, rendering the identification of a specific factor troublesome.

Several epidemiological studies in children and young adults, spending time in outdoor settings, report findings parallel to those of the experimental exposures. In summer camp studies, as in other epidemiological studies on ozone outdoor exposure in children and adults, repetitive daily exposures to ambient ozone concentrations were associated with lower levels of lung function (220–230). In most studies, the magnitude of reported changes was small and comparable with those demonstrated in controlled human exposure studies, although Spektor and colleagues reported greater lung function deficits in children spending a 4-week recreation at a New Jersey summer camp (220) and reductions in spirometry about twice as large as in chamber studies in adults engaged in regular outdoor exercise in Tuxedo, New York (224). Ambient cofactors may thus potentiate the response to ambient ozone exposure in certain environments. In Mexico City, where WHO and US ozone standards are regularly exceeded, schoolchildren exercising for 1 hr at high ambient levels above 0.15 ppm up to 0.36 ppm were studied (230). Although these children had been repeatedly exposed to high levels of ozone in their daily activities before testing, an acute response, comparable with results from chamber studies, was elicited. Decreases in lung function were transient and reversed with decreasing ambient ozone levels (222,226). The long-term significance of these findings thus remains to be established.

In asthmatic children, significant negative associations between peak flow measurements and levels of PM_{10} have been found in some (214,231), but not in all studies (233,234). In the Czech Republic, where SO_2 and PM_{10} still reach high levels, up to 0.172 ppm SO_2 and 171 $\mu g/m^3$ PM_{10}, children showed significant, although extremely small changes in lung function, but not in symptoms (235). SO_2 levels at 0.023 ppm produced just a 0.57% fall in peak flow. Adults remained unaffected by these exposures. One other study in adult asthmatic patients has shown negative associations between peak flow and both ozone and SO_2 (236).

IV. Initiation of Asthma

In theory, exposure to air pollution might induce new cases of asthma through damage of the airway epithelium, stimulation of inflammatory cell activity, increased release of inflammatory mediators, thereby, enhanced penetration of allergens through the airway epithelium. Furthermore, oxidant exposure may increase airway inflammation, and thereby induce bronchial hyperresponsiveness in susceptible (e.g., atopic) subjects and add to the prevalence of asthma in polluted areas.

Few surveys have specifically studied the prevalence of asthma and associated objective markers of disease, such as atopic sensitization and airway hyperresponsiveness, in areas exposed to a wide range of pollutant concentrations. Most population studies investigated the prevalence of respiratory symptoms with little information specific to asthma or other wheezing illnesses between a few areas with different pollution profiles. The limitations of this type of studies are manifold.

First, not all that wheezes is asthma. Airflow limitation secondary to damage of the airway epithelium, inflammation, increased sputum production, and disordered clearance of mucus in acute and chronic bronchitis may present as wheezing. Furthermore, the benign condition of transient early wheezing must be distinguished from childhood asthma. As long as no objective parameters closely related to childhood and adult asthma, such as atopy and BHR, are measured the etiology of wheezing symptoms remains obscure.

Second, differences in the prevalence of asthma between two areas may arise from variation in factors, other than air pollution, that determine the development of asthma and wheezing illnesses. Careful assessment of such confounding factors must occur and be considered when interpreting the findings. Ideally, multicenter studies of air pollution, including regions over a wide range of concentrations of one specific pollutant without significant variation of other pollutants or risk factors for asthma, would overcome some of the methodological limitations of two- or three-point comparisons.

There is no consistent evidence that the prevalence of wheezing illnesses is increased in polluted areas as compared with control areas. In Eastern Europe, a 1.5- to 2-fold higher prevalence of wheezing and wheeze in the past year was found in children living in the more polluted towns of Czechoslovakia, Romania, and Poland (236). In contrast, a similar prevalence of wheezing and asthma was found in polluted and nonpolluted areas in Western Europe (Denmark, The Netherlands, Greece, and Spain). In Italy, environmental air pollution was not associated with asthma and atopy, but with an increased prevalence of cough and phlegm, pneumonia, early respiratory infection, and rhinitis (237). Among already sensitized subjects, symptoms were more frequent in those children living in an industrialized area as compared with a rural area, suggesting that air pollution may be related to the development of respiratory symptoms among already sensitized individuals.

An extensive survey of respiratory health enrolling over 5000 schoolchildren was carried out in 1980–1981 in six cities of Eastern and Midwestern United States (238). Across these six cities a twofold variation in annual mean TSP and ozone levels, a threefold variation in NO_2, and an eightfold variation in mean SO_2 was found. There was no significant relation between the prevalence of wheeze with level of any pollutant. In contrast, the prevalence of diagnosed asthma increased significantly with rising ozone levels, but hay fever symptoms did not show the same trend. In Arizona, the prevalence of wheeze or asthma was not increased in children living in the vicinity of smelter mills, who were exposed long-term to brief peaks of high concentrations of SO_2 (> 0.280 ppm). In contrast, children from an industrial town in Israel exposed to increased levels of NO_2 and SO_2 showed a higher prevalence of most asthmatic symptoms as compared with children of a control area (239). None of these studies included objective measures of bronchial reactivity or atopic sensitization.

In adults, the prevalence of wheezing and "frequent chest illness" was almost twice as high in Glendora, Los Angeles County, California, an area with very high levels of oxidants, NO_2, and sulfates as in adults living in Lancaster, a nearby control area with low levels of most pollutants (240). Diagnosed asthma, bronchitis, or emphysema, however, were equally prevalent in these regions. Likewise, Linn and colleagues failed to show any relation between prevalence of wheeze and asthma in nonsmoking adult Seventh Day Adventists in California (241). However, when relating the incidence of new cases of asthma within this cohort, who were followed over 10 years to estimates of lifetime exposure to oxidant air pollution, the risk of developing asthma increased significantly with cultivate particulate exposure (RR = 1.74; 95% CI: 1.11–2.72/1000 hr per year in excess of 200 μg/m^3 TSP). Estimated personal exposures to particles and ozone were highly correlated (r = 0.72), and cumulative ozone exposure was also significantly related to incident asthma in men.

It appears thus impossible to distinguish the independent effect of each pollutant with certainty. A higher prevalence of wheeze on most days or nights among women exposed to increased levels of SO_2 and particulate pollution caused by coal-fired electricity-generating plants has furthermore been reported in Pennsylvania (242).

A unique opportunity to study the effects of air pollution on the development of childhood asthma and atopy are with the reunification of Germany. Genetically similar populations in both parts of the country had been exposed over more than 40 years to radically different environmental conditions. Industrial areas of the former German Democratic Republic experienced excessively high levels of winter SO_2 (0.105 ppm annual average) and particulate pollution (80 $\mu g/m^3$ annual average), whereas in the West German cities outdoor nitrogen dioxide concentrations (0.028 ppm annual average) tended to be higher, reflecting the much denser car traffic. Several studies in children, as in adults, have shown consistently that the prevalences of asthma, bronchial hyperresponsiveness, hay fever, and atopy were all significantly lower in the polluted cities of East Germany compared with Western German cities (243–247). Likewise, the prevalence of atopic sensitization and asthma was lower in schoolchildren living in the more-polluted eastern part of the Baltic Area as compared with western Sweden (248,249).

Conversely, the prevalence of childhood bronchitis and wheeze was higher in the eastern part of the country compared with the western side. In Leipzig, East Germany, air pollution levels were associated with the occurrence of upper respiratory tract symptoms in school-age children (250). Although in the winter period, daily mean concentrations of SO_2 and NO_2, and daily maximum levels of TSP significantly increased the risk of developing symptoms of the upper respiratory tract, only NO_2 levels remained significant predictors of symptoms during the summer. Thus, the higher prevalence of wheeze in polluted areas may reflect nonspecific, irritative damage of the airways, resulting in acute and chronic bronchitis, rather then the initiation of asthma and atopy.

High rates of road traffic impaired pulmonary function and increased respiratory symptoms in children living in Munich, West Germany (251). However, the prevalence of allergic rhinitis, asthma, BHR, and atopic sensitization was not associated with increasing car traffic counts. A few other surveys have investigated effects of exposure to vehicle emissions in Japan, Britain, and Germany. In Japanese women aged 40–59 years the prevalence of respiratory symptoms, such as wheeze, on most days and nights or wheeze apart from colds, and chronic cough or phlegm was related to living within 20 m of a busy road in Tokyo (252). Likewise, an increase in respiratory symptoms was found in Dutch girls, but not in boys living close to major roads (253). Neither study included objective measures of disease to distinguish between bronchitic and asthmatic symptoms. Two further German studies have linked self-reported symptoms of wheeze and allergic rhinitis in children to self-reported exposure to main roads or frequency of heavy goods vehicle traffic (254,255). This subjective way of exposure assessment may, however, introduce substantial bias because parents of affected children may tend to overreport traffic exposure and vice versa. In the United Kingdom, the prevalence of current wheeze and asthma was unrelated to motorway exposure (256), whereas preschool children admitted to the hospital because of asthma were significantly more likely to live in an area with high traffic flow (257). These findings were confirmed by Pershagen and colleagues in Sweden, who demonstrated a significant relation between hospital admissions for wheezing illnesses in preschool girls, but not in boys, and outdoor NO_2 exposure, resulting mainly from traffic emissions (258). In both studies a significant proportion of these children may have had benign transient early wheezing that is unrelated to the development of childhood asthma. Finally, a Japanese survey reported an increased prevalence of cedar pollinosis in areas with high traffic exposure and concomitant increased pollen counts (259). The results of this study should, however, be interpreted with caution because potential confounding factors, such as socioeconomic status, were not explored.

V. Conclusions

The weight of evidence argues against a causal relation between air pollution and the initiation of asthma. The geographic variation in the prevalence of asthma in children and adults does not coincide with variations in air pollution levels. Moreover, the increase in the prevalence of asthma seen over the last decades is unlikely to be the result of changes in air pollution. The emissions of SO_2 and particles from coal combustion have fallen markedly during the past 30 years in many Western countries, and there is no evidence for an increase in peak ozone concentrations over the past 15–20 years. Emissions from mobile sources of NO_x and particles have increased, but the results of epidemiological surveys and controlled human exposure studies do not support a causal link between exposure to these pollutants and the inception of asthma.

Among asthmatic subjects, exposure to sulfur dioxide, and in some asthmatic individuals to ozone, in concentrations encountered in ambient outdoor air, causes an increase in airway resistance in chamber studies. In panel studies, winter pollution episodes and ozone exposure reduce lung function in asthmatic children by a small amount, although an increase in symptoms is less likely. In adult asthmatic patients, the effects of exposure to both ozone and winter pollutants are less consistent, but point in the same direction. Several epidemiological surveys in eastern United States and Canada have furthermore found higher asthma admission rates on high ozone days, whereas no such correlation was found in the western United States. The summertime pollutant mixtures in eastern and western America may differ from each other and from mixtures occurring over Europe and other countries. Finally, exposure to ozone and possibly to nitrogen dioxide may enhance the response to allergen challenge in asthmatic subjects already sensitized to that allergen.

References

1. Ferris BG. Epidemiological standardisation project. Am Rev Respir Dis 1978; 118(suppl):7–53.
2. ISAAC Co-ordinating Committee. Manual for the International Study of Asthma and Allergies in Childhood (ISAAC). Bochum and Auckland: ISAAC Co-ordinating Committee, 1992.
3. Martinez FD, Wright AL, Taussig LM, Holberg CJ, Halonen M, Morgan WJ, GHMA personnel. Asthma and wheezing in the first six years of life. N Engl J Med 1995; 332:133–138.
4. Strachan DP. The prevalence and natural history of wheezing in early childhood. J R Coll Gen Pract 1985; 35:182–184.
5. Park ES, Golding J, Carswell F, Stewart-Brown S. Preschool wheezing and prognosis at 10. Arch Dis Child 1986; 61:642–646.
6. Martinez FD, Morgan WJ, Wright AL, Holberg C, Taussig LM, GHMA personnel. Diminished lung function as a predisposing factor for wheezing respiratory illness in infants. N Engl J Med 1988; 319:1112–1117.
7. Martinez FD, Morgan WJ, Wright AL, Holberg C, Taussig LM, GHMA personnel. Initial airway function is a risk factor for recurrent wheezing respiratory illnesses during the first three years of life. Am Rev Respir Dis 1991; 143:312–316.
8. Tager IB, Hanrhan JP, Tosteson TD, Castile RG, Brown RW, Weiss ST, Speizer FE. Lung function, pre- and post-natal smoke exposure, and wheezing in the first year of life. Am Rev Respir Dis 1993; 147:811–817.
9. Sporik R, Holgate ST, Cogswell JJ. Natural history of asthma in childhood—a birth cohort study. Arch Dis Child 1991; 66:1050–1053.
10. Hanrahan J, Tager I, Castile R, Segal M, Weiss S, Speizer FE. Pulmonary function measures in healthy infants. Am Rev Respir Dis 1990; 140:1127–1135.
11. Hanrahan JP, Tager IB, Segal MR, Tosteson TD, Castile RG, van Vunakis H, Weiss ST, Speizer FE. The effect of maternal smoking during pregnancy on early infant lung function. Am Rev Respir Dis 1992; 146:1129–1135.
12. Taylor B, Wadsworth J. Maternal smoking during pregnancy and lower respiratory tract illness in early life. Arch Dis Child 1987; 62:786–791.
13. Young S, Arnott J, Le Souef P, Landau LI. Flow limitation during tidal expiration in symptom-free infants and the subsequent development of asthma. J Pediatr 1994; 124:681–688.
14. Clarke JR, Reese A, Silverman M. Bronchial responsiveness and lung function in infants with lower respiratory tract illness over the first 6 months of life. Arch Dis Child 1992; 67:1454–1458.
15. Stick SM, Arnott J, Turner DJ, Young S, Landau LI, Le Souef PN. Bronchial responsiveness and lung function in recurrently wheezing infants. Am Rev Respir Dis 1991; 144:1012–1015.
16. Morgan WJ, Taussig LM. The chronic bronchitis complex in children. Pediatr Clin North Am 1984; 31:851–864.
17. Burrows B, Martinez FD, Halonen M, Barbee RA, Cline MG. Association of asthma with serum IgE levels and skin-test reactivity to allergens. N Engl J Med 1989; 320:271–277.
18. Sears MR, Burrows B, Flannery EM, Herbison GP, Hewitt CJ, Holdaway MD. Relation between airway responsiveness and serum IgE in children with asthma and in apparently normal children. N Engl J Med 1991; 325:1067–1071.
19. Clough JB, Williams JD, Holgate ST. Effect of atopy on the natural history of symptoms, peak expiratory flow, and bronchial responsiveness in 7- and 8-year-old children with cough and wheeze. Am Rev Respir Dis 1991; 143:755–760.
20. Kelly WJ, Hudson I, Phelan PD, Pain M, Olinsky A. Atopy in subjects with asthma followed to the age of 28 years. J Allergy Clin Immunol 1990; 85:548–557.
21. Van Asperen PP, Kemp AS, Mukhi A. Atopy in infancy predicts the severity of bronchial hyperresponsiveness in later childhood. J Allergy Clin Immunol 1990; 85:790–795.

22. Zimmerman B, Feanny S, Resiman J, Hak H, Rashed N, McLaughlin FJ, Levison H. Allergy in asthma. J Allergy Clin Immunol 1988; 81:63–70.
23. Peat JK, Salome CM, Woolcock AJ. Longitudinal changes in atopy during a 4-year period: relation to bronchial hyperresponsiveness and respiratory symptoms in a population sample of Australian schoolchildren. J Allergy Clin Immunol 1990; 85:65–74.
24. Sherrill DL, Martinez FD. On early sensitization to allergens and development of respiratory symptoms. Am J Respir Crit Care Med 1996; 153:A431.
25. Price IF, Hey EN, Soothill JF. Antigen provocation to the skin, nose and lung, in children with asthma; immediate and dual hypersensitivity reaction. Exp Immunol 1982; 47:587–594.
26. Warner JO. Significance of late reactions after bronchial challenge with house dust mite. Arch Dis Child 1976; 51:905–911.
27. Holgate ST, Kay AB. Mast cells, mediators and asthma. Clin Allergy 1985; 15:221–234.
28. O'Byrne PM, Dolovich J. Hargreave FE. Late asthmatic responses. Am Rev Respir Dis 1987; 136:740–751.
29. Drazen JM, Austen KF. Leukotrienes and airway responses. Am Rev Respir Dis 1981; 136:985–998.
30. Azzawi M, Bradley B, Jeffrey PK, Frew A, Wardlaw A, Knowles G, Assoufi B, Collins J, Durham S, Kay AB. Identification of activated T lymphocytes and eosinophils in bronchial biopsies in stable atopic asthma. Am Rev Respir Dis 1990; 142:1407–1413.
31. Robinson D, Hamid Q, Ying S, Tsicopoulos A, Barkans J, Bentley AM, Corrigan C, Durham SR, Kay AB. Predominant Th2-like bronchoalveolar T-lymphocyte population in atopic asthma. N Engl J Med 1992; 326:298–304.
32. Folkerts G, Verheyen AKCP, Geuens GMA, Folkerts HF, Nijkamp FP. Virus-induced changes in airway responsiveness, morphology, and histamine levels in guinea pigs. Am Rev Respir Dis 1993; 147:1569–1577.
33. Whincup PH, Cook DG, Strachan DP, Papacosta O. Time trends in respiratory symptoms in childhood over a 24 year period. Arch Dis Child 1993; 68:729–734.
34. Burr ML, Butland BK, King S, Vaughan-Williams E. Changes in asthma prevalence: two surveys 15 years apart. Arch Dis Child 1989; 64:1452–1456.
35. Burney PGJ, Chinn S, Rona RJ. Has the prevalence of asthma increased in children? Evidence from the national study of health and growth 1973–86. Br Med J 1990; 300:1306–1310.
36. Anderson HR, Butland BK, Strachan DP. Trends in prevalence and severity of childhood asthma. Br Med J 1994; 308:160–1604.
37. Ninan T, Russell G. Respiratory symptoms and atopy in Aberdeen schoolchildren: evidence from two surveys 25 years apart. Br Med J 1992; 304:873–875.
38. Gergen PJ, Mullally DI, Evans R III. National survey of prevalence of asthma among children in the United States, 1976 to 1980. Pediatrics 1988; 81:1–7.
39. Weitzman M, Gortmaker SL, Sobol AM, Perrin JM. Recent trends in the prevalence and severity of childhood asthma. JAMA 1992; 268:2673–2677.
40. Robertson CF, Heycock E, Bishop J, Nolan T, Olinsky A, Phelan PD. Prevalence of asthma in Melbourne schoolchildren: changes over 26 years. Br Med J 1991; 302:1116–1118.
41. Peat JK, van den Berg RH, Green WF, Mellis CM, Leeder SR, Woolcock AJ. Changing prevalence of asthma in Australian children. Br Med J 1994; 308:1591–1596.
42. Erzen D, Roos LL, Manfreda J, Anthonisen NR. Changes in asthma severity in Manitoba. Chest 1995; 108:16–23.
43. Health effects of outdoor air pollution. Part 1. Am J Respir Crit Care Med 1996; 153:3–50.
44. Health effects of atmospheric acids and their precursors. Report of the ATS Workshop on the Health Effects of Atmospheric Acids and Their Precursors. Am Rev Respir Dis 1991; 144:464–467.
45. Sandström T. Respiratory effects of air pollutants: experimental studies in humans. Eur Respir J 1995; 8:976–995.

46. Morgan DL, Wenzel DG. Cytotoxic action of rat alveolar macrophages for ozone-exposed lung fibroblasts. Toxicol Lett 1985; 26:37–42.
47. Goldstein BD, Lodi C, Collinson C, Balchum OJ. Ozone and lipid peroxidation. Arch Environ Health 1969; 18:631–635.
48. Bhalla DK, Young C. Effects of acute exposure to O_3 on rats: sequence of epithelial and inflammatory changes in the distal airways. Inhal Toxicol 1992; 4:17–31.
49. Koren HS, Devlin RB, Graham DE, Mann R, McGee MP, Horstman DH, Kozumbo WJ, Becker S, House DE, McDonnell WF, Bromberg PA. Ozone-induced inflammation in the lower airways of human subjects. Am Rev Respir Dis 1989; 139:407–415.
50. Gerrity TR, Weaver RA, Berntsen J, House DE, O'Neil JJ. Extrathoracic and intrathoracic removal of ozone in tidal breathing humans. J Appl Physiol 1988; 65:393–400.
51. Miller FJ, Overton JH, Jaskot RH, Menzel DB. A model of the regional uptake of gaseous pollutants in the lung. II. The sensitivity of the uptake of ozone in the human lung to lower respiratory tract reactions and exercise. Toxicol Appl Pharmacol 1985; 79:11–27.
52. Castelman WL, Dungworth DL, Schwartz LW, Tyler WS. Acute respiratory bronchiolitis. An ultrastructural and autoradiographic study of epithelial cell injury and renewal in rhesus monkeys exposed to ozone. Am J Pathol 1980; 98:811–840.
53. Tepper JS, Costa DL, Lehmann JR, Weber MF, Hatch GE. Unattenuated structural and biochemical alterations in the rat lung during functional adaptation to ozone. Am Rev Respir Dis 1989; 140:493–501.
54. Kerr HD, Kulle TJ, McIlhany ML, Swidersky P. Effects of ozone on pulmonary function in normal subjects: an environmental-chamber study. Am Rev Respir Dis 1975; 111.763–773.
55. McDonnell WF, Horstman DH, Hazucha MJ, Seal E Jr, Haak ED, Salaam SA, House DE. Pulmonary effects of ozone exposure during exercise: dose response characteristics. J Appl Physiol 1983; 5:1345–1352.
56. Kulle TJ, Sauder LR, Hebel JR, Chatham MD. Ozone response relationships in healthy nonsmokers. Am Rev Respir Dis 1985; 132:36–41.
57. Linn WS, Avol EL, Shamoo DA, Spier CE, Valencia LM, Venet TG, Fischer DA, Hackney JD. A dose–response study of healthy, heavily exercising men exposed to ozone at concentrations near the ambient air quality standard. Toxicol Ind Health 1986; 2:99–112.
58. Weinmann GG, Bowes SM, Gerbase MW, Kimball AW, Frank R. Response to acute ozone exposure in healthy men. Results of a screening procedure. Am J Respir Crit Care Med 1995; 151:33–40.
59. Horstman DH, Folinsbee LJ, Ives PJ, Abdul-Salaam S, McDonnell WF. Ozone concentration and pulmonary response relationships for 6.6-hour exposures with five hours of moderate exercise to 0.08, 0.10, and 0.12 ppm. Am Rev Respir Dis 1990; 142:1158–1163.
60. Hazucha MJ. Relationship between ozone exposure and pulmonary function changes. J Appl Physiol 1987; 62:1671–1680.
61. McDonnell WF, Horstman DH, Abdul-Salaam S, House DE. Reproducibility of individual responses to ozone exposure. Am Rev Respir Dis 1985; 131:36–40.
62. Gliner JA, Horvath SM, Folinsbee LJ. Pre-exposure to low ozone concentrations does not diminish the pulmonary function response on exposure to higher ozone concentration. Am Rev Respir Dis 1983; 127:51–55.
63. Emons K, Foster WM. Smoking cessation and acute airway response to ozone. Arch Environ Health 1991; 45:288–295.
64. McDonnell WF, Muller KE, Bromberg PA, Shy CM. Predictors of individual differences in acute response to ozone exposure. Am Rev Respir Dis 1993; 147:818–825.
65. Solic JJ, Hazucha MJ, Bromberg BA. The acute effects of 0.2 ppm ozone in patients with chronic obstructive pulmonary disease. Am Rev Respir Dis 1982; 125:664–669.
66. Linn WS, Fischer DA, Medway DA, Anzar UT, Spier CE, Valencia LM, Venet TG, Hackney JD. Short-term respiratory effects of 0.2 ppm ozone exposure in volunteers with chronic obstructive disease. Am Rev Respir Dis 1982; 125:658–663.

67. Holtzman MJ, Cunningham JH, Sheller JR, Irsigker GB, Nadel JA, Boushey HA. Effect of ozone on bronchial reactivity in atopic and nonatopic subjects. Am Rev Respir Dis 1979; 120:1059–1067.
68. Linn WS, Jones MP, Bachmayer EA, Spier CE, Mazur SF, Avol EL, Hackney JD. Short-term respiratory effects of polluted ambient air: laboratory study of volunteers in a high oxidant community. Am Rev Respir Dis 1980; 121:243–252.
69. Koenig JQ, Covert DS, Marshall SG, van Belle G, Pierson WE. The effects of ozone and nitrogen dioxide on pulmonary function in healthy and in asthmatic adolescents. Am Rev Respir Dis 1987; 136:1152–1157.
70. Holtzman MJ, Cunningham JH, Sheller JR, Irsigler GB, Nadel JA, Boushey HA. Effect of ozone on the bronchial reactivity in atopic and nonatopic subjects. Am Rev Respir Dis 1979; 120:1059–1067.
71. Linn WS, Buckley RD, Spier CE, Blessey RL, Jones MP, Fischer DA, Hackney JD. Health effects of ozone exposure in asthmatics. Am Rev Respir Dis 1978; 117:835–843.
72. Hazucha MJ. Relationship between ozone exposure and pulmonary function changes. J Appl Physiol 1987; 62:1671–1680.
73. Kreit JW, Gross KB, Moore TB, Lorenzen TJ, D'Arcy J, Eschenbacher WL. Ozone-induced changes in pulmonary function and bronchial responsiveness in asthmatics. J Appl Physiol 1989; 66:217–222.
74. Hazucha MJ, Silverman F, Parent C, Field S, Bates DV. Pulmonary function in man after short-term exposure to ozone. Arch Environ Health 1973; 27:183–188.
75. Kerr HD, Kulle TJ, McIlhany ML, Swidersky P. Effects of ozone on pulmonary function in normal subjects: an environmental-chamber study. Am Rev Respir Dis 1975; 111:763–773.
76. Folinsbee LJ, Bedi JF, Horvath SM. Pulmonary function changes after one hour continuous heavy exercise in 0.21 ppm ozone. J Appl Physiol Respir Environ Exerc Physiol 1984; 57:984–988.
77. McDonnell WF, Kehrl HR, Abdul Salaam S, Ives PJ, Folinsbee LJ, Devlin RB, O'Neil JJ, Horstman DH. Respiratory response of humans exposed to lower levels of ozone for 6.6 hours. Arch Environ Health 1991; 46:145–150.
78. Folinsbee LJ, McDonnell WF, Horstman DH. Pulmonary function and symptom responses after 6.6-hour exposure to 0.12 ppm ozone with moderate exercise. J Air Pollut Control Assoc 1988; 38:28–35.
79. Hostman DH, Folinsbee LJ, Ives PJ, Abdul-Salaam S, McDonnel WF. Ozone concentration and pulmonary response relationships for 6.6-hour exposures with five hours of moderate exercise to 0.08, 0.10, and 0.12 ppm. Am Rev Respir Dis 1990; 142:1158–1163.
80. Adams WC, Savin WM, Christo AE. Detection of ozone toxicity during continuous exercise via the effective dose concept. J Appl Physiol 1981; 51:415–422.
81. Hazucha MJ. Relationship between ozone exposure and pulmonary function changes. J Appl Physiol 1987; 62:1671–1680.
82. Golden JA, Nadel JA, Boushey HA. Bronchial hyperirritability in healthy subjects after exposure to ozone. Am Rev Respir Dis 1978; 118:287–294.
83. Jörres R, Nowak D, Magnussen H, Speckin P, Koschyk S. The effect of ozone exposure on allergen responsiveness in subjects with asthma or rhinitis. Am J Respir Crit Care Med 1996; 153:56–64.
84. Fernandes ALG, Molfino NA, McClean PA, Silverman F, Tarlo S, Raizenne M, Slutsky AS, Zamel N. The effect of pre-exposure to 0.12 ppm of ozone on exercise-induced asthma. Chest 1994; 106:1077–1082.
85. Weymer AR, Gong H, Lyness A, Linn WS. Pre-exposure to ozone does not enhance or produce exercise-induced asthma. Am J Respir Crit Care Med 1994; 149:1413–1419.
86. Molfino NA, Wright SC, Kazt I, Tarlo S, Silverman F, McClean PA, Szalai JP, Raizenne M, Slutsky AS, Zamel N. Effect of low concentrations of ozone on inhaled allergen responses in asthmatic subjects. Lancet 1991; 338:199–203.

87. Linn WS, Avol EL, Shamoo DA, Peng RC, Valencia LM, Little DE, Hackney JD. Repeated laboratory ozone exposures of volunteer Los Angeles residence: an apparent seasonal variation in response. Toxicol Ind Health 1988; 4:505–520.
88. Linn WS, Medway DA, Anzar UT, Valencia LM, Spier CE, Tsao FSD, Fischer A, Hackney JD. Persistence of adaptation to ozone in volunteers exposed repeatedly for six weeks. Am Rev Respir Dis 1982; 125:491–495.
89. Farrell BP, Kerr HD, Kulle TJ, Sauder LR, Young JL. Adaptation in human subjects to the effects of inhaled ozone after repeated exposure. Am Rev Respir Dis 1979; 119:725–730.
90. McDonnell WF, Horstman DH, Abdul-Salaam S, Raggio LJ, Green JA. The respiratory responses of subjects with allergic rhinitis to ozone exposure and their relationship to nonspecific airway reactivity. Toxicol Ind Health 1987; 3:507–517.
91. Dimeo MJ, Glenn MG, Holtzman MJ, Sheller JR, Nadel JA, Boushey HA. Threshold concentration of ozone causing an increase in bronchial reactivity in humans and adaptation with repeated exposures. Am Rev Respir Dis 1981; 124:245–248.
92. Folinsbee LJ, Horstman DH, Kehrl HR, Harder S, Abdul-Salaam S, Ives PJ. Respiratory responses to repeated prolonged exposure to 0.12 ppm ozone. Am J Respir Crit Care Med 1994; 149:98–105.
93. Kulle TJ, Sauder LR, Kerr HD, Farrell BP, Bermel MS, Smith DM. Duration of pulmonary function adaptation to ozone in humans. Am Ind Hyg Assoc J 1982; 43:832–837.
94. Hazucha MJ, Bates DV, Bromberg PA. Mechanism of action of ozone in the human lung. J Appl Physiol 1989; 67:1535–1541.
95. Beckett WS, McDonnell WF, Horstman DH, House DE. Role of the parasympathetic nervous system in acute lung response to ozone. J Appl Physiol 1985; 59:1879–1885.
96. Schelegle ES, Adams WC, Siefkin AD. Indomethacin pretreatment reduces ozone-induced pulmonary function decrements in human subjects. Am Rev Respir Dis 1987; 136:1350–1354.
97. Ying RL, Gross KB, Terzo TS, Eschenbacher WL. Indomethacin does not inhibit the ozone-induced increase in bronchial responsiveness in human subjects. Am Rev Respir Dis 1990; 142:817–821.
98. Basha MA, Gross KB, Gwizdala CJ, Haidar AH, Popovich J. Bronchoalveolar lavage neutrophilia in asthmatic and healthy volunteers after controlled exposure to ozone and filtered purified air. Chest 1994; 106:1757–1765.
99. Koren HS, Devlin RB, Graham DE, Mann R, McGee P, Horstman DH, Kozumbo WJ, Becker S, House DE, McDonnell WF, Bromberg PA. Ozone-induced inflammation in the lower airways of human subjects. Am Rev Respir Dis 1989; 139:407–415.
100. Devlin RB, McDonnell WF, Mann R, Becker S, House DE, Schreinemachers D, Koren HS. Exposure of humans to ambient levels of ozone for 6.6 hours causes cellular and biochemical changes in the lung. Am J Respir Cell Mol Biol 1981; 4:72–81.
101. Aris RM, Christian D, Hearne PQ, Kerr K, Finkbeiner WE, Balmes JR. Ozone-induced airway inflammation in human subjects as determined by airway lavage and biopsy. Am Rev Respir Dis 1993; 148:1363–1372.
102. Scannell C, Chen L, Aris RM, Tager I, Christian D, Ferrando R, Welch B, Kelly T, Balmes JR. Greater ozone-induced inflammatory responses in subjects with asthma. Am J Respir Crit Care Med 1996; 154:24–29.
103. Frank NR, Yoder RE, Brain JD, Yokoyama E. $^{35}SO_2$ absorption by the nose and mouth under conditions of varying concentration and flow. Arch Environ Health 1969; 18:315–322.
104. Alarie YC, Ulrich CE, Busey WM, Krumm AA, McFarland HN. Long-term continuous exposure to sulfur dioxide in cynomolgus monkeys. Arch Environ Health 1972; 24:115–128.
105. Kulle TJ, Sauder LR, Shanty F, Kerr HD, Farrell BP, Miller WR, Milman JH. Sulfur oxide and ammonium sulfate effects on pulmonary function and bronchial reactivity in human subjects. Am Ind Hyg Assoc J 1984; 45:156–161.

106. Bedi JF, Folinsbee LJ, Horvath SM. Pulmonary function effects of 1.0 and 2.0 ppm sulfur dioxide exposures in active young male nonsmokers. J Air Pollut Control Assoc 1984; 34:1117–1121.
107. Schachter EN, Witek TJ, Beck GJ, Hosein HR, Colice G, Leaderer BP, Cain W. Airway effects of low concentrations of sulfur dioxide: dose–response characteristics. Arch Environ Health 1984; 39:34–42.
108. Folinsbee LJ, Bedi JF, Horvath SM. Pulmonary response to threshold levels of sulfur dioxide (1.0 ppm) and ozone (0.3 ppm). J Appl Physiol 1985; 58:1783–1787.
109. Balmes JR, Fine JM, Sheppard D. Symptomatic bronchoconstriction after short-term inhalation of sulfur dioxide. Am Rev Respir Dis 1987; 136:1117–1121.
110. Koenig JQ, Piersson WE, Horike M, Frank R. Effects of inhaled sulfur dioxide (SO_2) on pulmonary function in healthy adolescents: exposure to SO_2 alone or SO_2 and sodium chloride droplet aerosol during rest and exercise. Arch Environ Health 1982; 37:15–19.
111. Roger LJ, Kehrl HR, Hazucha M, Hostman DH. Bronchoconstriction in asthmatics exposed to sulfur dioxide during repeated exercise. J Appl Physiol 1985; 59:784–791.
112. Sheppard D, Wong WS, Uehara CF, Nadel A, Boushe HA. Lower threshold and greater bronchomotor responsiveness of asthmatic subjects to sulfur dioxide. Am Rev Respir Dis 1980; 22:873–878.
113. Sheppard D, Saisho A, Nadel AJ, Boushey HA. Exercise increases sulfur dioxide-induced bronchoconstriction in asthmatic subjects. Am Rev Respir Dis 1981; 123:486–491.
114. Horstman DH, Seal EJ, Folinsbee LJ, Ives P, Roger LH. The relationship between exposure duration and sulfur dioxide-induced bronchoconstriction in asthmatic subjects. Am Ind Hyg Assoc J 1988; 49:38–47.
115. Kehlr HR, Roger LJ, Hazucha MJ, Horstman DH. Differing response of asthmatics to SO_2 exposure with continuous and intermittent exercise. Am Rev Respir Dis 1987; 135:350–355.
116. Sheppard D, Epstein J, Bethel RA, Nadel JA, Boushey HA. Tolerance to sulfur dioxide-induced bronchoconstriction in subjects with asthma. Environ Res 1983; 30:412–419.
117. Hackney JD, Linn WS, Bailey RM, Spier CE, Valencia LM. Time course of exercise-induced bronchoconstriction in asthmatics exposed to sulfur dioxide. Environ Res 1984; 34:321–327.
118. Linn WS, Avol EL, Shamoo DA, Venet TG, Anderson KR, Whynot JD, Hackney JD. Asthmatics' responses to 6-hour SO_2 exposures on two successive days. Arch Environ Health 1984; 39:313–319.
119. Linn WS, Venet TG, Shamoo DA, Valencia LM, Anzar UT, Spier CE, Hackney JD. Respiratory effects of sulfur dioxide in heavily exercising asthmatics. Am Rev Respir Dis 1983; 127:278–283.
120. Jaeger MJ, Tribble D, Wittig JH. Effect of 0.5 ppm sulfur dioxide on the respiratory function of normal and asthmatic subjects. Lung 1979; 156:119–127.
121. Sandstroem T, Kolmodin-Hedman B, Sternbjerg N, Andersson M-C, Loefvenius G. Challenge test for sulfur dioxide: symptom and lung function measurements. Scand J Work Environ Health 1988; 14:77–79.
122. Horstman DH, Seal EJ, Folinsbee LJ, Ives P, Roger LH. The relationship between exposure duration and sulfur dioxide induced bronchoconstriction in asthmatic subjects. Am Ind Hyg Assoc J 1988; 49:38–47.
123. Sheppard DW, Eschenbacher WL, Boushey HA, Bethel RA. Magnitude of the interaction between the bronchomotor effects of sulfur dioxide and those of cold (dry) air. Am Rev Respir Dis 1984; 130:52–55.
124. Linn WS, Shamoo DA, Anderson KR, Whynot JD, Avol EL, Hackney JD. Effects of heat and humidity on the responses of exercising asthmatics to sulfur dioxide exposure. Am Rev Respir Dis 1985; 131:221–225.
125. Tan WC, Cripps E, Douglas N, Sudlow MF. Protective effect of drugs on bronchoconstriction induced by sulphur dioxide. Thorax 1982; 37:671–676.

126. Briggs DF, Goel V. Mechanisms of action of sodium cromoglycate. Can J Physiol Pharmacol 1985; 63:760–765.
127. Myers DJ, Bigby BG, Calvayrac P, Sheppard D, Boushey HA. Interaction of cromolyn and a muscarinic antagonist in inhibiting bronchial reactivity to sulfur dioxide and to eucapnic hyperpnea alone. Am Rev Respir Dis 1986; 133:1154–1158.
128. Meyers DJ, Bigby BG, Boushey HA. The inhibition of sulfur dioxide-induced bronchoconstriction in asthmatic subjects by cromolyn is dose-dependent. Am Rev Respir Dis 1986; 133:1150–1153.
129. Sandström T, Stjernberg N, Andersson M-C, Kolmodin-Hedman B, Lundgren R, Rosenhall L, Angström T. Cell response in bronchoalveolar lavage fluid after exposure to sulfur dioxide: a time–response study. Am Rev Respir Dis 1989; 140:1828–1831.
130. Amdur MO, Bayles J, Urgo V, Underhill DW. Comparative irritant potency of sulfate salts. Environ Res 1978; 16:1–8.
131. Utell MJ, Morrow PE, Speers DM, Darling J, Hyde RW. Airway responses to sulfate and sulfuric acid aerosols in asthmatics: an exposure–response relationship. Am Rev Respir Dis 1983; 128:444–450.
132. Larson TV, Frank R, Covert DS, Holub D, Morgan MS. Measurements of respiratory ammonia and the chemical neutralization of inhaled sulfuric acid aerosol in anesthetized dogs. Am Rev Respir Dis 1982; 125:502–506.
133. Utell MJ, Morrow PE, Hyde RW. Airway reactivity to sulfate and sulfuric acid aerosols in normal and asthmatic subjects. J Aer Pollut Control Assoc 1984; 34:931–935.
134. Kulle TJ, Kerr HD, Farrell BP, Sauder LR, Bermel MS. Pulmonary function and bronchial reactivity in humans subjects with exposure to ozone and respirable sulfuric acid aerosol. Am Rev Respir Dis 1982; 126:996–1000.
135. Leikauf GD, Yeates DB, Wales KA, Spektor DM, Albert RE, Lippmann M. Effects of sulfuric acid aerosol on respiratory mechanics and mucociliary particle clearance in healthy nonsmoking adults. Am Ind Hyg Assoc J 1981; 42:273–282.
136. Sackner MA, Ford D, Fernandez R, Cipley R, Perez D, Kwoka M, Reinhart M, Michaelson ED, Schreck R, Wanner A. Effects of sulfuric acid aerosol on cardiopulmonary function in dogs, sheep, and humans. Am Rev Respir Dis 1978; 118:497–510.
137. Avol EL, Jones MP, Bailey RM, Chang NN, Kleinman MT, Linn WS, Bell KA, Hackney JD. Controlled exposures of human volunteers to sulfate aerosols. Am Rev Respir Dis 1979; 120:319–327.
138. Horstman D, Hazucha M, Haak E, Stacy R. Effects of submicronic sulfuric acid aerosol on human pulmonary function. Arch Environ Health 1982; 37:136–141.
139. Kerr HD, Kulle TJ, Farrell BP, Saunder LR, Young JL, Swift DL, Bourshok RM. Effects of sulfuric acid aerosol on pulmonary function in human subjects: an environmental chamber study. Environ Res 1981; 26:42–50.
140. Frampton MW, Voter KZ, Morrow PE, Roberts NJ Jr, Utell MJ. Sulfuric acid aerosol exposure in humans assessed by bronchoalveolar lavage. Am Rev Respir Dis 1992; 146:626–632.
141. Newhouse MT, Dolvich M, Obminski, Wolff RK. Effect of TLV levels of SO_2 and H_2SO_4 on bronchial clearance in exercising man. Arch Environ Health 1978; 33:24–32.
142. Koenig JQ, Pierson WE, Horike M. The effects of inhaled sulfuric acid on pulmonary function in adolescent asthmatics. Am Rev Respir Dis 1983; 128:221–225.
143. Koenig JQ, Covert DS, Pierson WE. Effects of inhalation of acidic compounds on pulmonary function in allergic adolescent subjects. Environ Health Perspect 1989; 79:173–178.
144. Morrow PE, Utell MJ, Bauer MA, Speers DM, Gibb FR. Effects of near ambient levels of sulfuric acid aerosol on lung function in exercising subjects with asthma and COPD. Ann Occup Hyg 1994; 38:933–938.
145. Aris RD, Christian D, Sheppard D, Balmes JR. Lack of bronchoconstrictor response to sulfuric acid aerosols and fogs. Am Rev Respir Dis 1991; 143:744–750.

146. Hanley QS, Koenig JQ, Larson TV, Anderson TL, van Belle G, Rebolledo V, Covert DS, Pierson WE. Response of young asthmatic patient to inhaled sulfuric acid. Am Rev Respir Dis 1992; 145:326–331.
147. Blames JR, Fine JM, Christian D, Gordon T, Sheppard D. Acidity potentiates bronchoconstriction induced by hypoosmolar aerosols. Am Rev Respir Dis 1988; 138:35–39.
148. Linn WS, Avol EL, Anderson KR, Shamoo DA, Peng R-C, Hackney JD. Effect of droplet size on respiratory responses to inhaled sulfuric acid in normal and asthmatic volunteers. Am Rev Respir Dis 1989; 140:161–166.
149. Aris D, Christian D, Sheppard D, Balmes JR. Acid fog-induced bronchoconstriction. The role of hydroxymethanesulfonic acid. Am Rev Respir Dis 1990; 141:546–551.
150. Frampton MW, Voter KZ, Morrow PE, Roberts NJ Jr, Culp DJ, Cox C, Utell MJ. Sulfuric acid aerosol exposure in humans assessed by bronchoalveolar lavage. Am Rev Respir Dis 1992; 146:626–632.
151. Health effects of outdoor air pollution. Part 2. Am J Respir Crit Care Med 1996; 153:477–498.
152. Anderson HR, Limb ES, Bland JM, Ponce de Leon A, Strachan DP, Bower JS. Health effects of an air pollution episode in London, December 1991. Thorax 1995; 50:1188–1193.
153. Gold DR. Indoor air pollution. Clin Chest Med 1992; 13:215–231.
154. Goldstein E, Peek NF, Parks NJ, Hines HH, Steffey EP, Trakington B. Fate and distribution of inhaled nitrogen dioxide in rhesus monkeys. Am Rev Respir Dis 1977; 115:403–412.
155. Bauer MA, Utell MJ, Morrow PE, Speers DM, Gibb FR. Inhalation of 0.30 ppm nitrogen dioxide potentiates exercise-induced bronchospasm in asthmatics. Am Rev Respir Dis 1986; 134:1203–1208.
156. Postlethwait EM, Bidani A. Reactive uptake governs the pulmonary air space removal of inhaled nitrogen dioxide. J Appl Physiol 1990; 68:594–603.
157. Mustafa MG, Tierny DF. Biochemical and metabolic changes in lung with oxygen, ozone and nitrogen dioxide toxicity. Am Rev Respir Dis 1978; 118:1061–1090.
158. Patel J, Block RE. Nitrogen dioxide-induced changes in cell membrane fluidity and function. Am Rev Respir Dis 1986; 134:1196–1202.
159. Pryor WA, Lightsey JW. Mechanisms of nitrogen dioxide actions, initiation of lipid peroxidation and the production of nitrous acid. Science 1981; 214:435–437.
160. Thomas T, Rhodes RA. C-1 palpitate incorporation by rat lung: effect of nitrogen dioxide. Proc Soc Exp Biol Med 1970; 108:1181–1183.
161. Greenberg SD, Györkey F, Jenkins D, Györkey P. Alveolar epithelial cells following exposure to nitric acid. Arch Environ Health 1971; 22:655–662.
162. Linn WS, Solomon JC, Trim SC, Spier CE, Shamoo DA, Venet TG, Avol EL, Hackney JD. Effects of exposure to 4 ppm nitrogen dioxide in healthy and asthmatic volunteers. Arch Environ Health 1985; 40:234–238.
163. Hackeny JD, Theide FC, Linn WS, Pedersen EE, Spier CE, Law DC, Fischer DA. Experimental studies on human health effects of air pollutants. Part IV. Short-term physiological and clinical effects of nitrogen dioxide exposures. Arch Environ Health 1978; 33:135–180.
164. Kerr HD, Kulle TJ, McIlhany ML, Swiderzsky. Effects of nitrogen dioxide on pulmonary function in human subjects: an environmental chamber study. Environ Res 1979; 19:392–404.
165. Mohsenin V. Effects of vitamin C on NO_2-induced airway hyperresponsiveness in normal subjects: a randomized double-blind experiment. Am Rev Respir Dis 1987; 136:1408–1411.
166. Mohsenin V. Airway responses to 2.0 ppm nitrogen dioxide in normal subjects. Arch Environ Health 1988; 43:242–246.

167. Hazucha MJ, Ginsberg JF, Mcdonnell WF, Haak ED Jr, Pimmel RL, Salaam SA, House DE, Bromberg PA. Effects of 0.1 ppm nitrogen dioxide on airways of normal and asthmatic subjects. J Appl Physiol 1983; 54:730–739.
168. Folinsbee LJ, Horvath SM, Bedi JF, Delehunt JC. Effect of 0.62 ppm NO_2 on cardiopulmonary function in young male nonsmokers. Environ Res 1978; 15:199–205.
169. Beil M, Ulmer WT. The acute effects of 5 ppm of NO_2 on the resistance of the human respiratory tract to breathing. Int Arch Occup Environ Health 1976; 38:31–44.
170. Bylin G, Lindvall T, Rehnt T, Sundin B. Effects of short-term exposure to ambient nitrogen dioxide concentrations on human bronchial reactivity and lung function. Eur J Respir Dis 1985; 66:205–217.
171. Frampton MW, Morrow PE, Cox C, Gibb FR, Speers DM, Utell MJ. Effects of nitrogen dioxide exposure on pulmonary function and airway reactivity in normal humans. Am Rev Respir Dis 1991; 143:522–527.
172. Oherek J, Massari JP, Gayrard P, Grimaud C, Charpin J. Effect of short-term, low-level nitrogen dioxide exposure on bronchial sensitivity of asthmatic patients. J Clin Invest 1976; 57:301–307.
173. Koenig JQ, Pierson WE, Marshall SG, Cover DS, Morgan MS, Van Belle G. The effects of ozone and nitrogen dioxide on lung function in healthy and adolescent asthmatics. Res Rep Health Eff Inst 1988; 14:5–24.
174. Linn WS, Shamoo DA, Avol EL, Whynot JD, Anderson KR, Venet TG, Hackney JD. Dose-response study of asthmatic volunteers exposed to nitrogen dioxide during intermittent exercise. Arch Environ Health 1986; 41:292–296.
175. Morrow PE, Utell MJ. Responses of susceptible subpopulations to nitrogen dioxide. Res Rep Health Eff Inst 1989; 23:1–44.
176. Roger LJ, Horstman DH, McConnell W, Kehrl H, Ives PJ, Seal E, Chapman R, Massaro EJ. Pulmonary function, airway responsiveness and respiratory symptoms in asthmatics following exercise in NO_2. Toxicol Ind Health 1990; 6:155–171.
177. Jörres R, Magnussen H. Effect of 0.25 ppm nitrogen dioxide on the airway response to methacholine in asymptomatic patients. Lung 1991; 169:77–85.
178. Kleinman MT, Bailey RM, Linn WS, Anderson KR, Whynot JD, Shamoo DA, Hackney JD. Effect of 0.2 ppm nitrogen dioxide on pulmonary function and response to bronchoprovocation in asthmatics. J Toxicol Environ Health 1983; 12:815–826.
179. Bauer MA, Utell MJ, Morrow PE, Speers DM, Gibb FR. Route of inhalation influences airway responses to 0.3 ppm nitrogen dioxide in asthmatic subjects [abstr]: Am Rev Respir Dis 1985; 133:A171.
180. Roger LJ, Horstman DH, McDonnell WF, Kehrl H, Seal E, Chapman RS, Massaro EJ. Pulmonary effects in asthmatics exposed to 0.3 ppm NO_2 during repeated exercise. Toxicologist 1985; 5:70.
181. Tunicliffe WS, Burge PS, Ayres JG. Effect of domestic concentrations of nitrogen dioxide on airway responses to inhaled allergen in asthmatic patients. Lancet 1994; 344:1733–1736.
182. Devalia JL, Rusnak C, Herdman MJ, Trigg CJ, Tarraf H, Davies RJ. Effect of nitrogen dioxide and sulphur dioxide on airway response of mild asthmatic patients to allergen inhalation. Lancet 1994; 344:1668–1671.
183. Frampton MW, Finkelstien JN, Roberts NJ Jr, Smelgin AM, Morrow PE, Utell MJ. Effects of nitrogen dioxide exposure on bronchoalveolar lavage proteins in humans. Am J Respir Cell Mol Biol 1989; 1:499–505.
184. Helleday R, Sandström T, Stjernberg N. Differences in bronchoalveolar cell response to nitrogen dioxide exposure between smokers and nonsmokers. Eur Respir J 1994; 7:1213–1220.
185. Sandström T, Andersson MC, Kolmodi-Hedman B, Stjernberg N, Angström T. Bronchoalveolar mastocytosis and lymphocytosis after nitrogen dioxide exposure in man: a time–kinetic study. Eur Respir J 1990; 3:138–143.

186. Sandström T, Stjernberg N, Eklund A, Ledin M-C, Bjermer L, Kolmodi-Hedman B, Lindström K, Rosenhall L, Angström T. Inflammatory cell response in bronchoalveolar lavage fluid after nitrogen dioxide exposure of healthy subjects: a dose–response study. Eur Respir J 1991; 3:332–339.
187. Rubinstein I, Reiss TF, Bigby BG, Stites DP, Boushey HA Jr. Effects of 0.6 ppm nitrogen dioxide on circulating and bronchoalveolar lavage lymphocyte phenotypes in healthy subjects. Environ Res 1991; 55:18–30.
188. Jörres R, Magnussen H. Airways response of asthmatics after a 30 min exposure, at resting ventilation, to 0.25 ppm NO_2 or 0.5 ppm SO_2. Eur Respir J 1990; 3:132–137.
189. Rubinstein I, Bigby BG, Reiss TF, Boushey HA. Short-term exposure to 0.3 ppm nitrogen dioxide does not potentiate airway responsiveness to sulfur dioxide in asthmatic subjects. Am Rev Respir Dis 1990; 141:381–385.
190. Koenig JQ, Covert DS, Smith MS, van Belle G, Pierson WE. The pulmonary effects of ozone and nitrogen dioxide alone and combined in healthy and asthmatic adolescent subjects. Toxicol Ind Health 1988; 3:521–532.
191. Follinsbee LJ, Bedi JF, Horvath SM. Combined effects of ozone and nitrogen dioxide on respiratory function in man. Am Ind Hyg Assoc J 1981; 42:534–541.
192. Adams WC, Brookes KA, Schelegle ES. Effects of NO_2 alone and in combination with O_3 on young men and women. J Appl Physiol 1987; 62:1698–1704.
193. Koenig JQ, Covert S, Hanley QS, van Belle G, Pierson WE. Prior exposure to ozone potentiates the subsequent response to sulfur dioxide in adolescent asthmatic subjects. Am Rev Respir Dis 1990; 141:377–380.
194. Stacy RW, Seal E Jr, House DE, Green J, Roger LJ, Raggio L. A survey of effects of gaseous and aerosol pollutants on pulmonary function of normal males. Arch Environ Health 1983; 38:104–115.
195. Kagawa J. Respiratory effects of two-hour exposures with intermittent exercise to ozone, sulfur dioxide and nitrogen dioxide alone and in combination in normal subjects. Am Ind Hyg Assoc J 1983; 44:14–20.
196. Bedi JF, Folinsbee LJ, Horvath SM, Ebenstein RS. Human exposure to sulfur dioxide and ozone: absence of a synergistic effect. Arch Environ Health 1979; 34:233–239.
197. Bedi JF, Horvath SM, Folinsbee LJ. Human exposure to sulfur dioxide and ozone in a high temperature-humidity system. Am Ind Hyg Assoc J 1982; 43:26–30.
198. Aris R, Christian D, Sheppard D, Balmes JR. The effects of sequential exposure to acidic fog and ozone on pulmonary function in exercising subjects. Am Rev Respir Dis 1991; 143:85–91.
199. Department of Health. Committee on the Medical Effects of Air Pollutants. Asthma and outdoor air pollution. HMSO, 1995.
200. Bates DV, Sizto R. Relationship between air pollutant levels and hospital admissions in southern Ontario. Can J Public Health 1983; 74:117–122.
201. Bates DV, Sizto R. Air pollution and hospital admissions in southern Ontario: the acid summer haze effect. Environ Res 1987; 43:317–331.
202. Bates DV, Sizto R. The Ontario air pollution study: identification of the causal agent. Environ Health Perspect 1989; 79:69–72.
203. Burnett RT, Dales RE, Raizenne ME, Krewski D, Summers PW, Roberts GR, Raad-Young M, Dann T, Brook J. Effects of low ambient levels of ozone and sulfates on the frequency of respiratory admissions to Ontario hospitals. Environ Res 1994; 65:172–194.
204. Thurston GD, Ito K, Hayes CG, Bates DV, Lippmann M. Respiratory hospital admissions and summertime haze air pollution in Toronto, Ontario: consideration of the role of acid aerosols. Environ Res 1994; 65:271–290.
205. Cody RP, Weisel CP, Birnbaum G, Lioy PJ. The effect of ozone associated with summertime photochemical smog on the frequency of asthma visits to hospital emergency departments. Environ Res 1992; 58:184–194.

206. Bates DV, Baker-Anderson M, Sizto R. Asthma attack periodicity: a study of hospital emergency visits in Vancouver. Environ Res 1990; 51:51–70.
207. Goldstein IF, Duberg E. Air pollution and asthma: search for a relationship. J Ann Pollut Control Assoc 1981; 31:370.
208. Ribon A, Glasser M, Sudhivoraseth N. Bronchial asthma in children and its occurrence in relation to weather and air pollution. Ann Allergy 1972; 30:276–281.
209. Goldstein IF, Weinstein AL. Air pollution and asthma: effects of exposures to short term sulfur dioxide peaks. Environ Res 1986; 40:332–345.
210. Goldstein IF, Rausch LE. Time series analysis of morbidity data for assessment of acute environmental health effects. Environ Res 1978; 17:266–275.
211. Walters S, Griffths RK, Ayres JG. Temporal association between hospital admissions for asthma in Birmingham and ambient levels of sulphur dioxide and smoke. Thorax 1994; 49:133–140.
212. Schwartz J, Slater D, Larson TV, Pierson WE, Koenig JE. Particulate air pollution and hospital emergency room visits for asthma in Seattle. Am Rev Respir Dis 1993; 147:826–831.
213. Delfino RJ, Becklake MR, Hanley JA. The relationship of urgent hospital admissions for respiratory illnesses to photochemical air pollution levels in Montreal. Environ Res 1994; 67:1–19.
214. Pope CA, Dockery DW. Acute health effects of PM_{10} on symptomatic and asymptomatic children. Am Rev Respir Dis 1992; 145:1123–1128.
215. Schwartz J. Air pollution and hospital admissions for the elderly in Detroit, Michigan. Am J Respir Crit Care Med 1994; 150:648–655.
216. Tseng RYM, Li CK, Spinks JA. Particulate air pollution and hospitalization for asthma. Ann Allergy 1992; 68:425–432.
217. Castellsague J, Sunyer J, Sáez M, Anto JM. Short-term association between air pollution and emergency room visits for asthma in Barcelona. Thorax 1995; 50:1051–1054.
218. Pope CA. Respiratory hospital admissions associated with PM_{10} pollution in Utah, Salt Lake and Cache valleys. Arch Environ Health 1991; 46:90–97.
219. Walters S, Phupinyokul M, Ayres J. Hospital admission rates for asthma and respiratory disease in the West Midlands: their relationship to air pollution levels. Thorax 1995; 50:948–954.
220. Spektor DM, Thurston GD, Mao J, He D, Hayes C, Lippmann M. Effects of single- and multi-day ozone exposures on respiratory function in active normal children. Environ Res 1991; 55:107–122.
221. Lippmann M, Lioy PJ, Leikauf G, Green KB, Baxter D, Morandi M, Pternack B, Fife D, Speizer FE. Effects of ozone on pulmonary function of children. Adv Mod Environ Toxicol 1983; 5:423–426.
222. Kinney PL, Ware JH, Spengler JD, Dockery DW, Speizer FE, Ferris BG Jr. Short-term pulmonary function change in association with ozone levels. Am Rev Respir Dis 1989; 139:56–61.
223. Lioy PJ, Vollmuth TA, Lippmann M. Persistence of peak flow decrement in children following ozone exposures exceeding the National Ambien Air Quality Standard. J Am Pollut Control Assoc 1985; 35:1068–1071.
224. Spektor DM, Lippmann M, Thurston GD, Lioy PJ, Stecko J, O'Connor G, Garschick E, Speizer FE, Hayes C. Effects of ambient ozone on respiratory function in healthy adults exercising outdoors. Am Rev Respir Dis 1988; 138:832–838.
225. Berry M, Lioy PJ, Gelperin K, Buckler G, Klotz J. Accumulated exposure to ozone and measurement of health effects in children and counselors at two summer camps. Environ Res 1991; 54:135–150.
226. Higgins IT, D'Arcy JB, Gibbons DI, Avol EL, Gross KB. Effect of exposures to ambient ozone on ventilatory lung function in children. Am Rev Respir Dis 1990; 141:1136–1146.
227. Castillejos M, Gold DR, Dockery D, Tosteson T, Baum T, Speizer FE. Effects of ambi-

ent ozone on respiratory function and symptoms in Mexico City schoolchildren. Am Rev Respir Dis 1992; 145:276–282.
228. Hoek G, Fischer P, Brunekreef B, Lebret E, Hofscreuder P, Mennen M. Acute effects of ambient ozone on pulmonary function of children in The Netherlands. Am Rev Respir Dis 1993; 147:111–117.
229. Avol EL, Linn WD, Venet TG, Shamoo DA, Hackney JD. Comparative respiratory effects of ozone and ambient oxidant pollution exposure during heavy exercise. J Am Pollut Control Assoc 1989; 34:804–809.
230. Castillejos M, Gold DR, Damokosh AI, Serrano P, Allen G, McDonnell WF, Dockery D, Velasco SR, Hernandez M, Hayes C. Acute effects of ozone on the pulmonary function of exercising schoolchildren from Mexico City. Am J Respir Crit Care Med 1995; 152:1501–1507.
231. Pope CA, Dockery DW, Spengler JD, Raizenne ME. Respiratory health and PM_{10} pollution. Am Rev Respir Dis 1991; 144:668–674.
232. Brown EB, Ipsen J. Changes in severity of symptoms of asthma and allergic rhinitis due to air pollutants. J Allergy 1968; 41:254–268.
233. Kurata KH, Glovsky M, Newcomb RL, Easton JG. A multi-factorial study of patients with asthma. Part 2: Air pollution, animal dander and asthma symptoms. Ann Allergy 1976; 37:398–409.
234. Peters A, Goldstein IF, Beyer U, Franke K, Heinrich J, Dockery DW, Spengler JD, Wichmann HE. Acute health effects of exposure to high levels of air pollution in Eastern Europe. Am J Epidemiol 1996; 144:570–581.
235. Forsberg B, Stjemberg N, Falk M, Lundback B, Wall S. Air pollution levels, meteorological conditions and asthma symptoms. Eur Respir J 1993; 6:1109–1115.
236. Colley JRT, Brasser LJ. Chronic respiratory disease in children in relation to air pollution: report on a WHO study. Copenhagen: WHO, 1980.
237. Corbo GM, Forastiere F, Dell'Orco V, Pistelli R, Agabati N, De Stefanis B, Ciappi G, Perucci CA. Effects of environment on atopic status and respiratory disorders in children. J Allergy Clin Immunol 1993; 92:616–623.
238. Dockery DW, Speizer FE, Stram DO, Ware JH, Spengler JD, Ferris BG. Effects of inhalable particles on respiratory health of children. Am Rev Respir Dis 1989; 139:587–594.
239. Goren AI, Hellmann S. Prevalence of respiratory symptoms and diseases in schoolchildren living in a polluted and in a low polluted area in Israel. Environ Res 1988; 45:28–37.
240. Detels R, Sayre JW, Coulson AH, Rokaw SN, Massey FJ, Tashkin DP, Wu MM. The UCLA population studies of chronic obstructive disease. IV: Respiratory effect of long-term exposure to photochemical oxidants, nitrogen dioxide and sulfates on current and never smokers. Am Rev Respir Dis 1981; 124:873–880.
241. Linn WS, Hackney JD, Pederson EE, Breisacher P, Patterson J, Mulry A, Coyle JF. Respiratory function and symptoms in urban office workers in relation to oxidant air pollution exposure. Am Rev Respir Dis 1976; 114:477–483.
242. Schenker MB, Speizer FE, Samet JM, Gruhl J, Batterman S. Health effects of air pollution due to coal combustion in the Chestnut Ridge region of Pennsylvania: results of a cross-sectional analysis in adults. Arch Environ Health 1983; 38:325–330.
243. von Mutius E, Frizsch C, Weiland SK, Roell G, Magnussen H. Prevalence of asthma and allergic disorders among children in united Germany: a descriptive comparison. Br Med J 1992; 305:1395–1399.
244. von Mutius E, Martinez FD, Fritzsch C, Nicolai T, Roell G, Thiemann HH. Prevalence of asthma and atopy in two areas of West and East Germany. Am J Respir Crit Care Med 1994; 149:358–364.
245. Nowak D, Heinrich J, Jörres R, Wassmer G, Berger J, Beck E, Boczor S, Claussen M, Wichmann HE, Magnussen H. Prevalence of respiratory symptoms, bronchial

hyperresponsiveness and atopy among adults: West and East Germany. Eur Respir J 1996; 9:2541–2552.

246. Kraemer U, Altus C, Behrendt H, Dolgner R, Gutsmuths FJ, Hille J, Hinricks J, Mangold M, Paetz B, Ranft U, Roepke H, Teichmann S, Willer HJ, Schlipköter HW. [Epidemiologic survey on the effect of air pollution on the health of schoolchildren] (in German). Forum Staedte-Hyg. 1992; 43:82–87.
247. Klein K, Data R, Goelwitz S, Jaeger L. Allergies—a comparison between two vocational schools in East and West Germany. Allergy 1992; 47(suppl):288.
248. Braback L, Breborowicz A, Dreborg S, Knutsson A, Pieklik H, Bjorksten B. Atopic sensitization and respiratory symptoms among Polish and Swedish school children. Clin Exp Allergy 1994; 24:826–835.
249. Braback L, Breborowicz A, Julge K, Knutsson A, Riikjarv MA, Vasar M, Bjorksten B. Risk factors for respiratory symptoms and atopic sensitisation in the Baltic area. Arch Dis Child 1995; 72:487–493.
250. von Mutius E, Sherrill DL, Fritzsch CH, Martinez FD, Lebowtz MD. Air pollution and upper respiratory symptoms in children from East Germany. Eur Respir J 1995; 8:723–728.
251. Wjst M, Reitmeir P, Dold S, Wulff A, Nicolai T, von Loeffelholz-Colberg E, von Mutius E. Road traffic and adverse effects on respiratory health in children. Br Med J 1993; 307:596–600.
252. Nitta H, Sato T, Nakai S, Maeda K, Aoki S, Ono M. Respiratory health associated with exposure to automobile exhaust. I. Results of cross-sectional studies in 1979, 1982, and 1983. Arch Environ Health 1993; 48:53–58.
253. Oosterlee A, Drijver M, Lebret E, Brunekreef B. Chronic respiratory symptoms in children and adults living along streets with high traffic density. Occup Environ Med 1996; 53:241–247.
254. Weiland SK, Mundt KA, Rückmann A, Keil U. Self-reported wheezing and allergic rhinitis in children and traffic density on street of residence. Ann Epidemiol 1994; 4:79–83.
255. Duhme H, Weiland SK, Keil U, Kraemer B, Schmid M, Stender M, Chambless L. The association between self-reported symptoms of asthma and allergic rhinitis and self-reported traffic density on street of residence in adolescents. Epidemiology 1996; 7:578–582.
256. Waldron G, Pottle B, Dod J. Asthma and the motorways—one district's experience. J Public Health Med 1995; 17:85–89.
257. Edwards J, Walters S, Griffiths RK. Hospital admissions for asthma in preschool children: relationship to major roads in Birmingham, United Kingdom. Arch Environ Health 1994; 49:223–227.
258. Pershagen G, Rylander E, Norberg S, Eriksson M, Nordvall SL. Air pollution involving nitrogen dioxide exposure and wheezing bronchitis in children. Int J Epidemiol 1995; 24:1147–1153.
259. Ishizaki T, Koizumi K, Ikemori R, Ishyama Y, Kushibiki E. Studies of prevalence of Japanese cedar pollinosis among the residents in a densely cultivated area. Ann Allergy 1987; 58:265–270.

32

The Genetic Basis of Allergy and Asthma

PAMELA J. AMELUNG and EUGENE R. BLEECKER

Center for the Genetics of Asthma and Complex Diseases
University of Maryland School of Medicine
Baltimore, Maryland

I. Introduction

Asthma is a respiratory disease that is characterized by variable airways obstruction, airway inflammation, and bronchial hyperresponsiveness (BHR; 1–3). Most patients with asthma have clinical and serological evidence of atopy, and the two disorders appear to be closely linked. The prevalence of asthma and allergic disorders has been increasing in recent years (4), as has the morbidity and mortality associated with this disease (5). There appears to be a significant heritable component to the development of asthma and atopy, for there is familial aggregation and increased risk to first-degree relatives. Asthma and other allergic disorders are not inherited in a simple mendelian fashion and, therefore, are "complex" genetic disorders. There are likely several genes involved in their development and, as with other complex diseases, the search for what determines genetic susceptibility to these disorders is complicated. The expression of clinical asthma and allergy appears to be determined by environmental factors, such as exposures to allergens, viral respiratory infections, air pollutants, and occupational factors (Fig. 1). Thus, important gene–gene and gene–environment interactions influence the progression of these diseases. Similar to other complex diseases, asthma is more prevalent in the general population than single-gene disorders. Because these disorders have widespread

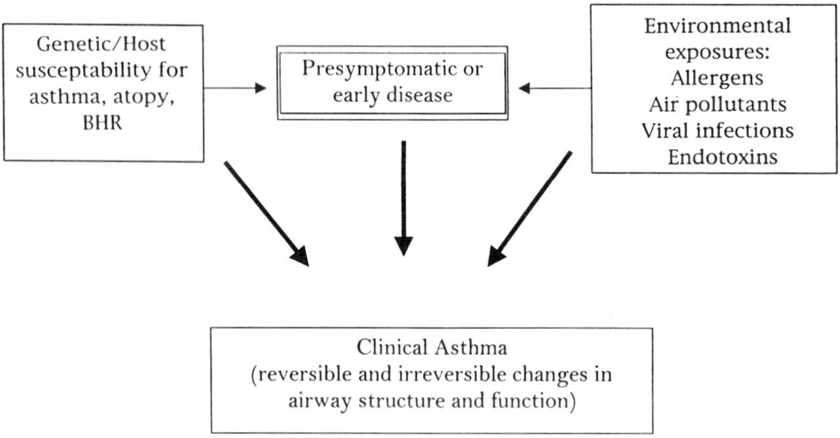

Figure 1 Gene–environment interactions in asthma.

public health significance, understanding the genetic basis of atopy and asthma is important because genetic approaches will elucidate new pathogenic disease mechanisms, may lead to the development of novel therapeutic interventions, and will facilitate presymptomatic and early disease diagnosis. This chapter will present the evidence for a genetic component in asthma, discuss the general approaches used in the study of complex genetic diseases, and summarize the progress that has been made in applying these techniques to the study of allergy and asthma.

II. Heriditary Contribution to Asthma

A. Family Studies

Numerous investigators have found a significant hereditary component in asthma and in phenotypes associated with asthma. These studies have reported an increased frequency of asthma and atopy in first-degree relatives of asthmatic subjects compared with those of control subjects (6–8). Familial aggregation may be due to common environmental factors, or to an interaction of environmental and genetic factors, that can influence the perceived pattern of inheritance. To test for familial aggregation, a comparison of disease frequencies in related individuals is performed, and compared with the disease frequency in the entire population. The excess risk for relatives is expressed as the *risk ratio* (λ), which is defined as the prevalence of the disorder in first-degree relatives, divided by the prevalence in the general population (9,10). The higher the value of λ, the greater the genetic contribution to the disorder. For asthma, λ has been estimated to be on the order of 5–6, assuming a population prevalence of 4% and a prevalence of 20–25% in first-degree relatives.

These figures may underestimate true prevalence because there have been worldwide trends showing increases in the prevalence of asthma and other allergic disorders (11). If one assumes that the genetic basis for these conditions is unchanged, then increases in prevalence are caused by changes in environmental factors that trigger the clinical expression of these diseases in susceptible hosts. Underestimates of the true prevalence of allergy and asthma can cause misclassification and affect the results of studies investigating their genetic basis.

B. Twin Studies

Twin studies can help determine the relative contributions of genes and the environment in complex genetic disorders. The difference between disease frequency in monozygotic (MZ) and dizygotic (DZ) twins provides an indication for heritability, whereas the difference between MZ twins may indicate environmental influences. Because MZ twins have identical genotypes and DZ twins, on average, share only 50% of their genes, a genetic disease would be expected to demonstrate a higher concordance rate in MZ than in DZ twins. In addition, twins usually share a common environment, which can limit the effect of environmental influences on phenotype, although this is less true for adult twins. Confining studies to same-sex twins is important in asthma and allergy because sex differences are reported in the prevalence of these disorders. Results from numerous twin studies have shown significant differences between monozygotic and dizygotic twin pairs, providing evidence for a genetic component in asthma and associated phenotypes, such as BHR, allergic skin test responses, and total serum IgE levels (12–14).

III. Environmental Contribution to Asthma

The prevalence of asthma differs among geographic areas of the world. Asthma is more frequent in economically developed communities, and an increase occurs in the offspring of first-generation migrants from rural to urban areas. These differences are likely due to environmental influences. One explanation for this increase is an increase in allergen exposure, especially to the house dust mite (15). Increases in cigarette smoking by women of childbearing age is another factor that has coincided with the rise in asthma and atopy in Western communities (16), and tobacco smoke increases serum IgE levels (17). Dietary sodium intake is correlated with bronchial hyperresponsiveness and adult male mortality from asthma (18–20). Respiratory viral infections, especially those with human rhinovirus, are associated with asthma exacerbations in children (21), but there are no studies to suggest these infections are important in the induction of asthma. Other, as yet not proved, environmental factors thought to contribute to the increased prevalence of asthma, are indoor and outdoor air pollutants and occupational exposure.

IV. Phenotype Definition

Precisely defining the asthma and allergic phenotype, as well as relevant intermediate phenotypes, is critical if one hopes to begin to dissect the genetic components of these conditions (22). The definition of asthma has changed dramatically throughout the years (3,23–25). Recently, inflammation has become the central feature of most definitions of asthma; however, there is no readily available validated marker of airway inflammation that can be used to differentiate asthma from closely related conditions, such as allergic rhinitis (3). Furthermore, clinical asthma can be a variable disease process over time; childhood asthma may resolve only to reappear in some persons later in life, whereas in others, asthma may not develop until later in life. Allergy is closely related to asthma, but allergic markers (serum IgE levels and skin tests responses) may decrease with aging, making understanding the relation of allergic factors and asthma more complicated (26–28). Bronchial hyperresponsiveness may change, depending on exposure to environmental triggers and the effects of therapeutic interventions (29–31). Thus, the clinical expression of asthma may change from a disease initially triggered by specific allergen exposures and viral infections in childhood, to a more irreversible airway disease in older patients, who may have experienced additional exposures to various environmental agents, such as tobacco smoke and air pollutants (32).

In a population of Dutch asthmatics, first studied in the 1960s and now restudied as part of a genetics of asthma project, approximately 10% of subjects had lost bronchial hyperresponsiveness to histamine. Others had increased airways obstruction and less reversible, or irreversible, airways obstruction. Finally, 15% had lost their atopic characteristics, in terms of either skin test reactivity or IgE levels. In this study, an algorithm, based on BHR, symptoms, smoking, 1-sec forced expiratory volume (FEV_1), and reversibility, was developed to classify individuals as "definite asthma," "probable asthma," "unable to classify or chronic obstructive pulmonary disease (COPD)," or "unaffected" [33]. Results of this algorithm showed that 16% of the offspring of a parent with asthma were classified as definite asthma, and only 60% of that group had a physician's diagnosis of asthma. This finding supports the importance of using objective testing as well as questionnaire data for classification of the asthma and allergy. Use of associated phenotypes that are often quantitative measures (total serum IgE levels, BHR, allergen skin testing) is an important approach for investigating the genetics of asthma and allergy (Table 1). Associated phenotypes, such as total serum IgE, correlate with the clinical expression of allergy as well as with BHR and asthma (34,35). In addition, use of quantitative measurements allowed most persons within a family or population to provide useful information for genetic analysis, as opposed to dichotomous traits (the presence or absence of wheeze), which provide useful information in a smaller percentage of the population. Results from family studies of asthma are difficult to compare because of the various definitions of asthma that are frequently used. Another

Table 1 Possible Phenotypes for Family Studies in Allergy and Asthma

Atopic parameters
Total serum IgE
Specific IgE levels
Allergen skin tests
Bronchial hyperresponsiveness
Direct methods (methacholine, histamine, etc.)
Indirect methods (adenosine, exercise, osmotic challenge, etc.)
Asthma
Physician diagnosis
Symptoms
Severity scores
Pulmonary function testing
Assessment of airflow obstruction
Bronchodilator reversibility
Peakflow variability
Combinations of "atopic" and "asthmatic" parameters

obstacle in these studies is that the clinical expression of asthma and related phenotypes may vary with age (33,36).

A. Serum IgE Levels

Total serum IgE levels correlate with clinical allergy and asthma, and immunological factors associated with an increase in total serum IgE levels are related to impaired pulmonary function (37). Despite the close relation among asthma, atopy, and total serum IgE levels, these traits are not interchangeable. However, both IgE levels and the diameter of allergy skin tests will increase from birth into young adulthood, followed by a decrease with aging (38). This may cause bias when family members from different generations are studied.

B. Bronchial Hyperresponsiveness

Bronchial hyperresponsiveness is another feature of asthma that appears to have a genetic component (7,14,39). In addition, several studies have shown an association between BHR and atopy (35,40), and virtually all asthmatics display BHR (41). In spite of this, the usefulness of BHR as a marker for asthma may be limited in that not all persons with BHR have evidence of clinical asthma. In addition, BHR is found in other conditions, such as cystic fibrosis, and may be found in normal persons after viral upper respiratory infections.

V. Approaches to Genetic Studies of Asthma

Mapping genes for complex diseases, such as asthma, involves two basic approaches: (1) complex segregation analysis, followed by linkage analysis using the best-fitting genetic model identified by the segregation analysis; and (2) linkage analysis using affected pairs of relatives without a specified model of inheritance (Fig. 2). In the first approach, segregation analysis is used to test explicit models of inheritance in families, using the qualitative or quantitative data on the trait, possible environmental factors, and family structure. It compares the observed number of affected individuals with the expected number, using various mendelian modes of inheritance (e.g., recessive, dominant, or polygenic). The best-fitting model can be determined by comparing the likelihoods from the models tested with the likelihood of a general model. Models that differ significantly from the general model can be rejected.

Segregation analysis of the asthma phenotype based on a physician's diagnosis has provided further evidence for genetic susceptibility caused by the presence of multiple genes (8). Townley and co-workers were the first to report the results of segregation analysis for bronchial responsiveness to methacholine (42). They were unable to exclude genetic and environmental models and concluded that the bimodal distribution of bronchial responsiveness was not due to segregation at a single autosomal locus. In another study, BHR was reported to be inherited as an autosomal dominant trait, with incomplete penetrance (7). Several studies on total serum IgE levels have demonstrated at least one major gene important in IgE regulation (43–46). In the Dutch family study recessive inheritance of high serum IgE levels was found, with the low and high groups showing levels of 38 and 437 international units (IU), respectively (47). Recently, Martinez and co-workers reported evidence for codominant inheritance in a large sample of families (48), and Xu and colleagues (49) have reported that major genes in at least two chromosomal regions may be important in the regulation of serum IgE levels. For linkage analysis, DNA marker data are used together with data on the trait and family structure. The purpose of linkage analysis is to delineate major genes by demonstrating cosegregation of the disease with polymorphic DNA markers. A polymorphic marker is usually not a specific disease gene, but is a chromosomal marker, with multiple alleles, that can be characterized in family members and traced through different generations. One can then test the hypothesis that a child with asthma inherited the same marker allele from his or her parent with asthma, and that children without asthma inherited the alternative allele. The maximum likelihood method of linkage analysis uses the model of inheritance obtained in segregation analysis and generates a logarithm of the odds (LOD) score. Usually, an LOD of 3 or higher (odds 1000:1) is considered evidence for linkage. In the second approach, linkage is analyzed without a specific model of inheritance, as is performed with sib-pair analysis. This analysis is based on the sharing of marker alleles identical by descent in sib pairs. In the presence of linkage, sibs who are identical by descent for a marker would be expected to have similar phenotypes (i.e., both have asthma or atopy).

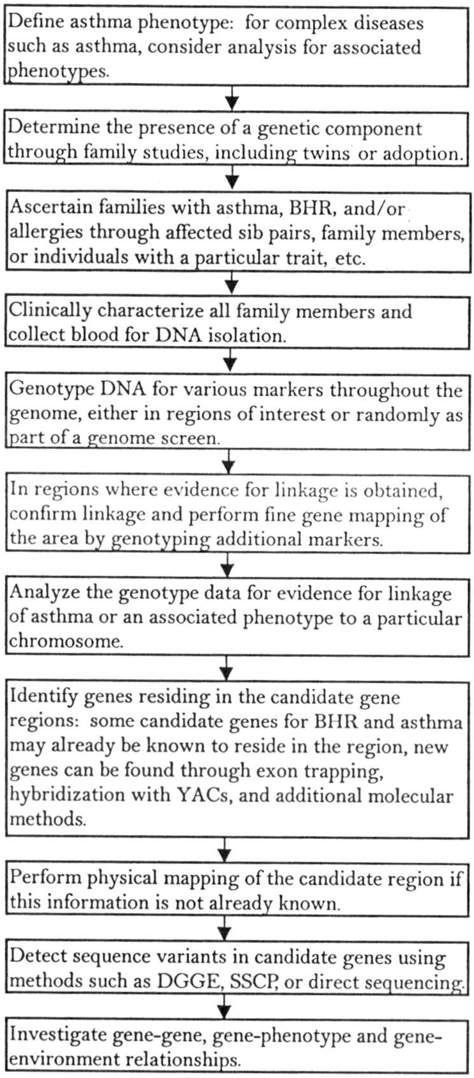

Figure 2 Methods for identification of disease or susceptibility genes for allergy and asthma.

Besides the LOD score and sib-pair analysis, association studies can be used to assess the importance of a candidate gene for a particular disease. These studies evaluate differences in relative risk of disease, associated with different alleles of a gene. Associations are sought because they may demonstrate important relations between the marker allele (or candidate gene allele) and the pathogenesis of the disorder. Another explanation of an observed association is linkage disequilibrium, which exists when alleles at two loci occur together on the same chromosome more often than predicted by chance alone. An association is observed in population studies because there is linkage between the disease locus and a common genetic background for the affected haplotype.

There are two general approaches for linkage analysis in asthma: a candidate gene approach in which specific chromosomal regions are studied, because of the presence of genes that are thought to be important in the pathogenesis of asthma (Table 2); and a genome-wide screen, in which evenly spaced markers throughout the entire genome are studied. Both approaches have been used in the search for asthma genes.

VI. Linkage Studies with Candidate Genes

A. Chromosome 11

Cookson et. al. (50) provided the first description of a genetic localization for inherited atopy. They reported mapping a major gene for atopy by showing linkage of the atopic phenotype with a marker on chromosome 11q, with a LOD of 5.58, using an autosomal dominant model for inheritance. Several investigators have been unable to replicate these findings (51–54). Additional studies by the original authors suggested that transmission of atopy was exclusively through the maternal line (55), and mutations of the β-subunit of the high-affinity IgE receptor (Fcε1R-β) were detected and were associated with atopy (56). Other linkage studies of the Fcε1R-β locus have produced conflicting results (57–60). Independent attempts to detect the variant of Fcε1R-β (Leu-181) described by the Oxford group (56) have been unsuccessful (61–63). The frequency of the mutation appears too low to explain the high prevalence of atopic disease, suggesting the presence of additional genes on other chromosomes. Recently, Doull and co-workers (64) found a significant asso-

Table 2 Proposed Chromosomal Locations for Susceptibility Gene for Asthma and Allergy

Chromosome 5q
Total serum IgE and bronchial hyperresponsiveness mapping to 5q, a region with multiple candidate genes (47,65–67)
Chromosome 6p
Associations between responses to specific allergens and HLA haplotypes (69)
Chromosome 11q
Maternal inheritance of atopy, proposed mutation in high affinity IgE receptor (56,59)
Chromosome 12q
Linkage of asthma phenotype to a region of candidate genes, including interferon gamma (70)
Chromosome 14q
Linkage of the T-cell receptor and skin test reactivity (71)

ciation between BHR and log [IgE] and two separate markers on chromosome 11q. These two markers were too distant from the gene encoding Fcε1R-β for a sequence variant in that gene to account for the association.

B. Chromosome 5

Chromosome 5q has been widely investigated for asthma and allergy genes owing to the presence there of multiple candidate genes, including several proinflammatory regulator cytokines and the β_2-adrenergic receptor. Evidence for linkage to chromosome 5q for a locus regulating total serum IgE levels has been observed in an isolated Amish population of 11 large families (65). By sib-pair analysis the strongest evidence for linkage was found near the interleukin (IL)-4 locus. There was also evidence for linkage by LOD score analysis using a model of dominant inheritance of high IgE levels. In a study of families from the Netherlands, ascertained through a parent with asthma originally studied 25–35 years ago, Meyers and coworkers (47) using a model of recessive inheritance of high IgE levels, found evidence for linkage of total serum IgE levels to 5q. In this study, the region with the best evidence for linkage was a region adjacent to the IL-4 cytokine locus near the β_2-adrenergic receptor gene. Further segregation analysis of IgE levels in this population showed evidence for a second major locus unlinked to chromosome 5.

By sib-pair analysis, evidence for linkage for BHR was also observed in the latter population in the same region on chromosome 5q31–33 (66). These studies show that susceptibility to BHR is coinherited at the same or nearby a major gene that controls total serum IgE levels in this population. Furthermore, evidence for linkage of the asthmatic phenotype has been reported in the same population (67). Additional evidence for linkage to this region has been observed in several studies, including randomly ascertained families for atopy, and in other populations ascertained for the asthmatic and allergic phenotypes (Table 3; 64).

C. Other Chromosomes of Interest

Multiple studies have shown a relation between specific immune responses and the human leukocyte antigen (HLA) loci on chromosome 6p. Specific immune responses

Table 3 Evidence for Linkage to the Allergic or Asthmatic Phenotype to Chromosome 5q

Old-Order Amish: atopy (65)
Dutch: atopy, BHR (47,66)
Southampton: atopy (64)
United States: asthma (73)
Australia: atopy (78)
Hutterites: asthma, BHR (79)

to highly purified allergens are strongly correlated with specific HLA haplotypes (DR and DQ; 68,69).

Evidence for linkage to chromosome 12q has been observed in studies of the Amish and an Afro-Caribbean population (70). Evidence for linkage near the T-cell receptor (TCR) α/δ locus on chromosome 14 to specific IgE responses to common inhaled allergens has been described in two populations (71), although this region did not show evidence for linkage with an atopic phenotype in a genome screen in a similar population (72). There are also many more known candidate genes in allergy and asthma yet to be investigated.

VII. Linkage Studies with Genome Screening

Two genome screens in atopic or asthmatic sib pairs have now been completed. Results from atopic sib pairs (72) and the Collaborative Study on the Genetics of Asthma (CSGA) asthmatic sib pairs have revealed additional regions with evidence for linkage (73). The CSGA has reported data on an initial genome-wide search for asthma susceptibility genes in 237 affected sib-pairs and their parents from three ethnic or racial groups. Sib-pair analysis has provided evidence for linkage with markers in six novel chromosomal regions: 5p and 17p-q in African Americans; 11p and 19q in Caucasian; and 2q and 21q in Hispanics. In addition, evidence for linkage was discovered in five regions previously reported to be linked to asthma or asthma-associated phenotypes, as outlined in the foregoing: 5q, 6p, 12q, 13q, and 14q in Caucasian sib pairs and 12q in Hispanic sib pairs. These data indicate that the number and relative importance of asthma genes may vary among ethnic groups and that many genes may influence asthma susceptibility. In 10 of these 11 chromosomal regions, there are candidate genes that are involved in T-cell biology or cytokine function, supporting the value of this approach in investigating the genetic basis of allergy and asthma.

VIII. Candidate Gene Mutational Analysis

Liggett and co-workers have investigated polymorphisms in the β_2-adrenergic receptor gene on chromosome 5q in unrelated patients (74). They discovered nine different point mutations, four of which caused changes in the encoded amino acids at residues 16, 27, 34, and 164. The most frequent polymorphisms were arginine-16 to glycine (Arg-16/Gly) and glutamine-27 to glutamic acid (Gln-27/Glu). None of these mutations was more prevalent in the asthmatic group when compared with the control group. However, in the asthma group the Arg-16/Gly mutation appeared to identify a subset of subjects with more severe asthma, in that they were more likely to be steroid-dependent. Thus, mutations at this locus do not appear to have a primary role in the development of asthma, but they may modulate the severity of the asthma phenotype. These investigators later went on to show that the glycine allele at position 16 caused enhanced downregulation of receptor after agonist exposure, providing a plausible explanation for the observed association of this mutation with severe asthma. This mutation is more prevalent in nocturnal asthmatics, compared with nonnocturnal asthmatics (75). Another variant, Glu-27, demonstrates attenuated downregulation of the receptor after long-term agonist exposure. This variant was associated with lower levels of airways hyperresponsiveness in a group of asthmatics (76). These studies suggest that β-adrenergic genotype is important in the expression of the asthmatic phenotype.

In other studies, In and colleagues (77) have examined the transcription factor-binding regions and the protein-encoding regions of the 5-lipoxygenase (5-LO) gene for mutations. 5-Lipoxygenase is the first committed enzyme in the synthesis of leukotrienes, catalyzing the formation of leukotriene A_4 from arachidonic acid. They discovered a family of alleles with variation in the number of tandem zinc finger-binding proteins (Sp1 and Egr-1) in the transcription factor-binding region. These alleles exhibit functional differences when compared with wild-type alleles. The authors concluded that these mutations could possibly modify gene transcription through differences in the zinc finger transcription-binding sites. This may explain the substantial heterogeneity observed among individual asthmatics in their therapeutic response to drugs that interrupt the 5-LO pathway.

IX. Future Applications

In recent years, there has been an explosion of information relating to potential genetic mechanisms that may partly contribute to the development of allergy and asthma. These studies may be useful in understanding basic mechanisms involved in the development and progression of asthma and allergy. Investigators have now discovered several potential areas of the genome that may be involved in these diseases. The identification of genes linked to asthma and allergy should enable the development of diagnostic and perhaps prognostic tests for these diseases. Such diagnostic testing may help patients avert potential harm by early medical intervention and by the avoidance of specific environmental factors. The discovery of genes that lead to a better understanding of the pathophysiology of asthma and allergic diseases may lead to the development of new treatment modalities. In addition, in the future, pharmacological decisions may be based on genotype information for specific genetic loci. For example, the decision to treat an asthmatic with long-acting β_2-agonists may rely on a patient's specific genetic sequence at the β_2-receptor gene locus.

X. Summary

Family and linkage studies of the genetics of allergy and asthma have made significant progress during the past few years. Investigators have now located several chromosomal regions of potential importance in these disorders. Confirmation of these findings and beginning the search for specific susceptibility genes in these areas is now essential. However, because it is clear that multiple genes, as well as environmental factors, are important in determining susceptibility, these studies will require the combined expertise of several fields, including clinical and molecular genetics and genetic epidemiology. An understanding of the genetic mechanisms responsible for allergy and asthma has widespread public health consequences because it may lead to a better understanding of the pathogenesis of asthma. These approaches should also lead to improved preventive measures and new therapeutic approaches. Identification of specific mutations or genetic variants in asthma could lead to the possibility of screening, with the potential to modify outcome by preventing exposure to certain allergens. In addition, there is the potential that pharmacological therapy will be influenced by sequence variants in genes that modulate therapeutic responses to specific drug therapy.

Acknowledgments

Supported by National Institute of Health R01 HL48341 and U01 HL49602.

References

1. Holgate ST, Beasley R, Twentyman OP. The pathogenesis and significance of bronchial hyperresponsiveness in airway disease. Clin Sci 1987; 73:561–572.
2. Beasley R, Roche WR, Roberts JA, Holgate ST. Cellular events in the bronchi in mild asthma before and after bronchial provocation. Am Rev Respir Dis 1989; 139:806–817.
3 Sheffer AL, Bailey WC, Bleecker ER, Busse WW, Ellis E, Evans D, Fanta CH, Janson-Bjerklie S, Malveaux FJ, Murphy SA, Nelson HS, Shapiro G. Guidelines for the diagnosis and management of asthma. J Allergy Clin Immunol 1991; 88:425–534.
4. Ninan TK, Russell G. Respiratory symptoms and atopy in Aberdeen school children: evidence from two surveys 25 years apart. Br Med J 1992; 304:873–875.
5. Gergen PJ, Weiss KB. The increasing problem of asthma in the United States. Am Rev Respir Dis 1992; 146:823–824.
6. Sibbald B, Horn MEZ, Brain EA. Genetic factors in childhood asthma. Thorax 1980; 35:671–674.
7. Longo F, Strinati R, Poli F, Fumi F. Genetic factors in non-specific bronchial hyperreactivity. Am J Dis Child 1987; 141:331–334.
8. Holberg CJ, Elston RC, Halonen M, Wright AL, Taussig LM, Morgan WJ, Martinez FD. Segregation analysis of physician-diagnosed asthma in Hispanic and non-Hispanic white families—a recessive component. Am J Respir Crit Care Med 1996; 154:144–150.
9. Risch N. Linkage strategies for genetically complex traits. II The power of affected relative pairs. Am J Hum Genet 1990; 46:229–241.
10. Risch N. Linkage models for genetically complex traits. I Multilocus models. Am J Hum Genet 1990; 46:222–228.
11. Bleecker ER, Postma DS, Meyers DA. Genetic susceptibility to asthma in a changing environment. In: The Rising Trends in Asthma. Ciba Foundation Symposium: London, 1997; pp. 90–105.
12. Edfors-Lub M. Allergy in 7000 twin pairs. Acta Allergol 1971; 26:249–285.

13. Duffy DL, Martin NG, Battistutta D, Hopper JL, Matthews JD. Genetics of asthma and hayfever in Australian twins. Am Rev Respir Dis 1990; 142:1351–1358.
14. Hopp RJ, Bewtra AK, Watt GD, Nair NM, Townley RG. Genetic analysis of allergic disease in twins. J Allergy Clin Immunol. 1984; 73:265–270.
15. Woolcock AH, Green W, Alpers MP. Asthma in a rural highland area of Papua New Guinea. Am Rev Respir Dis 1981; 123:565–567.
16. Burney PG, Chinn S, Rona RJ. Has the prevalence of asthma increased in children? Evidence from the national study of health and growth. Br Med J 1990; 300:1306–1310.
17. Burrows B, Halonen M, Barbee RA, Lebowitz MD. The relationship of serum immunoglobulin E to cigarette smoking. Am Rev Respir Dis 1981; 124:523–525.
18. Burney P. A diet rich in sodium may potentiate asthma. Chest 1987; 91:1435–1438.
19. Burney P, Britton JR, Chinn S, Tattersfield AE, Platt HS, Papacosta AO, Kelson MC. Response to inhaled histamine and 24 hour sodium excretion. Br Med J 1986; 292:1483–1486.
20. Burney P, Nield JE, Twort CHC, Chinn S, Jones TD, Mitchell WD, Bateman C, Cameron IR. The effect of changing dietary sodium on the bronchial response to histamine. Thorax 1989; 44:36–41.
21. Johnston SL, Pattemore PK, Sanderson G, Smith S, Campbell MJ, Josephs TLK, Cunningham A, Robinson BS, Myint SH, Ward ME, Tyrrell DA. The relationship between upper respiratory infections and hospital admissions for asthma: a time trend analysis. Am J Respir Crit Care Med 1996; 154:654–660.
22. Weisch DG, Meyers DA, Samet JM, et al. Classification of the asthma phenotype in genetic studies. In: Liggett S, Meyers DA, eds. Genetics of Asthma. New York: Marcel Dekker, 1996.
23. Ciba Guest Symposium. Terminology, definitions, and classification of chronic pulmonary emphysema and related conditions. Thorax 1959; 14:286–299.
24. American Thoracic Society. Definitions and classification of chronic bronchitis, asthma, and pulmonary emphysema. Am Rev Respir Dis 1962; 85:762–768.
25. Medical Research Council. Definition and classification of chronic bronchitis for clinical and epidemiological purposes. Lancet 1965; 1:775–779.
26. Panhuysen CIM, Bleecker ER, Koeter GH, Meyers DA, Postma DS. Characterization of obstructive airways disease in family members of probands with asthma: an algorithm for the diagnosis of asthma. Am J Respir Crit Care Med 1997; 157(6pt1):1734–1742.
27. Peat JK, Salome C, Berry G, Woolcock AJ. Relation of dose–response slope to respiratory symptoms in a population of Australian schoolchildren. Am Rev Respir Dis 1991; 144:663–667.
28. Sporik R, Holgate ST, Cogswell JJ. Natural history of asthma in childhood—a birth cohort study. Arch Dis Child 1991; 66:1050–1053.
29. Cartier A, Thompson NC, Frith PA, Roberts RS, Hargreave FE. Allergen-induced increase in bronchial responsiveness to histamine: relationship to the late asthmatic response and change in airway caliber. J Allergy Clin Immunol 1982; 70:170–177.
30. Hopp RJ, Bewtra AK, Nair NM, Townley RG. The effect of age on methacholine response. J Allergy Clin Immunol 1985; 76:609–613.
31. Platts-Mills TAE, Mitchell EB, Nock P, Tovey ER, Moszoro H, Wilkins SR. Reduction of bronchial hyperreactivity during prolonged allergen avoidance. Lancet 1982; 2:675–677.
32. Postma DS, de Vries K, Koeter GH, Sluiter HJ. Independent influence of reversibility of air-flow obstruction and non-specific hyperreactivity on the long-term course of lung function in chronic air-flow obstruction. Am Rev Respir Dis 1986; 134:276–280.
33. Panhuysen CIM, Vonk JM, Schouten JP, van Altena R, Bleecker ER, Koeter GH, Postma DS. Do adult patients outgrow their asthma. Am J Respir Cir Care Med 1997; 155:1267–1272.
34. Burrows B, Sears MR, Flannery EM, Herbison GP, Holdaway MD. Relationship of bronchial responsiveness assessed by methacholine to serum IgE, lung function, symptoms, and diagnoses in 11-year-old New Zealand children. J Allergy Clin Immunol 1992; 90:376–385.
35. Sears M, Burrows B, Flannery EM, Herbison GP, Hewitt CJ, Holdaway MD. Relation be-

tween airway responsiveness and serum IgE in children with asthma and in apparently normal children. N Engl J Med 1991; 325:1067–1071.
36. O'Connor GT, Sparrow D, Weiss ST. The role of allergy and nonspecific bronchial hyperresponsiveness in the pathogenesis of chronic obstructive pulmonary disease. Am Rev Respir Dis 1989; 140:225–252.
37. Burrows B, Martinez FD, Halonen M, Barbee RA, Cline MG. Association of asthma with serum IgE levels and skin-test reactivity to allergens. N Engl J Med 1989; 320:271–277.
38. Sibbald S, Strachan DP. Epidemiology of rhinitis. In: Busse WW, Holgate ST, eds. Asthma and Rhinitis. London: Blackwell Scientific, 1995:32–43.
39. Sibbald B, Turner-Warwick M. Factors influencing the prevalence of asthma among first degree relatives of extrinsic and intrinsic asthmatics. Thorax 1979; 34:332–337.
40. Burrows B, Sears MR, Flannery EM, Herbison GP, Holdaway MD. Relationship of bronchial responsiveness to allergy skin test reactivity, lung function, respiratory symptoms, and diagnosis in 13-year-old New Zealand children. J Allergy Clin Immunol 1995; 95:548–556.
41. Boushey HA, Holtzman MJ, Sheller JR, Nadel JA. Bronchial hyperresponsiveness. Am Rev Respir Dis 1980; 121:389–413.
42. Townley RG, Bewtra MD, Wilson AF, Hopp RJ, Elston RC, Nair NM, Watt GD. Segregation analysis of bronchial response to methacholine inhalation in families with and without asthma. J Allergy Clin Immunol 1986; 77:101–107.
43. Marsh DG, Bias WB, Ishizaka K. Genetic control of basal serum immunoglobulin E level and its effect on specific reagenic sensitivity. Proc Natl Acad Sci USA 1974; 71:3588–3592.
44. Gerrad JW, Rao DC, Morton NE. A genetic study of immunoglobulin E. Am J Hum Genet 1976; 30:46–58.
45. Blumenthal MN, Namboodiri KK, Mendell N, Gleich G, Elston RC, Yunis E. Genetic transmission of serum IgE levels. Am J Med Genet 1981; 10:219–228.
46. Meyers DA, Beaty TH, Freidhoff LR, Marsh DG. Inheritance of serum IgE (basal levels) in man. Am J Hum Genet 1987; 41:51–62.
47. Meyers DA, Postma DS, Panhuysen CIM, Xu J, Amelung PJ, Levitt RC, Bleecker ER. Evidence for a locus regulating total serum IgE levels mapping to chromosome 5. Genomics 1994; 23:464–470.
48. Martinez FD, Holberg CJ, Halonen M, Morgan W, J., Wright AL, Taussig LM. Evidence for Mendelian inheritance of serum IgE levels in Hispanic and non-Hispanic white families. Am J Hum Genet 1994; 55:555–564.
49. Xu J, Levitt RC, Panhuysen CIM, Postma DS, Taylor EW, Amelung PJ, Holroyd KJ, Bleecker ER, Meyers DA. Evidence for two unlinked loci regulating total serum IgE levels. Am J Hum Genet 1995; 57:425–430.
50. Cookson WOCM, Sharp PA, Faux JA, Hopkin JM. Linkage between immunoglobulin E responses underlying asthma and rhinitis and chromosome 11q. Lancet 1989 Jun 10; 1(8650) 1292–1295.
51. Lympany P, Welsh KL, Cochrane GM, Kemeny DM, Lee TH. Genetic analysis of the linkage between chromosome 11q and atopy. Clin Exp Allergy 1992; 22:1085–1092.
52. Amelung PJ, Panhuysen CIM, Postma DS, Levitt RC, Koeter GH, Francomano CA, Bleecker ER, Meyers DA. Atopy and bronchial hyperresponsiveness: exclusion of linkage to markers on chromosomes 11q and 6p. Clin Exp Allergy 1992; 22:1077–1084.
53. Rich SS, Romman-Johnson B, Greenberg B, Roberts S, Blumenthal MN. Genetic analysis of atopy in three large kindreds: no evidence of linkage to DS11S97. Clin Exp Allergy 1992; 22:1070–1076.
54. Hizawa N, Yamaguchi E, Ohe H, Itoh M, Furuya K, Ohnuma N, Kawakami Y. Lack of linkage between atopy and locus 11q13. Clin Exp Allergy 1992; 22:1065–1069.
55. Cookson WOCM, Young RP, Sanford AJ, Mofatt MF, Shirakawa T, Sharp PA, Faux JA, Julier C, Le Souef PN, Nakumura Y, Lathrop GM, Hopkin JM. Maternal inheritance of atopic IgE responsiveness on chromosome 11q. Lancet 1992; 340:381–384.
56. Shirakawa T, Li A, Dubowitz M, Dekker JW, Shaw AE, Faux JA, Ra C, Cookson WOCM,

Hopkin JM. Association between atopy and variants of the β-subunit of the high-affinity immunoglobulin E receptor. Nature Genet 1994; 7:125–130.
57. Brereton HM, Ruffin RE, Thompson RJ, Turner DR. Familial atopy in Australian pedigrees: adventitious linkage to chromosome 8 is not confirmed nor is there evidence of linkage to the high affinity IgE receptor. Clin Exp Allergy 1994; 24:868–877.
58. Collee JM, de Vries HG, Gerritsen J. Allele sharing on chromosome 11q13 in sibs with asthma. Lancet 1993; 342:936.
59. Shirakawa T, Morimoto K, Hasimito T, Furuyama J, Yamamoto M, Takai S. Linkage between atopic IgE responses and chromosome 11q in Japanese families. Clin Genet 1994; 46:228–232.
60. Coleman R, Trembath RC, Harper JI. Chromosome 11q13 and atopy underlying atopic eczema. Lancet 1993; 341:1121–1122.
61. Hizawa N, Yamaguchi E, Furuyama J, Ohnuma N, Kodama N, Kojima J, Ohe M, Kawakami Y. Association between high total serum IgE levels and D11S97 on chromosome 11q13 in Japanese subjects. J Med Genet 1995; 32:363–369.
62. Duffy DL, Healey SC, Chenevix-Trench G, Martin NG, Weger J, Lichter J. Atopy in Australia [letter; comment]. Nature Genet 1995; 10:260.
63. Martinati LC, Trabetti E, Casartelli A, Boner AL, Pignatti PF. Affected sib-pair and mutation analyses of the high affinity IgE receptor beta chain locus in Italian families with atopic asthmatic children. Am J Respir Crit Care Med 1996; 153:1682–1685.
64. Doull IJM, Lawrence S, Watson M, Begishvili T, Beasley RW, Lamp F, Holgate ST, Morton NE. Allelic association of gene markers on chromosomes 5q and 11q with atopy and bronchial hyperresponsiveness. Am J Respir Crit Care Med 1996; 153:1280–1284.
65. Marsh DG, Neely JD, Breazeale DR, Ghosh B, Freidhoff LOR, Ehlich-Kautzky E, Schou C, Krishnasawamy G, Beaty TH. Linkage analysis of IL4 and other chromosome 5q31.1 markers and total serum immunoglobulin E concentrations. Science 1994; 264:1162–1166.
66. Postma DS, Bleecker ER, Amelung PJ, Holroyd KJ, Xu J, Panhuysen CIM, Meyers DA, Levitt RC. Genetic susceptibility to asthma—bronchial hyperresponsiveness coinherited with a major gene for atopy. N Engl J Med 1995; 333:894–900.
67. Panhuysen CIM, Levitt RC, Postma DS, Xu J, Amelung PJ, Holroyd KJ, van Altena R, Koeter GH, Meyers DA, Bleecker ER. Evidence for a susceptibility locus for asthma mapping to chromosome 5q. Clin Res 1995; 43:281A.
68. Marsh DG, Meyers DA, Bias WB. The epidemiology and genetics of atopic allergy. N Engl J Med 1982; 305:1551–1559.
69. Blumenthal MN, Marcus-Bagley D, Awdeh B, Johnson B, Yunis E, Alper CA. HLA-DR2, [HLA-B7, SC31, DR2], and [HLA-B8, SC01, DR3] haplotypes distinguish subjects with asthma from those with rhinitis only in ragweed pollen allergy. J Immunol 1992; 148:411–416.
70. Barnes KC, Neely JD, Duffy DL, Freidhoff LR, Breazeale DR, Schou C, Naidu RP, Levett PN, Renault B, Kucherlapati R, Lozzino S, Ehrlich E, Beaty TH, Marsh DG. Linkage of asthma and total serum IgE concentration to markers on chromosome 12q: evidence from Afro-Caribbean and Caucasian populations. Genomics 1996; 37:41–50.
71. Moffatt MF, Cornelis F, Schou C, Faux JA, Young RP, James AL, Ryan G, le Souef P, Musk AW, Hopkin J, Cookson WOCM. Genetic linkage of T-cell receptor α/δ complex to specific IgE responses. Lancet 1994; 343:1597–1560.
72. Daniels SE, Bhattacharrya S, James A, Leaves NI, Young A, Hill MR, Faux JA, Ryan GF, LeSouef PN, Lathrop GM, Musk AW, Cookson WO. A genome-wide search for quantitative trait loci underlying asthma. Nature 1996; 383:247–250.
73. Collaborative Study on the Genetics of Asthma. A genome-wide search for asthma susceptibility loci in ethnically diverse populations. Nature Genet 1997; 15:389–392.
74. Reihsaus E, Innis M, MacIntyre N, Liggett SB. Mutations in the gene encoding for the β_2-adrenergic receptor in normal and asthmatic subjects. Am J Respir Cell Mol Biol 1993; 8:334–339.

75. Turki J, Pak J, Green SA, Martin RJ, Liggett SB. Genetic polymorphisms of the β_2-adrenergic receptor in nocturnal and non-nocturnal asthma. J Clin Invest 1995; 95:1635–1641.
76. Hall IP, Wheatley A, Wilding P, Liggett SB. Association of Glu 27 β_2-adrenoceptor polymorphism with lower airway reactivity in asthmatic subjects. Lancet 1995; 345:1213–1214.
77. In KH, Asano K, Beier D, Grobholz J, Finn PW, Silverman EK, Silverman ES, Collins T, Fischer AR, Keith TP, Serino K, Kim SW, DeSanctis GT, Yandava C, Pillari A, Rubin P, Kemp J, Isreal E, Busse W, Ledford D, Murray JJ, Segal A, Tinkleman D, Drazen JM. Naturally occurring mutations in the human 5-lipoxygenase gene promoter that modify transcription factor binding and reporter gene transcription. J Clin Invest 1997; 99:1130–1137.
78. Walley AJ, Bhattacharyya S, Leaves N, Daniels SE, Cookson WOCM. Linkage and allelic association of chromosome 5 microsattelite markers with atopic asthma phenotypes in a general population sample [abstr]. Am J Respir Crit Care Med 1997; 155:A257.
79. Ober C, Cox NJ, Parry RR, Di Rienzo A, Abney MA, Andal JA, Cosentino JF, Gidley H, Kurtz B, Lander ES, Petterson A, Richardson AR, Robertson AS, Schlenker EH, Summerhill E. Genome-wide search for asthma susceptibility loci in the Hutterites [abstr]. Am J Hum Genet 1997; 61:A41.

33

Gene Therapy Strategies for Asthma

PASCAL DEMOLY, DANY JAFFUEL, JEAN BOUSQUET, PHILIPPE GODARD, and FRANÇOIS-BERNARD MICHEL

Montpellier University and
Montpellier University Hospital
Service des Maladies Respiratoires–INSERM U454
Montpellier, France

MARC MATHIEU

Service des Maladies Respiratoires–INSERM U454
Montpellier University Hospital
Montpellier, France

I. Introduction

The prevalence and severity of asthma have continually increased since 1960 (1,2), despite great advances in the understanding of the physiological mechanisms of the disease and of better medical treatment. The major advance over the last few years has been the understanding of asthma as an inflammatory disease and the use of corticosteroids in its treatment. Although β_2 adrenergic agonists and inhaled corticosteroids are able to control the disease in most patients, this does not always hold in particular for those patients who also require daily doses of oral corticosteroids. New therapeutic strategies therefore, must be devised for these patients. A variety of gene-based strategies have recently been proposed for inflammatory and immunological disorders. Thus, it is the purpose of this review to consider its application to asthma therapy.

Existing knowledge does not yet allow us to identify molecular targets that are highly likely to be amenable to gene therapy. After a brief outline of the genetics of asthma, we will review its immunopathology, slanting the discussion toward the possibility of a gene-based treatment.

II. Genetics of Asthma

The clinical and biological manifestations of asthma are extremely heterogeneous, reflecting the multitude of causative and aggravating factors and, it would seem, the presence of many different underlying pathophysiological mechanisms that give rise to a common feature: bronchial inflammation (Fig. 1). Given this heterogeneity, it is likely that several genes are involved. Current molecular genetic data still cannot pinpoint an abnormal gene that is associated with asthma, such as the one for cystic fibrosis. However, certain gene products are clearly associated with the pathophysiology of asthma and so could be used as targets for a genetic therapy for this disease.

The genetic or familial component of asthma has long been known (3). The complexity of the asthmatic phenotype associated with both bronchial hyperreactivity and with allergy complicates the genetic studies in this area. Most genetic studies are focused on the genes involved in the immune response or the response to immunoglobulin E (IgE): these being genes of the class II major histocompatibility complex (MHC; on chromosome 6p) (4), the gene of the α-chain of the T-cell receptor (TCR; on chromosome 14) (5), the gene for interleukin (IL)-4 (on chromosome 5q) (6), and the gene for the β-chain of the high-affinity receptor for IgE (on chromosome 11q) (7), respectively. Such molecular genetic studies have already

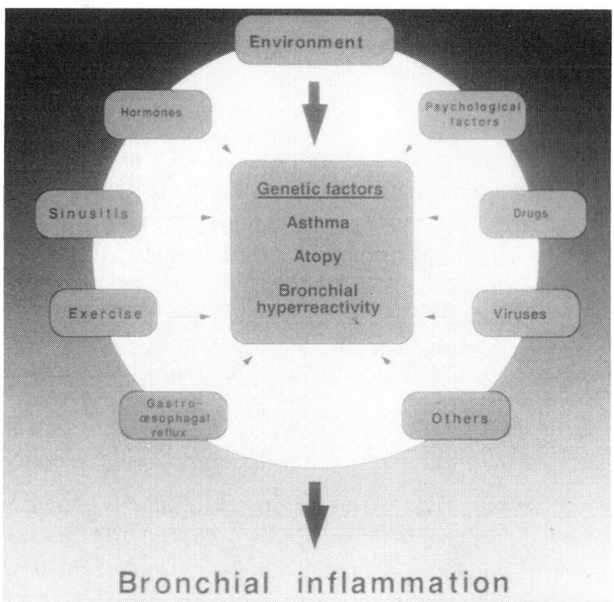

Figure 1 Main causative and aggravating factors underlying asthma.

made advances in this area. However, very little genetic information is currently available for severe asthma. Polymorphisms in certain genes (e.g., β-adrenergic receptor-coding sequences and IL-4 promoter sequences) have been found in severe asthma (8,9). However, a familial link with the severity of asthma has yet to be fully established. The development and the continuation of such studies, together with the human genome program, will allow us to envisage a future with research into the genetics of asthma and allergies in terms of fundamental research, of prevention, and of new therapeutic strategies (including gene therapy).

III. Strategies for Gene Transfer in Asthma

A. Vectors and Delivery Routes

Many systems for gene transfer are currently available. Their major advantages and disadvantages are outlined in Table 1. We will not explore this subject in greater depth and, instead, refer the readers to the excellent reviews available (10,11). We should, however, draw attention to the side effects and particularly the inflammation induced by these vectors, which must be taken into account in diseases such as asthma in which the major feature is bronchial inflammation. At present, the technology for using plasmids, either naked DNA plasmids or plasmids included into liposomes, or those associated with a receptor, such as the receptor for transferrin, do not appear to be transferable to the in vivo situation, except for DNA vaccines. The use of recombinant viruses is the oldest method, and more recent developments include the use of retroviruses, adenoassociated viruses, and recombinant adenoviruses. The major advantage of these latter viruses is that they are able to infect cells that are in a quiescent state (such as respiratory cells, in which less than 1% of cells are in the cycle; 12). The problem of vectorization is now a crucial problem in the domain of gene therapy, no matter what the illness. The objective is to improve the targeting of the vectors and, thereby, reach all cells, including refractory cells (polymorphonuclear cells and lymphocytes), with maximum safety. If we accept that the epithelium is the target site in asthma (the most efficacious medications being administered by aerosol), the precise cell that should be targeted remains unclear. Vectors have different efficacies, depending on the cell type involved. Thus, although adenovirus vectors may be employed for airway epithelial cells, they are much less effective for gene transfer to lymphocytes. Differentiated peripheral blood lymphocytes are a cell type that resists transfection; consequently, new strategies have to be evaluated. However, these cells could potentially be targeted through epithelial cells by transferring to this latter cell type the gene for a protein secreted into the local microenvironment and known to modulate lymphocytic function. The bronchial site of this inflammation means that full advantage can be taken of current in vivo technology with aerosols of the therapeutic gene(s); but, given the importance of the role of lymphocytes in the pathophysiology of asthma, ex vivo gene therapy should also be considered, with isolation, purification, genetic modification

Table 1 Advantages and Disadvantages of the Currently Available Gene Transfer Vectors

Vectors	Cellular specificity (range)	Capacity	Production titer	Subcellular localization	Transduction power
Viral vectors					
Retrovirus	Limited (dividing cells)	Limited (≈7–8 kb)	Low ($\leq 10^6$ pfu/mL)	Chromosomal	High
Adenovirus	Large	Limited (≈7–10 kb)	High (10^{11} pfu/mL)	Episomal	High
AAV[a]	Large	Limited (≈4.5 kb)	High in theory (usually low)	Chromosomal[b]; episomal[a,c]	High
Herpes virus	Large	Large (≈30 kb)	High	Episomal	Low
Poxvirus	Large	Large (≈30kb)	High	Episomal	High
Nonviral vectors					
Conjugates	Large	Large		Extrachromosomal	High
Liposomes	Large	Large		Extrachromosomal	Low

Note: [a]Wild-type AAV or adenoassociated viruses integrate the chromosomes of the [b]targeted cells. However, [c]AAV vectors seem to have an extra-chromosomal location.

in vitro, and reinfection of lymphocytes which, when they relocalize to the bronchial epithelium, could beneficially modulate the local immune response. Moreover, understanding the role played by cells of the monocyte–macrophage lineage in presenting antigens to lymphocytes, and with the easy access to alveolar macrophages by bronchoalveolar lavage and their privileged position in contact with the bronchial epithelium, a strategy targeting alveolar macrophages could also be applied. Thus, it is not impossible to envisage ex vivo gene therapy in asthma targeting alveolar macrophages that could be transfected in vitro and then reintroduced into the body to allow the in situ liberation of the recombinant protein, product of the therapeutic gene.

B. The Genes of Interest

Gene therapy in asthma cannot rely on data from molecular genetic studies because the gene(s) involved still remain to be determined. Therefore, gene therapy, such as that currently under trial in monogenetic diseases such as cystic fibrosis, cannot be envisaged. However, as a result of detailed studies on certain established mechanisms underlying the pathophysiology of asthma, we can suggest several possible lines of research. Although replacement a deficient gene is a "simple task" in the realms of gene therapy, to block the expression of this or that inflammatory or immunoregulatory protein requires sophisticated techniques, including those involving soluble receptors, negative dominants, ribosomes, single-chain intracellular antibodies, or antisense oligonucleotides. In asthma, no protein is truly repressed, but rather, there is a hypersecretion. However, the discovery of immunomodulating cytokines that may be anti-inflammatory, such as interferon (IFN)-γ, interleukin (IL)-10, and IL-12, opens new perspectives, which will be elaborated on in the following discussion.

Action on the Infiltration and Activation of Eosinophils

The targeting of eosinophils is a possible therapeutic strategy under consideration. These cells infiltrate the bronchial mucosa of asthmatic subjects, whether or not they are allergic, and are often degranulated and activated in terms of liberation of cytotoxic granule-derived proteins (such as eosinophil cationic protein [ECP] and major basic protein [MBP] and bronchoconstrictive lipid-derived mediators, such as platelet activating factor (PAF) and leukotriene (LT) C_4 (13). In addition, the numbers of eosinophils and their corresponding mediators are increased following allergic provocation (14). The eosinophilic infiltrate is correlated with the severity of the disease (13) and, sometimes, with the level of bronchial hyperreactivity. This infiltration is less marked or absent in asthmatic patients treated with inhaled or oral corticosteroids. The increased number of eosinophils could be due to an influx of cells from the peripheral circulation or to an increase in their survival time.

The recruitment of eosinophils from the blood involves several different processes (15). The initial adhesion and the passage across the endothelium brings into

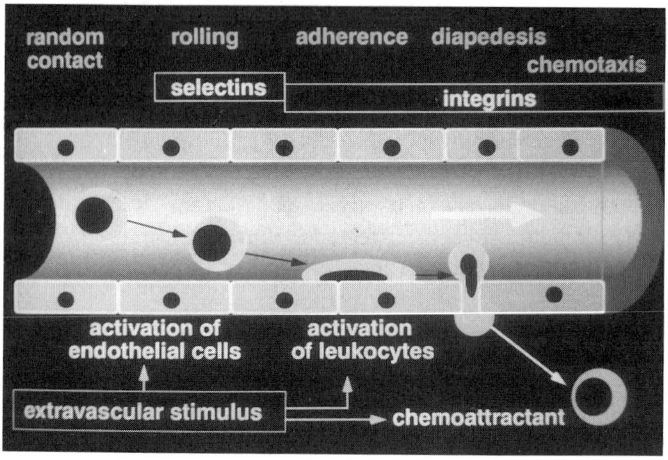

Figure 2 The stages of eosinophil recruitment: In their passage from the blood to the respiratory epithelium, polynuclear eosinophils use the adhesion molecule, L-selectin, Mac-1/LFA-1, ICAM-1, and VLA-4, for the adhesion to and the passage across the vascular endothelium and finally arrive at their destination at the site of inflammation after traversing the tissue matrix. These adhesion molecules often induce a "priming" or even activation of the cells.

play a cascade of various adhesion molecules (Fig. 2). The migration through the bronchial epithelium is probably under the command of chemoattractant factors, such as granulocyte–macrophage colony-stimulating factor (GM-CSF), C5a, PAF, IL-3, IL-5, monocyte chemoattractant protein (MCP)-3, macrophage inflammatory protein (MIP)-1α, RANTES, and IL-8, which are all chemotactic for eosinophils (16). GM-CSF for example, has several properties, and attracts, activates, and prolongs the survival of eosinophils. It is synthesized to a greater extent in the mucosa of asthmatic subjects and is found in higher levels in the bronchoalveolar lavage (BAL) fluid and occasionally in peripheral blood. The level of expression is correlated with the number of eosinophils, with the degree of bronchial hyperreactivity, and is decreased following oral corticosteroid therapy (17). IL-5 exhibits the same properties on the eosinophil. With in situ hybridization techniques, using cells obtained from bronchoalveolar lavage and bronchial biopsies, the number of cells transcribing the gene for IL-5 is increased in asthmatic subjects, as compared to normals, and this effect is correlated with the numbers of eosinophils present, the extent of obstruction, and degree of bronchial hyperreactivity (18,19). The feasibility of a therapy that appears to oppose the influx of eosinophils (again the major cause of lesions and of the increase in bronchial hyperreactivity) by the use of antibodies directed against cytokines and adhesion molecules has been demonstrated in mouse (20), guinea pig (21), rat (22), sheep (23), and monkey (24) models of asthma. The use of anti-IL-5 antibodies into mouse (20) and monkey (24) models reduces both the numbers of eosinophils and the associated bronchial hyperreactivity.

The absence of an eosinophilic infiltration and of increased bronchial hyperreactivity in mice sensitized to ovalbumin, but deficient in IL-4 (25,26) gives rise to a different target for the development of new treatments in asthma. However, the use of anti–IL-4 antibodies does not diminish the eosinophilic infiltration; except when administered during the sensitization phase. In addition, animal studies with blocking antibodies have demonstrated the role of adhesion molecules such as ICAM-1 (27), very late activation antigen (VLA)-4 (α4β1, CD49d/CD29) (21,22), and lymphocyte function-associated associated antigen (LFA)-l (CD11a/CD18) (22) in this eosinophil infiltration. The study of bronchial biopsies in asthmatics has shown an increased expression of Mac-1 (CDllb/CD18), LFA-1, VLA-4, ICAM-1, E-selectin (ELAM-1; endothelial leukocyte adhesion molecule-1; CD62E) and vascular cell adhesion molecule (VCAM)-1 (CD106) (28). Many of these molecules are common to all granulocytes, whereas others, such as VLA-4, are expressed only on eosinophils (29). Other authors have reported an increase in the levels of soluble E-selectin (30) and soluble ICAM-1 (31) in the bronchoalveolar lavage fluid of asthmatic patients 18 hr after allergen challenge; an increase in serum E-selectin and ICAM-1 values in acute asthma (32), and an increase in the expression of these two adhesion molecules in the bronchial microvasculature 6 hr after endobronchial allergen challenge (33). Some animal studies in sheep (23) and in ovalbumin-sensitized rats (34,35) have shown that injection of anti–ICAM-1 (34), anti–VLA-4 (24,36), anti–LFA-1 (35), or anti–Mac-1 (35) results in a significant reduction in bronchial hyperreactivity following allergen challenge, without affecting the influx of eosinophils and lymphocytes into the alveolar spaces and bronchoalveolar tissue. A daily parallel injection of anti-ICAM-1 antibodies in monkeys diminishes the supplementary influx of eosinophils and the associated nonspecific bronchial hyperreactivity (27), but it has no effect on the basal infiltration (36). These studies underline the important, but not exclusive, role of adhesion molecules in the phenomena surrounding cellular activation (37).

Animal studies have also demonstrated the feasibility of targeting proinflammatory cytokines that are able to activate endothelial cells and induce the expression of adhesion molecules. Thus, the use of a receptor antagonist for IL-1 in the guinea pig (38) and for the soluble receptor for tumor necrosis factor (TNF) in the mouse (16) has resulted in both cases in a decrease in the eosinophilic infiltrate. Thus, the blockage of cellular recruitment into the bronchial epithelium by targeting chemoattractants, their receptors, adhesion molecules, and the cytokines that induce the expression of these factors is a possible therapeutic strategy.

The use of a monoclonal antibody in humans induces a rapid immune response against these antibodies; however, the techniques of gene transfer represent a possible alternative. Deactivation of the eosinophils already present in the airways is another therapeutic strategy to investigate. As a matter of fact, the targeting of adhesion molecules involves this objective, and animal studies have already proved its potential usefulness (37). Thus, the administration of anti–VLA-4 antibodies to sensitized sheep diminishes the release of PAF-induced eosinophil peroxidase (EPO) in vitro (23). The binding of eosinophils to fibronectin by VLA-4 induces a secretion of LTC_4, ECP, and EPO (29). Lefort et al. (39) have recently shown that neutralization of endogenously secreted MBP, utilizing a specific antiserum, prevented antigen-induced bronchial hyperreactivity in ovalbumin-sensitized guinea pigs, without affecting the number of bronchoalveolar eosinophils.

To directly target the enzymes involved in the synthesis of lipid mediators, granular proteins, cytokines that activate eosinophils and their receptors is another strategy one might consider. In fact, numerous illnesses are associated with an infiltration of eosinophils into the lungs (e.g., drug allergies, eosinophil-associated pneumonia, and histocytosis X), but are not accompanied by asthma, which involves not only recruitment of these cells, but also an activation signal. The basis of this strategy was first outlined by White et al. (40). By chemically blocking human eosinophil phospholipase A_2 (PLA_2), these authors completely inhibited the liberation of EPO and blocked the arachidonic acid breakdown pathway. An action on the enzymes of the arachidonic acid cascade is already an objective of classic pharmalcological therapies (with, for example, the appearance of anti-5-lipoxygenases on the market). An enzyme of interest that could be inhibited by antisense therapy would be the cytosolic PLA_2, which is the rate-limiting enzyme for arachidonic acid production from membrane phospholipids (41). An action on enzymes that are involved in the later stages of the arachidonic acid cascade is likely be less efficient and would not allow a concomitant action on the granular protein pathway, as described in the foregoing.

Action on the Infiltration and Activation of T Lymphocytes

The targeting of T lymphocytes is another therapeutic possibility. In asthmatics, there is an increased number of activated T cells in the lamina propria and, occasionally in the epithelium. Many of these cells express membrane markers of activation, such as CD25 or HLA-DR (42,43). As for eosinophils, the degree of infiltration is variable from one subject to another. The infiltration is mainly composed of T helper cells ($CD4^+$), which are often said to be equivalent to the mouse Th2 lineage (demonstrated using in situ hybridization by the presence of mRNA for IL-4 and IL-5 in bronchoalveolar lavage cells (19) and in bronchial biopsies (18). These cells synthesize, at least in vitro, IL-3, IL-4, IL-5, IL-6, and GM-CSF, but not IFN-γ or IL-2. Thus, they control both the synthesis of IgE, chemotactism, proliferation, differentiation, or local activation, and possibly govern other cell types involved in asthma, such as eosinophils (IL-5, IL-3, GM-CSF . . .), mast cells and basophils (IL-1, IL-3, IL-4, IL-5, IL-10, GM-CSF), and cells of the monocyte–macrophage lineage (GM-CSF, IL-4, IFN-γ). This cellular infiltration is correlated with the number of eosinophils present, the level of bronchial obstruction and the bronchial hyperreactivity (19). Inhaled corticosteroids significantly decrease the numbers of T cells and other inflammatory cells, suggesting that T cells are likely to be the major target for these drugs.

An action on T cells would first of all reduce the infiltration of other inflammatory cells, particularly of eosinophils, as we have already discussed, and we shall see further examples. This action would also diminish the production of IgE. Two signals are necessary for the synthesis of IgE (44): IL-4 (and as shown more recently IL-13), which induces the isotype switch, the interaction between the T-cell receptor–CD3 complex and HLA-DR molecules on B cells. This interaction can equally occur through the intermediary of the CD40 ligand with CD40. IFN-γ, IFN-α, transforming growth factor (TGF)-β, IL-8, and IL-12 oppose the action of IL-4, whereas IL-6 and TGF-α stimulate IgE synthesis.

Let us now review some of the therapeutic interventions already attempted at the IgE synthesis level. The use of IL-4 receptors inhibits the synthesis of IL-4–dependent IgE production (45). Replacing tyrosine at position 124 of IL-4 with aspartic acid gives rise to a mutated form of the IL-4 protein. This Tyr–Asp–IL-4 mutant is capable of binding to the IL-4 receptor, but incapable of activating it. In an SCID mouse model, the Tyr–Asp–IL-4 mutant is able to inhibit the IL-4–or IL-13–induced synthesis of IgE both in vitro and in vivo (46). Injection of IFN-γ into human subjects with hyper-IgE syndrome, atopic eczema, allergic rhinitis, or steroid-dependent asthma, has no significant effect on serum levels of total or specific IgE, although occasionally a reduction in the spontaneous production of IgE by monocytes of treated patients has been reported (47–50). A clinical improvement has been observed in patients with atopic eczema who do not respond to conventional treatments. Side effects are notably nausea, vomiting, headaches, fever, fatigue, and occasionally a mild neutropenia. These effects are not seen when IFN-γ is administered by aerosol (51,52), underscoring the preference of local administration. When this cytokine was administered by aerosol to ovalbumin-sensitized mice, no inhibition of the IgE response was seen, unless the cytokine was given simultaneously with, or better 3 days before, allergen administration (53). This may only confirm in vivo, the in vitro data showing that the mouse Th2 cells do not revert, as opposed to those of humans. Even this local administration exposes the subject to certain theoretical risks, involving localized activation of the bronchial epithelium, with increased permeability of the epithelial barrier and induction of increased expression of HLA-DR, ICAM-1, and production of nitric oxide synthase.

A recent study involving five asthmatic subjects and five controls showed that 3 weeks of treatment with inhaled IFN-γ was well tolerated, but did not affect the respiratory parameters measured (bronchial hyperreactivity to methacholine, FEV_1, morning peak flow) or the expression of HLA-DR or ICAM-1 on the bronchial biopsies obtained (52). The possible modulation of the IgE response was not investigated in this study. A different strategy could be to used soluble forms of CD40 which, by inhibiting interactions between T and B lymphocytes, would result in the inhibition of IgE production (54). In consequence, modulation of IgE synthesis by acting on IL-4, although possible, is not simple; B lymphocytes apparently have no further need for IL-4 once they are committed to IgE production (44). Because most of the immune response that leads to the synthesis of IgE takes place in the pulmonary lymphatic ganglions, the problem of targeting these cells arises. Any therapy that aims to block the production of IL-4, either directly (antisense therapy) or indirectly (involving the use of immunomodulatory cytokines such as IFN-γ or IL-12), will intervene only in new sensitizations and has little or no effect on already-established responses. The production of IgE could also be modified by the removal of B lymphocytes, which express IgE on their surface. The feasibility of such a strategy has recently been described by Lustgarten and Eshar (55), who transfected T-lymphocyte cell lines with a chimeric T-cell receptor containing the variable region of a nonanaphylactic anti-IgE antibody directed against the binding zone of IgE with the high-affinity receptor. These cells were thus capable of being specifically activated and were able to synthesize IL-2 when placed in contact with B lymphocytes expressing IgE on their membrane surface. In this way, ex vivo manipulation of peripheral blood T lymphocytes would allow the continuous and long-lasting elimination of IgE-producing cells, without risk of anaphylaxis, as a result of mast cell activation. It would also overcome the problem of the incomplete and short-lived efficacy that arises if one tries to remove IgE-producing B lymphocytes by injection of anti-IgE antibodies whether these antibodies are used on their own or are coupled to ricin toxin A (55).

The last, but not the least, strategy aimed at reducing IgE synthesis is specific immunotherapy. Although classic immunotherapy with allergen extracts down-regulates the T-cell responses and has beneficial effects in highly selected asthmatic patients, more efficient and safe methods are being sought (56). Gene transfer technology (i.e., DNA vaccines) has recently been applied to allergen immunotherapy, as it is being evaluated in neoplastic and mainly infectious diseases (57). Balb/c mice immunized intradermally with a plasmid DNA encoding the *Escherichia coli* β-galactosidase (β-Gal) mounted a specific Thl response, whereas β-Gal protein immunization induced a Th2 response to the same antigen (58). Plasmid β-Gal DNA intradermal injections into β-Gal–sensitized mice caused a 66–75% reduction of the specific IgE level. Intramuscular injections of rats with a plasmid DNA encoding a house dust mite allergen also prevents aerosolized allergen-induced induction of IgE synthesis, histamine release in bronchoalveolar fluids, and airway hyperresponsiveness (53).

The targeting of other cytokines, such as IL-5, is a strategy (discussed earlier) that has been tested in the mouse (20) and the monkey (24) by the administration of monoclonal antibodies. The soluble receptors for the α- and β-chains of IL-5 (IL-5Rβ) or mutant inactive forms of IL-5 remain the subject of continuing research. The use of a soluble receptor IL-5Rβ would have the advantage that it could simultaneously decrease the levels of IL-3 and GM-CSF; these three cytokines possess a common β-chain in the heart of their receptors. This hypothesis would require confirmation using an experimental model. The use of receptor antagonists for IL-1 (IL-1R) in the guinea pig (38) and of soluble receptors for TNF-α in the mouse (16) has, in both cases, resulted in a decrease in eosinophil infiltration. In a human model of the cutaneous allergic reaction, the subcutaneous injection of IL-1R at the site of allergen injection in 15 allergic patients led to reduction, and even complete abolition, of the cutaneous response (60). In other inflammatory diseases, such as rheumatoid arthritis, the use of p55 TNF-α receptors has been efficacious and is currently the subject of a clinical trial (61).

Interleukin-12 is another candidate for such intervention. This cytokine is produced principally by cells of the monocyte–macrophage lineage and can direct the immune response towards a Th1 phenotype by favoring the proliferation of these cells and inhibiting the development of Th2 lymphocytes (62). This action is partly due to the induction, in synergy with IL-2, of the synthesis of IFN-γ and stimulation of natural killer (NK) cells. The feasibility of this form of therapy has recently been demonstrated in Balb/c mice that were sensitized to ragweed pollen (63). Intraperitoneal injections of IL-12 for several successive days before intratracheal challenge with the sensitizing allergen decreased the serum levels of specific IgE, the levels of IL-4 in bronchoalveolar lavage fluid, and the numbers of cells in this fluid that expressed the mRNA for the Th2 cytokines IL-4, IL-5, and IL-10. The levels of IFN-γ, the numbers of cells expressing mRNA for IFN-γ, and the numbers of eosinophils in the lavage fluid were also clearly decreased (63). However, it would be interesting to ascertain the effect of such a treatment administered after and not during the sensitization phase.

Another interesting immunomodulating candidate is IL-10 because of its inhibitory effects on the functions of monocytes–macrophages, lymphocytes, and eosinophils. IL-10 is produced by Th0 and Th2 cells, B lymphocytes, monocytes–macrophages, and bronchial epithelial cells (64,65). Moreover, IL-10 activates both B lymphocytes and mast cells in terms of proliferation and of viability (64). This cytokine is a powerful immunosuppressor of monocyte–macrophage and dendritic cell functions (including the synthesis of cytokines, the genesis of oxygen free radicals, and antigen presentation; 64). This latter effect is the means by which IL-10 has been shown to be an inhibitor of IL-4–induced IgE production (66). IL-10 inhibits the proliferation of Thl lymphocytes and neutrophils and the synthesis of their cytokines (IL-2, IFN-γ, IL-3, TNF, GM-CSF; 64). Finally, IL-10 inhibits eosinophil survival and cytokine production (GM-CSF, TNF-α, IL-8; 67). Intratracheal injection of IL-10 several minutes before allergenic provocation in ovalbumin-sensitized rats significantly inhibits the late-phase response, the influx of eosinophils and lymphocytes into the bronchoalveolar lavage fluid, and the degree of activation of cells in the lavage fluid in terms of release of oxygen free radicals, confirming the anti-inflammatory capabilities of this cytokine in vivo (68). Use of a recombinant adenovirus vector to transfer IL-10 intranasally to ovalbumin-sensitized mice, decreased total cell and eosinophil numbers and decreased IL-5 levels into the bronchoalveolar fluids (69).

To summarize, the different biological tools that are presently envisaged in asthma to block the activation of Th2 lymphocytes or to induce anergy or switch of Th2 cells toward the Thl phenotype are synthetic peptides, soluble CD40, soluble receptors (IL-4R, IL-IR, TNF), and immunomodulatory cytokines: IFN-γ, IL-10, IL-12, TGF-β, and Tyr–Asp–IL-4 mutant. There are indeed some promising data concerning gene therapy in animal models of asthma and allergy (58,59,69). Gene transfer techniques would prevent not only the rapid induction of an immune response directed against the therapeutic proteins that would be given in a purified form, but would also avoid their rapid degradation, allowing sustained levels in the airways, and the onset of systemic side effects that they could induce if administered systemically.

Action on Transcription Factors

The binding of cytokines to their membrane receptors provokes a cascade of enzymatic reactions that result in the activation of transcription factors, such as the AP-1 complexes (*jun/fos* or *jun/jun*) and nuclear factor-kappa B (NFκB). These two factors have the ability to inhibit the activation of transcription by the glucocorticoid receptor (GR) and vice versa (70). Usually, this mutual transrepression is mediated by a physical protein–protein interactions between the GR and AP-1 or the GR and NFκB. With the gene for proliferin, it appears that a "composite" responsive element of corticosteroids is able to fix both to the GR and AP-1, leading to the activation or suppression of transcription by corticosteroids, depending on the composition of the AP-1 complex (70). Importantly, AP-1 and NFκB induce the synthesis of numerous proinflammatory cytokines, such as TNF-α, IL-1, and IL-2, that in turn, can activate these transcription factors (70). It is likely that the corticosteroids break the cycle of inflammation by inhibiting the AP-1 or NFκB transcriptional activities. Hence, in steroid-resistant asthma, it logically follows that persistent inflammation may be due to a functional or quantitative deregulation either in the GR or in the interacting transcription factors. In agreement with this hypothesis, Adcock et al. (71) have found an increase in AP-1 complexes in nuclear extracts of peripheral blood lymphocytes obtained from steroid-resistant patients. Numerous possibilities for new therapeutic strategies at these levels could be envisaged. Recent data in the literature suggest that a modification in the local cytokine microenvironment could reverse a qualitative abnormality in the GR: the association between IL-2 and IL-4 decreases the affinity of the GR for the corticosteroids, and this effect can be reversed by IFN-γ (72). The strategies that can be envisaged here include an antisense gene therapy targeting the gene for IL-4, or a genetic immunomodulation that would favor the Thl phenotype over Th2 cells, this being achieved, for example, by the products of the genes for IFN-γ and IL-12 (as already described). Another strategy would be to restore the equilibrium between those transcription factors for which activity is modulated by the corticosteroids; for example, by transferring the genes of either anti-inflammatory transcription factors (such as GR mutants deleted from the ligand-binding domain, which are active even in the absence of the hormone) or antagonists of proinflammatory transcription factors (such as *fra*-1, a member of AP-1 protein family, which renders the fra-1–*jun* complex inactive, or IκB, which is a natural NFκB inhibitor). The use of such a strategy demands further evaluation because it would be an interesting alternative to oral corticosteroids, avoiding their side effects, which are sometimes very severe. As a first and convincing step toward this, Wrighton et al. (73) have constructed a recombinant adenovirus containing the IκBα gene fused to a nuclear localization signal. Infection of endothelial cells with this vector resulted in successful reduction of expression of numerous markers of endothelial activation following lipopolysaccharide stimulation, including VCAM- 1, IL-1, IL-6, IL-8, and tissue factor.

IV. The Most Severe Asthmatic Patients

Thus, the principal strategy in asthma, for which we have just detailed the available data, has been to inhibit the action of Th2 lymphocytes, of which the cortege of cytokines are responsible, at least partly, for the pathophysiology of the disease. There remain, however, numerous obstacles in designing a gene-based strategy, which are due to the incomplete nature of our knowledge of the pathophysiology of asthma, principally which genes to use, which cells to target, what delivery routes, and the possible side effects of the vectors currently available for gene transfer. It is also clear that even the most severe forms of asthma do not fulfill all the classic criteria for gene therapy: a potentially lethal disease, without alternative therapy, in which the responsible gene is known and completely characterized, and for which the product is nontoxic. Corticosteroid-dependent asthma may well fulfill some of these criteria.

It is true that therapeutic advances over the past two decades have enabled us to obtain satisfactory results both clinically and functionally in most patients. Corticosteroids are the most effective treatment for asthma and represent the only therapy that can significantly reduce bronchial inflammation. Although these drugs are generally administered by inhalation, long-term oral administration is sometimes required to control the disease (steroid-dependent patients). The small group of patients who require oral corticosteroids is very heterogeneous, both clinically and functionally (74); some are stable and have a quasi-normal lung function with a corticosteroids dose of about 10 mg/day, whereas others remain unstable despite taking much higher doses of these drugs. Particular attention is required owing to the potential side effects of this treatment (the possibility of stunted growth in children, steroid-induced osteoporosis, cutaneous fragility, an increase in the risk of infections, cataracts, and diabetes), and to the associated severe underlying bronchial inflammation (with increased risk of hospitalization and death). The corticosteroids appear to be less effective for the bronchial inflammation of steroid-dependent patients, although the reasons for this are ill-defined. Finally, there is an even smaller subgroup of patients who are completely resistant to corticosteroids (steroid-resistant patients). In both cases one can speak of “steroid-resistance” with certain differences in the degree of resistance. No epidemiological data are available, but these patients represent 0.1–0.01% of all asthmatic subjects (75). Numerous corticosteroid-sparing agents have been proposed, but without major success, irrespective of the particular drug tested, and severe side effects have been reported for some of them (methotrexate, chloroquine, dapsone, troleandomycin, or cyclosporine; 76). An alternative approach, therefore, is needed and will likely be based on the understanding of the mechanisms underlying steroid resistance.

Many hypotheses have been put forward to explain this resistance, but there is no consensus, and suggestions range from pharmacological explanations (increase in plasma clearance of cortisol, variations in the kinetics of corticosteroids) to cellular-based proposals [abnormalities in monocyte or lymphocyte function; 77–80)] or molecular-based proposals (abnormalities in the corticosteroid receptor or GR binding to its ligand and its DNA target; 71,72,81,82). Although pharmacological theories remain controversial and for some are largely based on the severity of the disease (75), cellular-based hypotheses have as yet no defined molecular basis. Nevertheless, it has repeatedly been stated that in steroid-resistant asthmatics there is a decrease in the effects of corticosteroids on the inhibition of phytohemagglutinin-induced blood monocyte maturation, on the inhibition of cytokine liberation from peripheral blood monocytes, on the decrease in activated eosinophils and T lymphocytes in bronchoalveolar lavage fluid, and on the cutaneous blanching when corticosteroids are applied topically (75,77,79,80). The increased inflammation observed in steroid-resistant patients is reflected functionally by an increase in nonspecific bronchial hyperreactivity (78), and, biologically, by T lymphocytes in peripheral blood and bronchoalveolar lavage fluid that express increased levels of membrane markers of inflammation (CD25 and HLA-DR); and mRNA for inflammatory cytokines (IL-2 and IL-4; 83). Studies so far published reveal two types of abnormalities of the GR in steroid-resistant asthma: a decrease in the affinity for the hormone (72,81) and a diminution in the numbers of receptors that bind with high affinity to the DNA (82), and this could be explained by an increase in AP-1–GR complexes (71). What are the molecular bases of these abnormalities? The primary structure of the GR does not seem to be a major cause because in six patients with steroid-resistance, chemical mutation analysis of the complementary DNA did not show any mutation (84). The presence of high concentrations of proinflammatory cytokines is often cited as being a major cause, particularly IL-2 and IL-4. A combination of the two cytokines induces and maintains a low affinity of the GR in T lymphocytes of both steroid-resistant subjects and in healthy volunteers ex vivo (72). IFN-γ negates the effect of the IL-2–IL-4 combination, probably by favoring the differentiation of Th1, rather than Th2 cells (72). Moreover, these patients have increased amounts of bronchoalveolar cells expressing IL-2 and IL-4 mRNA, suggesting that this phenomenon may happen in vivo (83). Thus, from a perspective for gene therapy in asthma, it would seem that the most severe steroid-dependent patients, and in particular, those who are steroid-resistant, should be considered the primary target for such therapeutic intervention.

V. Conclusion

In essence, a review of pathophysiology allows the definition of a range of therapeutic targets, each of which might or might not be susceptible to gene therapy. Which gene to choose and whether such an approach would work remains entirely speculative. In line with this there are four published works (55,58,59,69) that have direct bearing on gene therapy linked to asthma, and all the rest are only suggestive. It might thus be worthwhile to conduct studies to test the feasibility of such a step.

Acknowledgments

The authors wish to thank Dr. D. T. Curiel (Gene Therapy Program, University of Alabama at Birmingham, Birmingham, Alabama) for reviewing the manuscript. This work has been supported by the Fondation pour la Recherche Médicale, the European Allergy Institute—Fondation de France, and the Conseil Régional Languedoc-Roussillon.

References

1. Burr ML, Butland BK, King S, Vaughan WE. Changes in asthma prevalence: two surveys 15 years apart. Arch Dis Child 1989; 64:1452–1456.
2. Woolcock AJ. Worldwide differences in asthma prevalence and mortality. Chest 1986; 90:S40–S45.
3. Cooke RA, Van der Veer A. Human sensitization. J Immunol 1916; 1:201–305.
4. Marsh DG, Meyers DA, Bias WB. The epidemiology and genetics of atopic allergy. N Engl J Med 1981; 305:1551–1559.
5. Moffatt MF, Hill MR, Cornélis F, Scjou S, Faux JA, Young RP, James AL, Ryan G, le Souef P, Musk AW, Hopkin JM, Cookson WOCM. Genetic linkage of T-cell receptor alpha/delta complex to specific IgE responses. Lancet 1994; 343:1597–1600.
6. Marsh DG, Neely JD, Breazeale DR, Ghosh B, Freidhoff LR, Ehrlich-Kautzky E, Schou C, Krishnaswamy G, Beaty TH. Linkage analysis of IL4 and other chromosome 5q31.1 markers and total serum immunoglobulin E concentrations. Science 1994; 264:1152–1156.
7. Cookson WOCM, Sharp PA, Faux JA, Hopkin JM. Linkage between immunoglobulin E responses underlying asthma and rhinitis and chromosome 1lq. Lancet 1989; 1:1292–1295.
8. Turki J, Pak J, Green SA, Martin RJ, Liggett SB. Genetic polymorphisms of the beta(2)-adrenergic receptor in nocturnal and nonnoctumal asthma. Evidence that Glyl6 correlates with the nocturnal phenotype. J Clin Invest 1995; 95:1635–1641.
9. Rosenwasser L, Klemm DJ, Dresback JK, Inamura H, Mascali JJ, Klinnert M, Borish L. Promoter polymorphisms in the chromosome 5 gene cluster in asthma and atopy. Clin Exp Allergy 1995; 5:S74–S78.
10. Miller N, Vile R. Targeted vectors for gene therapy. FASEB 1995; 9:1900–1995.
11. Vos JMH. In: Vos JMH, ed. Viruses in Human Gene Therapy. Durham, SC: Academic Press, 1995.
12. Demoly P, Simony-Lafontaine J, Chanez P, Pujol JL, Lequeux N, Michel FB, Bousquet J. Cell proliferation in the bronchial mucosa of asthmatics and chronic bronchitics. Am J Respir Crit Care Med 1994; 150:214–217.

13. Bousquet J, Chanez P, Lacoste JY, Barnéon G, Ghavanian N, Enander I, Venge P, Ahlstedt A, Simony-Lafontaine J, Godard P, Michel FB. Eosinophilic inflammation in asthma. N Engl J Med 1990; 323:1033–1039.
14. Metzger WJ, Richerson HB, Worden K, Monick M, Hunninghake GW. Bronchoalveolar lavage of allergic asthmatic patients following allergen bronchoprovocation. Chest 1986; 89:477–483.
15. Resnick MB, Weller PF. Mechanisms of eosinophil recruitment. Am J Respir Cell Mol Biol 1993; 8:349–355.
16. Lukacs NW, Strieter RM, Kunkel SL. Leukocyte infiltration in allergic airway inflammation. Am J Respir Cell Mol Biol 1995; 13:1–6.
17. Woolley KL, Adelroth E, Woolley MJ, Jordana M, O'Byrne PM. Granulocyte–macrophage colony-stimulating factor, eosinophils and eosinophil cationic protein in subjects with and without mild, stable, atopic asthma. Eur Respir J 1994; 7:1576–1584.
18. Hamid Q, Azzawi M, Yin S, Moqbel R, Wardlaw AJ, Corrigan CJ, Bradley B, Durham SR, Collins JW, Jeffery PK, Quint DJ, Kay AB. Expression of mRNA for interleukin-5 in mucosal bronchial biopsies from asthma. J Clin Invest 1991; 87:1541–1546.
19. Robinson D, Hamid Q, Bentley A, Ying S, Kay AB, Durham SR. Activation of $CD4^+$ T cells, increased Th2-type cytokine mRNA expression and eosinophil recruitment in bronchoalveolar lavage after allergen inhalation challenge in patients with atopic asthma. J Allergy Clin Immunol 1993; 92:313–324.
20. Kung TT, Stelts DM, Zurcher JA, Adams GK III, Egan RW, Kreutner W, Watnick AS, Jones H, Chapman RW. Involvement of IL-5 in a murine model of allergic pulmonary inflammation: prophylactic and therapeutic effect of an anti-IL5 antibody. Am J Respir Cell Mol Biol 1995; 13:360–365.
21. Das AM, Williams TJ, Lobb R, Nourshargh S. Lung eosinophilia is dependent on IL-5 and the adhesion molecules CD18 and VLA-4, in a guinea-pig model. Immunology 1995; 84:41–46.
22. Laberge S, Rabb H, Issekutz TB, Martin JG. Role of VLA-4 and LFA-1 in allergen-induced airway hyperresponsiveness and lung inflammation in the rat. Am J Respir Crit Care Med 1995; 151:822–829.
23. Abraham WM, Sielczak MW, Ahmed A, Cortes A, Lauredo IT, Kim J, Pepinsky P, Benjamin CD, Leone DR, Lobb RR, Weller PF. α-4-Integrins mediate antigen-induced late bronchial responses and prolonged airway hyperresponsiveness in sheep. J Clin Invest 1994; 93:776–787.
24. Mauser PJ, Pitman AM, Fernandez X, Foran SK, Adams GK III, Kreutner W, Egan RW, Chapman RW. Effects of an antibody to IL-5 in a monkey model of asthma. Am J Respir Crit Care Med 1995; 152:467–472.
25. Coyle AJ, Le Gros G, Bertrand C, Tsuyuki S, Heusser CH, Kopf M, Anderson GP. Interleukin-4 is required for the induction of lung Th2 mucosal immunity. Am J Respir Cell Mol Biol 1995; 13:54–59.
26. Brusselle G, Kips J, Bluethmann H, Pauwels R. Allergen-induced airway inflammation and bronchial responsiveness in wild-type and interleukin-4–deficient mice. Am J Respir Cell Mol Biol 1995; 12:254–259.
27. Wegner CD, Gundel RH, Reilly P, Haynes N, Letts G, Rothlein R. Intercellular adhesion molecule-1 (ICAM-1) in the pathogenesis of asthma. Science 1990; 24:456–459.
28. Ohkawara Y, Yamauchi K, Maruyama N, Hoshi H, Iohno I, Honna M, Tanno Y, Tamura G, Shirato K, Ohtani H. In situ expression of the cell adhesion molecules in bronchial tissues from asthmatics with airflow limitation: in vivo evidence of VCAM-1/VLA-4 interaction in selective eosinophil infiltration. Am J Respir Cell Mol Biol 1995; 12:4–12.
29. Leff AR. Inflammatory mediation of airway hyperresponsiveness by peripheral blood granulocytes. The case of eosinophils. Chest 1994; 106:1202–1208.
30. Georas SN, Liu MC, Newman W, Beall LD, Stealey BA, Bochner BS. Alteres adhesion molecule expression and endothelial cell activation accompany the recruitment of human granulocytes to the lung after segmental allergen challenge. Am J Respir Cell Mol Biol 1992; 7:261–269.

31. Takahashi N, Liu MC, Proud D, Yu XY, Hasegawa S, Spannhake EW. Soluble intercellular adhesion molecule-1 in bronchoalveolar lavage fluid of allergic subjects following segmental antigen challenge. Am J Respir Crit Care Med 1994; 150:704–709.
32. Montefort S, Lai CKW, Kapahi P, Leung J, Lai KN, Chan HS, Haskard DO, Howarth PH, Holgate ST. Circulating adhesion molecules in asthma. Am J Respir Crit Care Med 1994; 149:1149–1152.
33. Montefort S, Gratziou C, Goulding D, Polosa R, Haskard DO, Howarth PH, Holgate ST, Caroll MP. Bronchial biopsy evidence for leukocyte infiltration and upregulation of leukocyte–endothelial cell adhesion molecules 6 hours after local antigen challenge of sensitized asthmatic airways. J Clin Invest 1994; 93:1411–1421.
34. Sun J, Elwood W, Haczku A, Bames PJ, Hellewell P G, Chung KF. Contribution of intercellular adhesion molecule-1 in allergen-induced airway hyperresponsiveness and inflammation in sensitized brown-Norway rats. Int Arch Allergy Immunol 1994; 104:291–295.
35. Rabb H, Olivenstein AR, Issekutz TB, Renzi PM, Martin JG, Pantano R, Seguin, S. The role of the leukocyte adhesion molecules VLA-4, LFA-1, and Mac-1 in allergic airway responses in the rat. Am J Respir Crit Care Med 1994; 149:1186–1191.
36. Gundel RH, Wegner CD, Torcellini CA, Letts LG. The role of intercellular adhesion molecule-1 in chronic airway inflammation. Clin Exp Allergy 1992; 22:569–575.
37. Pilewski JM, Abelda SM. Cell adhesion molecules in asthma: homing, activation and airway remodeling. Am J Respir Cell Mol Biol 1995; 12:1–3.
38. Watson ML, Smith D, Bourne AD, Thompson RC, Westwick J. Cytokines contribute to airway dysfunction in antigen-challenged guinea pigs: inhibition of airway reactivity, pulmonary eosinophil accumulation, and tumor necrosis factor generation by pretreatment with an interleukin-1 receptor antagonist. Am J Respir Cell Mol Biol 1994; 8:365–369.
39. Lefort J, Nahori MA, Ruffié C, Vargaftig B, Pretolani M. In vivo neutralization of eosinophil-derived major basic protein inhibits antigen-induced bronchial hyperreactivity in sensitized guinea pigs. J Clin Invest 1996; 97:1117–1121.
40. White SR, Strek ME, Kulp GV, Burch RA, Leff AR. Down-regulation of human eosinophil activation and degranulation by inhibition of phospholipase A_2. J Clin Invest 1993; 91:2118–2125.
41. Smith WL. Prostanoid biosynthesis and mechanisms of action. Am J Physiol 1992; 263:F181–F19l.
42. Djukanovic R, Roche WR, Wilson JW, Beasley CRW. Twentyman OP, Howarth PH, Holgate ST. State of the art: mucosal inflammation in asthma. Am Rev Respir Dis 1990; 142:434–457.
43. Kay AB. Asthma and inflammation. J Allergy Clin Immunol 1991; 87:893–910.
44. Geha RS. Regulation of IgE synthesis in humans. J Allergy Clin Immunol 1992; 90:143–150.
45. Maliszewski CR, Fanslow WC. Soluble receptors for IL-1 and IL-4: biological activity and therapeutic potential. Trends Biotechnol 1990; 8:324–329.
46. Carballido JM, Schols D, Namikawa R, Zurawski S, Zurawski G, Roncarolo MG, de Vries JE. IL-4 induces human B cell maturation and IgE synthesis in SCID-hu mice. Inhibition of ongoing IgE production by in vivo treatment with an IL-4/IL-13 receptor antagonist. J Immunol 1995; 155:4162–4170.
47. Boguniewicz M, Jaffe HS, Izu A, Sullinvan MJ, York D, Geha RS, Leung DYM. Recombinant IFN-γ in treatment of patients with atopic dermatitis and elevated IgE levels. Am J Med 1990; 88:365–370.
48. Li JTC, Yunginger JW, Reed CE, Jaffe HS, Nelson DR, Gleich GJ. Lack of suppression of IgE production by recombinant IFN-γ. A controlled trial in patients with allergic rhinitis. J Allergy Clin Inimunol 1990; 85:934–940.
49. Reinhold U, Wehrmann W, Kukel S, Kreysel HW. Recombinant interferon-γ in severe atopic dermatitis. Lancet 1990; 335:1282.
50. Boguniewicz M, Schneider IC, Milgrom H, Newell D, Jaffe HS, Izu AE, Bucalo LR, Leung DYM. Treatment of steroid-dependent asthma with recombinant interferon-gamma (rIFN-γ). J Allergy Clin Immunol 1992; 89:A288.

51. Jaffe HA, Buhl R, Mastrangelli A, Holroyd KJ, Saltini C, Czerski D, Jaffe HS, Kramer S, Sherwin S, Crystal RG. Organ specific cytokine therapy. Local activation of mononuclear phagocytes by delivery of an aerosol of recombinant IFN-γ to the human lung. J Clin Invest 1991; 88:297–302.
52. Boguniewicz M, Martin RJ, Martin BA, Torvik J, Celniker A, Williams M, Leung, DYM. Aerosolized recombinant interferon-gamma (rIFN-γ) in normal subjects and asthmatics. J Allergy Clin Immunol 1993; 91:A226.
53. Lack G, Renz H, Saloza J, Bradley KL, Loader J, Leung DYM, Larsen G, Gelfand EW. Nebulized but not parenteral IFN-γ decreases IgE production and normalizes airway function in a murine model of allergen sensitization. J Immunol 1994; 152:2546–2554.
54. Fanslow WCDM, Anderson DM, Grabstein KH, Clark EA, Cosman D, Armitage RJ. Soluble forms of CD40 inhibit biologic responses of human B cells. J Immunol 1992; 149:655–660.
55. Lustgarten J, Esshar Z. Specific elimination of IgE production using T cell lines expressing chimeric T cell receptor genes. Eur J Immunol 1995; 25:2985–2991.
56. Bousquet J, Michel FB. Specific immunotherapy in asthma: is it effective? J Allergy Clin Immunol 1994; 94: 1-11.
57. McDonnel WM, Askari FK. DNA vaccines. N Engl J Med 1996; 334:42–45.
58. Raz E, Tighe H, Sato Y, Corr M, Dudler JA, Roman M, Swain SL, Spiegelberg HL, Carson DA. Preferential induction of a Th1 immune response and inhibition of specific IgE antibody formation by plasmid DNA immunization. Proc Natl Acad Sci USA 1996; 93:5141–5145.
59. Hsu CH, Chua KY, Tao MH, Lai YL, Wu HD, Huang SK, Hsieh KH. Immunoprophylaxis of allergen-induced immunoglobulin E synthesis and airway hyperresponsiveness in vivo by genetic immunization. Nature Med 1996; 2:540–544.
60. Mullarkey MF, Leiferman KM, Peters MS, Caro I, Roux ER, Hanna RK, Rubin AS, Jacobs CA. Human cutaneous allergic late-phase response is inhibited by soluble IL-1 receptor. J Immunol 1994; 152:2033–2041.
61. Haak-Frendscho M, Marsters SA, Mordenti J, Brady S, Gillett NA, Chen SA, Ashkenazi A. Inhibition of TNF by a TNF receptor immunoadhesin. Comparison to an anti-TNF monoclonal antibody. J Immunol 1994; 152:1347–1351.
62. Manetti R, Parronchi P, Giudizi MG, Piccinni MP, Maggi E, Trinchieri G, Romagnani S. Natural killer cell stimulatory factor (interleukin 12 [IL-12]) induces T helper type 1 (Thl)-specific immune responses and inhibits the development of IL-4-producing Th cells. J Exp Med 1993; 177:1199–1204.
63. Sur S, Lam J, Sigounas A, Holbert D, Metzger WJ. IL-12 decreases allergen induced eosinophil recruitment and Th2 cytokine mRNA expression in BAL cells. Allergy 1996; 51:23.
64. Howa M, O'Garra A, Ishida H, de Waal Malefyt HR, de Vries J. Biological properties of interleukin 10. J Clin Immunol 1992; 12:239–247.
65. Bonfield TL, Konstan MW, Burfeind P, Panuska JR, Hillirad JB, Berger M. Normal bronchial epithelial cells constitutively produce the anti-inflammatory cytokine interleukin-10, which is downregulated in cystic fibrosis. Am J Respir Cell Mol Biol 1995; 13:257–261.
66. Punnonen J, de Waal Malefyt R, van Vlasselaer P, Gauchat JF, de Vries JE. IL-10 and viral IL-10 prevent IL-4-induced IgE synthesis by inhibiting the accessory cell function of monocytes. J Immunol 1993; 151:1280–1289.
67. Takanashi S, Nonaka R, Xing Z, O'Byrne PM, Dolovich J, Jordana M. Interleukin 10 inhibits lipopolysaccharide-induced survival and cytokine production by human peripheral blood eosinophils. J Exp Med 1994; 180:711–715.
68. Wooley MJ, Wooley KL, Otis J, Conlon PD, O'Byrne PM, Jordana M. Inhibitory effects of IL-10 on allergen-induced airway inflammation and airway responses in brown Norway rats. Am J Respir Crit Care Med 1994; 148:A760.
69. Ohkawara Y, Xing Z, Gauldie J, Jordana M. Adenovirus vector-mediated gene transfer of murine interleukin-10 [mIL-10] inhibits antigen induced airways inflammation in sensitized mice. Am J Respir Crit Care Med 1996; 152:A143.

70. Gronemeyer H. Control of transcription activation by steroid hormone receptors. FASEB J 1992; 6:2524–2529.
71. Adcock IA, Lane SJ, Brown CR, Lee TH, Barnes PJ. Abnormal glucocorticoid receptor/AP1 interaction in steroid-resistant asthma. J Exp Med 1995; 182:1951–1958.
72. Kam JC, Szefler SJ, Surs W, Sher ER, Leung DYM. Combination IL-2 and IL-4 reduces glucocorticoid receptor-binding affinity and T cell response to glucocorticoids. J Immunol 1993; 151:3460–3466.
73. Wrighton CJ, Hofer-Warbinek R, Moll T, Eytner R, Bach FH, de Martin R. Inhibition of endothelial cell activation by adenovirus-mediated expression of IκBα, an inhibitor of the transcription factor NFκB. J Exp Med 1996; 183:1013–1022.
74. Paradis L, Des Roches A, Vignola AM. Godard P, Bousquet J, Chanez P. Heterogeneity of glucocorticosteroid (GCs) dependent asthmatics. Am J Respir Crit Care Med 1995; 151:A675.
75. Barnes PJ, Greening AP, Crompton GK. Glucocorticoid resistance in asthma. Am J Respir Crit Care Med 1995; 152:S125-S142.
76. Moss RB. Alternative pharmacotherapies for steroid-dependent asthma. Chest 1995; 107:817–825.
77. Wilkinson JR, Lane SJ, Lee TH. Effects of corticosteroids on cytokine generation and expression of activation antigens by monocytes in bronchial asthma. Int Arch Allergy Appl Immunol 1991; 94:220–221.
78. Carmichael J, Paterson IC, Diaz P, Crompton GK, Kay AB, Grant IWB. Corticosteroid resistance in chronic asthma. Br Med J 1982; 282:1419–1422.
79. Corrigan CJ, Brown PH, Barnes NC, Tsai JJ, Frew AJ, Kay AB. Glucocorticoid resistance in chronic asthma. Peripheral blood T lymphocyte activation and comparison of the T lymphocyte inhibitory effects of glucocorticoids and cyclosporin A. Am Rev Respir Dis 1991; 144:1026–1032.
80. Alvarez J, Surs W, Leung DY, Ikle D, Gelfand EW, Szefler SJ. Steroid-resistant asthma: immunologic and pharmacologic features. J Allergy Clin Immunol 1992; 89:714–721.
81. Sher E, Leung DYM, Surs W, Kam JC, Zieg G, Kamada AK, Szefler SJ. Steroid resistant asthma. Cellular mechanisms contributing to inadequate response to glucocorticoid therapy. J Clin Invest 1994; 93:33–39.
82. Adcock IA, Lane SJ, Brown CR, Peters MJ, Lee TH, Barnes PJ. Differences in binding of glucocorticoid receptor to DNA in steroid-resistant asthma. J Immunol 1995; 154:3500–3505.
83. Leung DYM, Martin RJ, Szefler SJ, Sher ER, Ying S, Kay AB, Hamid Q. Dysregulation of interleukin 4, interleukin 5, and interferon γ gene expression in steroid-resistant asthma. J Exp Med 1995; 181:33–40.
84. Lane SJ, Arm JP, Staynov DZ, Lee TH. Chemical mutational analysis of the human glucocorticoid receptor cDNA in glucocorticoid-resistant bronchial asthma. Am J Respir Cell Mol Biol 1994; 11:42–48.

AUTHOR INDEX

Italic numbers give the page on which the complete reference is listed.

A

B

D

E

G

H

I

J

M

N

O

Q

R

S

X

Y

SUBJECT INDEX

Page numbers followed by "t" indicate tables.

B

C

D

E

F

Q

R

S